Evidence-based Pediatric Infectious Diseases

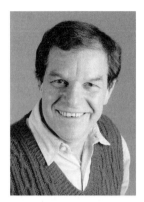

Professor David Isaacs

Evidence-based Pediatric Infectious Diseases

By

David Isaacs

Clinical Professor of Paediatric Infectious Diseases
University of Sydney and Senior Staff Physician
in Pediatric Infectious Diseases and Immunology
The Children's Hospital at Westmead
Sydney
Australia

Consultant Editors:
Elizabeth Elliott
Ruth Gilbert
Virginia Moyer
Michael Pichichero

BMJ|Books

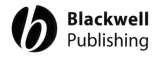
Blackwell
Publishing

© 2007 David Isaacs
Published by Blackwell Publishing
BMJ Books is an imprint of the BMJ Publishing Group Limited, used under licence

Blackwell Publishing, Inc., 350 Main Street, Malden, Massachusetts 02148-5020, USA
Blackwell Publishing Ltd, 9600 Garsington Road, Oxford OX4 2DQ, UK
Blackwell Publishing Asia Pty Ltd, 550 Swanston Street, Carlton, Victoria 3053, Australia

First published 2007

1   2007

Library of Congress Cataloging-in-Publication Data

Isaacs, David, MD.
   Evidence-based pediatric infectious diseases / by David Isaacs ; with consultants, Elizabeth Elliott ... [et al.].
      p. ; cm.
   "BMJ books."
   Includes bibliographical references and Index.
ISBN 978-1-4051-4858-0 (pbk. : alk. paper)
1. Communicable diseases in children.   2. Evidence-based pediatrics.
I. Elliott, Elizabeth J. II. Title.
[DNLM: 1. Communicable Diseases–Handbooks.   2. Adolescent.   3. Child.
4. Evidence-Based Medicine–Handbooks.   WC 39 I73e 2007]

RJ401.I83 2007
618.92′9–dc22

                                                    2007008364

ISBN: 978-1-4051-4858-0

A catalogue record for this title is available from the British Library

Set in 9.5/12pt Minion by Aptara Inc., New Delhi, India
Printed and bound in Singapore by Utopia Press Pte Ltd

Commissioning Editor: Mary Banks
Editorial Assistant: Victoria Pittman
Development Editor: Lauren Brindley
Production Controller: Rachel Edwards

For further information on Blackwell Publishing, visit our website:
http://www.blackwellpublishing.com

The publisher's policy is to use permanent paper from mills that operate a sustainable forestry policy, and which has been manufactured from pulp processed using acid-free and elementary chlorine-free practices. Furthermore, the publisher ensures that the text paper and cover board used have met acceptable environmental accreditation standards.

Contents

About the authors, vii

Preface, viii

Acknowledgements, x

Abbreviations, xii

1 Evidence-based practice, 1

2 Rational antibiotic use, 9

3 Cardiac infections, 14

4 Cervical infections, 29

5 Eye infections, 40

6 Fever, 55

7 Gastrointestinal infections, 74

8 HIV infection, 102

9 Immune deficiency, 117

10 Meningitis and central nervous system
    infections, 132

11 Osteomyelitis and septic arthritis, 156

12 Respiratory infections, 166

13 Sexually transmitted and genital infections, 211

14 Skin and soft tissue infections, 224

15 Systemic sepsis, 243

16 Tropical infections and travel, 256

17 Urinary tract infections, 271

18 Viral infections, 283

Appendix 1 Renal impairment and
    antimicrobials, 299

Appendix 2 Aminoglycosides: dosing and
    monitoring blood levels, 301

Appendix 3 Antimicrobial drug dose
    recommendations, 306

Index, 321

About the authors

David Isaacs is a senior staff physician in pediatric infectious diseases and immunology at The Children's Hospital at Westmead, Sydney, and Clinical Professor of Paediatric Infectious Diseases at the University of Sydney. He has published 10 books and over 200 peer-reviewed publications. His research interests are neonatal infections, respiratory virus infections, immunizations, and ethics. He has published also on medical ethics and several humorous articles. Professor Isaacs is on multiple national and international committees on infectious diseases and immunizations and is a reviewer for the Cochrane Collaboration.

Elizabeth Elliott is Professor of Paediatrics and Child Health, University of Sydney; Consultant Paediatrician, The Children's Hospital at Westmead; Director, Centre for Evidence Based Paediatrics, Gastroenterology and Nutrition; and Practitioner Fellow, National Health and Medical Research Council of Australia. She is Director of the Australian Paediatric Surveillance Unit and past Convenor of the International Network of Paediatric Surveillance Units. She is Senior Associate Editor and co-author of *Evidence Based Pediatrics and Child Health* (Moyer V, ed., BMJ Books 2000, 2nd edition, 2004).

Ruth Gilbert is Reader in Clinical Epidemiology at the Institute of Child Health, London, having completed her training in pediatrics. She has published extensively on the epidemiology of infectious diseases, both original papers and textbooks. She coordinates research programs on the evaluation of screening and diagnostic tests and treatment for congenital toxoplasmosis, and for neonatal group B streptococcal infection. She is coauthor of *Evidence-Based Pediatrics and Child Health*, by Moyer V et al. Ruth teaches evidence-based medicine, has published Cochrane reviews, and is a reviewer for the Cochrane Collaboration.

Michael E. Pichichero is Professor of Microbiology and Immunology, Pediatrics and Medicine at the University of Rochester in New York. He is board certified in pediatrics, in adult and pediatric allergy and immunology, and in pediatric infectious disease. Dr. Pichichero is a partner in the Elmwood Pediatric Group; a recipient of numerous awards, he has over 500 publications in infectious disease, immunology, and allergy. His major practice and research interests are in vaccine development, streptococcal infections, and otitis media.

Virginia Moyer is Professor of Pediatrics and Section Head, Academic General Pediatrics at Baylor College of Medicine and Texas Children's Hospital in Houston, Texas. Dr. Moyer has particular interests in teaching clinical epidemiology and studying the use of diagnostic tests in clinical care. She is a member of the Evidence-Based Medicine Working Group, the United States Preventive Services Task Force, and the International Advisory Board for the Cochrane Collaboration Child Health Field. She is Editor in Chief of the book *Evidence-Based Pediatrics and Child Health* (2nd edition), and the journal *Current Problems in Pediatrics and Adolescent Health Care*, and is a founding Associate Editor of *Evidence-Based Child Health: A Cochrane Review Journal*.

Preface

Some books provide comprehensive recommendations without giving the evidence. Some books provide comprehensive evidence without giving any recommendations.

There is a tension between providing useful management recommendations and between providing detailed evidence that allows clinicians to make their own decisions. Books on managing infections, like the excellent Antibiotic Guidelines[1] and the Red Book,[2] give recommendations about which antibiotics to use and the doses, but not the evidence supporting the recommendations. This is deliberate, to keep the books to a manageable length. In contrast, books such as that edited by Virginia Moyer[3] attempt to analyze the evidence for clinical decisions in depth. Sources of summarized evidence, such as the BMJ's important Clinical Evidence series, provide detailed evidence without recommendations and leave it to the busy clinician to weigh the evidence presented and decide about treatment. While helpful, the depth of the analysis of the evidence means that these sources can deal only with a limited number of clinical situations.

The fundamental principle of the current book is to combine the strengths of both approaches, by analyzing the evidence on management (treatment and, where relevant, diagnosis and prevention) if this is controversial or uncertain, presenting the evidence briefly and then our recommendations about management. The busy clinician can then weigh up the strength of the evidence for our recommendations, and decide how to act. Clinicians can also review the literature themselves, if they have time.

Evidence-based medicine (EBM) has great strengths. For years, many of us thought we were practising EBM, but the best evidence was not easily accessible. That has changed with increasing emphasis on randomized controlled trials, meta-analyses of randomized controlled trials, systematic reviews of the evidence and the rigorous approach to assessing the quality of randomized controlled trials included in the Cochrane reviews, and with the availability of electronic search engines to find the evidence.

Some have espoused EBM wholeheartedly and even, dare one say it, some have advocated it uncritically. It has been fun to satirize this overemphasis on EBM.[4,5] In reality, EBM has strengths and weaknesses. We should use its strengths while acknowledging its weaknesses.

When evidence is lacking, we still need to decide what to do with our patient. In infectious diseases, do we give antibiotics now or watch carefully? What about adjunctive therapy, steroids, or intravenous immunoglobulin, which might help in critical situations? Reading any of the spate of Practice Guidelines published recently is sobering, because so many of the recommendations are based on "consensus expert opinion" in the absence of good trial data.

In this book we present the evidence for management of many pediatric infectious diseases affecting children in industrialized and developing countries, travelers, and refugees. Our recommendations are based on current evidence about efficacy and safety, but also the likely effects on antibiotic resistance, the costs, adverse effects, ethical and any other relevant considerations.

David Isaacs

References

1 Therapeutic Guidelines Ltd. *Therapeutic Guidelines: Antibiotic*, 13th edn. Melbourne: Therapeutic Guidelines Ltd., 2006.

2 American Academy of Pediatrics. In: Pickering LK (ed.), *Red Book: 2003 Report of the Committee on Infectious Diseases*, 26th edn. Elk Grove Village, IL: American Academy of Pediatrics, 2003.

3 Moyer VA, (ed). *Evidence-Based Pediatrics and Child Health*, 2nd edn. London: BMJ Books, 2004.

4 Isaacs D, Fitzgerald D. Seven alternatives to evidence-based medicine. *BMJ* 1999;319:1618.

5 Smith GCS, Pell JP. Parachute use to prevent death and major trauma related to gravitational challenge: systematic review of randomised controlled trials. *BMJ* 2003;327:1459–61.

Acknowledgements

We would like to thank the following for reading chapters and for their helpful comments: Henry Kilham, general pediatrician at The Children's Hospital at Westmead (CHW), Sydney, Australia; Elisabeth Hodson and Jonathan Craig, pediatric nephrologists at CHW; David Schell, pediatric intensivist at CHW; Alyson Kakakios and Melanie Wong, pediatric immunologists at CHW; Alison Kesson, microbiologist and infectious diseases specialist at CHW; Peter Shaw, oncologist at CHW; Paul Tait, child protection specialist at CHW; Chris Blyth, pediatric immunology and infectious diseases physician at Sydney Children's Hospital; Rana Chakraborty, pediatric infectious diseases specialist at St George's Hospital, London; Mary Isaacs (nee Cummins), general pediatrician at Ealing Hospital, UK; Anna Isaacs, medical student at Sydney University and Emily Isaacs, medical student at Birmingham University, UK.

DI has been a member of the writing group for the book *Therapeutic Guidelines: Antibiotic* (TGA) from 1994, when the 8th edition was published until now, the 13th edition having been published in 2006. These books are the work of Therapeutic Guidelines Limited, a non-profit-making organization, which publishes evidence-based guideline books on many different areas of medicine. The first edition of TGA was published in 1978, and was the origin of Therapeutic Guidelines Limited. The aim of TGA, then and now, is to promote good antibiotic prescribing, which includes making recommendations that will minimize antibiotic resistance, and also, though less importantly, consider cost as a factor. A committee of experts, drawn from the fields of infectious diseases, microbiology, tropical medicine, general practice, and pharmacology, meets regularly to review the evidence and discuss treatment.

The recommendations in TGA focus almost entirely on antimicrobial use, rather than diagnosis or other aspects of management. While the book you are currently reading has considered the evidence independently of TGA, and also addresses diagnosis and adjunctive therapies, the presentation of antibiotic doses given in boxed format uses an almost identical format to that used by TGA, and we would like to acknowledge this. We have adopted this format, which has evolved over 28 years, because it expresses so clearly and unambiguously which antibiotics should be prescribed and how often. In addition, the actual pediatric doses we recommend are similar but not always identical to those used in TGA. DI would like to acknowledge his indebtedness to his colleagues on the TGA committees for their wisdom and experience, shared so selflessly. While hesitating to single out any one colleague, DI would like particularly to acknowledge Professor John Turnidge from Adelaide, for his advice on antibiotic use in children. DI would also like to acknowledge the staff of Therapeutic Guidelines Limited, notably Jonathan Dartnell and Jenny Johnstone for their expert support and assistance and Mary Hemming for her open support. Therapeutic Guidelines Limited has given permission for us to use their material to help direct our thinking and for us to include some of their antibiotic guidelines, and we gratefully acknowledge their generosity.

Therapeutic Guidelines: Antibiotic, Version 13, 2006 (ISBN 9780975739341 and ISSN 1329-5039), is published in print and electronically and distributed by Therapeutic Guidelines Limited, 23-47 Villiers St, North Melbourne, Vic 3051, Australia.

Telephone: 613 9329 1566
Fax: 613 9326 5632
E-mail: sales@tg.com.au
Website: www.tg.com.au

Abbreviations

These abbreviations are used frequently in this book.

CI = Confidence Interval: a way of expressing uncertainty in measurements; the 95% CI tells you that 95% of the time the true value will lie within this range. For example, if you are told that a treatment compared with placebo has a relative risk of 0.50 (95% CI 0.31–0.72) that means the treatment reduces the risk by 50%, and 95% of the time it will reduce the risk by somewhere between 31 and 72%.

NNT = Number Needed to Treat: the number of patients you need to treat in order to achieve one extra favorable outcome. For example, if 9 of 10 patients treated with antibiotics for an infection get better compared with 7 of 10 treated with placebo, 2 extra patients get better for every 10 treated and so the NNT is 10/2 or 5.

OR = Odds Ratio: the ratio of the odds of having the outcome in the treated group compared to the odds of having it in the control group. For example:
· If 10 of 100 treated patients have persistent symptoms, the odds of persistent symptoms are 10/90 or 0.11 (11%).
· If 30 of 100 untreated/placebo patients in the same study have persistent symptoms, the odds are 30/70 or 0.43 (43%).
· The odds ratio is 0.11/0.43, which is 0.26.

RR = Relative Risk or Risk Ratio: the ratio of the risk in the treated group to the risk in the control group. For example:
· If 10 of 100 treated patients have persistent symptoms, the risk of persistent symptoms is 10/100 or 0.1 (10%).
· If 30 of 100 untreated/placebo patients in the same study have persistent symptoms, the risk is 30/100 or 0.3 (30%).
· The relative risk or risk ratio is 0.1/0.3, which is 0.33.
[When the event rate is 10% or lower, the OR and RR are similar. For more common events, the difference between OR and RR becomes wider, with the RR always closer to 1. In general, it is preferable to use RR.]

RCT = Randomized controlled trial: participants are randomly allocated to an experimental or control group and the outcome measured.

CHAPTER 1
Evidence-based practice

1.1 Why evidence-based practice?

We all like to think we are practicing medicine based on the best evidence available. However, we sometimes do things in medicine for one or more of the following reasons:

· "It has always been done that way"
· "Everyone does it that way"
· "The consultant says so"
· "The protocol says so"

We tend not to challenge the dogma because we are too busy or because we do not know how to find the evidence or because we think we know the evidence. If doctors are asked what are the main obstacles to them in trying to review the literature, the commonest answers are lack of time,[1–5] followed by lack of knowledge.[4,5] However, innovations have made it much easier and quicker to search the literature.

Sometimes the best evidence available for a clinical decision will be a high-quality systematic review of several good RCTs on patients like yours (see Section 1.5, p. 2). At other times, there may be no trials and the only evidence will be from observational studies, such as case series or even case reports. A clinician making the clinical decision will find it helpful to know the strength of the evidence and the degree of uncertainty in making that decision.

Young doctors should be encouraged to challenge dogma and to ask for the evidence supporting management whenever possible. Senior doctors should be quick to ask the young doctors to look it up themselves and return with the evidence. We should all be open-minded enough to accept that our current practices may be wrong and not supported by the evidence.

In the past our attempts to practice in an evidence-based way were hampered by difficulty in getting easy access to the evidence. Literature searches were cumbersome and evidence was rarely presented to us in a convenient or easily digestible way. That is no longer an excuse. Anyone with Internet access has immediate access to the best evidence and can review the recent literature in a few minutes.

The concept of evidence-based medicine (EBM) was developed by Sackett and colleagues at McMaster University in Canada during the 1980s and 1990s. They defined EBM as the integration of the best research evidence with clinical expertise and patient values.[6] Our ability to practice EBM has been enhanced by the development of systematic ways of reviewing the literature and the availability of search engines to find the evidence.

1.2 The Cochrane Library

The Cochrane Collaboration has revolutionized the way we look at evidence. The Cochrane Collaboration was founded in 1993 and named for the British epidemiologist Archie Cochrane. It is an international non-profit-making organization that produces systematic reviews (see Section 1.5, p. 2) of health-care interventions and makes sure they are updated regularly. We consider that a good Cochrane systematic review provides the best available evidence on interventions. This is because a Cochrane review involves a formalized process of finding all published and unpublished studies, assessing their quality, selecting only those studies that meet predetermined criteria, and performing a meta-analysis when possible. A meta-analysis is a way of combining the results from several studies to get an overall mathematical summary of the data.

Cochrane reviews are only about interventions, which often but not always involve treatment. Cochrane reviews on treatment usually include only RCTs because an RCT is the best study design for avoiding bias when assessing treatment. When considering the evidence for any intervention, it is almost always worth searching the Cochrane Library before looking else-where.

A Cochrane review takes on average 700 hours of work, so we are privileged to have ready access to such information, presented clearly in the Cochrane Library. Even if the Cochrane reviewers find no RCTs or only one, the knowledge that there is only scanty evidence on which to base clinical decisions is itself valuable.

The Cochrane Library is free in developing countries and in the UK, where the National Health Service (NHS) pays for it. It requires a subscription in the USA and Australia, but many libraries and hospitals subscribe. Abstracts of Cochrane reviews are available free to all through PubMed. The Web site for the Cochrane Library is http://www.thecochranelibrary.com/.

1.3 Clinical evidence

Another extremely useful resource is Clinical Evidence, which is a collection of systematic reviews from the BMJ. Clinical evidence is free in developing countries and in the UK, where the NHS pays for it. It requires a subscription in the USA, but many libraries subscribe, and it is currently distributed free to US primary care physicians through an American foundation. The Web site is http://www.clinicalevidence.com/.

1.4 Medline and PubMed

PubMed is a means of easy access to Medline, the comprehensive database provided free to all users by the US National Library of Medicine and the National Institutes of Health. It allows access to the abstracts of thousands of publications from many scientific journals. In addition, if when looking at the abstract the journal logo appears on the right side of the screen, clicking the logo often allows free access to the whole paper. The Web site is http://www.pubmed.gov/.

1.5 Hierarchy of evidence

For studies relating to treatment, which will be the most frequent scenario in this book, there is an accepted hierarchy of evidence, based on study design. This is because any studies where patients are not randomly allocated to one or other treatment (randomized) are likely to be affected by bias. This is not to say there is intentional bias. However, in a non-randomized study,

the groups may differ significantly. One group may be more severely affected than the other. An example is preadmission antibiotics for suspected meningococcal infection. A cohort study compared the outcome in a non-randomized group of patients with suspected meningococcal infection given preadmission antibiotics to the outcome in patients not given antibiotics.[7] Patients given antibiotics were more likely to die than patients not given antibiotics. It might appear that antibiotics increase mortality, but the patients given antibiotics are likely to have been sicker than those not given antibiotics. Thus there was bias and the groups were not truly comparable. Studies that do not involve randomized patients are sometimes called "observational studies."

In general, a Cochrane review (see Section 1.2, p. 1) will give better evidence than a non-Cochrane systematic review and so on, although it is important for you to assess the quality of any evidence, including that from Cochrane and non-Cochrane systematic reviews. Weak data can lead to misleading conclusions.

1 *Cochrane review:* A peer-reviewed systematic review, usually of RCTs, using explicit methods and published in the Cochrane Library's Database of Systematic Reviews.

[A Cochrane review is only as good as the quality of the studies included. In many reviews, a meta-analysis is possible, summarizing the evidence from a number of trials.]

2 *Systematic review (non-Cochrane):* A review that systematically searches for all primary studies on a question, appraises, and summarizes them. Systematic reviews that evaluate treatment usually include RCTs rather than other study types.

[The abstracts of non-Cochrane systematic reviews can be found in PubMed under "Clinical Queries," and the abstracts of good-quality systematic reviews are in the Cochrane Library's Database of Abstracts of Reviews of Effectiveness.]

3 *Meta-analysis:* A meta-analysis is a mathematical summary in which the results of all the relevant studies are added together and analyzed, almost as if it had been one huge trial.

4 *RCT:* Subjects are randomly allocated to an experimental (treatment) group or a control (placebo or different treatment) group and the outcome studied.

5 *Cohort study:* A non-randomized study of two groups of patients. One group receives the exposure of interest (e.g., a treatment) and the other does not. The study on preadmission antibiotics for meningococcal infection[7] is an example.

6 *Case-control study:* Patients with the outcome being studied are matched with one or more controls without the outcome of interest and compared regarding different exposures to look for risk factors for or predictors of the outcome. For example, a group of children with a rare outcome, say tuberculous meningitis (TBM), could be compared with matched controls without TBM with regard to BCG vaccination, contact with TB, socioeconomic factors, etc., to determine factors that appear to protect against TBM (such as BCG) and risk factors (such as contact with TB and possibly socioeconomic status).

7 *Case series:* Reports of a series of patients with a condition but no controls.

8 *Case reports:* Reports of one or more patients with a condition.

The hierarchy of evidence of studies does not apply to evidence about etiology, diagnosis, and prognosis:

The best evidence about **etiology** is from large cohort studies or case-control studies or sometimes RCTs.

The best evidence about **diagnosis** is from large cross-sectional studies in a similar population to yours, because the results will be most relevant to your clinical practice. In these studies, the test or tests you are interested in is compared to a reference test or "gold standard." For example, a new test like polymerase chain reaction for respiratory syncytial virus might be compared to viral culture.

The best evidence about **prognosis** is from large cohort studies, in a population like yours, followed over time. The no-treatment or placebo groups from large RCTs can provide excellent data on prognosis also.

The hierarchy of evidence is an oversimplification. It is also important to decide how the results apply to your patients. In general, you need to think whether there are biological reasons why the treatment effect could differ in your patients. Often there are more data for adults than children, as in the Cochrane systematic review of sore throat[8] we discuss later. Should you ignore data from adult studies or are these relevant? For example, is the biology of appendicitis so different in adults compared with children that you can learn no relevant information from studies done entirely in adults?

The other question you always need to consider is "What is the baseline risk in my population?" in order to work out how much your particular patient will benefit. For example, how likely is my patient to have prolonged symptoms from acute otitis media, and by how much would this be reduced by applying the relative risk for antibiotic treatment (measured as a relative risk or odds ratio)?

1.6 Searching the literature

The busy clinician will save time by looking for sources of summarized evidence first. If you have access to the Internet, the easiest initial approach is to look first in the Cochrane Library if available (for systematic reviews and RCTs), then in Clinical Evidence if available, and then in Medline via PubMed. If the programs are not already available on your computer, you can find them by going straight to the Web sites http://www.thecochranelibrary.com for the Cochrane Library, http://www.clinicalevidence.com/ for Clinical Evidence, and http://www.pubmed.gov/ for PubMed. The Web addresses can then be saved as favorites.

Framing the question

The next step is to decide on search terms. It will be a lot easier to search the literature if you can frame the question well.[9] Most questions about treatment in this book are framed in the classic evidence-based PICO format,[9] where P = Population, I = Intervention, C = Comparison, and O = Outcome. Suppose you are interested in whether or not antibiotics are indicated for sore throat in children (see Figure 1.1). Framing the question in the PICO format, you ask "For children with sore throats (Population), do antibiotics (Intervention) compared to no antibiotics or placebo (Comparison) reduce the duration of illness or reduce the frequency of complications (Outcome)?"

Searching for a Cochrane systematic review

You type the search terms "tonsillitis child" or "sore throat" or "sore throat child" into the Cochrane Library search window (where it says "Enter search term" in Figure 1.2) and find that there is a Cochrane systematic review by Del Mar et al.[8] The Cochrane reviewers

Frame the question:	Population	Intervention	Comparison	Outcome
	Children with sore throat or tonsillitis	Antibiotics	No antibiotics or placebo	Duration of illness or frequency of complications
Search the literature:	Cochrane Library: find a Cochrane review of antibiotics for sore throat in adults and children			
Assess the evidence:	Results: • Six patients need to be treated with antibiotics to cure one extra sore throat at day 3 • Antibiotics reduce the frequency of complications • Antibiotics more effective when patient has group A streptococcal infection • Difficult to distinguish between adults and children in the studies, and no subgroup analysis of children was possible • The evidence is most relevant for children 3 years and older, because the benefits of antibiotics will be less for younger children, who are much more likely to have viral infection causing their sore throat			
Decide on action:	Decide if your patient is similar to those studied. If your patient is more likely to have group A streptococcal infection, the benefits of starting antibiotics immediately are likely to be greater			

Figure 1.1 Answering a clinical question about treatment.

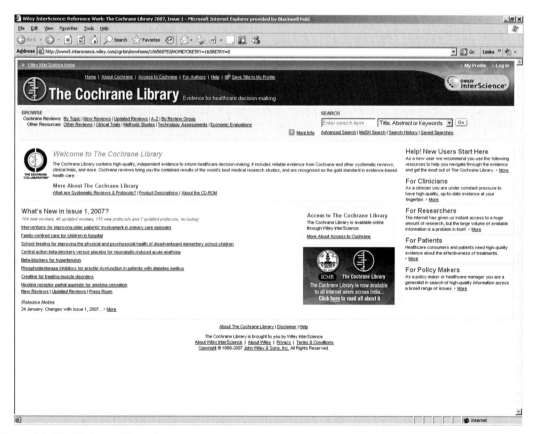

Figure 1.2 The Cochrane Library home page.

include 27 RCTs, perform a meta-analysis, and present conclusions about the benefits and risks of treating sore throats with antibiotics based on current evidence.[8] When you assess the relevance of the Cochrane review to your patient(s), you note that very few of the studies were performed only in children and the studies that include adults and children do not separate them out clearly. This is a common problem when searching the literature for evidence about children. You search the evidence further for variations in etiology and find that case series show a low incidence of group A streptococcal infection and a high incidence of viral infection in children younger than 3 years with tonsillitis. You make a clinical decision for your patient(s) based on your assessment of the literature (see also p. 176).

Searching for a non-Cochrane systematic review

If you do not find a Cochrane systematic review, you may find a systematic review in Clinical Evidence. If neither is successful, you may still find a quick answer to your clinical question. For example, you see a patient with hepatitis A. The books tell you to give normal human immunoglobulin to household contacts, but you wonder about the strength of the evidence. When you enter "hepatitis A" into the Cochrane Library search, you get 53 "hits," but most are about hepatitis B and hepatitis C. You find a Cochrane systematic review on vaccines for hepatitis A, and a protocol for immunoglobulin and hepatitis A but no data. There is nothing in Clinical Evidence on hepatitis A.

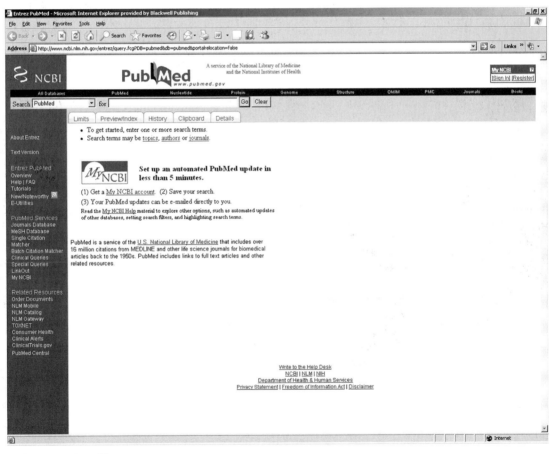

Figure 1.3 PubMed home page.

You turn to Medline using PubMed to look for a systematic review first. The best way to search rapidly for these is to use the "Clinical Queries" option. When you click "Clinical Queries," under PubMed services on the left-hand side of the PubMed home page (Figure 1.3), a new screen appears (Figure 1.4). There is an option "Find systematic reviews." When you enter "hepatitis A" into the box and click "Enter," you get 77 hits. But if you enter "hepatitis A immunoglobulin," you get 15 hits, of which the third is a systematic review of the effectiveness of immune globulins in preventing infectious hepatitis and hepatitis A. The systematic review says post-exposure immunoglobulin was 69% effective in preventing hepatitis A infection (RR 0.31, 95% CI 0.20–0.47).[10]

Searching for a meta-analysis

Suppose your search does not reveal a systematic review. For example, you want to know if immunoglobulin can prevent measles. You find no systematic reviews in the Cochrane Library, Clinical Evidence, or PubMed. Your next question is whether there is a meta-analysis. You can look for a meta-analysis in PubMed using the "Limits" option, at the top left hand of the home page screen (Figure 1.3). You enter the search term "measles," click "Limits," and a number of options appear. Down the bottom of the page on the left is the heading "Type of Article." You click "Meta-Analysis," then click "Go," and find there are 16 meta-analyses of measles listed, mostly about immunization and vitamin A, but none is relevant to your question.

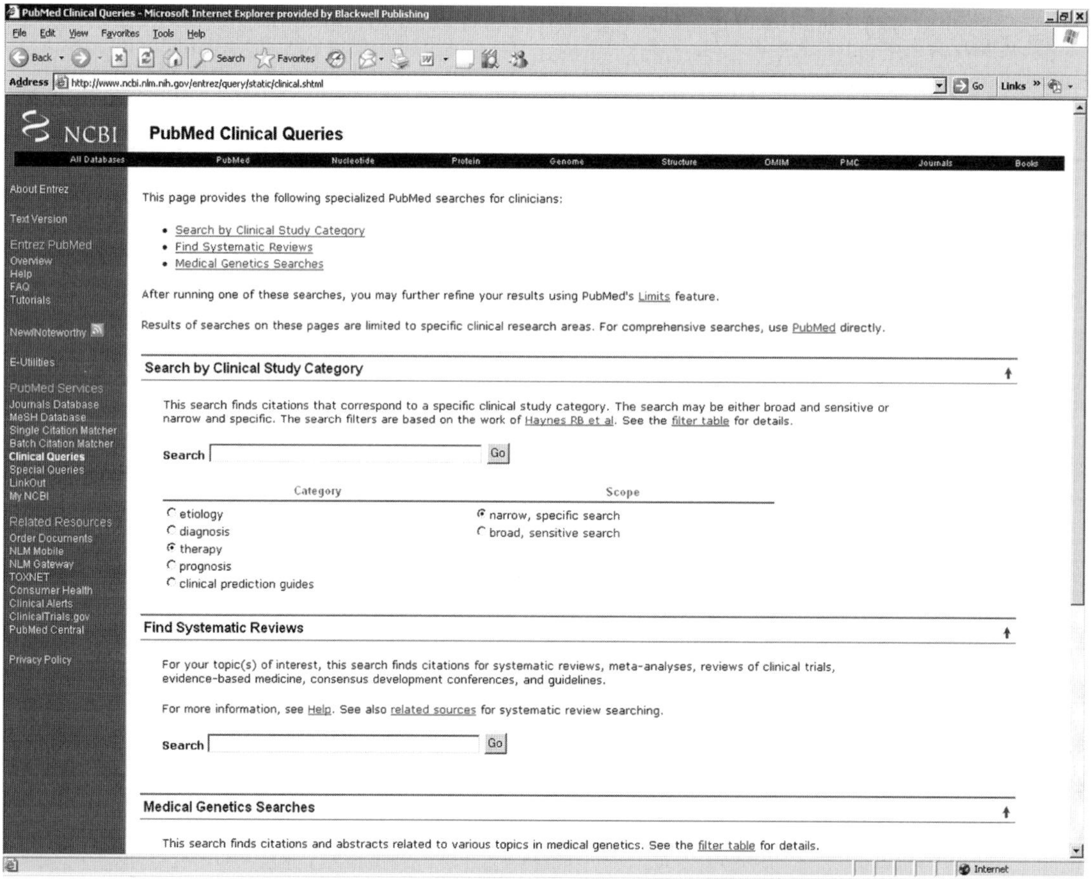

Figure 1.4 PubMed "Clinical Queries" page.

Searching for RCTs

If there is no systematic review and no meta-analysis, are there any RCTs? The best way to search rapidly for these is to use the "Clinical Queries" option again, but this time use the "Search by Clinical Study Category" option (the top box on Figure 1.4). You note this is already set on "therapy" and a "narrow, specific search," because these settings automatically find all RCTs, the commonest type of clinical query. When you put in your search term "measles and (immunoglobulin or immune globulin)" and click "Go," the program comes up with 94 RCTs. Most of the studies are irrelevant and can be ignored (this always tends to be the case). When you scan the titles and the abstracts, only one is helpful, and this shows that post-exposure prophylaxis with immunoglobulin could not be shown to be effective, reducing the risk of infection by only 8% with wide confidence intervals (less than 0–59%) that crossed zero, so the result is not statistically significant.[11] The study does not tell you whether immunoglobulin reduced severity. You conclude that there is no good evidence that giving post-exposure immunoglobulin prevents measles, and you can find no RCT data to say whether or not it reduces severity.

If you find no RCTs, you may need to try different search terms to make sure that it is not because you are asking the wrong question. There is a lot of trial and error in searching the literature and you will improve with practice.

Searching for non-randomized studies

If you use "Clinical Queries" but change from a "narrow, specific search" to a "broad, sensitive search," this gives you all clinical trials on the topic, not just RCTs.

Searching for questions about diagnosis

You can also use PubMed to search for questions about diagnosis, such as the best tests available to diagnose a condition. It is best to use "Clinical Queries" again, but this time when you get to the "Clinical Queries" page (Figure 1.4) select "diagnosis" before or after entering your search terms. This automatically takes you

Table 1.1 Relationship between question type, study type, and best source of evidence.

Question Type	Information Sought	Study Type	Best Source of Evidence
Treatment	Comparison of current best practice with a new therapy or comparison of new therapy with placebo	Systematic reviews of RCTs (with or without meta-analysis); RCTs; clinical practice guidelines (if based on a systematic review of the literature and an assessment of the quality of the evidence)	Cochrane Library Clinical Evidence Clinical practice guidelines Medline (PubMed) Evidence-based Web sites
Baseline risk (frequency)	Disease incidence; or disease prevalence; or frequency of complications	Population-based studies or cohort studies	Medline (PubMed) Review articles Textbooks
Etiology	Cause of disease	Cohort studies; case-control studies; RCTs when the question is about an adverse effect of an intervention	Cochrane Library Clinical Evidence Medline (PubMed)
Diagnosis	Information about the accuracy of a test, its capacity to identify a specific disorder and to distinguish the disorder from other disorders, and the applicability of a test to a particular patient population	The best studies allow an independent blind comparison between the test and the reference ("gold") standard for diagnosis	Cochrane Library Medline (PubMed)
Prognosis	Outcomes of disease: short and long term	Cohort studies or no treatment/placebo arm of RCTs	Medline (PubMed) Textbooks

to studies that give specificity (if you stay on "narrow, specific search") or sensitivity and specificity (if you select "broad, sensitive search").

Table 1.1 gives a guide to the most likely places to find the evidence you are seeking depending on the type of question. For a more comprehensive description of EBM and its application to clinical practice, we refer you to recent comprehensive but readable books.[9,12]

The sort of quick search described above should take you 10–15 minutes. You will improve with practice. If you are scared of trying, you will never know how easy and satisfying it is to scan the literature and find quite good evidence you never knew existed.

References

1 Dawes M, Sampson U. Knowledge management in clinical practice: a systematic review of information seeking behavior in physicians. *Int J Med Inform* 2003;71:91–5.

2 Riordan FAI, Boyle EM, Phillips B. Best paediatric evidence: is it accessible and used on-call? *Arch Dis Child* 2004;89:469–71.

3 D'Alessandro DM, Kreiter CD, Peterson MW. An evaluation of information-seeking behaviors of general pediatricians. *Pediatrics* 2004;113:64–9.

4 Ely JW, Osheroff JA, Ebell MH, Chambliss ML, Vinson DC. Obstacles to answering doctors' questions about patient care with evidence: qualitative study. *BMJ* 2002;324:1–7.

5 Coumou HC, Meijman FJ. How do primary care physicians seek answers to clinical questions? A literature review. *J Med Libr Assoc* 2006;94:55–60.

6 Sackett DL, Strauss SE, Richardson WS, Rosenberg W, Haynes RB. *Evidence-Based Medicine: How To Practice and Teach EBM*, 2nd edn. Edinburgh: Churchill Livingstone, 2000.

7 Norgard B, Sorensen HT, Jensen ES, Faber T, Schonheyder HC, Nielsen GL. Pre-hospital parenteral antibiotic treatment of meningococcal disease and case fatality: a Danish population-based cohort study. *J Infect* 2002;45:144–51.

8 Del Mar CB, Glasziou PP, Spinks AB. Antibiotics for sore throat. *The Cochrane Database of Systematic Reviews* 2006;(4):Art. No. CD000023.

9 Strauss SE, Richardson WS, Glasziou P, Haynes RB. *Evidence-Based Medicine: How To Practice and Teach EBM*, 3rd edn. Edinburgh: Churchill Livingstone, 2005:13–30.

10 Bianco E, De Masi S, Mele A, Jefferson T. Effectiveness of immune globulins in preventing infectious hepatitis and hepatitis A: a systematic review. *Dig Liver Dis* 2004;36:834–42.

11 King GE, Markowitz LE, Patriarca PA, Dales LG. Clinical efficacy of measles vaccine during the 1990 measles epidemic. *Pediatr Infect Dis J* 1991;10:883–8.

12 Moyer VA (ed). *Evidence-Based Pediatrics and Child Health*, 2nd edn. London: BMJ Books, 2004.

Rational antibiotic use

Rational antibiotic use requires accurate diagnosis and appropriate antibiotic use. Antibiotics have radically improved the prognosis of infectious diseases. Infections that were almost invariably fatal are now almost always curable if treatment is started early. Antibiotics are among our most valuable resources, but their use is threatened by the emergence of resistant strains of bacteria. Physicians need to use antibiotics wisely and responsibly. This means that when deciding which antibiotic to use, we need to consider the likelihood that an antibiotic will induce resistance, as well as traditional evidence-based comparisons of efficacy.

2.1 Antibiotic resistance

Antibiotic use selects for antibiotic-resistant bacteria.[1–5] This is an example of rapid Darwinian natural selection in action: naturally occurring genetic variants that are antibiotic-resistant are selected by the use of antibiotics which kill off antibiotic-sensitive strains. It occurs in hospitals with the use of parenteral antibiotics[1–3] and in the community with oral antibiotics.[4,5] When penicillin was first used in the 1940s and 1950s, *Staphylococcus aureus* was always exquisitely sensitive to benzylpenicillin. The antibiotic pressure exerted by widespread penicillin use selected naturally occurring, mutant strains of *S. aureus*, which were inherently resistant to penicillin. Within a very short period of time, most disease-causing strains of *S. aureus* were penicillin-resistant.

Antibiotic resistance is a highly complex subject and many factors drive resistance, including the nature of the antibiotic, the organism, the host, and the environment.[6] What are some of the most important factors leading to antibiotic resistance and what is the evidence that they can be changed?

Broad- and narrow-spectrum antibiotics

Broad-spectrum antibiotics might be expected to be more potent selectors of antibiotic resistance than narrow-spectrum antibiotics, and this has indeed proved to be the case in clinical practice.[1–3] Furthermore, exposure to broad-spectrum antibiotics can select for resistance to multiple antibiotics. The third-generation cephalosporins (e.g., cefotaxime, ceftazidime, ceftriaxone) have been shown to be associated with resistance to multiple antibiotics, including selection for organisms with inducible resistance (the organisms exist naturally and multiply during antibiotic treatment) and for extended spectrum beta-lactamase (ESBL)-producing gram-negative bacilli. If the cephalosporins are stopped and the "antibiotic pressure" driving resistance is removed, the situation improves. In an important study of neonatal units in the Netherlands, de Man et al[1] showed that empiric therapy using "narrow-spectrum" antibiotics, penicillin and tobramycin, was significantly less likely to select for resistant organisms than using "broad-spectrum" amoxicillin and cefotaxime. The precise distinction between narrow-spectrum and broad-spectrum antibiotics can be debated, but the most obvious distinction is whether prolonged use is associated with the selection of organisms resistant to multiple antibiotics.

On the other hand, the evidence that broad-spectrum antibiotics are a major problem is rather weak. If a broad-spectrum antibiotic is used for as short a time as possible, it is much less likely to drive resistance. The use of antibiotics such as azithromycin, which has a long half-life, is far more likely to cause problems than short-term use of cephalosporins for sore throat. Indeed, when a single dose of azithromycin was given to Australian Aboriginal children with trachoma, the proportion of children colonized with azithromycin-resistant *Streptococcus pneumoniae* strains increased from 1.9% before treatment to up to 54.5% at follow-up.[7] The evidence suggested that the selective effect of azithromycin allowed the growth and transmission of preexisting, azithromycin-resistant strains.[7]

Population antibiotic use

It might seem self-evident that the sheer volume of antibiotic use is important in resistance: if we use more antibiotics in a population, then we ought to be more likely to select for resistant organisms. This might be through taking antibiotics more often, e.g., for upper respiratory tract infections (URTIs), or taking them for longer or at higher dose. It has been very difficult, however, to find evidence to support this theory. A study looking at antibiotic use in different European countries showed a correlation between high rates of antibiotic resistance and high consumption of broad-spectrum, oral antibiotics in the community.[5] Beta-lactam antibiotic use is associated with increased colonization with penicillin-insensitive pneumococci, both at an individual level (children who had recently received a beta-lactam antibiotic were more likely to be colonized[8]) and a population level.[9] Note that the term penicillin-insensitive is used, because pneumococci are often relatively insensitive to penicillin, but not absolutely resistant, so most pneumococcal infections except meningitis can be cured by increasing the dose of penicillin.

There is some evidence that widespread antibiotic resistance is reversible. Nationwide reduction in macrolide consumption in Finland was associated with a significant decline in erythromycin resistance of group A streptococci.[10] A French controlled intervention study showed a modest reduction in penicillin-insensitive pneumococci associated with reducing the number of prescriptions for URTIs, but not with education on dose and duration.[11] On the other hand, there are situations where decreased use of antibiotics has not been associated with a reduction in antibiotic resistance.

Antibiotic dose and duration

Intuitively, one would think that the dose and duration of antibiotic use would be an important determinant of resistance. Treatment with sub-optimal doses or for long periods might be expected to select for re-sistant organisms. Indeed, a French study of antibiotic use in children found that both dose and duration were important.[12] Not only was oral beta-lactam use associated with a threefold increased risk of carriage of penicillin-insensitive pneumococci, but children treated with lower than recommended doses of oral beta-lactam had an almost sixfold greater risk of carriage of these organisms than children treated with the recommended dose.[12] Treatment with a beta-lactam for longer than 5 days was also associated with an increased risk of carriage.[12] The results suggest that either low daily dose or long duration of treatment with an oral beta-lactam can contribute to the selective pressure in promoting pharyngeal carriage of penicillin-insensitive pneumococci.

Relatively long-term use of a quinolone antibiotic like ciprofloxacin has also been associated with the emergence of ciprofloxacin-resistant strains of MRSA[13] and *Pseudomonas aeruginosa*.[14]

A study on the long-term use of prophylactic antibiotics to prevent urinary tract infection found no statistically significant correlation between the emergence of resistant *Escherichia coli* and the consumption of trimethoprim-sulfamethoxazole, amoxicillin-clavulanate, and a number of other antibiotics, but did find highly statistically significant correlations between consumption of broad-spectrum penicillins and quinolones and resistance to ciprofloxacin and nalidixic acid.[15] Quinolone consumption was associated with resistance to gentamicin and nitrofurantoin. Strains of *E. coli* with multiple antimicrobial resistance were significantly more common in countries with high total antimicrobial consumption.[15]

Topical antibiotics

Sub-therapeutic concentrations of antibiotics select for resistant strains of bacteria in vitro, and there is evidence that inappropriately low doses of oral antibiotics are associated with resistance in vivo (see above, Antibiotic dose and duration). Another situation where sub-therapeutic antibiotic concentrations are likely is the use of topical antibiotics. In practice, the actual antibiotic is important: in a study comparing vaginal antibiotics, topical clindamycin but not topical metronidazole was associated with the emergence of resistant strains.[16] While one study showed that topical ciprofloxacin was superior to framycetin in the short-term treatment of recurrent otorrhea,[17] a recent report found that 17 children with recurrent otorrhea treated with topical ciprofloxacin were colonized with multidrug resistant *Pseudomonas* strains.[18] A randomized trial found that selective decontamination of the intestinal tract with antibiotics, a form of prolonged topical treatment, was associated with a significant increase in resistance of *S. aureus* to oxacillin and ciprofloxacin.[19]

Mucosal penetration

The factors leading to antibiotic resistance are not always predictable. Sometimes explanations have to be sought for clinical observations. For example, macrolides were found in Spain to be stronger selectors for penicillin-resistant pneumococci than beta-lactam antibiotics.[20] It has been suggested that one explanation could be the greater mucosal penetration of macrolides,[6] although another possible explanation is that azithromycin, the macrolide used, is bacteriostatic for *S. pneumoniae*.

2.2 Combating antibiotic resistance

There are several measures we can use to try to prevent and to reduce antibiotic resistance, a problem that has been with us ever since antibiotics were first used therapeutically. These can be instituted in hospital and in the community.

Question | For hospital doctors, do antibiotic restriction policies compared with no policy reduce inappropriate prescribing? Do they reduce antibiotic resistance?

Literature review | We found a Cochrane review of 66 studies, which were a combination of RCTs, controlled before and after studies and interrupted time series, of varying quality.[21]

A Cochrane review[21] of interventions to improve hospital prescribing of antibiotics found that interventions mainly aimed at limiting inappropriate prescribing usually led to decreased treatment (81% of studies) and improved microbiologic outcomes, such as antibiotic resistance (75%). Three of 5 studies showed that instituting antibiotic policies was associated with a reduction in the incidence of *Clostridium difficile* diarrhea.

The measures recommended in Box 2.1 follow from the likely mechanisms of resistance described above.

Box 2.1 Recommendations on antibiotic use: eight steps to reduce antibiotic resistance.

1 Do not use antibiotics unless there is good evidence that they are beneficial in this situation
2 Use the narrowest spectrum antibiotic that will work
3 Use antibiotics at the appropriate dose
4 Use one antibiotic unless it has been shown that two or more are superior
5 Use antibiotics for as short as possible
6 Do not use prophylactic antibiotics, unless there is good evidence of benefit
7 Do not use topical antibiotics if possible, or if you must then prefer ones which are not also used systemically
8 Try to prevent infection, through immunization, infection control, and hygiene measures

Are antibiotics needed?

There are many situations where antibiotics are prescribed against all evidence. A classic example is viral URTIs. Repeated studies and one Cochrane review[22] have shown no benefit and often adverse effects from antibiotics given for URTI, yet repeated studies in general practice, private practice, and hospital practice have shown that antibiotics are prescribed for up to 90% of children with viral URTI.[22]

Narrow versus broad spectrum

In this book, we will tend to prefer the use of a narrow-spectrum antibiotic to a broad-spectrum antibiotic, particularly for prolonged use in an intensive care setting. This is not merely because of price (broad-spectrum antibiotics are usually much more expensive than narrow-spectrum antibiotics).

It is now widely accepted that education about appropriate antibiotic use is important, both in hospitals and in the community. Hospital antibiotic prescribing often needs reinforcing with more formal mechanisms for ensuring rational antibiotic use, which may involve constraining antibiotic use by rationing it to appropriate situations. By their use of parenteral antibiotics, particularly in oncology and in intensive care, hospitals are major drivers of antibiotic resistance. Policies to restrict important antibiotics, such as vancomycin (to prevent the emergence of vancomycin-resistant enterococci and vancomycin-intermediate *S. aureus*) or carbapenems and third-generation cephalosporins (to try to prevent selection for extended-spectrum beta-lactamase producing Gram-negative bacilli, ESBL), need to be reinforced with antibiotic approval systems. There are prescriber support systems to help doctors use the most appropriate antibiotics. Electronic databases are increasingly popular.[23] The mere presence of an approval system, however, does not ensure better prescribing, and antibiotic use still requires auditing. Sometimes an audit will even show that antibiotic prescribing deteriorated despite the introduction of an approval system,[24] indicating that more stringent policing of antibiotic use is needed.

On a national basis, some countries are able to limit the use of broad-spectrum antibiotics by having a limit on the number of antibiotics available or a limit on the number whose cost is subsidized by the government.

Single versus multiple antibiotics

For a small number of infections, multiple antimicrobials are clearly superior to one, most notably in the treatment of slow-growing organisms with a propensity for resistance, such as tuberculosis and HIV. Some antibiotics should not be used on their own because of the rapid development of resistance through a one-step mutation; e.g., fusidic acid or rifampicin should not be used alone to treat *S. aureus* infections. In general, however, it is better to use one antibiotic rather than two, unless there is good evidence. For staphylococcal osteomyelitis, for example, it is not uncommon for children to be prescribed fusidic acid as well as flucloxacillin, although there is no evidence that the combination is better than flucloxacillin alone. This risks increased toxicity as well as an increased chance of resistance, without likely clinical benefit.

Oral versus parenteral

Some oral antibiotics are extremely well absorbed and can be used as effectively as parenteral antibiotics. Absorption of antibiotics is erratic in the neonatal period, when parenteral antibiotics should be used for serious infections. For some infections, such as endocarditis, high levels of antibiotics need to be maintained and prolonged parenteral therapy is recommended. For osteomyelitis, in contrast, pediatric studies have shown that children can be treated effectively with short courses of parenteral antibiotics followed by long oral courses.

Duration

For some infections, such as osteomyelitis and endocarditis, where tissue penetration is a problem, there is evidence that using shorter courses than those usually recommended is associated with unacceptable rates of relapse. In other situations, such as urinary tract infection, short courses of antibiotics have been shown to be as effective as longer courses. In many situations, there is no good evidence about the optimal duration of antibiotic use, and it is usually considered safe to stop antibiotics once the patient is clinically better. Prolonged antibiotic use without evidence of benefit should be discouraged because of the risk of resistance (see p. 10).

Many doctors now use electronic ordering of drugs, including antibiotics. One danger is that current software systems are more likely to order repeat, computer-generated, antibiotic prescriptions than happens with handwritten prescriptions.[23,24] Use of computer-generated prescriptions is estimated to result in 500,000 unnecessary prescriptions of amoxicillin, amoxicillin-clavulanate, cefaclor, or roxithromycin annually in Australia.[25]

Topical antibiotic use

Because of the risks of inducing antibiotic resistance, topical antibiotics should not be used unless absolutely necessary. Antiseptics such as chlorhexidine may be just as effective. If topical antibiotics are used in situations where benefit has been proved, e.g., for chronically discharging ears, then topical antibiotics that are not used systemically, such as mupirocin or framycetin, are generally preferable to ones, such as quinolones, that are more likely to drive antibiotic resistance.

Prevention

Immunization against resistant strains of bacteria can help reduce antibiotic resistance. A classic example is the introduction of pneumococcal conjugate vaccines that include the serotypes of pneumococcus, which are most likely to be resistant to penicillin. Use of these vaccines has been associated with a significant reduction in carriage of penicillin-resistant pneumococci.[26]

There is an increased incidence of infections in child-care facilities, often with resistant organisms. Hygiene measures can reduce the incidence of infections and the need for antibiotics.[27]

References

1 de Man P, Verhoeven BA, Verbrugh HA et al. An antibiotic policy to prevent emergence of resistant bacilli. *Lancet* 2000;355:973–8.

2 Ariffin H, Navaratnam P, Kee TK, Balan G. Antibiotic resistance patterns in nosocomial gram-negative bacterial infections in units with heavy antibiotic usage. *J Trop Pediatr* 2004;50:26–31.

3 Isaacs D. Unnatural selection: reducing antibiotic resistance in neonatal units. *Arch Dis Child Fetal Neonatal* 2006;91:F72–4.

4 Lee SO, Lee ES, Park SY, Kim SY, Seo YH, Cho YK. Reduced use of third-generation cephalosporins decreases the acquisition of extended-spectrum beta-lactamase-producing *Klebsiella pneumoniae. Infect Control Hosp Epidemiol* 2004;25:832–7.

5 Goossens H, Ferech M, Stichele RV et al. Outpatient antibiotic use in Europe and association with resistance: a cross-national database study. *Lancet* 2005;365:579–87.

6 Turnidge J, Christiansen K. Antibiotic use and resistance—proving the obvious. *Lancet* 2005;365:548–9.

7 Leach AJ, Shelby-James TM, Mayo M et al. A prospective study of the impact of community-based azithromycin treatment of trachoma on carriage and resistance of *Streptococcus pneumoniae. Clin Infect Dis* 1997;24:356–62.

8 Nasrin D, Collignon PJ, Roberts L, Wilson EJ, Pilotto LS, Douglas RM. Effect of beta lactam antibiotic use on pneumococcal resistance to penicillin: prospective cohort study. *BMJ* 2002;324:28–30.

9 Arason VA, Kristinsson KG, Sigurdsson JA, Stefansdottir G, Molstad S, Gudmundsson S. Do antimicrobials increase the carriage rate of penicillin resistant pneumococci in children? Cross sectional prevalence study. *BMJ* 1996;313:387–91.

10 Seppala H, Klaukka T, Vuopio-Varkila et al. The effect of changes in the consumption of macrolide antibiotics on erythromycin resistance in group A streptococci in Finland. *N Engl J Med* 1997;337:441–6.

11 Guillemot D, Varon E, Bernede C et al. Reduction of antibiotic use in the community reduces the rate of colonization with penicillin G-nonsusceptible *Streptococcus pneumoniae. Clin Infect Dis* 2005;41:930–8.

12 Guillemot D, Carbon C, Balkau B et al. Low dosage and long treatment duration of beta-lactam: risk factors for carriage of penicillin-resistant *Streptococcus pneumoniae. JAMA* 1998;279:365–70.

13 Peterson LR, Quick JN, Jensen B et al. Emergence of ciprofloxacin resistance in nosocomial methicillin-resistant *Staphylococcus aureus* isolates. Resistance during ciprofloxacin plus rifampin therapy for methicillin-resistant *S. aureus* colonization. *Arch Intern Med* 1990;150:2151–5.

14 Pitt TL, Sparrow M, Warner M, Stefanidou M. Survey of resistance of *Pseudomonas aeruginosa* from UK patients with cystic fibrosis to six commonly prescribed antimicrobial agents. *Thorax* 2003;58:794–6.

15 Kahlmeter G, Menday P, Cars O. Non-hospital antimicrobial usage and resistance in community-acquired *Escherichia coli* urinary tract infection. *J Antimicrob Chemother* 2003; 52:1005–10.

16 Austin MN, Beigi RH, Meyn LA, Hillier SL. Microbiologic response to treatment of bacterial vaginosis with topical clindamycin or metronidazole. *J Clin Microbiol* 2005;43:4492–7.

17 Couzos S, Lea T, Mueller R, Murray R, Culbong M. Effectiveness of ototopical antibiotics for chronic suppurative otitis media in Aboriginal children: a community-based, multicentre, double-blind trial. *Med J Aust* 2003;179: 185–90.

18 Jang CH, Park SY. Emergence of ciprofloxacin-resistant *Pseudomonas* in paediatric otitis media. *Int J Pediatr Otorhinolaryngol* 2003;67:313–6.

19 Lingnau W, Berger J, Javorsky F, Fille M, Allerberger F, Benzer H. Changing bacterial ecology during a five-year period of selective intestinal decontamination. *J Hosp Infect* 1998;39:195–206.

20 Garcia-Rey C, Aguilar L, Baquero F, Casal J, Dal-Re R. Importance of local variations in antibiotic consumption and geographic differences for erythromycin and penicillin resistance in *Streptococcus pneumoniae. J Clin Microbiol* 2002;40:2959–63.

21 Davey P, Brown E, Fenelon L et al. Interventions to improve antibiotic prescribing practices for hospital inpatients. *The Cochrane Database of Systematic Reviews* 2005;(4):Art. No. CD003543.

22 Arroll B, Kenealy T. Antibiotics for the common cold and acute purulent rhinitis. *The Cochrane Database of Systematic Reviews* 2005;(3):Art. No. CD000247.

23 Grayson ML, Melvani S, Kirsa SW et al. Impact of an electronic antibiotic advice and approval system on antibiotic prescribing in an Australian teaching hospital. *Med J Aust* 2004;180:455–8.

24 Bolon MK, Arnold AD, Feldman HA, Goldmann DA, Wright SB. An antibiotic order form intervention does not improve or reduce vancomycin use. *Pediatr Infect Dis J* 2005;24:1053–8.

25 Newby DA, Fryer JL, Henry DA. Effect of computerised prescribing on use of antibiotics. *Med J Aust* 2003;178:210–3.

26 Whitney CG, Klugman KP. Vaccines as tools against resistance: the example of conjugate pneumococcal vaccine. *Semin Pediatr Infect Dis* 2004;15:86–93.

27 Uhari M, Mottonen M. An open randomized controlled trial of infection prevention in child day-care centers. *Pediatr Infect Dis J* 1999;18:672–7.

CHAPTER 3
Cardiac infections

3.1 Infective endocarditis

Clinical features of infective endocarditis

Infective endocarditis is a rare condition, and is rarer in children than in adults.[1,2] The major risk factor for infective endocarditis for children in industrialized countries is congenital heart disease.[2] In developing countries, valve lesions secondary to rheumatic heart disease remain an important risk factor.[2] Long-term central indwelling catheters, particularly intracardiac ones, are also a risk factor, particularly when used to infuse parenteral nutrition. In adults and some adolescents, intravenous drug use is a risk factor. About 10% of children develop infective endocarditis on an apparently previously normal heart valve (native valve endocarditis).[2]

The clinical presentation relates to one of four phenomena: bacteremic (or fungemic), valvulitic, immunologic, and embolic. Most childhood cases of infective endocarditis present indolently (so-called subacute endocarditis) with prolonged low-grade fever and one or more of malaise, lethargy, pallor, weakness, arthralgias, myalgias, weight loss, sweating, and rigors.[2] Splenomegaly and new heart murmurs are the most common signs.[2] Extracardiac manifestations such as petechiae or purpura, which can be raised, hemorrhages, necrotic lesions, Roth spots (retinal hemorrhages), Janeway lesions (macules on the palms or soles), and Osler nodes (tender finger palp nodules) are less common in children than adults.[2] Hematuria and/or abnormal renal function can result from glomerulonephritis or renal infarct. Children may occasionally present with stroke because of rupture of a mycotic aneurysm caused by CNS emboli. Other embolic phenomena (to abdominal viscera or to the heart causing ischemia) occur rarely.[2] Children occasionally present acutely ill from fulminant endocarditis, usually caused by *Staphylococcus aureus*, with high, spiking fevers and rapidly evolving heart murmurs and signs.[2,3]

Many children with endocarditis do not have the classic cutaneous stigmata, and clinical suspicion needs to be high to avoid missing the diagnosis.

Organisms causing infective endocarditis

The major organisms causing infective endocarditis are shown in Box 3.1.

Various studies in children have shown that about 50% of all episodes of infective endocarditis, whether

---

Box 3.1 Organisms isolated from children with infective endocarditis (in approximate order of frequency[2,4,5]).

- Viridans streptococci
- *Staphylococcus aureus*
- Enterococci
- HACEK group of Gram-negative bacilli:
  Haemophilus aphrophilus
  Actinobacillus acinetomycetemcomitans
  Cardiobacterium hominis
  Eikenella corrodens
  Kingella kingae
- Non-toxigenic *Corynebacterium diphtheriae* (diphtheroids)
- Other Gram-negative bacilli, e.g., salmonella, haemophilus
- Coagulase negative staphylococci
- Miscellaneous (*Streptococcus pneumoniae*, fungi, *Bartonella*, *Coxiella*, etc.)
- Culture negative

The antibiotics and doses recommended in this chapter are based on those in *Therapeutic Guidelines: Antibiotic*, 13th edn, Therapeutic Guidelines Ltd, Melbourne, 2006.

or not associated with congenital heart disease,[4] are caused by so-called viridans or alpha-hemolytic streptococci.[2,4,5] These include *S. sanguis, S. oralis* (or *S. mitis*), *S. salivarius, S. mutans,* and *Gemella morbillorum* (previously *S. morbillorum*). Members of the *S. anginosus* group (*S. intermedius, S. anginosus,* and *S. constellatus*) are sometimes called the *S. milleri* group. These latter organisms can cause endocarditis, but are more likely to cause abscesses. The alpha-hemolytic streptococci are usually sensitive to penicillin, although some are relatively insensitive.[2] *S. bovis* is a non-enterococcal penicillin-susceptible group D streptococcus.

The HACEK group of organisms are fastidious Gram-negative bacilli which are low-grade commensals of the mouth and upper respiratory tract. They virtually never cause bacteremia except in patients with endocarditis.[2,4,5]

Staphylococci, both *S. aureus* and coagulase negative staphylococci, are more likely to be associated with indwelling vascular catheters and following heart surgery. *S. aureus* infection should be suspected in a child who has skin sepsis (boils, pyoderma) as well as endocarditis.

In the newborn and in children with central catheters, particularly if on long-term parenteral nutrition, *S. aureus* and *Candida* are the commonest causes of endocarditis.[2,4,5]

Diagnosis of infective endocarditis

Blood cultures

The greater the number of blood cultures sent, the greater the yield.[1,2,4,5] Ideally, we recommend sending at least three blood cultures from separate venepunctures from patients with suspected endocarditis before giving antibiotics.[1] This should be possible even in fulminant infection, where it is important to start antibiotics as soon as possible. Once a bacterium has been cultured, the laboratory should be requested to measure the minimum inhibitory concentration (MIC) of the antibiotic which will inhibit growth of that bacterium, because this will guide treatment.[2]

Echocardiography

The echocardiogram is central to the diagnosis of infective endocarditis. In adults, transesophageal echocardiography (TEE) is more sensitive than transthoracic echocardiography (TTE).[6] No such studies have been published in children.[2] In children, trans-thoracic is generally preferred to TEE, because the quality of images with TTE is relatively good in children[1,2] and because a general anesthetic may be necessary to obtain a TEE in a young child. TEE may be helpful when ultrasound penetration is poor, e.g., in obese children, muscular adolescents, post-cardiac surgery, and children with pulmonary hyperinflation.[2]

Other tests

A number of non-specific findings may support a diagnosis of infective endocarditis, but their absence does not exclude the diagnosis. These include anemia, leukocytosis, thrombocytopenia, elevated ESR and acute phase proteins, hematuria, proteinuria, and renal insufficiency.[2]

The modified Duke criteria

Question | For children with suspected endocarditis are the modified Duke criteria sensitive and specific enough for clinical use?

Literature review | We found two studies comparing the use of the Duke criteria with other diagnostic criteria for children with proven endocarditis.[7,8]

Because of the difficulties in defining endocarditis when clinical signs are absent, diagnostic schemes have been developed. In 1994, a team from Duke University developed the Duke criteria, which classified cases as "definite" (proved at surgery or autopsy), "possible" (not meeting the criteria), or "rejected" because no evidence of endocarditis was found or another diagnosis was far more likely.[7] Subsequently, the Duke criteria have been modified so that "definite" cases include clinically diagnosed cases, with positive blood cultures with characteristic organisms and echocardiographic evidence, as well as pathologically diagnosed cases.[9] The modified Duke criteria take into account that some organisms, such as the HACEK group of fastidious Gram-negative bacilli, virtually never cause bacteremia unless the patient has endocarditis, whereas others such as *S. aureus* may cause bacteremia with or without endocarditis.[3] The modified Duke criteria are recommended as the main basis for diagnosis in adults,[1,10] and a simplified summary is given in Box 3.2.

Box 3.2 Simplified version of modified Duke criteria for definition of infective endocarditis.[1,9]

Pathologic criteria
Microorganisms by culture or histology from a vegetation or intracardiac abscess
or
Vegetation or intracardiac abscess confirmed histopathologically

Clinical criteria
Definite: 2 major; or 1 major + 3 minor; or 5 minor criteria
Possible: 1 major + 1 minor; or 3 minor criteria
Major criteria:
a. Blood culture grows typical microorganisms from two or more separate specimens
b. One blood culture positive for *Coxiella burnetii* or positive serology for *C. burnetii*
c. Echocardiogram positive
Minor criteria:
a. Predisposing feature (heart condition, IV drug user)
b. Fever
c. Vasculitic or other embolic or hemorrhagic clinical features, e.g., Janeway lesions
d. Immunologic phenomena, e.g., nephritis, Osler's nodes, Roth spots
e. Blood culture positive, but not enough to meet major criterion above
Rejected: Does not meet criteria for possible infective endocarditis and/or firm alternate diagnosis

The modified Duke criteria have been evaluated in children and compared to preexisting criteria, the von Reyn[7] and Beth Israel criteria.[8] In these studies, children with proven endocarditis were assessed retrospectively to see if they fulfilled Duke[9] or modified Duke criteria.[10] All 149 children fulfilled Duke criteria for definite or possible infection and none was rejected by Duke criteria, although some cases were missed using the older criteria.[7,8] We conclude that the modified Duke criteria have good sensitivity and specificity for endocarditis in children. However, the modified Duke criteria were developed for epidemiologic comparisons and for clinical research. They are a clinical guide for diagnosis, and a clinician may judge that it is wise to treat a child for endocarditis even if the child does not meet the Duke criteria. The decision to treat may be appropriate even if the risk of the child having endocarditis is relatively low, if the consequences of missing the diagnosis would be disastrous.

Treatment of infective endocarditis

Surgery for infective endocarditis
Reviews[1,2] have reported echocardiographic features that suggest surgical intervention should be considered, although these are based on expert opinion rather than controlled trials (see Box 3.3).

Antimicrobials for infective endocarditis
The general principles of the antimicrobial treatment of infective endocarditis are that the dose should be high enough and duration long enough to sterilize the heart valves. Organisms in vegetations are embedded in a fibrin-platelet matrix and exist in very large numbers with a low metabolic rate, all of which decreases susceptibility to antimicrobials.[2] It is recommended that treatment is given intravenously for the entire duration of each antibiotic course, except for occasional very rare infections, like Q fever. Oral antibiotics have only ever been studied in adult IV drug users with right-sided endocarditis, and the results cannot be extrapolated to children. They are not recommended in children because of concerns about achieving adequate blood levels with oral treatment.[1,2]

For fulminant infections, infections of prosthetic valves, and persistent infections, we recommend consulting a cardiovascular surgeon.

Box 3.3 Echocardiographic features indicating possible need for surgery.[1,2]

Vegetation
  Persistent vegetation after systemic embolus or emboli
  Large vegetation of anterior mitral leaflet (particularly > 10 mm)
  Increasing size of vegetation
Valve
  Acute aortic or mitral regurgitation with heart failure
  Resistant heart failure
  Valve perforation, rupture, dehiscence, or fistula
Endocardium
  New heart block
  Large abscess

Question | For children with infective endocarditis is any one antibiotic regimen more effective than others?

Literature review | We found one small non-randomized study in children.[11] We found six RCTs in adults, five of staphylococcal endocarditis and only one of streptococcal endocarditis.[12] We found one meta-analysis of the role of adding aminoglycosides to a beta-lactam.[13] We found treatment guidelines for adults[1] and children[2] based on best available evidence and expert consensus where evidence was not available.

We found no useful data for children. The only study was a non-randomized study of 10 children who received cefotaxime plus an aminoglycoside compared with 10 children who received different beta-lactams plus an aminoglycoside for longer time.[11] The outcome was equivalent.

In adults, the data were also very limited. A meta-analysis of four RCTs and one retrospective study involving 261 patients did not find that the addition of aminoglycosides to a beta-lactam improved outcome.[13] However, the quality of the studies was weak, and the confidence intervals wide.[13] In the only RCT of the treatment of penicillin-susceptible streptococcal endocarditis, once daily ceftriaxone for 4 weeks was equivalent to 2 weeks of ceftriaxone plus gentamicin.[12]

For short course therapy for right-sided *S. aureus* endocarditis in intravenous drug-users, cloxacillin alone was as effective as cloxacillin plus an aminoglycoside.[14]

The current recommendation for the initial empirical treatment of endocarditis is to use once-daily dosing of gentamicin, in case the patient has Gram-negative sepsis, pending blood culture results. If endocarditis is subsequently proven to be streptococcal or enterococcal, thrice-daily low-dose gentamicin is often recommended for synergy, although the evidence is weak.[12–14]

The antibiotic regimens recommended below are, therefore, based mainly on expert opinion.[1,2,15,16]

Empiric treatment of endocarditis, unknown organism

For empiric therapy to cover streptococcal, staphylococcal, and Gram-negative endocarditis, we recommend:

benzylpenicillin 60 mg (100,000 U)/kg (max 2.4 g or 4 million U) IV, 4-hourly PLUS

di/flucl/oxa/nafcillin 50 mg/kg (max 2 g) IV, 4-hourly PLUS
gentamicin <10 years: 7.5 mg/kg; ≥10 years: 6 mg/kg IV, daily OR
gentamicin 2.5 mg/kg IV, 8-hourly

[NB: See Appendix 2 for advice on the prolonged use of gentamicin.]

We recommend initial empiric therapy using vancomycin and gentamicin in any of the following circumstances:

· prosthetic cardiac valve;
· hospital-acquired infection;
· anaphylactic penicillin allergy;
· community-associated MRSA (cMRSA) infection suspected on epidemiologic grounds, such as ethnicity, although skin and soft tissue infections due to cMRSA are far more common than endocarditis.

When using vancomycin, we recommend:

vancomycin 12 years or older: 25 mg/kg (max 1 g); child <12 years: 30 mg/kg (max 1 g) IV, 12-hourly PLUS
gentamicin <10 years: 7.5 mg/kg; ≥10 years: 6 mg/kg IV, daily OR
gentamicin 2.5 mg/kg IV, 8-hourly

[NB: See Appendix 2 for advice on the prolonged use of gentamicin.]

The antibiotics should be changed, if necessary, to the most appropriate regimen as soon as the organism and its susceptibility pattern are known.

Streptococcal endocarditis due to highly penicillin-sensitive organisms

Viridans streptococci are usually highly susceptible to benzylpenicillin (defined as MIC ≤0.12 mg/L). The MIC for penicillin should be measured, as this determines treatment. Low-dose aminoglycoside is added for synergy.[12]

For **uncomplicated endocarditis** due to streptococci which are highly susceptible to benzyl penicillin (MIC ≤0.12 mg/L), we recommend:

gentamicin 1 mg/kg IV, 8-hourly for 14 days PLUS EITHER
benzylpenicillin 45 mg (75,000 U)/kg (max 1.8 g or 3 million U) IV, 4-hourly for 14 days OR
ceftriaxone 100 mg /kg (max 4g) IV, 24-hourly for 14 days

[NB: For low-dose 8-hourly synergistic dosing, measure only trough levels and keep level <1 mg/L to minimize toxicity (see Appendix 2).]

Alternatively, as a single drug, use:

benzylpenicillin 45 mg (75,000 U)/kg (max 1.8 g or 3 million U) IV, 4-hourly OR
ceftriaxone 100 mg/kg (max 4g) IV, 24-hourly for 4 weeks

Adults at low risk for severe disease may be managed successfully as outpatients after initial inpatient therapy (usually for at least 1 to 2 weeks),[15] although use of an established outpatient intravenous antibiotic therapy program is recommended.[16] For suitable patients, a proven treatment course is ceftriaxone 2 g IV daily to complete a 4-week course. Limited evidence supports the use of a continuous infusion of benzylpenicillin to treat adults at home using the same total daily dose as intermittent therapy outlined above.[15,16] Such management in children should only be contemplated in special circumstances.

For **complicated endocarditis** (large vegetation, multiple emboli, symptoms longer than 3 months, secondary septic events), we recommend treatment in hospital with:

benzylpenicillin 60 mg (100,000 U)/kg (max 2.4 g or 4 million U) IV, 4-hourly for 4 weeks PLUS
gentamicin 1 mg/kg IV, 8-hourly for 14 days

[NB: For low-dose 8-hourly synergistic dosing, measure only trough levels and keep level <1 mg/L to minimize toxicity (see Appendix 2).]

Streptococci relatively resistant to benzylpenicillin (MIC >0.12 to ≤0.5 mg/L)

For endocarditis due to streptococci relatively resistant to benzylpenicillin (MIC >0.12 to ≤0.5 mg/L), we recommend:

gentamicin 1 mg/kg IV, 8-hourly for 14 days PLUS EITHER
benzylpenicillin 60 mg (100,000 U)/kg (max 2.4 g or 4 million U) IV, 4-hourly for 4 weeks OR
ceftriaxone 100 mg/kg (max 4 g) IV, 24-hourly for 4 weeks

[NB: For low-dose 8-hourly synergistic dosing, measure only trough levels and keep level <1 mg/L to minimize toxicity (see Appendix 2).]

Streptococci resistant to benzylpenicillin (MIC >0.5 to <4 mg/L)

To treat endocarditis due to streptococci resistant to benzylpenicillin, follow the treatment recommendations for penicillin-susceptible enterococcal endocarditis (see enterococcal endocarditis, below).

The susceptibility of *Abiotrophia defectiva*, *Granulicatella* (previously called nutritionally variant streptococci), and *Gemella* species is often difficult to determine and unreliable.[1] They should be treated as for enterococci (see below).

Streptococci highly resistant to benzylpenicillin (MIC ≥4 mg/L)

There is no established regimen for endocarditis due to highly benzylpenicillin-resistant streptococci (MIC ≥4 mg/L).[1] Animal data and case reports[1,2] favor the use of the following regimen:

vancomycin <12 years: 30 mg/kg (max 1 g) IV, 12-hourly, 12 years and older: 25 mg/kg (max 1 g) IV, 12-hourly PLUS
gentamicin 1 mg/kg IV, 8-hourly for 4 weeks

[NB: For low-dose 8-hourly synergistic dosing, measure only trough levels and keep level <1 mg/L to minimize toxicity (see Appendix 2).]

Enterococcal endocarditis

Organisms such as *Enterococcus faecalis* and *Enterococcus faecium* are relatively difficult to treat with penicillin, even when reported to be susceptible to penicillin (MIC 0.5–2 mg/L).[17] It is always recommended to give concomitant gentamicin for optimal bactericidal activity,[17] although there are no studies.[13] Antibiotic resistance is an increasing problem.[1,2] All isolates should undergo testing for penicillin MIC and high-level aminoglycoside resistance. Enterococci are inherently resistant to third-generation cephalosporins, which should not be used to treat them.[17]

For susceptible infections, use:

gentamicin 1 mg/kg IV, 8-hourly for 6 weeks PLUS EITHER
benzylpenicillin 60 mg (100,000 U)/kg (max 2.4 g or 4 million U) IV, 4-hourly for 6 weeks OR
amoxi/ampicillin 50 mg/kg (max 2 g) IV, 4-hourly for 6 weeks

[NB: For low-dose 8-hourly synergistic dosing, measure only trough levels and keep level <1 mg/L to minimize toxicity (see Appendix 2).]

For patients with short-term symptoms (<3 month) the duration of treatment may be shortened to 4 weeks.[1,2]

For aminoglycoside-sensitive enterococci with high-level penicillin resistance, we recommend:

vancomycin <12 years: 30 mg/kg (max 1 g) IV, 12-hourly, 12 years and older: 25 mg/kg (max 1 g) IV, 12-hourly PLUS
gentamicin 1 mg/kg IV, 8-hourly for 4 weeks

[NB: For low-dose 8-hourly synergistic dosing, measure only trough levels and keep level <1 mg/L to minimize toxicity (see Appendix 2).]

For enterococci with high-level aminoglycoside resistance, we recommend seeking advice on alternative regimens and considering surgery.[1,2] Vancomycin-resistant enterococci usually exhibit penicillin and high-level aminoglycoside resistance. Treatment is recommended with combination regimens including linezolid and/or quinupristin+dalfopristin, often with surgery.[17]

Staphylococcus aureus endocarditis

S. aureus endocarditis is significantly more common in perioperative endocarditis, in cyanotic patients and in infants <1 year old.[4] At present, almost all community-acquired *S. aureus* endocarditis is susceptible to methicillin, while cMRSA tend to cause soft tissue infections but not endocarditis. However, community-associated MRSA may become more virulent, and cMRSA endocarditis may become more common. Surgery is often needed and we recommend early consultation with a cardiac surgeon.

For methicillin-susceptible staphylococci, we recommend:

di/flucl/oxa/nafcillin 50 mg/kg (max 2 g) IV, 4-hourly for 4–6 weeks

Routine coadministration of gentamicin (as for streptococcal endocarditis) is not supported by evidence[14] and is not recommended.

Four weeks of therapy appears to be sufficient in uncomplicated cases,[2] including in intravenous drug users (IVDU) with right-sided endocarditis, but at least 6 weeks is recommended for complications, such as perivalvular abscess, osteomyelitis, or septic metastatic complications.[16]

For methicillin-resistant staphylococci, we recommend:

vancomycin <12 years: 30 g/kg (max 1 g) IV, 12-hourly, 12 years and older: 25 mg/kg (max 1 g) IV, 12-hourly

S. aureus with intermediate susceptibility to vancomycin have been described (vancomycin-intermediate *S. aureus*, VISA). Successful treatment with linezolid has been described in case reports,[18,19] but experience is limited.

Endocarditis caused by the HACEK group

The HACEK group of oral Gram-negative bacilli (see Box 3.1) often grow poorly on traditional culture media and may require specialized microbiologic techniques. Although many strains are susceptible to penicillin, susceptibility testing may be difficult, and the HACEK group should be treated as if they are penicillin-resistant.[1] We recommend:

ceftriaxone 50 mg/kg (max 2 g) IV, daily for 4 weeks OR
cefotaxime 50 mg/kg (max 2 g) IV, 8-hourly for 4 weeks

Cat scratch endocarditis

For cat scratch endocarditis, we recommend:

doxycycline >8 years: 2.5 mg/kg (max 100 mg) orally, 12-hourly for 6 weeks PLUS EITHER
gentamicin 1 mg/kg IV, 8-hourly for 14 days OR
rifampicin 7.5 mg/kg (max 300 mg) orally, 12-hourly for 14 days

[NB: For low-dose 8-hourly synergistic dosing, measure only trough levels and keep level <1 mg/L to minimize toxicity (see Appendix 2).]

Prosthetic material endocarditis

The mortality of endocarditis involving prosthetic material is high, particularly when infection is with *S. aureus*. Observational studies in adults suggest mortality rates may be decreased with a combined medical–surgical approach, using early replacement of infected valves or synthetic material.[20–22]

For empiric therapy, until a definitive diagnosis is made, we recommend:

vancomycin <12 years: 30 mg/kg (max 1 g) IV, 12-hourly, 12 years and older: 25 mg/kg (max 1 g) IV, 12-hourly PLUS

gentamicin <10 years: 7.5 mg/kg; ≥10 years: 6 mg/kg IV, daily OR

gentamicin 2.5 mg/kg IV, 8-hourly

[NB: See Appendix 2 for advice on the prolonged use of gentamicin.]

Endocarditis caused by other bacteria

Endocarditis may rarely be caused by other bacteria. Non-toxin-producing strains of *Corynebacterium diphtheriae* (i.e., diphtheroids, not diphtheria-causing strains) are frequent contaminants of blood cultures, but can also cause endocarditis, including in children.[23] *Neisseria gonorrhoeae* is another uncommon cause of endocarditis.[24] *Pseudomonas aeruginosa* and Gram-negative enteric bacilli (other than HACEK) are rare causes of endocarditis that usually requires prolonged therapy for at least 6 weeks and sometimes surgery.[2,25]

Fungal endocarditis

Fungal endocarditis is rare, occurring mostly in neonates, immunocompromised patients with indwelling catheters, and children on long-term parenteral nutrition through a central catheter.[2] Medical therapy alone is usually unsuccessful, and most patients need surgery as well as antifungal agents.[2] We recommend:

amphotericin B deoxycholate 1 mg/kg IV daily PLUS

flucytosine (5-FC) 25 mg/kg (max 1g) orally, 6-hourly (if susceptible)

Liposomal amphotericin may be considered in patients with moderate to severe renal impairment or unacceptable infusion-related toxicities.

Amphotericin B remains the first-line antifungal agent for medical therapy, although it does not penetrate vegetations well. Although the imidazoles, such as fluconazole, have no proven efficacy in human fungal endocarditis, long-term suppressive therapy with fluconazole could be considered for patients with suscep-tible organisms who are not able to undergo curative surgery.[2]

Culture-negative endocarditis

Endocarditis may be culture-negative because of prior antibiotic therapy or when caused by one of a number of microorganisms, such as *Bartonella* species (including *B. henselae* which causes cat scratch disease), *C. burnetii* (Q fever), *Legionella* species (in adults), or fungi, including *Candida albicans*.[26] Molecular methods, such as polymerase chain reaction for microbial 16S ribosomal RNA genes and sequencing of the product, may allow a specific organism to be identified.[27]

Patients with culture-negative endocarditis should be treated empirically with benzylpenicillin plus gentamicin, as for enterococcal endocarditis (see p. 18) unless there is a strong reason to suspect an alternate diagnosis such as Q fever or fungal infection. In a retrospective review of 348 culture-negative endocarditis cases referred to a French reference center, 48% had Q fever and 28% had *Bartonella* infection.[28] Q fever endocarditis requires a long course (at least 18 months) of combined therapy using doxycycline (>8 years) and hydroxychloroquine.[29]

Penicillin allergy

For patients with penicillin allergy, we recommend consulting an infectious diseases physician or clinical microbiologist. For patients with non-anaphylactic allergy, ceftriaxone can usually be substituted for benzylpenicillin in the treatment of streptococcal endocarditis, and cephalothin or cephazolin for di/flucloxacillin when treating staphylococcal infection. For patients with anaphylactic penicillin allergy, vancomycin alone can be used for either streptococcal or staphylococcal infection. Vancomycin plus gentamicin is the only alternative available for enterococcal endocarditis, apart from desensitizing the patient to penicillin.

Teicoplanin is an alternative antibiotic for streptococcal endocarditis, but is not recommended for staphylococcal endocarditis, because the relapse rate is high.

Failure rates with clindamycin and lincomycin are unacceptably high for all types of endocarditis, and it is recommended not to use these antibiotics to treat endocarditis.

Monitoring antibiotic levels when treating endocarditis

Gentamicin

When using low-dose gentamicin (1 mg/kg 8-hourly), we recommend measuring trough levels, maintaining the level <1 mg/L. The aim is to minimize the risk of ototoxicity and nephrotoxicity (see also Appendix 2).

For once-daily gentamicin, levels should be monitored using the area-under-the-curve method (see Appendix 2). Older children on long-term gentamicin (>1 week) should ideally be monitored for vestibular and auditory ototoxicity.

Vestibular toxicity can occur even when drug levels are within the normal therapeutic range, and may be irreversible.[30] Toxicity may present early during treatment, or weeks after completing therapy.

If indicated, baseline audiometry should be performed as soon as possible after starting therapy, and repeated regularly if aminoglycosides are continued >14 days.

Glycopeptides (vancomycin and teicoplanin)

Trough levels of the glycopeptides, vancomycin or teicoplanin, should be monitored to reduce toxicity and ensure adequate levels for killing. For maximal efficacy, the target trough levels are 10–20 mg/L for vancomycin and >20 mg/L for teicoplanin.

Di/flucl/oxa/nafcillin

Monitoring of di/flucl/oxa/nafcillin levels is not indicated with intermittent intravenous dosing. It may be considered in patients receiving flucloxacillin by continuous intravenous infusion.

Monitoring blood parameters when treating endocarditis

It is extremely common for patients on long-term treatment with beta-lactam antibiotics for endocarditis to have delayed adverse events, notably fever, rash, and/or neutropenia, often with eosinophilia. In an 8-year prospective study, 33% of adults treated for endocarditis with beta-lactams developed significant adverse effects.[31] Furthermore, 51% of those treated with penicillin G for more than 10 days developed any adverse event and 14% had neutropenia.[31] Di/flucl/oxa/nafcillin can also cause fever and neutropenia.[31] Flucloxacillin can cause cholestatic hepatitis, though mainly in adults, while dicloxacillin can cause interstitial nephritis.[32]

We recommend monitoring the differential white cell count for neutropenia and eosinophilia when patients are receiving beta-lactam antibiotics.

Prevention of endocarditis: antibiotic chemoprophylaxis

Question | For children with preexisting heart disease, do prophylactic antibiotics compared with no antibiotics or placebo reduce the risk of endocarditis?

Literature review | We found only one case-control study in adults and children.[33]

Despite the well-recognized association between recent dental work and endocarditis, it is not absolutely certain that the dental work causes the endocarditis. People who require dental work may already be at higher risk of endocarditis because of their bad teeth. It is known that children develop a transient bacteremia about half of the time when they brush their teeth.[34] Thus, it seems logical that dental work might increase the risk of bacteremia and endocarditis in persons with predisposing heart conditions.

It has been recommended for many years to give prophylactic antibiotics to adults and children known to be at increased risk for endocarditis when they have a procedure that is likely to cause bacteremia, such as dental work and some other surgical procedures. The evidence for this practice is extremely weak. A Cochrane systematic review[35] found no RCTs, although that is hardly surprising, because it is rare to get endocarditis after a procedure and an RCT would need very large numbers of patients. More surprisingly, the review found only one case-control study,[33] which included all the cases of endocarditis in the Netherlands over 2 years. No significant effect of penicillin prophylaxis on the incidence of endocarditis was seen.[33]

Despite the lack of good evidence, all authorities involved with children and adults at risk for endocarditis continue to recommend antibiotic chemoprophylaxis for certain procedures. The groups known to be at increased risk for endocarditis have been reviewed[36] and guidelines have been developed by the American Medical Association.[37] These have been modified for children[38] and for the Australian Indigenous population (see Table 3.1).[39]

Table 3.1 Cardiac conditions and risk for infective endocarditis.

High-risk Conditions	Medium-risk Conditions	Low-risk Conditions
Prosthetic cardiac valves (including bioprosthetic and homograft)	Congenital cardiac malformations, other than those defined as high or low risk	Surgical repair of atrial septal defect (ASD), venticular septal defect or patent ductus arteriosus
Previous infective endocarditis	Hypertrophic cardiomyopathy	Isolated secundum ASD
Complex cyanotic congenital heart disease (single ventricle, transposition of great arteries, tetralogy of Fallot)	Acquired valvular dysfunction (e.g., rheumatic heart disease) in non-indigenous patients	Previous coronary artery bypass grafts or stents
Surgically constructed systemic-pulmonary shunts or conduits	Mitral valve prolapse with valvular regurgitation or thickened leaflets	Mitral valve prolapse without regurgitation
Acquired valvular dysfunction (e.g., rheumatic heart disease) in indigenous patients	Significant valvular/hemodynamic dysfunction associated with septal defects	Previous Kawasaki disease without valve dysfunction
	Severe pulmonary stenosis	Previous rheumatic fever without valve dysfunction
		Cardiac pacemakers and implanted defibrillators
		Mild or moderate pulmonary stenosis
		Physiologic, functional, or innocent heart murmur

Adapted from References 37–39.

Dental procedures for which chemoprophylaxis is recommended,[38] on the basis of the likelihood of causing bacteremia, are dental extractions, periodontal procedures, including scaling, probing, and routine maintenance as well as initial placement of orthodontic bands but not brackets, and prophylactic cleaning of teeth or implants during which bleeding is expected.[38]

The recommendations for non-dental procedures are given in Table 3.2. They are based on likely risk of bacteremia, but there have been no studies to show efficacy.

If it is decided to give antibiotic prophylaxis, it is recommended to give a single dose of antibiotic before the procedure. There is no proven value to giving a follow-up dose 6 hours later, and this is no longer recommended.[37–39] The recommended regimens are given in Table 3.3.

3.2 Acute rheumatic fever

Acute rheumatic fever is an acute inflammatory condition that occurs subsequent to group A streptococcal (GAS) infection. The inflammation can affect joints, skin, central nervous system, and particularly the heart. Rheumatic heart disease is an autoimmune disease in which T-cell damage to the endocardium occurs as a result of mimicry between streptococcal M protein and cardiac myosin.[40] Carditis can occur with the first attack of acute rheumatic fever, or later with recurrences. Lasegue wrote, more than 100 years ago, that rheumatic fever "licks at the joint but bites at the heart."

Traditional teaching is that the GAS infection is usually of the throat (streptococcal tonsillitis and/or pharyngitis),[41] and this is supported by evidence from a meta-analysis of studies that antibiotic treatment of sore throats reduces the incidence of subsequent

Table 3.2 Recommendations on procedures and endocarditis prophylaxis.

Site	Recommended: High Risk	Not Recommended: Low Risk
Respiratory tract	Tonsillectomy and/or adenoidectomy Surgery involving respiratory mucosa Rigid bronchoscopy	Endotracheal intubation Flexible bronchoscopy Insertion of tympanostomy tubes (grommets)
Gastrointestinal tract	Biliary tract surgery Esophageal surgery Surgery involving intestinal mucosa	Endoscopy without biopsy Transesophageal echocardiography
Genitourinary tract	Cystoscopy Urethral dilatation	Urethral catheterization (if no infection) Vaginal procedures
Other		Cardiac catheterization Balloon angioplasty Circumcision

Adapted from Reference 38.

Table 3.3 Recommendations on antibiotic regimens for endocarditis prophylaxis.[38]

Condition	Situation	Antibiotic Regimen
Dental, oral, respiratory tract, or esophageal procedures	Standard general prophylaxis	Amoxicillin 50 mg/kg (max 2 g) orally, 1 hour before procedure
Dental, oral, respiratory tract, or esophageal procedures	Unable to take medication orally	Ampicillin 50 mg/kg (max 2 g) IV or IM, up to 30 min before procedure
Dental, oral, respiratory tract, or esophageal procedures	Allergic to penicillin	Clindamycin 20 mg/kg (max 600 mg) orally, 1 hour before procedure (same dose IV up to 30 min before if cannot take orally) *OR* Cephalexin 50 mg/kg (max 2 g) orally, 1 h before procedure (or cefazolin 25 mg/kg IM or IV, up to 30 min before)
Gastrointestinal or genitourinary tract procedures	High risk	Ampicillin 50 mg/kg IV or IM (max 2 g) *plus* gentamicin 1.5 mg/kg (max 120 mg) IV or IM, up to 30 min before procedure
Gastrointestinal or genitourinary tract procedures	Moderate risk	Amoxicillin 50 mg/kg (max 2 g) orally, 1 hour before procedure *OR* Ampicillin 50 mg/kg (max 2 g) IV or IM, up to 30 min before procedure
Gastrointestinal or genitourinary tract procedures	Allergic to ampicillin	Vancomycin 25 mg/kg (max 1 g), infused IV over 1–2 h, finishing up to 30 min before procedure If high risk, also give gentamicin 1.5 mg/kg (max 120 mg) IV or IM, up to 30 min before procedure

rheumatic fever.[42] Recent data suggest that in Australian Aboriginal children who have a rate of rheumatic fever >300 cases per 100,000 persons per year (among children 5–14 years old) compared to <5 cases per 100,000 persons per year in the non-Aboriginal Australian population, acute rheumatic fever occurs as a result of GAS skin infections (pyoderma or impetigo) and not throat infection.[43,44] Similar high rates of pyoderma and low rates of sore throat in association with acute rheumatic fever have been reported from Ethiopia, Jamaica, and southern India.[45]

Rheumatic fever is very much a disease of poverty. Another major risk factor is overcrowding, and outbreaks of rheumatic fever have traditionally been reported in boarding schools and army barracks.[46] However, as recently as the 1980s, there was a resurgence of acute rheumatic fever in middle class children in the mid-western USA.[47] This suggests that factors related to the virulence of the organism, the environment, and the host are all important in the etiology of rheumatic fever.

Diagnosis of acute rheumatic fever

Rheumatic fever usually presents acutely with fever, evanescent large joint polyarthritis or arthralgia, sometimes with the urticarial rash of erythema marginatum, sometimes with subcutaneous nodules, and sometimes with evidence of acute carditis.[46] Children with Sydenham's chorea often present much more indolently, with unusual choreiform movements that disappear at night, often involving just one limb, and with a labile affect, but without fever or laboratory evidence of inflammation and often without a history suggesting recent streptococcal infection.[46] Acute rheumatic fever can mimic a number of other conditions, both infective and non-infective, including infective endocarditis, viral infections, juvenile idiopathic arthritis, and Kawasaki disease. In 1944, Duckett Jones published criteria for the diagnosis of acute rheumatic fever,[48] and these have been modified by the American Heart Association.[46] They are useful for decisions about acute treatment and long-term prophylaxis (see below). It can be particularly difficult to decide about the management of children with post-streptococcal arthralgia or arthritis who may or may not be at risk for later carditis. The modified Jones criteria are shown in Table 3.4.

Table 3.4 Modified Duckett Jones criteria for diagnosing acute rheumatic fever.[46]

Major criteria	Acute carditis
	Polyarthritis
	Chorea
	Erythema marginatum
	Sub-cutaneous nodules
Minor criteria	Arthralgia
	Fever
	Elevated ESR or serum C-reactive protein
	Prolonged PR interval (first-degree heart block)
Evidence of GAS infection	Positive culture or rising antibody titer (antistreptolysin O = ASOT or anti-deoxyribonuclease B = anti-DNase B)
Diagnosis	Need evidence of streptococcal infection plus either two major *or* one major and two minor criteria (and no other diagnosis)

Acute rheumatic carditis can affect the endocardium, the myocardium, or the pericardium but usually all three (pancarditis).[46,49] If there is endocarditis, the mitral valve is most commonly affected, followed by the aortic valve. Valvular insufficiency is usual, but mitral stenosis due to thickening of the valve may develop early in young children.[46,49] Clinically, children with carditis present with cardiomegaly and heart failure, with tachycardia, with murmurs (e.g., a high-pitched pansystolic murmur radiating to the axilla of mitral incompetence or the Carey Coombs diastolic murmur of mitral stenosis), and rarely with arrhythmias due to myocarditis or with a rub and/or muffled heart sounds due to pericarditis.[46,49]

Prevention of acute rheumatic fever

Antibiotic treatment of sore throat
A Cochrane review of the treatment of acute sore throat found that antibiotics reduced acute rheumatic fever by more than three quarters (RR 0.22, 95% CI 0.02–2.08).[42] Prompt treatment of streptococcal sore throat is important,[50] but not all children who develop rheumatic fever have an identifiable sore throat, and some may have skin sepsis instead.[43–45]

Treatment of skin sepsis
Although it has not been proven that reducing skin sepsis in Aboriginal children prevents acute rheumatic

fever, it has been shown that the incidence of impetigo and pyoderma can be reduced by using permethrin to treat scabies.[51] Pyoderma was also reduced, but only temporarily, when Aboriginal children were given a single dose of azithromycin in a trachoma program.[52]

Treatment of acute rheumatic fever

Children with evidence of active infection should be treated with antibiotics to eradicate group A streptococcus (see p. 178).

The mainstay of anti-inflammatory treatment of acute rheumatic fever has been the use of aspirin, and it has been reported that the rapid defervescence of fever soon after starting aspirin is virtually diagnostic.[53] A Cochrane review of different anti-inflammatory drugs in acute rheumatic fever, however, found no RCTs comparing aspirin with placebo, so this observation is anecdotal.[54]

The Cochrane review included eight RCTs involving 996 people, and comparing different steroids (ACTH, cortisone, hydrocortisone, dexamethasone, and prednisone) and intravenous immunoglobulin with aspirin, placebo, or no treatment.[54] Six of the trials were conducted between 1950 and 1965. Overall there was no significant difference in the risk of cardiac disease at 1 year between the corticosteroid-treated and aspirin-treated groups (RR 0.87, 95% CI 0.66–1.15). Similarly, use of prednisone (RR 1.78, 95% CI 0.98–3.34) or intravenous immunoglobulins (RR 0.87, 95% CI 0.55–1.39) did not reduce the risk of developing heart valve lesions at 1 year compared to placebo.[54]

The optimal management of inflammation in acute rheumatic fever remains uncertain. In one study, naproxen was found to be as effective as aspirin, and substantially less likely to be associated with elevated liver enzymes.[55] The role of corticosteroids remains unclear.

Antibiotic prophylaxis of rheumatic fever

Question | For patients with a history of rheumatic fever do long-term prophylactic antibiotics, compared with no antibiotics or placebo, reduce the incidence of recurrent attacks of rheumatic fever and/or exacerbation of existing rheumatic heart disease, or the development of new rheumatic heart disease?

Literature review | We found 10 studies on penicillin prophylaxis with highly variable design, and 2 meta-analyses,[56,57] including a Cochrane review.[56]

The Cochrane review[56] did not pool the 9 studies found, because of heterogeneity and different study design. Three trials, with 1301 patients, compared penicillin to placebo. Only 1 of these 3 studies found that penicillin reduced rheumatic fever recurrence (RR 0.45, 95% CI 0.22–0.92) and streptococcal throat infection (RR 0.84, 95% CI 0.72–0.97). Four trials ($n = 1098$) compared long-acting IM penicillin with oral penicillin: all showed that IM penicillin reduced rheumatic fever recurrence and streptococcal throat infections compared to oral penicillin. It is not clear whether this is because of better compliance or because better antibiotic levels can be achieved with long-acting IM penicillin. One trial ($n = 360$) comparing 2-weekly with 4-weekly IM penicillin found 2-weekly was better at reducing rheumatic fever recurrence (RR 0.52, 95% CI 0.33–0.83) and streptococcal throat infections (RR 0.60, 95% CI 0.42–0.85). One trial ($n = 249$) showed 3-weekly IM penicillin reduced streptococcal throat infections (RR 0.67, 95% CI 0.48–0.92) compared to 4-weekly IM penicillin.[56]

The Cochrane review authors concluded that IM penicillin seemed to be more effective than oral penicillin in preventing rheumatic fever recurrence and streptococcal throat infections, and that 2-weekly or 3-weekly IM injections appeared to be more effective than 4-weekly injections.[56] However, they state that the evidence is based on poor-quality trials.

A more recent meta-analysis included 10 trials ($n = 7665$) and agreed that, in general, the methodologic quality of the studies was poor.[57] All the included trials were conducted during the period 1950–1961, and in 8 of the trials the study population was young adult males living on United States military bases. The meta-analysis revealed an overall protective effect for the use of antibiotics against acute rheumatic fever of 68% (RR 0.32, 95% CI = 0.21–0.48). When meta-analysis was restricted to trials evaluating penicillin, the protective effect was 80% (RR 0.20, 95% CI = 0.11–0.36). They concluded that 60 children with rheumatic fever needed to be treated with prophylactic penicillin to prevent one case of rheumatic carditis (number needed to treat, NNT = 60).[57]

Table 3.5 Duration of prophylaxis for rheumatic fever.[38,48]

Condition	Recommended Duration
Rheumatic fever with no carditis	For 5 years, or until 21 years old (whichever is longer)
Rheumatic fever with carditis, but with no residual valve disease	For 10 years or well into adulthood (whichever is longer)
Rheumatic fever with carditis, with residual valve disease	For at least 10 years after last episode, and until at least 40 years old, but sometimes lifelong

The WHO has recommended that registers be set up to monitor compliance in areas with a high prevalence of rheumatic fever.[58] There is observational evidence, particularly from New Zealand, that these registers improve delivery.[59]

We recommend continuous antimicrobial prophylaxis against *S. pyogenes* infection for patients with a well-documented history of rheumatic fever. IM administration of long-acting penicillin is preferred, especially in remote areas, as it is more effective and usually leads to better adherence: We prefer 3-weekly injections, but will give 4-weekly if it improves compliance. We recommend that treatment be given in a convenient site, such as a health center or in the patient's home.

Because compliance is so important and IM penicillin so painful, the rheumatic fever service in the Northern Territory of Australia mixes each 2 mL IM injection of benzathine penicillin with 0.5 mL of lignocaine (J. Carapetis, personal communication, 2006). Although we can find no evidence regarding safety and efficacy of this practice, we recommend using this regimen if compliance is likely to depend on it.

We recommend:

> **benzathine penicillin: adult and child ≥20 kg: 900 mg (=1.5 million units); child <20 kg: 450 mg (=750,000 units) IM, every 3 or 4 weeks**

If IM penicillin absolutely cannot be given, usually due to adherence problems, we recommend:

> **phenoxymethyl penicillin (all ages) 250 mg orally, 12-hourly**

For patients with anaphylactic penicillin allergy, we recommend:

> **erythromycin 250 mg orally, 12-hourly OR erythromycin ethyl succinate 400 mg orally, 12-hourly (all ages)**

The duration of prophylaxis is given in Table 3.5.

References

1 Baddour LM, Wilson WR, Bayer AS et al. Infective endocarditis: diagnosis, antimicrobial therapy, and management of complications. A statement for healthcare professionals from the Committee on Rheumatic Fever, Endocarditis, and Kawasaki Disease, Council on Cardiovascular Disease in the Young, and the Councils on Clinical Cardiology, Stroke, and Cardiovascular Surgery and Anesthesia, American Heart Association: endorsed by the Infectious Diseases Society of America. *Circulation* 2005;111:e394–434.

2 Ferrieri P, Gewitz MH, Gerber MA et al. Unique features of infective endocarditis in childhood. *Circulation* 2002;105:2115–27.

3 Sarli Issa V, Fabri J, Jr, Pomerantzeff PM, Grinberg M, Pereira-Barreto AC, Mansur AJ. Duration of symptoms in patients with infective endocarditis. *Int J Cardiol* 2003;89:63–70.

4 Ishiwada N, Niwa K, Tateno S et al. Causative organism influences clinical profile and outcome of infective endocarditis in pediatric patients and adults with congenital heart disease. *Circ J* 2005;69:1266–70.

5 Niwa K, Nakazawa M, Tateno S, Yoshinaga M, Terai M. Infective endocarditis in congenital heart disease: Japanese national collaboration study. *Heart* 2005;91:795–800.

6 Reynolds HR, Jagen MA, Tunick PA, Krouzon I. Sensitivity of trans-thoracic versus transesophageal echocardiography for the detection of native valve vegetations in the modern era. *J Am Soc Echocardiogr* 2003;16:67–70.

7 Del Pont JM, De Cicco LT, Vartalitis C et al. Infective endocarditis in children. *Pediatric Infect Dis J* 1995;14:1079–86.

8 Stockheim JA, Chadwick EG, Kessler S et al. Are the Duke criteria superior to Beth Israel criteria for the diagnosis of infective endocarditis in children? *Clin Infect Dis* 1998;27:1451–6.

9 Durack DT, Lukes AS, Bright DK. New diagnostic criteria for diagnosis of infective endocarditis: utilization of specific echocardiographic findings. Duke Endocarditis Service. *Am J Med* 1994;96:200–9.

10 Li JS, Sexton DJ, Mick N et al. Proposed modifications to the Duke criteria for the diagnosis of infective endocarditis. *Clin Infect Dis* 2000;30:633–8.

11 Felipe Flores L, Leon S, Casanova JM, Reyes PA. The treatment of infectious endocarditis. Cefotaxime versus "traditional" medical management [in Spanish]. *Arch Inst Cardiol Mex* 1993;63:47–51.

12 Sexton DJ, Tenenbaum MJ, Wilson WR et al., for the Endocarditis Treatment Consortium Group. Ceftriaxone once

daily for four weeks compared with ceftriaxone plus gentamicin once daily for two weeks for treatment of endocarditis due to penicillin-susceptible streptococci. *Clin Infect Dis* 1998;27: 1470–4.

13 Falagas ME, Matthaiou DK, Bliziotis IA. The role of aminoglycosides in combination with a beta-lactam for the treatment of bacterial endocarditis: a meta-analysis of comparative trials. *J Antimicrob Chemother* 2006;57:639–47.

14 Ribera E, Gomez-Jimenez J, Cortes E et al. Effectiveness of cloxacillin with and without gentamicin in short-term therapy for right-sided *Staphylococcus aureus* endocarditis: a randomized, controlled trial. *Ann Intern Med* 1996;125:969–74.

15 Stamboulian D, Bonvehi P, Arevalo C et al. Antibiotic management of outpatients with endocarditis due to penicillin-susceptible streptococci. *Rev Infect Dis* 1991;13(suppl 2): S160–3.

16 Therapeutic Guidelines Ltd. Cardiovascular infections. In: *Therapeutic Guidelines: Antibiotic*, version 13. Melbourne: Therapeutic Guidelines Ltd, 2006:49–60.

17 McDonald JR, Olaison L, Anderson DJ et al. Enterococcal endocarditis: 107 cases from the international collaboration on endocarditis merged database. *Am J Med* 2005;118:759–66.

18 Howden BP, Ward PB, Charles PG et al. Treatment outcomes for serious infections caused by methicillin-resistant *Staphylococcus aureus* with reduced vancomycin susceptibility. *Clin Infect Dis* 2004;38:521–8.

19 Leung KT, Tong MK, Siu YP, Lam CS, Ng HL, Lee HK. Treatment of vancomycin-intermediate *Staphylcoccus aureus* endocarditis with linezolid. *Scand J Infect Dis* 2004;36:483–5.

20 John MDV, Hibberd PL, Karchmer AW, Sleeper LA, Calderwood SB. *Staphylococcus aureus* prosthetic valve endocarditis: optimal management and risk factors for death. *Clin Infect Dis* 1998;26:1302–9.

21 Wolff M, Witchitz S, Chastang C, Regnier B, Vachon F. Prosthetic valve endocarditis in the ICU: prognostic factors of overall survival in a series of 122 cases and consequences for treatment decisions. *Chest* 1995;108:688–94.

22 Yu VL, Fang GD, Keys TF et al. Prosthetic valve endocarditis: superiority of surgical valve replacement versus medical therapy alone. *Am Thorac Surg* 1994;58:1073–7.

23 Belko J, Wessel DL, Malley R. Endocarditis caused by *Corynebacterium diphtheriae*: case report and review of the literature. *Pediatr Infect Dis J* 2000;19:159–63.

24 Thompson EC, Brantley D. Gonococcal endocarditis. *J Natl Med Assoc* 1996;88:353–6.

25 Geraci JE, Wilson WR. Endocarditis due to Gram-negative bacteria: report of 56 cases. *Mayo Clin Proc* 1982;57:145–8.

26 Moreillon P, Que YA. Infective endocarditis. *Lancet* 2004;363:139–49.

27 Millar BC, Moore JE. Current trends in the molecular diagnosis of infective endocarditis. *Eur J Clin Microbiol Infect Dis* 2004;23:353–65.

28 Houpikian P, Raoult D. Blood culture-negative endocarditis in a reference center: etiologic diagnosis of 348 cases. *Medicine (Baltimore)* 2005;84:162–73.

29 American Academy of Pediatrics. Q fever. In: Pickering LK (ed.), *Red Book: 2003 Report of the Committee on Infectious Diseases*, 26th edn. Elk Grove Village, IL: American Academy of Pediatrics, 2003:512–4.

30 Minor LB. Gentamicin-induced bilateral vestibular hypofunction. *JAMA* 1998;279:541–4.

31 Olaison L, Belin L, Hogevik H, Alestig K. Incidence of beta-lactam-induced delayed hypersensitivity and neutropenia during treatment of infective endocarditis. *Arch Intern Med* 1999;159:607–15.

32 Devereaux BM, Crawford DH, Purcell P, Powell LW, Roeser HP. Flucloxacillin associated cholestatic hepatitis: an Australian and Swedish epidemic? *Eur J Clin Pharmacol* 1995;49:81–5.

33 Van der Meer JTM, van Wijk W, Thompson J, Vandenbroucke JP, Valkenburg HA, Michel MF. Efficacy of antibiotic prophylaxis for prevention of native-valve endocarditis. *Lancet* 1992;339:135–9.

34 Bhanji S, Williams B, Sheller B, Elwood T, Mancl L. Transient bacteremia induced by toothbrushing: a comparison of the Sonicare toothbrush with a conventional toothbrush. *Pediatr Dent* 2002;24:295–9.

35 Oliver R, Roberts GJ, Hooper L. Penicillins for the prophylaxis of bacterial endocarditis in dentistry. *The Cochrane Database of Systematic Reviews* 2004;(2):Art No CD003813.

36 Steckelberg JM, Wilson WR. Risk factors for infective endocarditis. *Infect Dis Clin North Am* 1993;7:9–19.

37 Dajani AS, Taubert KA, Wilson W et al. Prevention of bacterial endocarditis: recommendations by the American Heart Association. *JAMA* 1997;277:1794–1801.

38 American Academy of Pediatrics. Antimicrobial prophylaxis. In: Pickering LK (ed.), *Red Book: 2003 Report of the Committee on Infectious Diseases*, 26th edn. Elk Grove Village, IL: American Academy of Pediatrics, 2003:778–87.

39 Therapeutic Guidelines Ltd. Prophylaxis: medical. In: *Therapeutic Guidelines: Antibiotic*, version 13. Melbourne: Therapeutic Guidelines Ltd, 2006:177–86.

40 Ellis NM, Li Y, Hildebrand W, Fischetti VA, Cunningham MW. T cell mimicry and epitope specificity of cross-reactive T cell clones from rheumatic heart disease. *J Immunol* 2005;175:5448–56.

41 Siegel AC, Johnson EE, Stollerman GH. Controlled studies of streptococcal pharyngitis in a paediatric population. 1: Factors related to the attack rate of rheumatic fever. *N Engl J Med* 1961;265:559–65.

42 Del Mar CB, Glasziou PP, Spinks AB. Antibiotics for sore throat. *The Cochrane Database of Systematic Reviews* 2006;(4):Art No CD000023.

43 Carapetis JR, Wolff DR, Currie BJ. Acute rheumatic fever and rheumatic heart disease in the Top End of Australia's Northern Territory. *Med J Aust* 1996;164:146–9.

44 McDonald MI, Towers RJ, Andrews RM, Benger N, Currie BJ, Carapetis JR. Low rates of streptococcal pharyngitis and high rates of pyoderma in Australian aboriginal communities where acute rheumatic fever is hyperendemic. *Clin Infect Dis* 2006;43:683–9.

45 Steer AC, Carapetis JR, Nolan TM, Shann F. Systematic review of rheumatic heart disease prevalence in children in developing countries: the role of environmental factors. *J Paediatr Child Health* 2002;38:229–34.

46 Special Writing Group of the Committee on Rheumatic Fever, Endocarditis, and Kawasaki Disease of the Council on Cardiovascular Disease in the Young of the American Heart Association. Guidelines for the diagnosis of rheumatic fever: Jones Criteria, 1992 update. *JAMA* 1992;268:2069–73.

47 Veasy LG, Wiedmeier SE, Orsmond GS et al. Resurgence of acute rheumatic fever in the intermountain area of the United States. *N Engl J Med* 1987;316:421–7.

48 Jones TD. The diagnosis of rheumatic fever. *JAMA* 1944;126: 481–6.

49 Lennon D. Acute rheumatic fever in children: recognition and treatment. *Paediatr Drugs* 2004;6:363–73.

50 Dajani A, Taubert K, Ferrieri P, Peter G, Shulman S, for the Committee on Rheumatic Fever, Endocarditis, and Kawasaki Disease of the Council on Cardiovascular Disease in the Young, the American Heart Association. Treatment of acute streptococcal pharyngitis and prevention of rheumatic fever: a statement for health professionals. *Pediatrics* 1995;96: 758–64.

51 Carapetis JR, Connors C, Yarmirr D, Krause V, Currie BJ. Success of a scabies control program in an Australian aboriginal community. *Pediatr Infect Dis J* 1997;16:494–9.

52 Shelby-James TM, Leach AJ, Carapetis JR, Currie BJ, Mathews JD. Impact of single dose azithromycin on group A streptococci in the upper respiratory tract and skin of Aboriginal children. *Pediatr Infect Dis J* 2002;21:375–80.

53 Stollerman GH. Treatment and prevention of rheumatic fever and rheumatic heart disease. *Pediatr Clin North Am* 1964;11:213–28.

54 Cilliers AM, Manyemba J, Saloojee H. Anti-inflammatory treatment for carditis in acute rheumatic fever. *The Cochrane Database of Systematic Reviews* 2003;(2):Art No CD003176.

55 Hashkes PJ, Tauber T, Somekh E et al. Naproxen as an alternative to aspirin for the treatment of arthritis of rheumatic fever: a randomized trial. *J Pediatr* 2003;143:399–401.

56 Manyemba J, Mayosi BM. Penicillin for secondary prevention of rheumatic fever. *The Cochrane Database of Systematic Reviews* 2002;(3):Art No CD002227.

57 Robertson KA, Volmink JA, Mayosi BM. Antibiotics for the primary prevention of acute rheumatic fever: a meta-analysis. *BMC Cardiovasc Disord* 2005;5:11.

58 World Health Organization. Strategy for controlling rheumatic fever/rheumatic heart disease, with emphasis on primary prevention: memorandum from a joint WHO/ISFC meeting. *Bull World Health Organ* 1995;73:583–7.

59 McDonald M, Brown A, Noonan S, Carapetis JR. Preventing recurrent rheumatic fever: the role of register based programmes. *Heart* 2005;91:1131–3.

CHAPTER 4
Cervical infections

4.1 Cervical lymphadenopathy

Children often have palpable, and sometimes visible, lymph nodes. In a study of over 3500 healthy 8–9-year-old Swedish schoolchildren, 27.6% had palpable submandibular, cervical, and/or supraclavicular lymph nodes.[1] The most common location was submandibular. In 8.7% of children, the lymph nodes were 5 mm or greater in diameter. Boys had a significantly higher prevalence of palpable lymph nodes than girls. There was also seasonal variation. Children who had positive skin-prick testing to atypical mycobacteria (*Mycobacterium avium* or *Mycobacterium scrofulaceum*) did not have a higher prevalence of palpable lymph nodes than those not infected.[1]

What is pathological? The term cervical lymphadenopathy is often reserved for lymph nodes >1 cm in diameter,[2–4] although a cutoff of 1.5 cm or greater has been used for Kawasaki disease,[5] while cutoffs from 1 to 2.5 cm have been used to define enlarged lymph nodes in different studies. Clearly, the reported incidence of lymphadenopathy will vary according to the definition.

Children with small lymph nodes who are otherwise well do not need any investigation. Their lymph nodes are thought to be minimally enlarged in response to common viral respiratory infections, which are the commonest cause of minor cervical lymphadenopathy in young children.[2–4]

Causes of cervical lymphadenopathy

The causes of cervical lymphadenopathy are myriad. Their frequency depends on various factors, the most important of which are the child's age and whether the child is from a rich, industrialized country with a temperate climate or from a poor, tropical country. In the former situation, most studies have found that *Staphylococcus aureus* is the most common cause of cervical lymphadenitis, particularly in infancy, followed by group A streptococcus and atypical mycobacterial infection.[6–12] In the latter, impoverished situation, *M. tuberculosis*, and HIV infection are now among the most important causes of lymphadenopathy, although pyogenic infection is also extremely common.[13–15]

S. aureus probably reaches the lymph nodes through the skin, although there may be no obvious abrasion. Other organisms, such as group A streptococcus, drain to the regional lymph nodes from the nasopharynx. *M. tuberculosis*, and less common causes of lymphadenitis, such as *Streptococcus pneumoniae*[16] and group B streptococcus, may spread via the bloodstream or locally from the nasopharynx.[17]

Table 4.1 summarizes some of the more important of the myriad causes of cervical lymphadenopathy, as reported in the literature.[1–15] We have deliberately excluded some of the rarer causes, which may be found in review articles.[4] A long list of the causes is not very helpful, so we have combined the underlying pathology with the usual clinical presentation.

Cervical lymphadenopathy: the history

Acute or chronic presentation

There is an important distinction between children who present with acute neck swelling, which is often tender and associated with fever, and children who present with a more gradual onset of non-tender swelling in the neck, often without fever. The former presentation is suggestive of an acute suppurative process, as with bacterial adenitis (including cat scratch), or suggestive of Kawasaki disease (see Section 6.9, p. 63). In contrast, children with lymphadenitis due to mycobacterial infection, either *M. tuberculosis* or atypical mycobacteria, tend to present in a far more indolent way. Although children with TB lymphadenitis may have systemic symptoms of fever, night sweats, and weight loss, it is far more common for them to be afebrile and well, and present just with enlarging or discharging neck glands.[13,14]

Table 4.1 Some of the more common causes of cervical lymphadenopathy in children.

Underlying Pathology	Usual Clinical Presentation	Cause
Acute bacterial suppurative lymphadenitis	Fever, tenderness, red, inflamed	*Staphylococcus aureus* Group A streptococcus Cat scratch (*Bartonella henselae*) Anaerobes
Chronic bacterial lymphadenitis	Fever may or may not be present, non-tender, reddish-purple skin discoloration, may suppurate	*Mycobacterium tuberculosis* Atypical mycobacteria
Acute viral	Fever, tenderness, may have palatal petechiae, eyelid edema, splenomegaly	EBV
Chronic viral	Other features of HIV infection	HIV
Inflammatory	Fever, tenderness, nodes usually unilateral and may resemble cervical abscess	Kawasaki disease
Protozoal	Asymptomatic or chronic illness with weakness and debility	*Toxoplasma gondii* (NB: CMV and EBV can present this way)
Malignancy	Fever, night sweats, weight loss	Lymphoma

Toxoplasmosis also tends to present indolently in older children and adolescents, with isolated cervical or occipital lymphadenopathy.[18] The lymph nodes are not tender, do not suppurate, are usually discrete, and stay enlarged for less than 4–6 weeks.[18] A form of the disease characterized by chronic lymphadenopathy has been described, and lymph-node enlargement can fluctuate for months, associated with weakness and debility.[19]

Malignancy is a relatively rare cause of cervical lymphadenopathy, usually in older children.[6–12]

Unilateral or bilateral lymphadenopathy
· Bilateral cervical lymphadenitis is most commonly seen with group A streptococcal infection and with viral infections, such as EBV.
· Cat scratch disease is almost always unilateral, and Kawasaki disease usually unilateral.
· Mycobacterial infections can be unilateral or bilateral.[4]

Site of neck swelling
The site of lymph node swelling can be helpful[4]:
· Post-erior cervical lymphadenopathy (occipital nodes) occurs acutely with rubella and EBV infection, and chronically with malignancy.

· Cat scratch usually causes preauricular or submandibular swelling.
· Malignancy is more likely to affect supraclavicular nodes (or post-erior nodes) than anterior nodes.
· Acute bilateral parotid swelling (the parotid overlies the mandible) suggests mumps.
· Chronic bilateral parotid swelling may be due to HIV infection or Sjögren disease.
· Acute, unilateral parotid swelling, particularly if recurrent, suggests recurrent parotitis of childhood.[20]

History of cat contact
A history of exposure to cats, and particularly to kittens or a sick cat, can help suggest a diagnosis of cat scratch disease[21] (see also Section 6.10, p. 66). There may be a nodule at the site of a previous scratch, which is likely to be on the face to cause cervical lymphadenopathy (scratches on the hand give rise to epitrochlear or axillary lymphadenopathy and on the leg give rise to inguinal lymphadenopathy). On the other hand, *B. henselae* can be transmitted by a lick from a cat, so a history of close contact alone is sufficient to raise suspicion of the diagnosis in a child with fever and cervical lymphadenopathy.[21] In addition, children with cat scratch lymphadenopathy may have a granulomatous

conjunctivitis (Parinaud oculoglandular syndrome) with granulomata visible on the palpebral conjunctiva.

Toxoplasma infection has also been associated with cat contact as well as with eating undercooked meat.[16]

History of exposure to infection

It is obviously important to ask about exposure to possible infections, such as TB, group A streptococcal infection, and viral infections. Some families will hide a family history of TB because of the stigma.

Dental infections

· Dental abscess and periodontal infection can be associated with acute lymphadenitis due to anaerobes.[7,9]
· Dental infection may result in Ludwig angina, a brawny induration of the floor of the mouth and suprahyoid region (bilaterally), presenting acutely with fever, neck swelling, bilateral submandibular swelling, or midline swelling under the jaw and elevation of the tongue[22] (see Section 4.5, p. 36).
· Actinomycosis is a chronic infection that can result from chronic dental and/or jaw infection and presents with chronic, unilateral, brawny sub-mandibular swelling[23] (see Section 4.2, p. 35).

Age

The age of the child often gives a clue to the likely cause of lymphadenopathy.[1–19] As stated above, the etiology is likely to be different if the child presents with acute, tender enlargement of the cervical nodes with overlying redness (see Table 4.2) or with sub-acute, non-tender neck swelling (see Table 4.3).

Neonates and young infants

Neonates and young infants can present with facial cellulitis and cervical adenitis due to group B streptococcal infection.[17] In one small study, the mean age of babies with group B streptococcal infection was 5 weeks, infected babies were more likely to be boys presenting with poor feeding and irritability, and sometimes ipsilateral otitis media, as well as with facial or submandibular cellulitis.[17] Most babies were bacteremic.[17]

Older children

Significant cervical lymphadenitis is less common in older children and adolescents. Other diagnoses such as

Table 4.2 Age and likely diagnosis for acutely inflamed, tender lymphadenopathy.

Age Group	Most Common Diagnoses
Neonate (< 1 month)	*Staphylococcus aureus* Group B streptococcus
Infant (1 month – 1 year)	*Staphylococcus aureus* Group A streptococcus Adenovirus or HSV infection Kawasaki disease
Young child (1–4 years)	*Staphylococcus aureus* Group A streptococcus Adenovirus, HSV, or EBV infection Kawasaki disease Cat scratch disease
Older child (> 4 years)	Cat scratch disease EBV infection Anaerobic bacteria (periodontal disease)

systemic lupus erythematosus and drug-induced lymphadenopathy (e.g., phenytoin, isoniazid) may need to be considered,[4] as well as the diagnoses in Tables 4.2 and 4.3.

Examination of child with cervical lymphadenitis

The general physical examination is important to look for signs of malnutrition or poor growth that would raise the possibility of TB, HIV infection, immunocompromise, or malignancy.

The color of the overlying skin may help. Erythema and warmth suggests a pyogenic process or Kawasaki

Table 4.3 Age and likely diagnosis for sub-acute, non-tender neck swelling.

Age Group	Most Common Diagnoses
Neonate (< 1 month)	Congenital lesion (branchial cleft cyst, cystic hygroma)
Infant (1 month – 1 year)	Congenital lesion TB (in endemic region)
Older child (> 4 years)	Toxoplasmosis TB Malignancy

disease. The skin overlying atypical mycobacterial infection often has a purplish discoloration, but it may look identical in TB lymphadenitis.

The character of the lymph nodes is important (see Table 4.1). Fluctuance suggests pus formation and the need for drainage by needle aspiration or surgical intervention. Malignant nodes are usually hard and often fixed to underlying tissues.

Investigation of cervical lymphadenitis

Hematology
Laboratory parameters may be diagnostically useful in infectious mononucleosis (showing atypical lymphocytes), or in malignancy (blast cells, pancytopenia), and helpful in suspected Kawasaki disease (neutrophilia, etc.; see Section 6.9, p. 63).

Fine needle aspiration
Fine needle aspiration (FNA) can be used to diagnose both pyogenic infections[9] and mycobacterial infections (see p. 33). Needle aspiration is therapeutically useful for draining small abscesses, and can avoid the need for surgery.[9]

In an observational study from Kentucky of 119 children undergoing FNA, 5 aspirates revealed malignancy and 8 grew a microorganism.[24] The remaining children were diagnosed as having a benign process, most commonly reactive lymphadenitis. The accuracy was 98%, and the procedure usually obviated the need for an excisional biopsy.[24]

Investigations for suspected mycobacterial infection

Tuberculin skin testing
In a situation of endemic TB, a simple clinical algorithm that identified children with persistent (>4 weeks) cervical lymphadenopathy, no visible local cause such as superficial pyoderma, no response to antibiotics against pyogenic organisms, and a cervical mass 2 cm in diameter or greater identified over 98% of cases, without the need for tuberculin skin testing.[13]

For children with suspected tuberculous or atypical mycobacterial infection, in an industrialized country where TB is relatively uncommon, skin-prick testing can be extremely helpful. If a child with cervical lymphadenitis has a negative tuberculin skin test (TST)

with human purified protein derivative (PPD), this virtually excludes TB.[25] The only exceptions would be a child who is extremely unwell, in which case TSTs can be negative due to anergy, or if the test is not performed adequately.

Some countries have skin tests for atypical mycobacterial infection, using avian PPD or sensitin (purified from *M. avium*) or *M. scrofulaceum* PPD or sensitin (from *M. scrofulaceum*).[1,25] In one study, 59 children with culture-proven non-tuberculous mycobacterial infection also had differential skin testing performed with avian and human PPD.[26] A positive response to avian PPD ($\geq$10 mm) correctly identified 58 of 59 infected children (98.3%).

There is cross-reaction between avian and human responses, and so children with a positive avian skin test often have positive TSTs using human PPD. In children with proven avian disease, the avian response is almost always greater than the human response: it was at least 2 mm greater in 55 cases (93%) in the study[26] shown in Figure 4.1. Ten children (17%) with atypical mycobacterial infection had a negative human Mantoux. No patient had both a negative human and avian Mantoux. Thus, if avian or scrofulaceum PPD is not available, a positive human Mantoux is helpful, but could be due to cross-reaction or true human TB, while

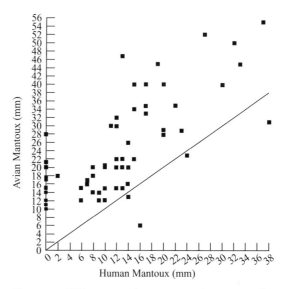

Figure 4.1 TST responses (Mantoux tests) to avian and human PPD in children with proven non-tuberculous mycobacterial infection (line of identity drawn). (Reprinted with permission from Reference 26.)

a negative human Mantoux does not exclude atypical mycobacterial infection but makes it less likely.

Fine needle aspiration for mycobacterial infection

Definitive diagnosis of mycobacterial infections, both human and atypical, can be made using material obtained either by surgical excision or by fine needle aspiration (FNA).[14,27] While it is often quoted that the definitive treatment of atypical mycobacterial infection is total excision of infected nodes,[28] there are no RCTs of the treatment of atypical mycobacterial infection comparing total excision with needle aspiration alone or with needle aspiration plus antimicrobials. The extremes of outcome of atypical mycobacterial infection are spontaneous resolution and chronic, discharging sinuses. We currently recommend referring all children with suspected mycobacterial lymphadenitis to an experienced pediatric surgeon (see Definitive surgery, below).

Polymerase chain reaction (PCR)

Question | In children with suspected mycobacterial lymphadenitis, is PCR a sensitive and specific test for diagnosing and excluding infection?

Literature review | We found 10 studies comparing PCR with culture, histopathology or ELISA.[29–38]

PCR has been used on lymph node aspirates to diagnose mycobacterial infections. The sensitivity of PCR for detecting TB in high-risk populations varied from 55% on FNAs and 68% on biopsy specimens to up to 96% on excised nodes.[29–38] PCR was found to be at least as sensitive as existing techniques of Ziehl–Neelsen stain and histopathology, but did not alter treatment in a high-risk setting.[29–38] False-positive tests were sometimes a problem, with the specificity reported from 38 to 86%.[29–38]

One advantage of PCR is that if a positive result is obtained, the product can be sequenced to distinguish between *M. tuberculosis* and atypical mycobacteria.[39] This is important because culture takes weeks, and is particularly useful in a developed country setting, where both *M. tuberculosis* and atypical mycobacterial infection are seen and they are difficult to distinguish clinically. Another advantage, is that when there is widespread resistance to antituberculous drugs, PCR techniques can be used to look for mutations predicting resistance.[40]

Treatment of cervical lymphadenopathy

Fine needle aspiration

The potential therapeutic role of FNA, in addition to its diagnostic role, for pyogenic and mycobacterial infections, has been discussed in sections above.

Definitive surgery

Surgical excision may be necessary to obtain an adequate diagnostic specimen and for therapeutic reasons in managing large abscesses and mycobacterial infections.

Antibiotics for pyogenic infections

Obviously it is best to base antibiotic treatment on microbiologic information from gram stain or culture. Where this is not possible, antibiotic therapy is based on the likely organisms, staphylococci and streptococci.

If oral therapy is possible, we recommend:

> **cephalexin 25 mg/kg (max 1 g) orally, 6-hourly** OR
> **di/flucl/oxa/nafcillin 25 mg/kg (max 1 g) orally, 6-hourly** OR
> **clindamycin 10 mg/kg (max 400 mg) orally, 8-hourly**

Clindamycin is recommended if, because of ethnicity or local epidemiology, there is a high likelihood of community-acquired MRSA infection.

For more severe infections, we recommend:

> **di/flucl/oxa/nafcillin 50 mg/kg (max 2 g) IV, 6-hourly** OR
> **cefazolin 25 mg/kg (max 1 g) IV, 6-hourly** OR
> **clindamycin 10 mg/kg (max 400 mg) IV, 8-hourly**

We recommend clindamycin or the combination of penicillin and metronidazole for dental-associated infections, because of the likelihood of anaerobic infection.

Treatment for tuberculous cervical lymphadenitis

The treatment of childhood cervical TB is with antituberculous drugs. A systematic review concluded that short-course therapy (6 months) has a low relapse rate, and is as effective as prolonged therapy.[41]

Daily regimen

For the daily regimen, we recommend

> **isoniazid 10 mg/kg (max 300 mg) orally, daily for 6 months** PLUS
> **rifampicin 10 mg/kg (max 600 mg) orally, daily for 6 months** PLUS
> **pyrazinamide 25 mg/kg (max 2 g) orally, daily for 2 months**

Because of concerns about its effect on vision, ethambutol is not recommended for children <6 years old. If used for older children instead of or as well as pyrazinamide, the dose is 15 mg/kg daily for 2 months, but we recommend stopping earlier if the organism is shown to be sensitive to isoniazid and rifampicin.

Three-times-weekly regimen (with directly observed therapy)

For the three-times-weekly regimen, we recommend:

> **isoniazid 15 mg/kg (max 600 mg) orally, three times weekly for 6 months** PLUS
> **rifampicin 15 mg/kg (max 600 mg) orally, three times weekly for 6 months** PLUS
> **pyrazinamide 50 mg/kg (max 3 g) orally, three times weekly for 2 months**

Because of concerns about its effect on vision, ethambutol is not recommended for children <6 years old. If used for older children instead of or as well as pyrazinamide, the dose is 30 mg/kg three-times weekly for 2 months, but we recommend stopping earlier if the organism is sensitive to isoniazid and rifampicin.

Children's enlarged lymph nodes may shrink and disappear on antituberculous drugs initially, but enlarge again while still on therapy. If therapy is directly observed, by far the most likely explanation is paradoxical enlargement due to an immune reaction to TB proteins, which typically occurs about 2 months into therapy.[42]

Treatment for atypical mycobacterial infections

Surgical excision of infected nodes is usually curative.[43] Most experts advocate early excisional biopsy to maximize the ability to recover the causative organism; to prevent further cosmetic damage; to remove infected tissue before more extensive spread occurs, making later surgery more difficult; and to cure the disease.[43] Surgery can be difficult, but complications, particularly facial nerve damage, are uncommon when the procedure is performed by an experienced surgeon. Most surgeons use dissection and/or curettage to remove infected tissue. In one study, 8 of 11 patients who initially underwent an incisional biopsy or incision and drainage developed a recurrence or draining sinus tract requiring a second surgical procedure, compared with only 1 of 15 patients who initially underwent a complete excision.[44] Recurrences can occur usually within 3 months of the initial surgery, but sometimes many months later, even when seemingly curative surgery has been performed.[45,46] This is usually due to leaving a deep collection behind, sometimes called a collarstud abscess, which can break through to the surface later.

Newer antituberculous drugs, notably clarithromycin and azithromycin, have some activity against atypical mycobacteria. There have been no RCTs comparing surgery with medical therapy.[40] A retrospective study reviewed 19 patients with presumed or proven atypical mycobacterial lymphadenitis: 9 were cured by immediate surgical excision, whereas 10 were treated initially with macrolide-containing chemotherapy. Of these 10 patients, 5 were cured with chemotherapy alone and 5 required subsequent surgical excision.[47] Thus, drug regimens effective against atypical mycobacteria can be tried if surgery is contraindicated. There are no data on whether it is better to use azithromycin or clarithromycin alone or two or three drugs, but data on respiratory infections with atypical mycobacteria favor the use of two or three drugs (see p. 202)

Treatment of lymphadenitis due to cat scratch disease

Cat scratch disease (*B. henselae* infection) is self-limiting in immunocompetent patients, and most cases do not require antibiotic therapy (see Section 6.10, p. 66). Antibiotic treatment, with azithromycin, is recommended for immunocompetent patients with lymphadenopathy which has not resolved after a month, or when the lymphadenopathy is associated with significant morbidity.[48]

For treatment of cat scratch disease, we recommend:

> **azithromycin 10 mg/kg (max 500 mg) orally, on day 1, then 5 mg/kg (max 250 mg) orally, daily for 4 more days**

4.2 Cervicofacial actinomycosis

Actinomycosis is a chronic, granulomatous infection caused by *Actinomyces* species. These are filamentous, branching, slow-growing, gram-positive anaerobic bacilli found as commensals in the human oropharynx and gastro-intestinal tract. Actinomyces do not invade normal tissues and require trauma to the mucous surface to cause disease. Cervicofacial actinomycosis is the most common form and usually arises from the teeth or mandible. It is rare in children and we could find only case reports and one small case series.[49] It causes a perimandibular abscess with a characteristic woody feel, due to fibrosis. There may be sinus discharge of yellow sulfur granules. The diagnosis is mainly clinical, usually but not always backed up by microbiologic confirmation. In children, actinomycosis can rarely cause chronic osteomyelitis of the mandible.[50]

Infection is indolent, and classic teaching is that therapy is with high-dose intravenous penicillin for 2–6 weeks, followed by oral penicillin or amoxicillin for a period of 6–12 months. A recent paper described 2 adults whose cervical actinomycosis responded to much shorter courses of IV and oral penicillin.[51] The authors review the literature, which shows weak, observational evidence for prolonged courses. They argue that treatment should be individualized and each patient's response monitored.[51] We agree with this approach, and recommend:

> **benzylpenicillin 30 mg (50,000 U)/kg (max 1.2 g or 2 million U) IV, 4-hourly for 1–2 weeks** THEN **amoxicillin 15 mg/kg (max 500 mg) orally, 8-hourly until resolved**

4.3 Nocardiosis

Both immunocompetent and immunocompromised patients can rarely develop lymphocutaneous infection due to the opportunist saprophytic soil organism, *Nocardia*.[52,53] An initial traumatic lesion on the face develops over 1–2 weeks into a popular lesion, with fever and a unilateral enlarged, tender submaxillary gland.[52,53] Prolonged therapy with cotrimoxazole or a sulfonamide is recommended (6–12 weaks for immunocompetent and 6–12 months for immunocompromised children).[54]

4.4 Deep neck infections

Deep neck or deep cervical fascial space infections generally result from contiguous spread from the respiratory tract or periodontal region, although hematogenous spread may occur. These infections are rare, but potentially life-threatening. The major deep neck infections are peritonsillar abscess (or quinsy), retropharyngeal abscess, and lateral pharyngeal abscess; some refer to these generically as parapharyngeal abscesses.

The characteristic features are shown in Table 4.4.

There are some general management points that apply to all three:

· **All can cause acute airway obstruction, which may require immediate airway management.**

· Frank pus generally forms on about the fifth day of infection.[55]

· If antibiotic treatment is started early, generally within the first 24–48 hours following the onset of pain when the infection is at the stage of cellulitis, the condition may resolve by fibrosis without abscess formation and without the need for surgery.[55]

Table 4.4 Clinical features of deep neck abscesses.[50]

Infection	Location	Peak Age	Clinical Features
Peritonsillar abscess	Tonsillar capsule	> 5 years	Unilateral swelling around tonsil, displacement of uvula; trismus
Retropharyngeal abscess	Between post-erior pharynx and prevertebral fascia	< 4 years	Neck pain, limited neck extension, torticollis. *Variable*: stridor, drooling, respiratory distress, visible post-erior pharyngeal bulging
Lateral pharyngeal abscess	Anterior and post-erior pharyngomaxillary space	> 8 years	Trismus, swelling in the parotid area, or tonsillar fossa

Peritonsillar abscess (quinsy)

Peritonsillar abscess is a complication of tonsillopharyngitis. The organisms responsible are predominantly aerobic streptococci, including group A streptococcus, and anaerobes.[55] The diagnosis is usually apparent clinically, although trismus may make it difficult to look in the mouth.

Although there have been anecdotal reports of cure with medical treatment alone, there is consensus that surgery is necessary. Initial studies concluded that immediate tonsillectomy was superior in terms of duration of illness to immediate surgical drainage and delayed (interval) tonsillectomy.[56,57] Subsequently, studies compared needle drainage with incision and drainage. Results were conflicting, with some finding needle aspiration to be highly effective[58,59] and others finding that abscesses often recurred following needle aspiration.[60] A meta-analysis found five RCTs on surgical technique, which indicated that needle aspiration, incision and drainage, and quinsy tonsillectomy are all effective for initial management, but could not say that any one was superior.[61]

For antibiotic therapy, we recommend:

> **benzylpenicillin 30 mg/kg (max 1.2 g) IV, 6-hourly** PLUS
> **metronidazole 7.5 mg/kg (max 500 mg) IV, 12-hourly**

or alternatively, on its own:

> **clindamycin 10 mg/kg (max 450 mg) IV, 8-hourly**

Once improving, treatment can be continued with oral amoxicillin-clavulanate or clindamycin.

Retropharyngeal abscess

Retropharyngeal abscess follows infection of the nasopharynx, paranasal sinuses, or middle ear, and trauma can predispose. It can occur as early as the neonatal period,[62] but the peak incidence is about 3 years.[55,62–64] Some reports emphasize that children often present with respiratory obstruction and stridor,[62,63] some that the presentation can mimic epiglottitis,[63] while others find that stridor and respiratory distress are rare.[64] The clinical presentation is age-dependent.[55] Older children are more likely to complain of neck pain, sore throat, and difficulty swallowing, while younger children are more likely to have stridor, refusal to swallow, dysphonia, drooling, and neck extension.[55,62–64]

Plain neck radiographs show widening of the prevertebral space in many patients, as many as 83% in one study.[65] CT scan with contrast has been reported as 81–100% accurate in some studies,[65,66] but other studies which compared CT with operative findings found a far lower sensitivity of 43–61%.[67,68]

Many children can be managed medically without the need for surgical drainage.[66–68] Some authorities advocate CT-guided drainage,[53] but there are no RCTs comparing medical and surgical management. Retropharyngeal abscesses are usually polymicrobial, with anaerobes, streptococci, *S. aureus*, and Gram-negative bacilli all common.

We recommend:

> **clindamycin 10 mg/kg (max 450 mg) IV, 8-hourly** PLUS
> **gentamicin <10 years: 7.5 mg/kg; ≥10 years: 6 mg/kg IV, daily**

or alternatively,

> **cefotaxime 25 mg/kg (max 1 g) IV, 8-hourly** PLUS
> **metronidazole 7.5 mg/kg (max 500 mg) IV, 12-hourly**

Lateral pharyngeal abscess

The organisms causing lateral pharyngeal abscess are mouth flora, as for peritonsillar abscess.[55] The same strictures apply with regard to diagnosis, early antibiotic treatment using the same antibiotics as for peritonsillar abscess above, and the need for drainage if there is frank pus and/or failure to respond to medical treatment.[55]

4.5   Ludwig angina

Ludwig angina is a rapidly progressive cellulitis and edema of the soft tissues of the neck and floor of the mouth, which results in swelling of the anterior neck below the lower jaw and swelling and elevation of the tongue. It originates in the region of the submandibular gland, and is usually odontogenic. Many adult patients with Ludwig angina are debilitated due to chronic diseases like diabetes, alcoholism or HIV infection.[69] In contrast, affected children are often otherwise healthy.[69,70]

Early signs and symptoms of obstruction may be subtle. Early recognition of the disease and appropriate airway management is vital, because airway compromise is the leading cause of death.[69]

For immediate, empiric antibiotic treatment, because infection is usually odontogenic, we recommend:

benzylpenicillin 30 mg/kg (max 1.2 g) IV, 6-hourly PLUS
metronidazole 7.5 mg/kg (max 500 mg) IV, 12-hourly

or alternatively, use on its own:

clindamycin 10 mg/kg (max 450 mg) IV, 8-hourly

4.6 Lemierre syndrome

Lemierre syndrome is a rare, aggressive, oropharyngeal infection consisting of pharyngitis, bacteremia, and suppurative thrombophlebitis of the internal jugular vein, often complicated by metastatic septic emboli. The most common cause is *Fusobacterium necrophorum*, a Gram-negative, non-spore-forming, obligate anaerobe, which is part of the normal oral flora. Other organisms, mainly anaerobes, may be isolated alone or with *Fusobacterium* from children with Lemierre syndrome.[71–73]

The septic emboli may cause pulmonary involvement with cavitating pneumonia, empyema, and lung abscess, although in one review, the most common finding on chest X-ray at presentation was pulmonary infiltrates in the absence of cavitation. The second most common site of septic embolization is the joints, with the hip, shoulders, and knees most frequently involved. Hepatic or splenic abscesses can occur rarely.[71–73]

The management is with antibiotics. The use of heparin is controversial. We recommend:

benzylpenicillin 30 mg/kg (max 1.2 g) IV, 6-hourly PLUS
metronidazole 7.5 mg/kg (max 500 mg) IV, 12-hourly

or alternatively, on its own:

clindamycin 10 mg/kg (max 450 mg) IV, 8-hourly

References

1 Larsson LO, Bentzon MW, Berg Kelly K et al. Palpable lymph nodes of the neck in Swedish schoolchildren. *Acta Paediatr* 1994;83:1091–4.

2 Leung AK, Robson WL. Cervical lymphadenopathy in children. *Can J Pediatr* 1991;3:10–17.

3 Margileth AM. Lymphadenopathy: when to diagnose and treat. *Contemp Pediatr* 1995;12:71–91.

4 Leung AK, Robson WL. Childhood cervical lymphadenopathy. *J Paediatr Health Care* 2004;18:3–7.

5 Newburger JW, Takahashi M, Gerber MA et al. Diagnosis, treatment, and long-term management of Kawasaki disease: a statement for health professionals from the Committee on Rheumatic Fever, Endocarditis, and Kawasaki Disease, Council on Cardiovascular Disease in the Young, American Heart Association. *Pediatrics* 2004;114:1708–33.

6 Yamauchi T, Ferrieri P, Anthony BF. The aetiology of acute cervical adenitis in children: serological and bacteriological studies. *J Med Microbiol* 1980;13:37–43.

7 Brook I. Aerobic and anaerobic bacteriology of cervical adenitis in children. *Clin Pediatr (Phila)* 1980;19:693–6.

8 Simo R, Hartley C, Rapado F, Zarod AP, Sanyal D, Rothera MP. Microbiology and antibiotic treatment of head and neck abscesses in children. *Clin Otolaryngol* 1998;23:164–8.

9 Lane RJ, Keane WM, Potsic WP. Pediatric infectious cervical lymphadenitis. *Otolaryngol Head Neck Surg* 1980;88:332–5.

10 Sundaresh HP, Kumar A, Hokanson JT, Novack AH. Etiology of cervical lymphadenitis in children. *Am Fam Physician* 1981;24:147–51.

11 Wright JE, Reid IS. Acute cervical lymphadenitis in children. *Aust Paediatr J* 1987;23:193–5.

12 Ahonkhai VI, Omokoku B, Rao M. Acute cervical lymphadenitis in hospitalized pediatric patients: predominance of *Staphylococcus aureus* in infancy. *J Natl Med Assoc* 1984;76:367–9.

13 Marais BJ, Wright CA, Schaaf HS et al. Tuberculous lymphadenitis as a cause of persistent cervical lymphadenopathy in children from a tuberculosis-endemic area. *Pediatr Infect Dis J* 2006;25:142–6.

14 McMaster P, Ezeilo N, Freisen H, Pomat N, Vince JD. Ten-year experience with paediatric lymph node tuberculosis in Port Moresby. *J Trop Pediatr* 2001;47:160–4.

15 Bern C. Human immunodeficiency virus-positive tuberculous lymphadenitis in Central Africa: clinical presentation of 157 cases. *Int J Tuberc Lung Dis* 1997;1:215–9.

16 Medina M, Goldfarb J, Traquina D, Seeley B, Sabella C. Cervical adenitis and deep neck infection caused by *Streptococcus pneumoniae*. *Pediatr Infect Dis J* 1997;16:823–4.

17 Baker CJ. Group B streptococcal cellulitis–adenitis in infants. *Am J Dis Child* 1982;136:631–3.

18 Montoya JG, Liesenfeld O. Toxoplasmosis. *Lancet* 2004;363:1965–76.

19 Durlach RA, Kaufer F, Carral L, Hirt J. Toxoplasmic lymphadenitis—clinical and serologic profile. *Clin Microbiol Infect* 2003;9:625–31.

20 Leerdam CM, Martin HC, Isaacs D. Recurrent parotitis of childhood. *J Paediatr Child Health* 2005;41:631–4.

21 Margileth AM. Recent advances in diagnosis and treatment of cat scratch disease. *Curr Infect Dis Rep* 2000;2:141–6.

22 Srirompotong S, Art-Smart T. Ludwig's angina: a clinical review. *Eur Arch Otorhinolaryngol* 2003;260:401–3.

23 Stewart MG, Sulek M. Pediatric actinomycosis of the head and neck. *Ear Nose Throat J* 1993;72:614–9.

24 Buchino JJ, Jones VF. Fine needle aspiration in the evaluation of children with lymphadenopathy. *Arch Pediatr Adolesc Med* 1994;148:1327–30.

25 Rose DN, Schechter CB, Adler JJ. Interpretation of the tuberculin skin test. *J Gen Intern Med* 1995;10:635–42.

26 Daley AJ, Isaacs D. Differential avian and human tuberculin skin testing in non-tuberculous mycobacterial infection. *Arch Dis Child* 1999;80:377–9.

27 Cheng AG, Chang A, Farwell DG, Agoff SN. Auramine orange stain with fluorescence microscopy is a rapid and sensitive technique for the detection of cervical lymphadenitis due to mycobacterial infection using fine needle aspiration cytology: a case series. *Otolaryngol Head Neck Surg* 2005;133:381–5.

28 American Academy of Pediatrics. Diseases caused by non-tuberculous mycobacteria. In: Pickering LK (ed.), *Red Book: 2003 Report of the Committee on Infectious Diseases*, 26th edn. Elk Grove Village, IL: American Academy of Pediatrics, 2003:661–6.

29 Vishnevskii BI, Mirlina ED, Bellendir EN et al. [Sensitivity and specificity of polymerase chain reaction based test in the diagnosis of peripheral lymph node tuberculosis]. *Probl Tuberk* 1998;4:41–4.

30 Manitchotpisit B, Kunachak S, Kulapraditharom B, Sura T. Combined use of fine needle aspiration cytology and polymerase chain reaction in the diagnosis of cervical tuberculous lymphadenitis. *J Med Assoc Thai* 1999;82:363–8.

31 Singh KK, Muralidhar M, Kumar A et al. Comparison of in house polymerase chain reaction with conventional techniques for the detection of Mycobacterium tuberculosis DNA in granulomatous lymphadenopathy. *J Clin Pathol* 2000;53:355–61.

32 Baek CH, Kim SI, Ko YH, Chu KC. Polymerase chain reaction detection of Mycobacterium tuberculosis from fine-needle aspirate for the diagnosis of cervical tuberculous lymphadenitis. *Laryngoscope* 2000;110:30–4.

33 Goel MM, Ranjan V, Dhole TN et al. Polymerase chain reaction vs. conventional diagnosis in fine needle aspirates of tuberculous lymph nodes. *Acta Cytol* 2001;45:333–40.

34 Aljafari AS, Khalil EA, Elsiddig KE et al. Diagnosis of tuberculous lymphadenitis by FNAC, microbiological methods and PCR: a comparative study. *Cytopathology* 2004;15:44–8.

35 Jain A, Verma RK, Tiwari V, Goel MM. Dot-ELISA vs. PCR of fine needle aspirates of tuberculous lymphadenitis: a prospective study in India. *Acta Cytol* 2005;49:17–21.

36 Pahwa R, Hedau S, Jain S et al. Assessment of possible tuberculous lymphadenopathy by PCR compared to non-molecular methods. *J Med Microbiol* 2005;54:873–8.

37 Chakravorty S, Sen MK, Tyagi JS. Diagnosis of extrapulmonary tuberculosis by smear, culture, and PCR using universal sample processing technology. *J Clin Microbiol* 2005;43:4357–62.

38 Osores F, Nolasco O, Verdonck K et al. Clinical evaluation of a 16S ribosomal RNA polymerase chain reaction test for the diagnosis of lymph node tuberculosis. *Clin Infect Dis* 2006;43:855–9.

39 Roth A, Reischl U, Streubel A et al. Novel diagnostic algorithm for identification of mycobacteria using genus-specific amplification of the 16S-23S rRNA gene spacer and restriction endonucleases. *J Clin Microbiol* 2000;38:1094–104.

40 Gong G, Lee H, Kang GH, Shim YH, Huh J, Khang SK. Nested PCR for diagnosis of tuberculous lymphadenitis and PCR-SSCP for identification of rifampicin resistance in fine-needle aspirates. *Diagn Cytopathol* 2002;26:228–31.

41 McMaster P, Isaacs D. Critical review of evidence for short course therapy for tuberculous adenitis in children. *Pediatr Infect Dis J* 2000;19:401–4.

42 Cheng VC, Lee RA, Chan KS et al. Clinical spectrum of paradoxical deterioration during anti-tuberculous therapy in non-HIV-infected patients. *Eur J Clin Microbiol Infect Dis* 2002;21:803–9.

43 Starke JR. Management of non-tuberculous mycobacterial cervical adenitis. *Pediatr Infect Dis J* 2000;19:674–5.

44 Stewart MG, Starke JR, Coker NJ. Non-tuberculous mycobacterial infections of the head and neck. *Arch Otolaryngol Head Neck Surg* 1994;120:873–6.

45 Tunkel DE, Romaneschi KB. Surgical treatment of cervicofacial non-tuberculous mycobacterial adenitis in children. *Laryngoscope* 1995;105:1024–8.

46 Suskind DL, Handler SD, Tom LW et al. Non-tuberculous mycobacterial cervical adenitis. *Clin Pediatr* 1997;36:403–9.

47 Hazra R, Robin CD, Perez-Atayde AR et al. Lymphadenitis due to non-tuberculous mycobacteria in children: presentation and response to therapy. *Clin Infect Dis* 1999;28:123–9.

48 Bass JW, Freitas BC, Freitas AD et al. Prospective randomized double blind placebo-controlled evaluation of azithromycin for treatment of cat-scratch disease. *Pediatr Infect Dis J* 1998;17:447–52.

49 Foster SV, Demmler GJ, Hawkins EP, Tillman JP. Pediatric cervicofacial actinomycosis. *South Med J* 1993;86:1147–50.

50 Robinson JL, Vaudry WL, Dobrovolsky W. Actinomycosis presenting as osteomyelitis in the pediatric population. *Pediatr Infect Dis J* 2005;24:365–9.

51 Sudhakar SS, Ross JJ. Short-term treatment of actinomycosis: two cases and a review. *Clin Infect Dis* 2004;38:444–7.

52 Lampe RM, Baker CJ, Septimus EJ, Wallace RJ, Jr. Cervicofacial nocardiosis in children. *J Pediatr* 1981;99:593–5.

53 Schwartz JG, McGough DA, Thorner RE, Fetchick RJ, Tio FO, Rinaldi MG. Primary lymphocutaneous *Nocardia brasiliensis* infection: three case reports and a review of the literature. *Diagn Microbiol Infect Dis* 1988;10:113–20.

54 American Academy of Pediatrics. Nocardiosis. In: Pickering LK (ed.), *Red Book: 2003 Report of the Committee on Infectious Diseases*, 26th edn. Elk Grove Village, IL: American Academy of Pediatrics, 2003:445–6.

55 Brook I. Microbiology and management of peritonsillar, retropharyngeal, and parapharyngeal abscesses. *J Oral Maxillofac Surg* 2004;62:1545–50.

56 Chowdhury CR, Bricknell MC. The management of quinsy—a prospective study. *J Laryngol Otol* 1992;106:986–8.

57 Fagan JJ, Wormald PJ. Quinsy tonsillectomy or interval tonsillectomy—a prospective randomised trial. *S Afr Med J* 1994;84:689–90.

58 Nagy M, Pizzuto M, Backstrom J, Brodsky L. Deep neck infections in children: a new approach to diagnosis and treatment. *Laryngoscope* 1997;107:1627–34.

59 Maharaj D, Rajah V, Hemsley S. Management of peritonsillar abscess. *J Laryngol Otol* 1991;105:743–5.

60 Wolf M, Even-Chen I, Kronenberg J. Peritonsillar abscess: repeated needle aspiration versus incision and drainage. *Ann Otol Rhinol Laryngol* 1994;103:554–7.

61 Johnson RF, Stewart MG, Wright CC. An evidence-based review of the treatment of peritonsillar abscess. *Otolaryngol Head Neck Surg* March 2003;128(3):332–43.

62 Coulthard M, Isaacs D. Retropharyngeal abscess. *Arch Dis Child* 1991;66:1227–30.

63 Craig FW, Schunk JE. Retropharyngeal abscess in children: clinical presentation, utility of imaging, and current management. *Pediatrics* 2003;111:1394–8.

64 Lee SS, Schwartz RH, Bahadori RS. Retropharyngeal abscess: epiglottitis of the new millennium. *J Pediatr* 2001;138:435–7.

65 Nagy M, Backstrom J. Comparison of the sensitivity of lateral neck radiographs and computed tomography scanning in pediatric deep-neck infections. *Laryngoscope* 1999;109:775–9.

66 Daya H, Lo S, Papsin BC, Zachariasova A et al. Retropharyngeal and parapharyngeal infections in children: the Toronto experience. *Int J Pediatr Otorhinolaryngol* 2005;69:81–6.

67 Vural C, Gungor A, Comerci S. Accuracy of computerized tomography in deep neck infections in the pediatric population. *Am J Otolaryngol* 2003;24:143–8.

68 Al-Sabah B, Bin Salleen H, Hagr A, Choi-Rosen J, Manoukian JJ, Tewfik TL. Retropharyngeal abscess in children: 10-year study. *J Otolaryngol* 2004;33:352–5.

69 K Saifeldeen, R Evans. Ludwig's angina. *Emerg Med J* 2004; 21:242–3.

70 Britt JC, Josephson GD, Gross CW. Ludwig's angina in the pediatric population: report of a case and review of the literature. *Int J Pediatr Otorhinolaryngol* 2000;52:79–87.

71 Brook I. Microbiology and management of deep facial infections and Lemierre syndrome. *ORL J Otorhinolaryngol Relat Spec* 2003;65:117–20.

72 Ramirez S, Hild TG, Rudolph CN et al. Increased diagnosis of Lemierre syndrome and other *Fusobacterium necrophorum* infections at a children's hospital. *Pediatrics* 2003;112:e380.

73 Chirinos JA, Lichtstein DM, Garcia J, Tamariz LJ. The evolution of Lemierre syndrome: report of 2 cases and review of the literature. *Medicine (Baltimore)* 2002;81:458–65.

CHAPTER 5
Eye infections

5.1 Cellulitis around the eye (periocular cellulitis)

It is common to define cellulitis around the eye in terms of the orbital septum, the thin fascia that separates the eyelid from the orbit. Infections are called "preseptal" if they are anterior to the orbital septum and "orbital" if they are post-erior (i.e., inside the orbit). While this is anatomically logical, there is not much evidence that the distinction is valid clinically. Furthermore, preseptal cellulitis is also sometimes called periorbital cellulitis, so that the term "periorbital cellulitis" (literally around the orbit) is used to refer to cellulitis only in front of the septum, while the term "orbital cellulitis" is used for cellulitis within the orbit. It is not surprising that physicians get confused.

It is probably more useful for clinicians to think of cellulitis around the eye (periocular cellulitis) in terms of the likely cause and the severity, since these will determine treatment. Cellulitis around the eye may be secondary to trauma (a scratch, insect bite, or penetrating skin injury), may spread from infected skin (impetigo, pyoderma, chicken pox), may be bloodborne (as with Hib infections), or may spread from the paranasal sinuses. These generally have distinct clinical presentations.[1–3] We will defy convention, and define cellulitis around the eye in terms of the likely etiology, based on the clinical presentation.

Local periocular cellulitis

Cellulitis of the eyelid, without proptosis or ophthalmoplegia, and without high fever or systemic illness, is likely to be caused by local introduction of organisms through trauma or spread from infected skin. Most children are <5 years old, and the most common

organisms are *Staphylococcus aureus* and *Streptococcus pneumoniae* (group A streptococcus).[1–3]

If the child is well, and has been immunized against Hib, we recommend:

> **cefuroxime 10 mg/kg (max 500 mg) orally 12-hourly** OR
> **cephalexin 25 mg/kg (max 1 g) orally, 8-hourly** OR
> **amoxicillin+clavulanate 22.5 + 3.2 mg/kg (max 875 + 125 mg) orally, 12-hourly**

If the child is ill enough to require parenteral therapy, we recommend to take blood cultures (to exclude hematogenous spread) and perform a CT scan to exclude sinusitis-associated infection.

We recommend:

> **cefotaxime 50 mg/kg (max 2 g) IV, 8-hourly** OR
> **ceftriaxone 50 mg/kg (max 2 g) IV, daily**

When improved, we recommend:

> **amoxicillin+clavulanate 22.5 + 3.2 mg/kg (max 875 + 125 mg) orally, 12-hourly** OR
> **clindamycin 10 mg/kg (max 450 mg) orally, 8-hourly**

If the child needs parenteral therapy and if, because of a local lesion such as a stye, dacryocystitis, impetigo, or a wound, staphylococcal infection is suspected, we recommend:

> **di/flucl/oxa/nafcillin 50 mg/kg (max 2 g) IV, 6-hourly** OR
> **cefazolin 15 mg/kg (max 600 mg) IV, 8-hourly** OR (if cMRSA likely)
> **clindamycin 10 mg/kg (max 450 mg) IV, 8-hourly**

Deep orbital (sinusitis-associated) cellulitis

The paranasal sinuses surround the orbit: the roof of the orbit is the floor of the frontal sinus, the floor

---

The antibiotics and doses recommended in this chapter are based on those in *Therapeutic Guidelines: Antibiotic*, 13th edn. Therapeutic Guidelines Ltd: Melbourne, 2006.

of the orbit is the roof of the maxillary sinus, and the ethmoid and sphenoid sinuses are the sides. Infection of the sinuses can readily spread through the bones to the orbit behind the eye. Here they cause erythema, swelling, pain and may or may not cause fever and systemic toxicity.[1-4] The classical clinical presentation is with proptosis, ophthalmoplegia, particularly of upward gaze, chemosis, and often reduced visual acuity.[1-4] Because the paranasal sinuses are rudimentary in infancy, and develop later, most affected children are >5 years old.[1-4] Affected children commonly have a sub-periosteal abscess, adjacent to the ethmoid sinus in young children and to the frontal sinus in older children.[2,3]

The diagnosis is initially clinical, but CT scan is necessary to determine whether or not there is an associated sub-periosteal abscess and the need for drainage.[1,2] In addition, there may be intracranial extension (see Section 10.2, p. 142).

Drainage of the sinuses or of an orbital, subperiosteal, or intracranial abscess may be required, and we recommend consulting an ENT surgeon, and if necessary a neurosurgeon.

Causative agents include untypeable *Haemophilus influenzae*, *S. pneumoniae*, *S. aureus*, aerobic Gramnegative bacteria, and anaerobes.[1,2]

We recommend:

> **di/flucl/oxa/nafcillin 50 mg/kg (max 2 g) IV, 6-hourly** OR
> **cefazolin 25 mg/kg (max 1 g) IV, 8-hourly** (OR if cMRSA likely)
> **clindamycin 10 mg/kg (max 450 mg) IV, 8-hourly** PLUS EITHER
> **ceftriaxone 50 mg/kg (max 2 g) IV, daily** OR
> **cefotaxime 50 mg/kg (max 2 g) IV, 8-hourly**

When improved, use:

> **amoxicillin+clavulanate 22.5 + 3.2 mg/kg (max 875 + 125 mg) orally, 12-hourly** OR
> **clindamycin 10 mg/kg (max 450 mg) orally, 8-hourly**

Bacteremia-associated periocular cellulitis

In the days before *H. influenzae* type b (Hib) immunization, and in countries where Hib vaccine is not routine, the most common presentation of cellulitis around the eye was in association with Hib bacteremia. Children were usually infants <1 year old, and almost always <4 years, and presented with swelling around the eye with a peculiar purple ("violaceous") color.[1-3,5] They were usually highly febrile, toxic, and had high peripheral blood white cell counts. Hib was by far the most common cause, not uncommonly associated with Hib meningitis.[1-3,5] Hib cellulitis has virtually disappeared following the introduction of universal Hib immunization.[5]

An identical clinical picture can be seen rarely with *S. pneumoniae*.[6] In the post-Hib immunization era, bacteremia-associated periocular cellulitis is described rarely with *S. pneumoniae*, group A streptococcus, other streptococci, and untypeable *H. influenzae*.[7,8] Where bacteremia seems clinically likely, we recommend taking blood cultures and admitting the child to hospital for IV antibiotics.

We recommend:

> **cefotaxime 50 mg/kg (max 2 g) IV, 8-hourly** OR
> **ceftriaxone 50 mg/kg (max 2 g) IV, daily**

Recurrent eyelid swelling

It is rare to get recurrent infectious cellulitis. Recurrent eyelid swelling is often diagnosed and treated as recurrent cellulitis. It is, however, much more likely to have an allergic basis, either as a manifestation of allergic conjunctivitis and/or as a form of angioedema.[9,10] We advise referral to an allergist for investigation for atopy.

5.2 Conjunctivitis in infants and children

Acute conjunctivitis is the most common disorder of the eye seen by the primary care practitioner.[2,11] We will consider neonatal conjunctivitis separately (see Section 5.3, p. 45). Several studies have documented that bacterial conjunctivitis, with or without otitis media, predominantly occurs in children <6 years of age.[11-16] It is difficult to distinguish viral from bacterial conjunctivitis clinically.

Organisms causing acute conjunctivitis in children

Outside the neonatal period, the commonest pathogens detected from children with acute conjunctivitis are untypeable *H. influenzae* (42-52%), adenovirus

(13–20%), and *S. pneumoniae* (7–17%).[11–16] A Gram stain and culture is necessary to distinguish and identify bacterial conjunctivitis, while special tests are needed to identify adenoviruses or herpes simplex virus (HSV) rapidly.

Clinical features of acute conjunctivitis in children

Most childhood conjunctivitis is mild, self-resolving, and viral, and requires no treatment. There are some recognizable clinical syndromes, however, which have treatment or public health implications.

Acute hemorrhagic conjunctivitis

Acute hemorrhagic conjunctivitis is most commonly caused by enteroviruses, including Coxsackieviruses, but can also be caused by adenovirus type 11. It is a highly contagious infection and usually occurs in epidemics.[16] Most reported cases occur in Asia, but several epidemics have been reported in Africa, the Caribbean, South America, Central America, and North America.[16] Patients present with sudden development of hyperemic conjunctiva, sub-conjunctival hemorrhages, chemosis of the conjunctiva, lid swelling, excessive tearing, photophobia, and pain. The major symptoms last 3–5 days, and resolve over 10 days. Neurologic complications have been reported in about 1 in 10,000 cases of enterovirus type 70 infection, ranging from transient, mild cranial nerve palsies to permanent flaccid paralysis of a limb (monoplegia) or limbs resembling poliomyelitis.[16]

Conjunctivitis-otitis syndrome

H. influenzae (untypeable) is the commonest organism isolated, and can be grown from the eyes of 42–52% of children with acute conjunctivitis.[12–16] Clinically it can cause the "conjunctivitis–otitis syndrome." Children characteristically develop low grade fever and mild respiratory symptoms, including cough and mucopurulent nasal discharge, followed after several days, by eye pain and discharge. Some children develop ear pain, but otitis is asymptomatic in about 60% of children.[11,17] Sometimes a child presents with otitis media and develops purulent conjunctivitis later.[11,17] In one study, *H. influenzae* was isolated from 73% of conjunctival cultures taken from children with both otitis and conjunctivitis.[17]

Gonococcal conjunctivitis

Gonococcal conjunctivitis is well recognized in neonates, but the diagnosis may not be considered in older children. Patients present with an abrupt onset of copious, purulent discharge; eyelid edema; and fever.[18] As in neonates, this organism can cause ulceration and perforation of the cornea, leading to blindness.[16,18] Because the organism is usually transmitted through sexual contact, all under-age children with gonococcal conjunctivitis should be investigated for possible sexual abuse. An outbreak of gonococcal conjunctivitis occurred when urine was applied to the eyes of patients with enteroviral conjunctivitis as a folk remedy.[19] Sexually active adolescents can contract gonococcal conjunctivitis and should be evaluated for other sites of infection, as well as for other sexually transmitted diseases.[20]

HSV conjunctivitis

HSV conjunctivitis may occur with primary infection or with recurrence. The peak age of primary infection is 1–5 years.[16,21] Neonatal HSV conjunctivitis is an emergency because of the risk of encephalitis (see p. 145). Recurrent HSV infections typically occur in older children and adults.[16] The diagnosis is most likely to be made if there are vesicles on the lid or face, or gingivostomatitis or keratitis. Corneal involvement with the classic dendritic appearance is present in 50% of patients.[16] The diagnosis can usually be made clinically, but if the diagnosis is in question, viral cultures and antigen detection tests (immunofluorescence, ELISA, polymerase chain reaction [PCR]) can be performed.[16]

Meningococcal conjunctivitis

Two types of meningococcal conjunctivitis have been described: primary, which can be invasive or noninvasive, and secondary, which occurs after systemic infection.[22,23] Complications of primary meningococcal conjunctivitis include corneal ulceration, keratitis, sub-conjunctival hemorrhage, iritis, and systemic meningococcal disease.[22,23] Patients present with acute, purulent discharge, and sometimes fever, similar to gonococcal conjunctivitis.[22,23] The Gram stain reveals Gram-negative diplococci.[22,23] In a review of children and adults with meningococcal conjunctivitis,[22] two-thirds of which was unilateral, 18% of patients developed systemic infection, which had a mortality over 13%. Systemic antibiotics should be administered, because topical antibiotics are ineffective,[22,23] and chemoprophylaxis should be offered to contacts (see p. 138).

Pharyngoconjunctival fever

Adenovirus is identified as the pathogen in about 20% of cases of conjunctivitis.[11-16] It can be detected by culture, immunofluorescence, ELISA or PCR,[16,24] but as the tests are not routinely performed, the true incidence may be higher than 20%. Adenovirus infection may be associated with either pharyngoconjunctival fever or epidemic keratoconjunctivitis. Outbreaks of pharyngoconjunctival fever have been associated with swimming in poorly chlorinated swimming pools and contaminated ponds. It manifests with high fever, pharyngitis, follicular conjunctivitis with chemosis and hyperemia, and bilateral preauricular adenopathy. It typically takes between 4 days and 2 weeks for symptoms to resolve.[16,24] Epidemic keratoconjunctivitis is a conjunctivitis with keratitis, and sometimes small, petechial hemorrhages, which presents with pain, photophobia and decreased vision, and sometimes associated pharyngitis and rhinitis.[16,24] Hazy, grayish-white subepithelial infiltrates can be found later in the course of illness, and may not resolve for several months. The conjunctival and eyelid swelling can be marked, and patients with severe cases may develop inflammatory pseudomembranes.[16,19] Severe cases may be mistaken for preseptal or periorbital cellulitis.[16,24]

Brazilian purpuric fever

H. aegyptius can cause conjunctivitis associated with overwhelming septicemia with purpura, indistinguishable from meningococcal infection. It has only been described in South America and Australia.[25]

Treatment of acute conjunctivitis in children

Question | For children beyond the neonatal period with acute conjunctivitis do topical antibiotics, compared with no treatment or placebo, hasten recovery?

Literature review | We found six RCTs, although only two were in children, and a Cochrane review.[26]

In considering topical antibiotic use, we need to distinguish children with proven bacterial conjunctivitis from those who present to their primary care physician with acute conjunctivitis.

A study of 102 children with bacterial conjunctivitis (61 *H. influenzae*, 22 *S. pneumoniae*) found that 62% of the children given topical polymyxin-bacitracin but only 28% of the placebo group had resolved at 3–5 days. By 8–10 days, 91 and 72% respectively had resolved, a difference which was not statistically significant although the organism persisted longer in the placebo group.[27]

An RCT in general practice found that antibiotics did not affect the severity of symptoms of acute infective conjunctivitis in adults and children, but antibiotics did reduce the duration of moderate symptoms from 4.8 to 3.3 days.[28] In the same study, only 53% of patients used antibiotics if a delayed prescription was given, yet the duration of symptoms in the delayed group was 3.9 days, suggesting this is a reasonable compromise between immediate and no antibiotics.

In contrast, an RCT of 326 children presenting to their family doctor with acute conjunctivitis and randomized to topical chloramphenicol or placebo found that 86 and 83% had resolved by 7 days, with no significant difference between treatment groups.[29] Recurrences within 6 weeks were equally common in each group.[29]

A Cochrane review[26] of the treatment of bacterial conjunctivitis in adults and children found that topical antibiotics were of benefit early (days 2–5) in improving clinical (RR 1.24, 95% CI 1.05–1.45) and microbiological (RR 1.77, 95% CI 1.23–2.54) remission rates. These early advantages were reduced by days 6–10, but still significant. Most cases, however, resolved spontaneously, with clinical remission being achieved by days 2–5 in 65% (95% CI 59–70) of those receiving placebo. No serious outcomes were reported in either the active or placebo arms of these trials, indicating that important, sight-threatening complications are an infrequent occurrence.

Question | In children beyond the neonatal period with acute conjunctivitis do oral antibiotics compared with topical antibiotics or placebo hasten recovery and/or prevent otitis media?

Literature review | We found one RCT comparing oral with topical antibiotics[30] and one RCT of oral antibiotics versus placebo.[31]

An RCT of 80 children found that 3 days of oral cefixime was not more effective than 7 days of topical polymyxin-bacitracin in either the eradication of conjunctival colonization with respiratory pathogens or the prevention of acute otitis media in children with acute bacterial conjunctivitis.[30]

An RCT of children with conjunctivitis found that oral amoxicillin reduced the proportion infected with untypeable *H. influenzae* who developed acute otitis media, but did not eradicate the organism.[31] The study did not evaluate duration of eye symptoms.

> **We recommend topical antibiotics for proven bacterial conjunctivitis, but not routinely for childhood conjunctivitis.**

Treatment of viral and presumed viral conjunctivitis

For most viral conjunctivitis, including adenoviral and enteroviral conjunctivitis, treatment is supportive.[16] Cold compresses, artificial tears, and topical vasoconstrictors may provide comfort. Studies comparing antiviral agents and anti-inflammatory medications with artificial tears show no significant difference between these medications and artificial tears.[32,33] Topical steroids should be avoided because they have significant side effects, such as superinfection, glaucoma, and cataract.[32] Topical steroids also may exacerbate a missed diagnosis of herpes conjunctivitis, may enhance adenoviral replication, and may increase the duration of adenoviral shedding.[32] Topical antibiotics are usually unnecessary, as secondary bacterial infections are rare.[16,32] We recommend using saline washes alone for mild cases of childhood conjunctivitis.

Specific therapy is available for conjunctivitis due to HSV or associated with zoster (see below).

Treatment of HSV conjunctivitis

Topical antiviral agents, such as acyclovir, are typically used to treat HSV conjunctivitis occurring in children well beyond the neonatal period[16,21] (for neonates, systemic therapy is essential). Oral or IV acyclovir can be used in severe cases or to suppress recurrent lesions,[34] but recurrent HSV keratoconjunctivitis is much more common in adults.[16,33] Steroids should be avoided, as they can aggravate the infection.[16]

Treatment of ophthalmic varicella zoster virus (VZV) infection

A mild conjunctivitis is frequent with chicken pox (primary infection with VZV) and usually requires no specific treatment.

Ophthalmic zoster (herpes zoster ophthalmicus) results from reactivation of latent VZV in the first branch of the trigeminal nerve (Vth nerve). It accounts for approximately 15% of all zoster cases. Without specific treatment 50–70% of patients with ophthalmic zoster will develop ocular complications from direct viral invasion (superficial keratitis including punctate and dendritic keratitis and conjunctivitis), secondary inflammation and alteration of autoimmune mechanisms (stromal keratitis, uveitis, scleritis, and episcleritis), or neurotrophic disorders (neurotrophic keratitis).[35,36]

Treatment should be with oral or IV antivirals and should be started as soon as the diagnosis is suspected. Oral acyclovir is highly effective in decreasing pain and in reducing the incidence of ocular complications, such as corneal damage and anterior uveitis.[37] Oral famciclovir[38] and oral valaciclovir[39] are as effective in adults as oral acyclovir, but are not recommended for children <12 years. Topical acyclovir alone is insufficient.[40] An ophthalmologist should be consulted.

For children, we recommend hospital admission for an ophthalmologic opinion and for IV therapy:

> **acyclovir 10 mg/kg IV, 8-hourly**

For older children and where compliance is good, it is possible to use:

> **acyclovir 20 mg/kg (max 800 mg) orally, 5 times daily for 7 days** OR
> **famciclovir (12 years or older) 250 mg orally, 8-hourly for 7 days** OR (if immunocompromised)
> **famciclovir 500 mg orally, 8-hourly for 10 days** OR
> **valaciclovir (12 years or older) 1 g orally, 8-hourly for 7 days**

Treatment of bacterial and presumed bacterial conjunctivitis

For severe cases, and where bacterial conjunctivitis is confirmed,[26–29] we recommend:

chloramphenicol 0.5% eye drops, 1–2 drops 2–6-hourly, for 2–3 days OR
chloramphenicol 1% eye ointment 1.5 cm 3-hourly or at bedtime (drops by day) OR
polymyxin, neomycin, bacitracin eye ointment 6–12-hourly OR
framycetin 0.5% eye drops, 2 drops every 1–2 hours initially, then 8-hourly as infection improves

Gentamicin, tobramycin, and quinolone eye drops are sub-stantially more expensive than the recommended drugs and are generally unnecessary for empiric treatment.

Treatment of gonococcal conjunctivitis

Gonococcal conjunctivitis can occur in older children and adolescents sporadically and in epidemics. The rare sporadic cases outside these areas should be treated in consultation with an ophthalmologist, and the possibility of child sexual abuse must be considered. Topical antimicrobial treatment alone is ineffective and topical antibiotics are not required when systemic therapy is used, although saline irrigation reduces discomfort and purulent discharge. For systemic therapy, because of penicillin resistance, we recommend:

ceftriaxone 50 mg/kg (max 1 g) IM or IV, as a single dose

Treatment of meningococcal conjunctivitis

For the treatment of acute meningococcal conjunctivitis, systemic antibiotics should be administered, because topical antibiotics are ineffective, and chemoprophylaxis should be offered to contacts (see p. 138). (see p. 138) We recommend:

benzylpenicillin 30 mg (50,000 U)/kg (max 1.2 g or 2 million U) IV, 4-hourly for 5 days

For patients with penicillin allergy (excluding anaphylactic allergy), we recommend:

ceftriaxone 100 mg/kg (max 4 g) IV, daily for 5 days OR
cefotaxime 50 mg/kg (max 2 g) IV, 6-hourly for 5 days

For patients with anaphylactic allergy to penicillin and/or cephalosporins, we recommend:

ciprofloxacin 10 mg/kg (max 400 mg) IV, 12-hourly for 5 days

5.3 Neonatal eye infections

Most neonatal conjunctivitis in industrialized countries is chemical, due to prophylaxis or other irritants.[16,41] On the other hand, there are four major diagnoses not to be missed in the newborn baby presenting with conjunctivitis: gonorrhea, chlamydia, HSV, and panophthalmitis.

Chemical conjunctivitis in neonates

Conjunctivitis occurring within the first 24 hours of life is most likely an irritant reaction to ocular prophylaxis.[16,41] This is most often seen with silver nitrate and less often with erythromycin or tetracycline prophylaxis.[16,41] The typical clinical course of chemical conjunctivitis is presentation of mild, purulent conjunctivitis within the first 24 hours of life and resolution within 48 hours. Gram stain of conjunctival scrapings shows no bacteria.[16,41] No specific treatment is needed.[16,41]

Gonococcal ophthalmia neonatorum

The typical presentation of gonococcal conjunctivitis is with sudden, severe, grossly purulent conjunctivitis in the first 3–5 days of life and sometimes at birth.[16,41] There may or may not be a history of maternal vaginal discharge. If not recognized, this organism can rapidly progress within 24 hours to ulceration and perforation of the globe.[16,41] If gonococcus is suspected, a culture and Gram stain of conjunctival scrapings should be obtained. Concomitant specimens for *Chlamydia* should also be obtained.[16,41] A presumptive diagnosis of gonococcal conjunctivitis is made by identifying Gram-negative diplococci in conjunctival scrapings and treatment should be started.[16,41]

We recommend:

ceftriaxone 25–50 mg/kg (max 125 mg) IV or IM, as single dose (unless jaundiced)

Ceftriaxone displaces bilirubin from albumin and can exacerbate jaundice. If jaundiced, we recommend:

cefotaxime 25 mg/kg IV, 6-hourly for 7 days

Topical antibiotic therapy alone is not sufficient and is unnecessary.[16,41] The eyes should be irrigated with saline several times a day until the purulence subsides. The mother and her sexual contacts should be treated for gonorrhea.[16,41] The patient also should be evaluated for disseminated infection, such as arthritis, meningitis, or sepsis.[16,41] Coinfection with *Chlamydia trachomatis* and *Neisseria gonorrhoeae* is common in some areas, and we recommend testing any baby with gonorrhea for chlamydia also.[16,41]

Neonatal chlamydia conjunctivitis

C. trachomatis can cause unilateral or bilateral mucopurulent neonatal conjunctivitis, classically at 5–14 days old, although extremes of 1–60 days have been described.[16,41] The presentation can vary from mild to moderate conjunctival erythema and from scant, mucoid discharge to copious, purulent discharge. Eyelid edema, chemosis, or pseudomembrane formation may also be present.[16,41] Corneal involvement is unusual initially, although untreated chlamydia conjunctivitis can result in varying degrees of conjunctival scarring and corneal infiltrates.[16,41]

The diagnosis can be made by both culture and rapid techniques. Special Dacron-tipped swabs are needed for culture, and epithelial cells must be collected, not just exudate.[16,41] Other tests using rapid techniques like PCR or ELISA are sensitive and specific.[42,43]

Up to half of untreated children with chlamydia ophthalmitis will develop chlamydia pneumonia,[44,45] and so the recommended treatment is with oral not topical antibiotics.[16,40,44,45] A preliminary study of azithromycin for neonatal disease had treatment failures and was inconclusive.[46] We recommend:

erythromycin base or ethylsuccinate 10 mg/kg orally, 6-hourly for 14 days

There have been unproven concerns about the relationship between erythromycin and pyloric stenosis,[47] but even if erythromycin genuinely causes pyloric stenosis in a proportion of babies, this may be a class effect of macrolides. The seriousness of chlamydia eye and pulmonary disease is a major consideration in our recommendation.

Sometimes a second course of erythromycin is needed, as the efficacy of erythromycin is approximately 80%.[16,41] Topical antibiotics are ineffective and unnecessary.[16,41,44,45] The mother and her sexual contacts should be treated for chlamydia.[16,41,44,45]

Neonatal HSV conjunctivitis

Neonatal HSV conjunctivitis classically presents from day 5 to day 14, but can be present at birth. Clinically, it can be unilateral or bilateral and there may be ipsilateral eyelid edema and serous discharge. If characteristic, blistering herpetic lesions develop on the lid or face, or if there are lesions in the mouth, or if there are corneal lesions, the diagnosis may be apparent. Otherwise, there are no clinical distinguishing features of HSV conjunctivitis.[48] Without treatment, however, 70% of neonates with HSV disease restricted to the skin, eye, or mouth (SEM) will progress to disseminated and/or CNS infection with a 50–85% mortality by 1 year of age.[48] With early diagnosis, HSV conjunctivitis is usually restricted to local disease. The prognosis of local (SEM) HSV infection is far better, but 2–12% still have neurologic impairment, indicating occult CNS disease or treatment failure.[48] Clearly, it is vital to make the diagnosis and treat as early as possible.

We recommend:

acyclovir 20 mg/kg, IV, 8-hourly for 14 days (21 days when CNS involvement proven)

Neonatal conjunctivitis from *Staphylococcus aureus* and other bacteria

Many other organisms can be grown from the eyes of babies with ophthalmia neonatorum, including *S. aureus*, *S. pneumoniae*, viridans streptococci, other *Streptococcus* species, *H. influenzae*, *Escherichia coli*, *Pseudomonas* species, *Klebsiella* species, *Enterobacter* species, *Proteus* species, viruses, and others.[16,41] Their role in neonatal conjunctivitis is controversial, and particularly that of *S. aureus*, which can be cultured frequently from the eyes of asymptomatic neonates.[16,41] Most infections caused by these organisms can be treated with topical antibiotics alone or even with saline without antibiotics.[41]

Pseudomonas aeruginosa needs special consideration. *P. aeruginosa* conjunctivitis can be mild (sticky eye), or babies can present with edema and erythema of the eyelids and purulent discharge, which can be associated with pannus formation and with endophthalmitis.[41] For babies with mild conjunctivitis associated with *Pseudomonas*, it is possible to use topical antibiotics, but an ill baby should be treated with systemic antibiotics.[49,50] On the other hand, isolation of *P. aeruginosa* from the eyes of a well neonate with mild conjunctivitis is not an indication for systemic antibiotics, because the risk of progression is extremely low.[49,50]

Other organisms apart from *Pseudomonas* that can cause neonatal endophthalmitis include group B streptococcus, other Gram-negative bacilli, and fungi, notably *Candida*.[49,50] The organism may be isolated from eye swab, blood, orcerebrospinal fluid, but if there is doubt, it may be necessary to take an intravitreal specimen from the eye for Gram stain and culture. An ophthalmologic consultation is obviously essential for diagnosis and treatment, which may involve subconjunctival or intravitreal injections, in addition to systemic antibiotics, because of poor penetration.[49,50]

5.4 Chronic conjunctivitis in neonates and older children

Nasolacrimal duct obstruction

Congenital nasolacrimal duct obstruction affects up to 20% of all newborns and is the commonest cause of chronic eye discharge in babies.[51–53] Affected children present with epiphora (excessive tearing), chronic or recurrent conjunctivitis, or eye discharge, which may progress to frank cases of acute dacryocystitis. Management ranges from watchful waiting to simple probing to probing with Silastic intubation to dacryocystorhinostomy. An observational study found that 964 of 4792 infants (20%) had evidence of defective lacrimal drainage (documented with a fluorescein disappearance test) and 95% of these babies were symptomatic with epiphora during the first month of life.[53] Spontaneous remission of epiphora occurred throughout the year, and 96% of cases had resolved before patients reached the age of 1 year.[53]

It is often recommended that most babies with nasolacrimal duct obstruction can be treated with massage alone, although there are no RCTs to say whether this actually speeds resolution.[53–56] More severe cases may need probing or saline irrigation by an ophthalmologist, which have been shown to be as effective as each other.[56] By the second year of life, probing has marginally better efficacy than watchful waiting, but 60% still resolve spontaneously.[57]

Chronic dacryocystitis

Chronic dacryocystitis means chronic inflammation of the lacrimal sac. It is really just a rather grand name for children with congenital nasolacrimal duct obstruction, but with chronic mucopurulent discharge. In a paper from Austria, bacteria could be grown from 73% of babies with chronic dacryocystitis; the organisms grown most frequently were *S. pneumoniae* (35%) and *H. influenzae* (20%), followed by *Pseudomonas*, viridans streptococci, and *Moraxella*.[58] No staphylococci were isolated. In contrast, a recent Polish paper[59] found staphylococci (*S. aureus* and coagulase negative staphylococci) were the commonest isolates. There are no RCTs of antibiotic therapy, but in the Austrian paper, initial therapy with topical bacitracin and neomycin was associated with resolution in 82.5% obreak patients.[58]

Trachoma (chronic *Chlamydia trachomatis* conjunctivitis)

Chronic *C. trachomatis* infection can produce trachoma, a form of chronic conjunctivitis which is a leading cause of blindness in the developing world. Trachoma is a disease of poverty that thrives in remote, marginalized, and displaced populations. Clinically, trachoma can be divided into its acute (active) and chronic or late-stage manifestations, but acute and chronic signs can occur at the same time in the same individual. In areas where it is endemic, repeated episodes of active disease occur, particularly during childhood, and are probably required for later development of the chronic sequelae. Following repeated infections, the upper tarsal conjunctiva becomes scarred. As scar tissue contracts, it shortens the inner surface of the upper lid, causing the eyelashes to turn in (entropion) and brush against the transparent cornea. This contact between eyelashes and the surface of the eye is called trichiasis: movement of the eye or eyelids damages the corneal epithelium. Corneal opacification and resulting blindness probably develops primarily as a result of this trauma and secondary bacterial corneal infection.

A Cochrane review of antibiotic treatment of trachoma found 15 RCTs with a total of 8678 participants.[61] The review did not show immediate benefit in the resolution of active trachoma from either oral or topical antibiotics compared with placebo/no treatment, but did show reduced infection at both 3 and 12 months after treatment.[61] Oral antibiotics were no more effective than topical antibiotics.[61]

A Gambian RCT involved 1803 villagers, 16% of whom had active trachoma.[62] They were randomized to receive either three doses of azithromycin at weekly intervals or daily topical tetracycline over 6 weeks. Two months after treatment, the prevalence of trachoma was 4.6 and 5.1% in the azithromycin and the tetracycline groups, respectively (OR 1.09; 95% CI 0.53–2.02). However, 12 months post-treatment there were fewer new prevalent cases, 7.7%, in the azithromycin group compared to 16% in the tetracycline group (OR 0.52; 95% CI 0.34–0.80) and trachoma resolution was significantly better with azithromycin (OR 2.02; 95% CI 1.42–3.50). The authors concluded that azithromycin is easy to administer and may be more successful in trachoma than prolonged topical treatment.

There is evidence that insecticide spray as a fly control measure reduces the incidence of trachoma significantly,[63] while face-washing may be beneficial.[64]

The diagnosis is primarily clinical, because growing the organism or detecting it by antigen detection, PCR, or ligase chain reaction tests is too expensive in the field. Clinical grading with the WHO simplified system can be highly repeatable provided graders are adequately trained and standardized.[65]

For neonates (inclusion conjunctivitis) and children under 6 kg, treat with oral erythromycin as shown above (see p. 46).

For children over 6 kg with acute or chronic trachoma, we recommend:

azithromycin 20 mg/kg (max 1 g) orally, as a single dose

The WHO has set a target of global elimination of trachoma as a public health problem by the year 2020.[61,62] Community screening programs have been instituted but are difficult because trachoma typically affects the most medically underserved populations.[65,66]

Chronic or recurrent keratoconjunctivitis

Keratitis is a sight-threatening condition, most commonly caused by HSV, and far more common in adults than children. Other causes include VZV, bacteria such as *S. aureus*, *S. pyogenes*, *S. pneumoniae*, Enterobacteriaceae, and *P. aeruginosa* (in contact lens users). Keratitis due to fungi, mycobacteria, or *Acanthamoeba* can also occur with contact lenses. Prompt ophthalmologic consultation and intervention is essential.

5.5   Infections of the eyelids

Blepharitis

Blepharitis is an inflammation of the lid margins. It occurs most commonly as a complication of seborrheic dermatitis of the scalp and eyebrows. Treatment of the seborrhea, e.g., with coal tar, is usually sufficient.

Blepharitis can be associated with culture of *S. aureus* and other staphylococci, but their role is uncertain. There are no RCTs comparing treatment with placebo, but we found two RCTs comparing different topical antibiotics for bacterial blepharitis.[67,68] Topical ciprofloxacin is superior to topical rifamycin[67] or topical fusidic acid.[68] For acute bacterial blepharitis, we recommend:

ciprofloxacin ophthalmic solution 0.3% one drop to each eye 2-hourly while awake for 2 days, then 4-hourly while awake for 5 days

Blepharokeratoconjunctivitis

Chronic or recurrent blepharitis is often associated with keratoconjunctivitis. Blepharokeratoconjunctivitis is a chronic inflammatory disorder of children, causing a spectrum of clinical manifestations, from chronic eyelid inflammation, recurrent chalazia, and conjunctival and corneal phylctenules to neovascularization and scarring.[69,70] It is sometimes called phlyctenular conjunctivitis.[69,70]

There are no RCTs comparing the use of topical antibiotics with placebo or with oral antibiotics. There are only observational reports of the use of oral erythromycin[71] or tetracyclines.[72] The antibiotics may be acting as anti-inflammatory agents, since topical and even oral corticosteroids are often used and appear to control inflammation.[69,70]

Chalazion

A chalazion is a sterile lipogranulomatous inflammatory mass, which causes a bulge in the eyelid.[67] It is non-tender and persists for 2 weeks or more. It is not infectious.

Dacryoadenitis

Dacryoadenitis is an infected lacrimal gland, causing swelling of the outer portion of the upper eyelid.[73,74] It can be associated with viral infections including EBV, when it causes characteristic bilateral, painless swelling of the upper lids (Hoagland's sign).[73,74] Bacterial dacryoadenitis, usually due to *S. aureus*, can present as an acute, painful inflammation, and the eyeball may be red and swollen.[73] Children with severe infections may require hospital admission. For severe infections, we recommend:

> di/flucl/oxa/nafcillin 25 mg/kg (max 1 g) orally or IV, 6-hourly OR
> cephalexin 25 mg/kg (max 1 g) orally, 8-hourly OR
> cefazolin 15 mg/kg (max 600 mg) IV, 8-hourly

Dacryocystitis

Acute dacryocystitis, which is an infection of the lacrimal sac, can cause a red, painful swelling of the medial canthus.[74] Children may be systemically very unwell and need hospitalization. The commonest cause is *S. aureus*, but *S. pyogenes*, Gram-negative and anaerobic organisms are described.[74] Referral to an ophthalmologist and consideration of duct probing or external drainage is recommended. Systemic antibiotic therapy is indicated and is best guided by results of Gram stain and culture.

Pending results, we recommend:

> di/flucl/oxa/nafcillin 50 mg/kg (max 2 g) IV, 6-hourly OR
> cefazolin 15 mg/kg (max 600 mg) IV, 8-hourly

Meibomian abscess (internal hordeolum)

Meibomian abscess (internal hordeolum) is an infection, usually a staphylococcal abscess, of a long sebaceous gland in the eyelid called a meibomian gland.[73] As these abscesses seldom discharge spontaneously, warm compresses and oral anti-staphylococcal antibiotics are recommended, particularly if there is accompanying cellulitis. Surgical incision and curettage may also be necessary. Topical antibiotics are not indicated. We recommend:

> di/flucl/oxa/nafcillin 12.5 mg/kg (max 500 mg) orally, 6-hourly OR

> cephalexin 12.5 mg/kg (max 500 mg) orally, 6-hourly

Stye (external hordeolum)

A stye is a bacterial infection of a hair follicle on the eyelid, usually caused by *S. aureus*.[73] Treatment is not usually necessary as it is self-limiting and annoying rather than painful. Warm compresses may soothe. If infection persists, we recommend:

> polymyxin, neomycin, bacitracin eye ointment 6–12-hourly OR
> framycetin 0.5% eye drops, 2 drops every 1–2 hours initially, then 8-hourly as infection improves

5.6 Infections of the globe

Endophthalmitis

Endophthalmitis almost always occurs as a result of one of three mechanisms: following surgery, from a penetrating injury, or from metastatic bacteremic spread.[75]

In adults, surgery is the commonest cause of endophthalmitis, mostly cataract surgery. In children, post-surgical endophthalmitis is rare,[76] but can be sight- and even life-threatening.[77]

Endophthalmitis can follow penetrating injuries. In one series, good results were obtained (visual acuity 20/200 in 67% of eyes) with early aggressive therapy, which included intravitreal antibiotics, and vitrectomy in two-thirds of cases.[78] The commonest organisms were streptococci, staphylococci, and Gram-negative bacilli.[78]

Endogenous bacterial endophthalmitis is rare, and occurs when bacteria from the bloodstream of a bacteremic person cross the blood-ocular barrier and multiply within the eye. The most common Gram-positive organisms from blood cultures are *S. aureus*, group B streptococci, *S. pneumoniae*, and *Listeria monocytogenes*. The most common Gram-negative organisms are *Klebsiella* spp., *E. coli*, *P. aeruginosa*, and *Neisseria meningitidis*.[79,80] Gram-negative organisms are responsible for the majority of cases reported from East Asian hospitals,[80] but Gram-positive organisms are more common in North America and Europe.[79] The visual outcome is poor with most cases leading to blindness in the affected eye. Many patients have extraocular foci of infection, with an associated mortality rate of 5%. The condition is often misdiagnosed, and the outcome of endogenous bacterial endophthalmitis has not improved in 55 years.[79]

Various forms of antibiotic therapy have been used including topical, intravenous, sub-conjunctival, and intravitreal.[75] There have been few trials of prophylaxis or treatment. One RCT showed that giving prophylactic intravitreal vancomycin (1 mg) and ceftazidime (2.25 mg) at the time of operation compared with no intravitreal antibiotics improved the outcome for patients undergoing primary repair for globe injuries.[81] Both groups received IV ciprofloxacin. The incidence of endophthalmitis was significantly lower in the intravitreal group (6%) than the control group (18%).[81] A second RCT of prophylactic intraocular injection of clindamycin and gentamicin for penetrating eye injury was underpowered and showed only a trend to reduced endophthalmitis.[82]

A multicenter RCT studied patients with a distinct clinical entity, post-cataract endophthalmitis. In this study, 420 patients with clinical endophthalmitis <6 weeks after cataract surgery or secondary intraocular lens implantation found that systemic antibiotics (ceftazidime and amikacin) did not improve visual acuity or media clarity at 9 months, compared with vitreal tap or vitrectomy. Vitrectomy was of no benefit, except in the sub-group of patients with initial light perception-only vision.[83]

Patients with penetrating eye injuries and/or endophthalmitis require specialized management by an ophthalmologist, possibly including intravitreal antibiotics (see below). Antibiotic therapy should be guided by Gram stain of material obtained urgently at operation. If there is to be significant delay before obtaining advice or admitting the patient to a specialized unit, we recommend:

> **ciprofloxacin 15 mg/kg (max 750 mg) orally, as a single dose** PLUS
> **vancomycin <12 years: 30 mg/kg; >11 years: 25 mg/kg (max 1.5 g) IV, as a single dose by slow infusion**

Regimens that have been used for intravitreal therapy in adults include:

> **vancomycin 1 mg by intravitreous injection**
> **ceftazidime 2.25 mg by intravitreous injection**

> **amikacin 0.4 mg by intravitreous injection**
> **amphotericin B 0.005 mg by intravitreous injection**

The dose is repeated if there is not a complete response after 24–48 hours. A study suggested that the addition of intravitreal dexamethasone 0.4 mg to intravitreal antibiotic therapy might improve the outcome for post-operative endophthalmitis, although the difference did not reach statistical significance.[84]

Uveitis

Uveitis refers to any intraocular inflammation. It may be anterior, involving the iris and ciliary body (iridocyclitis), or post-erior, involving the choroid and retina (chorioretinitis or choroidoretinitis).

Iridocyclitis

Iridocyclitis, particularly when chronic, is usually associated with juvenile arthritis and other inflammatory conditions, not infections.[85] Rare exceptions of infections that can cause acute or chronic iridocyclitis include herpes viruses (EBV, HSV, HHV-6, VZV), borrelia (Lyme disease), and mycobacteria (*Myobacterium tuberculosis*, *Myobacterium leprae*).

Chorioretinitis

Infectious chorioretinitis (or choroidoretinitis or retinochoroiditis) is most commonly due to infections acquired prenatally. The prenatal infections classically described as causing congenital chorioretinitis are toxoplasmosis,[86] cytomegalovirus (CMV),[87] and rubella,[88] although congenital infection with lymphocytic choriomeningitis virus[89] can also cause chorioretinitis. The chorioretinitis is usually associated with other signs of infection, such as intracerebral calcification and microcephaly or hydrocephalus.[86–89]

Cytomegalovirus chorioretinitis

Congenital CMV chorioretinitis is usually present at birth, often in association with microcephaly and periventricular calcification, and almost always carries a grave neurologic prognosis.[90] Its presentation may be delayed or it may reactivate later.[91] Although ganciclovir treatment of CMV-infected neonates may reduce the incidence of deafness, it has no effect on retinitis.[92]

CMV retinitis rarely occurs in immunocompromised patients with HIV infection, transplant recipients, and patients with cancer. Oral valganciclovir is as effective as IV ganciclovir as induction therapy for HIV-infected adults with CMV retinitis,[93] and can be used for maintenance therapy. There are no data yet on valganciclovir in children. Intraocular ganciclovir implants are effective in adults with HIV and CMV retinitis,[94] but have not been studied in children.

For induction therapy in children we recommend:

ganciclovir 5 mg/kg IV, 12-hourly for 14–21 days

For adolescents, we recommend:

valganciclovir 900 mg orally, 12-hourly for 14 to 21 days

For maintenance therapy, we recommend specialist advice.

Toxoplasma chorioretinitis

Toxoplasma gondii is an ubiquitous human parasite that can be ingested in undercooked meat or in contaminated soil or water. Infection of the retina results in acute intraocular inflammation (chorioretinitis) and the formation of a retinal scar. Congenital toxoplasmosis has an incidence of 1 in 1000 to 1 in 10,000 and is an important cause of chorioretinitis. Chorioretinitis can recur at any time, often years after the first infection. The mechanism of damage may be infective due to the local release of *T. gondii* parasites from cysts in the retina or inflammatory due to an immune response to retinal antigens normally hidden from immune surveillance and released due to cyst reactivation.[95] Chorioretinitis can also result from post-natally acquired toxoplasmosis, which is at least as common as chorioretinitis from congenital infection.[96] The diagnosis of toxoplasma infection is usually made clinically by the ophthalmologist, on the basis of a classic raised chorioretinitis with pigmentation.

There is good evidence in favor of treating congenital toxoplasmosis, including babies with toxoplasma chorioretinitis, which will not be covered here.

A Cochrane review of antibiotic therapy for toxoplasma chorioretinitis found three eligible trials, all methodologically poor, which randomized a total of 173 participants.[97] The authors concluded that there is a lack of evidence to support routine antibiotic treatment for acute toxoplasma chorioretinitis, although weak evidence to suggest that long-term treatment of patients with chronic recurrent toxoplasma chorioretinitis may reduce the risk of recurrence.[97] Nevertheless, based on accumulated experience, most uveitis specialists agree that treatment of acute toxoplasma chorioretinitis is warranted, although there is no consensus regarding the best treatment regimens.[98] An RCT found that 6 weeks treatment for acute toxoplasma chorioretinitis with trimethoprim-sulfamethoxazole was virtually identical to pyrimethamine and sulfadiazine in terms of resolution and adverse reactions.[99]

Possible regimens, to be continued for 6 weeks, are:

trimethoprim+sulfamethoxazole 4 + 20 mg/kg (max 160 + 800 mg) orally 12-hourly OR
*pyrimethamine 2.5 mg /kg (max 100 mg) orally, once daily for 2 days, followed by 1 mg/kg (max 25 mg) orally, daily, for a total of 6 weeks PLUS EITHER
sulfadiazine 50 mg/kg (max 1.5 g) orally, 6-hourly OR
clindamycin 10 mg/kg (max 450 mg) orally, 8-hourly

[*Patients on long-term pyrimethamine need to be given daily folate or folinic acid supplements (adult dose 5 mg).]

Adjunctive corticosteroid therapy is often used to reduce the duration and severity of acute symptoms due to intraocular inflammation, but there are no RCTs of their use. It is recommended that they not be given without concomitant antimicrobials, because of anecdotal reports of fulminant infection.[100]

References

1 Wald ER. Periorbital and orbital infections. *Pediatr Rev* 2004;25:312–20.
2 Baum J. Infections of the eye. *Clin Infect Dis* 1995;21:479–86.
3 Weiss A, Friendly D, Eglin K, Chang M, Gold B. Bacterial periorbital and orbital cellulitis in childhood. *Ophthalmology* 1983;90:195–203.
4 Powell KR, Kaplan SB, Hall CB, Nasello MA, Jr, Roghmann KJ. Periorbital cellulitis. Clinical and laboratory findings in 146 episodes, including tear countercurrent immunoelectrophoresis in 89 episodes. *Am J Dis Child* 1988;142:853–7.
5 Ambati BK, Ambati J, Azar N, Stratton L, Schmidt EV. Periorbital and orbital cellulitis before and after the advent of *Haemophilus influenzae* type B vaccination. *Ophthalmology* 2000;107:1450–3.
6 Thirumoorthi MC, Asmar BI, Dajani AS. Violaceous discoloration in pneumococcal cellulitis. *Pediatrics* 1978;62:492–3.

7 Donahue SP, Schwartz G. Preseptal and orbital cellulitis in childhood. A changing microbiologic spectrum. *Ophthalmology* 1998;105:1902–5.

8 Schwartz GR, Wright SW. Changing bacteriology of periorbital cellulitis. *Ann Emerg Med* 1996;28:617–20.

9 Ono SJ, Abelson MB. Allergic conjunctivitis: update on pathophysiology and prospects for future treatment. *J Allergy Clin Immunol* 2005;115:118–22.

10 Fonacier L, Luchs J, Udell I. Ocular allergies. *Curr Allergy Asthma Rep* 2001;1:389–96.

11 Wald ER. Conjunctivitis in infants and children. *Pediatr Infect Dis J* 1997;16(2, suppl):S17–20.

12 Bodor FF. Conjunctivitis–otitis syndrome. *Pediatrics* 1982; 69:695–8.

13 Gigliotti F, Williams WT, Hayden FG, Hendley JO. Etiology of acute conjunctivitis in children. *J Pediatr* 1981;98:531–6.

14 Weiss A, Brinser JH, Nazar-Stewart V. Acute conjunctivitis in childhood. *J Pediatr* 1993;122:10–14.

15 Vichyanond P, Brown Q, Jackson D. Acute bacterial conjunctivitis: bacteriology and clinical implications. *Clin Pediatr* 1986;25:506–9.

16 Teoh DL, Reynolds S. Diagnosis and management of pediatric conjunctivitis. *Pediatr Emerg Care* 2003;19:48–55.

17 Bodor FF. Systemic antibiotics for treatment of the conjunctivitis–otitis media syndrome. *Pediatr Infect Dis J* 1989;8:287–90.

18 Lewis LS, Glauser TA, Joffe MD. Gonococcal conjunctivitis in prepubertal children. *Am J Dis Child* 1990;144:546–8.

19 Alfonso E, Friedland B, Hupp S et al. *Neisseria gonorrhoeae* conjunctivitis: an outbreak during an epidemic of acute hemorrhagic conjunctivitis. *JAMA* 1983;250:794–5.

20 Pellerano RA, Bishop V, Silber TJ. Gonococcal conjunctivitis in adolescents: recognition and management. *Clin Pediatr* 1994;33:114–6.

21 Dawson CR. Ocular herpes simplex infections. *Clin Dermatol* 1984;2:56–66.

22 Barquet N, Gasser I, Domingo P, Moraga FA, Macaya A, Elcuaz R. Primary meningococcal conjunctivitis: report of 21 patients and review. *Rev Infect Dis* 1990;12:838–47.

23 Pomeranz HD, Storch GA, Lueder GT. Pediatric meningococcal conjunctivitis. *J Pediatr Ophthalmol Strabismus* 1999; 36:161–3.

24 Langley JM. Adenoviruses. *Pediatr Rev* 2005;26:244–9.

25 The Brazilian Purpuric Fever Study Group. Brazilian purpuric fever identified in a new region of Brazil. *J Infect Dis* 1992;165(suppl 1):S16–9.

26 Sheikh A, Hurwitz B. Antibiotics versus placebo for acute bacterial conjunctivitis. *The Cochrane Database of Systematic Reviews* 2006;(2):Art No CD001211.

27 Gigliotti F, Hendley JO, Morgan J, Michaels R, Dickens M, Lohr J. Efficacy of topical antibiotic therapy in acute conjunctivitis in children. *J Pediatr* 1984;104:623–6.

28 Everitt HA, Little PS, Smith PWF. A randomized controlled trial of management strategies for acute infective conjunctivitis in general practice. *BMJ* 2006;333:321–6.

29 Rose PW, Harnden A, Brueggemann AB et al. Chloramphenicol treatment for acute infective conjunctivitis in children in primary care: a randomised double-blind placebo-controlled trial. *Lancet* 2005;366:37–43.

30 Wald ER, Greenberg D, Hoberman A. Short term oral cefixime therapy for treatment of bacterial conjunctivitis. *Pediatr Infect Dis J* 2001;20:1039–42.

31 Harrison CJ, Hedrick JA, Block SL, Gilchrist MJ. Relation of the outcome of conjunctivitis and the conjunctivitis–otitis syndrome to identifiable risk factors and oral antimicrobial therapy. *Pediatr Infect Dis J* 1987;6:536–40.

32 Shiuey Y, Ambati BK, Adamis AP et al. A randomized, double-masked trial of topical ketorolac versus artificial tears for treatment of viral conjunctivitis. *Ophthalmology* 2000;107:1512–7.

33 Ward JB, Siojo LG, Waller SG. A prospective, masked clinical trial of trifluridine, dexamethasone, and artificial tears in the treatment of epidemic keratoconjunctivitis. *Cornea* 1993;12:216–21.

34 Herpetic Eye Disease Study Group. Acyclovir for the prevention of recurrent herpes simplex virus eye disease. *N Engl J Med* 1998;339:300–6.

35 Karbassi M, Raizman MB, Schuman JS. Herpes zoster ophthalmicus. *Surv Ophthalmol* 1992;36:395–410.

36 Cobo M, Foulks GN, Liesegang T et al. Observations on the natural history of herpes zoster ophthalmicus. *Curr Eye Res* 1987;6:195–9.

37 Cobo LM, Foulks GN, Liesegang T et al. Oral acyclovir in the treatment of acute herpes zoster ophthalmicus. *Ophthalmology* 1986;93:763–70.

38 Tyring S, Engst R, Corriveau C et al. Famciclovir for ophthalmic zoster: a randomised aciclovir controlled study. *Br J Ophthalmol* 2001;85:576–81.

39 Colin J, Prisant O, Cochener B, Lescale O, Rolland B, Hoang-Xuan T. Comparison of the efficacy and safety of valaciclovir and acyclovir for the treatment of herpes zoster ophthalmicus. *Ophthalmology* 2000;107:1507–11.

40 Neoh C, Harding SP, Saunders D et al. Comparison of topical and oral acyclovir in early herpes zoster ophthalmicus. *Eye* 1994;8688–91.

41 O'Hara MA. Ophthalmia neonatorum. *Pediatr Clin North Am* 1993;40:715–25.

42 Elnifro EM, Storey CC, Morris DJ, Tullo AB. Polymerase chain reaction for detection of *Chlamydia trachomatis* in conjunctival swabs. *Br J Ophthalmol* 1997;81:497–500.

43 Hammerschlag MR, Roblin PM, Gelling M, Tsumura N, Jule JE, Kutlin A. Use of polymerase chain reaction for the detection of *Chlamydia trachomatis* in ocular and nasopharyngeal specimens from infants with conjunctivitis. *Pediatr Infect Dis J* 1997;16:293–7.

44 Schachter J, Grossman M, Sweet RL, Holt J, Jordan C, Bishop E. Prospective study of perinatal transmission of *Chlamydia trachomatis*. *JAMA* 1986;255:3374–7.

45 Jain S. Perinatally acquired *Chlamydia trachomatis* associated morbidity in young infants. *J Matern Fetal Med* 1999;8:130–3.

46 Hammerschlag MR, Gelling M, Roblin PM et al. Treatment of neonatal conjunctivitis with azithromycin. *Pediatr Infect Dis J* 1998;17:1049–50.

47 Patole S, Rao S, Doherty D. Erythromycin as a prokinetic agent in preterm neonates: a systematic review. *Arch Dis Child Fetal Neonatal Ed* 2005;90:F301–6.

48 Kimberlin DW. Herpes simplex virus infections in neonates and early childhood. *Semin Pediatr Infect Dis* 2005;16:271–81.

49 Lohrer R, Belohradsky BH. Bacterial endophthalmitis in neonates. *Eur J Pediatr* 1987;146:354–9.

50 Isaacs D, Moxon ER. *Handbook of Neonatal Infections: A Practical Guide.* London: WB Saunders, 1999.

51 Robb RM. Congenital nasolacrimal duct obstruction. *Ophthalmol Clin North Am* 2001;14:443–6.

52 Tan AD, Rubin PA, Sutula FC, Remulla HD. Congenital nasolacrimal duct obstruction. *Int Ophthalmol Clin* 2001; 41:57–69.

53 MacEwen CJ, Young JDH. Epiphora during the first year of life. *Eye* 1991;5:596–600.

54 Kushner BJ. Congenital nasolacrimal system obstruction. *Arch Ophthalmol* 1982;100:597–600.

55 Kim YS, Moon SC, Yoo KW. Congenital nasolacrimal duct obstruction: irrigation or probing? *Korean J Ophthalmol* 2000;14:90–6.

56 Young JD, MacEwen CJ, Ogston SA. Congenital nasolacrimal duct obstruction in the second year of life: a multicentre trial of management. *Eye* 1996;10:485–91.

57 Kuchar A, Lukas J, Steinkogler FJ. Bacteriology and antibiotic therapy in congenital nasolacrimal duct obstruction. *Acta Ophthalmol Scand* 2000;78:694–8.

58 Huber-Spitzy V, Steinkogler FJ, Haselberger C. [The pathogen spectrum in neonatal dacryocystitis]. *Klin Monatsbl Augenheilkd* 1987;190:445–6.

59 Gerkowicz M, Koziol-Montewka M, Pietras-Trzpiel M, Kosior-Jarecka E, Szczepanik A, Latalska M. [Identification of bacterial flora of conjunctival sac in congenital nasolacrimal duct obstruction in children]. *Klin Oczna* 2005; 107:83–5.

60 Mabey D, Fraser-Hurt N, Powell C. Antibiotics for trachoma. *The Cochrane Database of Systematic Reviews* 2005,;(2):Art No CD001860.

61 Fraser-Hurt N, Bailey RL, Cousens S, Mabey D, Faal H, Mabey DC. Efficacy of oral azithromycin versus topical tetracycline in mass treatment of endemic trachoma. *Bull World Health Organ* 2001;79:632–40.

62 Rabiu M, Alhassan M, Ejere H. Environmental sanitary interventions for preventing active trachoma. *The Cochrane Database of Systematic Reviews* 2005;(2):Art No CD004003.

63 Ejere H, Alhassan MB, Rabiu M. Face washing promotion for preventing active trachoma. *The Cochrane Database of Systematic Reviews* 2004:(3):Art No CD003659.

64 Solomon AW, Peeling RW, Foster A, Mabey DC. Diagnosis and assessment of trachoma. *Clin Microbiol Rev* 2004; 17:982–1011.

65 World Health Organization. Planning for the global elimination of trachoma (GET): report of a W.H.O. consultation (W.H.O./PBL/97.60). Geneva, Switzerland: World Health Organization, 1997.

66 Adenis JP, Colin J, Verin P, Saint-Blancat P, Malet F. Ciprofloxacin ophthalmic solution versus rifamycin ophthalmic solution for the treatment of conjunctivitis and blepharitis. *Eur J Ophthalmol* 1995;5:82–7.

67 Adenis JP, Colin J, Verin P, Riss I, Saint-Blancat P. Ciprofloxacin ophthalmic solution in the treatment of conjunctivitis and blepharitis: a comparison with fusidic acid. *Eur J Ophthalmol* 1996;6:368–74.

68 Viswalingam M, Rauz S, Morlet N, Dart JK. Blepharokeratoconjunctivitis in children: diagnosis and treatment. *Br J Ophthalmol* 2005;89:400–3.

69 Farpour B, McClellan KA. Diagnosis and management of chronic blepharokeratoconjunctivitis in children. *J Pediatr Ophthalmol Strabismus* 2001;38:207–12.

70 Meisler DM, Raizman MB, Traboulsi EI. Oral erythromycin treatment for childhood blepharokeratitis. *J AAPOS* 2000;4:379–80.

71 Zaidman GW, Brown SI. Orally administered tetracycline for phlyctenular keratoconjunctivitis. *Am J Ophthalmol* 1981;92:178–82.

72 Boruchoff SA, Boruchoff SE. Infections of the lacrimal system. *Infect Dis Clin North Am* 1992;6:925–32.

73 Marchese-Ragona R, Marioni G, Staffieri A, de Filippis C. Acute infectious mononucleosis presenting with dacryoadenitis and tonsillitis. *Acta Ophthalmol Scand* 2002;80:345–6.

74 Hurwitz JJ, Rodgers KJ. Management of acquired dacryocystitis. *Can J Ophthalmol* 1983;18:213–6.

75 Kresloff MS, Castellarin AA, Zarbin MA. Endophthalmitis. *Surv Ophthalmol* 1998;43:193–224.

76 de Sa L, Hoyt CS, Good WV. Complications of pediatric ophthalmic surgery. *Int Ophthalmol Clin* 1992;32:31–9.

77 Al-Torbak AA, Al-Shahwan S, Al-Jadaan I, Al-Hommadi A, Edward DP. Endophthalmitis associated with the Ahmed glaucoma valve implant. *Br J Ophthalmol* 2005;89:454–8.

78 Alfaro DV, Roth DB, Laughlin RM, Goyal M, Liggett PE. Paediatric post-traumatic endophthalmitis. *Br J Ophthalmol* 1995;79:888–91.

79 Jackson TL, Eykyn SJ, Graham EM, Stanford MR. Endogenous bacterial endophthalmitis: a 17-year prospective series and review of 267 reported cases. *Surv Ophthalmol* 2003;48:403–23.

80 Wong JS, Chan TK, Lee HM, Chee SP. Endogenous bacterial endophthalmitis: an east Asian experience and a reappraisal of a severe ocular affliction. *Ophthalmology* 2000;107:1483–91.

81 Narang S, Gupta V, Gupta A, Dogra MR, Pandav SS, Das S. Role of prophylactic intravitreal antibiotics in open globe injuries. *Indian J Ophthalmol* 2003;51:39–44.

82 Soheilian M, Rafati N, Peyman GA. Prophylaxis of acute post-traumatic bacterial endophthalmitis with or without combined intraocular antibiotics: a prospective, double-masked randomized pilot study. *Int Ophthalmol* 2001; 24:323–30.

83 Endophthalmitis Vitrectomy Study Group. Results of the Endophthalmitis Vitrectomy Study. A randomized trial of immediate vitrectomy and of intravenous antibiotics for the

treatment of post-operative bacterial endophthalmitis. *Arch Ophthalmol* 1995;113:1479–96.

84 Gan IM, Ugahary LC, van Dissel JT et al. Intravitreal dexamethasone as adjuvant in the treatment of post-operative endophthalmitis: a prospective randomized trial. *Graefes Arch Clin Exp Ophthalmol* 2005;243:1200–5.

85 Levy-Clarke GA, Nussenblatt RB, Smith JA. Management of chronic pediatric uveitis. *Curr Opin Ophthalmol* 2005;16:281–8.

86 Montoya JG, Rosso F. Diagnosis and management of toxoplasmosis. *Clin Perinatol* 2005;32:705–26.

87 Ross SA, Boppana SB. Congenital cytomegalovirus infection: outcome and diagnosis. *Semin Pediatr Infect Dis* 2005;16:44–9.

88 Banatvala JE, Brown DW. Rubella. *Lancet* 2004;363:1127–37.

89 Barton LL, Mets MB. Congenital lymphocytic choriomeningitis virus infection: decade of rediscovery. *Clin Infect Dis* 2001;33:370–4.

90 Jones CA, Isaacs D. Predicting the outcome of symptomatic congenital cytomegalovirus infection. *J Paediatr Child Health* 1995;31:70–71.

91 Boppana S, Amos C, Britt W, Stagno S, Alford C, Pass R. Late onset and reactivation of chorioretinitis in children with congenital cytomegalovirus infection. *Pediatr Infect Dis J* 1994;13:1139–42.

92 Kimberlin DW, Lin CY, Sanchez PJ et al. Effect of ganciclovir therapy on hearing in symptomatic congenital cytomegalovirus disease involving the central nervous system: a randomized, controlled trial. *J Pediatr* 2003;143:16–25.

93 Martin DF, Sierra-Madero J, Walmsley S et al. A controlled trial of valganciclovir as induction therapy for cytomegalovirus retinitis. *N Engl J Med* 2002;346:1119–26.

94 Musch DC, Martin DF, Gordon JF, Davis MD, Kuppermann BD, for the Ganciclovir Implant Study Group. Treatment of cytomegalovirus retinitis with a sustained-release ganciclovir implant. *N Engl J Med* 1997;337:83–90.

95 Holland GN. Ocular toxoplasmosis: a global reassessment. Part 1: Epidemiology and course of disease. *Am J Ophthalmol* 2003;136:973–88.

96 Gilbert R, Tan HK, Cliffe S, Guy E, Stanford M. Symptomatic toxoplasma infection due to congenital and post-natally acquired infection. *Arch Dis Child* 2006;91:495–8.

97 Gilbert RE, See SE, Jones LV, Stanford MS. Antibiotics versus control for toxoplasma retinochoroiditis. *The Cochrane Database of Systematic Reviews* 2002;(1):Art No CD002218.

98 Holland GN. Ocular toxoplasmosis: a global reassessment. Part II: Disease manifestations and management. *Am J Ophthalmol* 2004;137:1–17.

99 Soheilian M, Sadoughi MM, Ghajarnia M et al. Prospective randomized trial of trimethoprim/sulfamethoxazole versus pyrimethamine and sulfadiazine in the treatment of ocular toxoplasmosis. *Ophthalmology* 2005;112:1876–82.

100 Silveira C, Belfort R, Jr, Muccioli C et al. The effect of long-term intermittent trimethoprim/sulfamethoxazole treatment on recurrences of toxoplasmic retinochoroiditis. *Am J Ophthalmol* 2002;134:41–6.

CHAPTER 6
Fever

Fever is a common symptom in childhood, usually but not always indicating an infection. The physician or pediatrician assessing a febrile child needs to consider some important questions:

1 Is it likely this child has a viral infection, and if so, is it safe to watch the child at home?

2 Does this child have a bacterial infection that can be treated with oral antibiotics at home?

3 Does this child need hospital admission for observation and/or antibiotics?

4 Does this child have a non-bacterial, treatable cause of fever, such as Kawasaki disease?

5 Does this child have life-threatening bacterial infection, so that I need to give the child immediate antibiotic treatment?

Assessment of the febrile child can be greatly assisted by clinical and epidemiologic considerations, which in themselves help predict the likelihood that any particular child has a serious bacterial infection (SBI).

Key factors in the assessment are:
· the child's age;
· height of temperature;
· presence or absence of a focus of infection;
· presence or absence of "toxicity."

6.1   What constitutes a fever?

This deceptively simple question defies a simple answer. The normal body temperature is subject to diurnal variation, and temperature may vary with age. The measured temperature varies depending on the site of temperature measurement (see below) and physical activity.

A study of 691 apparently well babies aged 0–3 months attending a well baby clinic[1] found a mean rectal temperature of 37.5°C, with standard deviation (SD) 0.3°C. Using these data, if a fever is defined as 2 SD above the mean, a baby aged 0–3 months would be defined as febrile if the rectal temperature exceeded 38.1°C.

For older children, the normal rectal temperature is often quoted as 37°C. We found numerous comparisons of temperatures measured in different ways, but no study exclusively of normal children's temperature.[2] The definition of fever employed will determine what is considered "abnormal," but conventionally children are usually defined as febrile if their core temperature exceeds 38°C, while studies of "highly febrile" children take a cutoff of 39°C, 39.5°C, or even 40°C.

The cutoff used for defining fever will thus determine the characteristics of the febrile children included in any study.

6.2   Measurement of temperature

Question | For determining a child's temperature, are axillary, tympanic, or oral temperature measurements sensitive and specific compared to rectal temperature measurement?

Literature review | We found three systematic reviews that reviewed different techniques in terms of accuracy[3–5] and acceptability.[3]

It is not possible to measure "core" temperature non-invasively. The best approximation to core temperature is the rectal temperature. There is debate about the optimum way of measuring a child's temperature, taking into account sensitivity and specificity but also acceptability to the child, the family, and health care professionals. A systematic review of optimal methods of temperature measurement found 33 primary research studies (10 graded as superior and 23 as average quality).[3] The following were the conclusions:

· Electronic digital and disposable crystal thermometers were as accurate as mercury glass (2 studies).

· Axillary temperatures were inaccurate, inconsistent, and insensitive in children >1 month (11 studies).

· Infrared tympanic temperatures were inaccurate, inconsistent, and insensitive at all ages (20 studies).

· Parents and staff preferred infrared tympanic thermometers for speed, hygiene, and safety (4 studies).

A subsequent systematic review[2] comparing axillary and rectal temperatures found that axillary temperatures were on average 0.17°C lower than rectal temperatures in neonates and 0.92°C lower in older children and "young people." There was wide variation across studies. The authors concluded that this has implications for clinical situations where temperature needs to be measured with precision.[2]

The same authors performed a systematic review comparing infrared ear thermometry with rectal thermometry.[4] Their conclusion from 22 comparisons involving 2679 children was that the mean difference was smaller than for axillary temperature at 0.29°C, but the confidence intervals were very wide, meaning that ear temperature could not be considered a good approximation of rectal temperature.[3] Although others have argued in favor of infrared thermometry[5] on grounds of acceptability and adequate accuracy, a review suggested that infrared ear thermometry would fail to diagnose fever (>38°C) in 3 or 4 out of every 10 febrile children.[6] This suggests that tympanic membrane measurement is not sufficiently accurate for excluding fever in children.

There is a paucity of data on oral temperature measurement.[3] At present, rectal temperatures represent the "gold standard" in day-to-day clinical practice. If temperature is measured in the axilla or ear, it should be with the knowledge that the axillary temperature is likely to be about 1°C lower than the rectal temperature and that the ear temperature will miss fever in 30–40% of children. We recommend the use of rectal or axillary temperature measurement when it is important to rule in or rule out fever.

6.3   Height of fever

Question | In a population of febrile children, are children with higher fever more likely than less febrile children to have serious bacterial infection (SBI)?

Literature review | We found 20 papers that examined the relation between height of fever and incidence of bacterial infection. We found a systematic review for infants <3 months old[7] and another for children aged 3–36 months.[8]

In a retrospective study of infants aged 4–8 weeks, the rate of SBI increased in direct proportion to fever height, being 3.2% in those with a temperature 38.1–38.9°C, 5.2% in those with a temperature 39–39.9°C, and 26% in those with a temperature >39.9°C.[9] On the other hand, a systematic review[7] found four other studies that looked at predictors of bacteremia in infants <3 months and included temperature as a variable. None found a relationship between the height of fever and the risk of SBI.[7]

A systematic review of height of temperature in children aged 3–36 months found 14 studies. These showed that the risk of pneumococcal bacteremia, which was the commonest outcome studied, increased with the height of temperature. In the era before pneumococcal immunization, the incidence of pneumococcal bacteremia in children aged 3–36 months increased progressively from 1.2% for temperature <39.5°C to 4.4% for a temperature of 40.5°C or above.[8] In the era before Hib immunization, the height of fever did not correlate with the risk of Hib bacteremia.[10] There are no data correlating height of fever with risk of bacteremia due to other organisms.[8]

6.4   Age of the febrile child

Febrile neonate

The younger the febrile child, the greater is the incidence of SBI. For febrile neonates the risk of SBI is 12–32%.[7,11,12] Studies have shown that even if neonates are identified as being at relatively low risk using the Rochester criteria (see Section 6.5, p. 57, and Table 6.2), 3–6% of supposedly low-risk neonates would have an SBI and 2% will have bacteremia.[7,11,12] This means it will be necessary to treat 17–33 "low-risk" febrile neonates with empiric parenteral antibiotics to avoid missing one baby with SBI. Because of the high risk that a neonate with SBI will deteriorate, we recommend admitting all febrile neonates, taking appropriate cultures, and starting antibiotics. The antibiotics can be stopped usually after 48 hours if cultures are negative.

> **Recommendation: All febrile neonates (0–28 days) with temperature >38°C should be admitted to hospital and investigated and treated empirically for bacterial infection, until culture results are available.**

Infant aged 1–3 months

For febrile infants aged 1–3 months, the risk of SBI, in the era before pneumococcal immunization, was about

15–21%,[7,13,14] which is higher than for children aged 3–36 months.[8]

Is it possible to identify a sub-population of infants aged 1–3 months at low risk for SBI who might be managed as outpatients?

6.5 Clinical assessment of the febrile child

Question | In febrile infants aged 28–90 days, can clinical assessment identify a sub-population of infants at low risk of SBI who might be managed safely as outpatients?

Literature review | We identified 16 studies and 2 systematic reviews[15,16] which identified infants at low risk for SBI.

Dagan and colleagues have developed criteria, known as the Rochester criteria, which describe babies <2 months old (60 days) with fever but at low risk for SBI.[17,18] The Rochester criteria are shown in Box 6.1.

In one systematic review,[15] the likelihood that infants aged 1–3 months, defined as low risk using the Rochester criteria, had SBI was 0.9% and had bacteremia was 0.65%. Using a broader definition of low risk, the authors found that the risk of SBI was 1.4%, of bacteremia was 1.1%, and of meningitis was 0.5%.[15] Another systematic review[16] of 10 studies concluded that if the Rochester criteria were satisfied, the probability of an infant having SBI was reduced from 7 to 0.2%. In contrast, a more recent review[7] estimated that the overall probability of bacteremia for a low-risk febrile infant was 0.8% and of SBI was 2%.

Box 6.1 Rochester criteria for low risk-febrile babies aged <60 days.[17,18]

· Infant appears well and not toxic
· Previously healthy
· Born at term
· No antenatal or perinatal antibiotics
· Not treated for prolonged jaundice
· Not in hospital longer than the mother after birth
· Not hospitalized sub-sequently
· No recent antibiotics
· No evidence of bacterial infection (skin, soft tissue, bone, joint, ear)

It is arguable whether or not these data support management of low-risk infants as outpatients. In the era prior to immunization with pneumococcal conjugate vaccine, it was common practice to give low-risk infants and children a dose of IM ceftriaxone and to send them home. This practice is less common and less justifiable in places where universal pneumococcal immunization has resulted in pneumococcal bacteremia being extremely rare; in a recent US study the rate was 0.2% of febrile children aged 3–36 months.[19]

In our algorithm shown in Figure 6.1, we suggest that all febrile children aged <3 months at high risk for SBI (see Box 6.1 for low-risk criteria) should be admitted to hospital for empiric antibiotic treatment. An alternative that avoids hospital admission is to identify babies at low risk for SBI using the Rochester criteria, take cultures, give an IM or IV dose of a long-acting antibiotic such as ceftriaxone, and review the next day.

Toxicity

Question | In children with fever, can clinical examination predict reliably which babies have sepsis?

Literature review | We found 4 studies and 1 systematic review[7] in babies <3 months old and 19 studies and 1 review[8] in children 3–36 months old.

Pediatricians often use a term, "toxicity," or talk about a "toxic child," to describe febrile children who are non-specifically unwell, based on assessment of the child's level of activity, responsiveness, feeding, and peripheral perfusion. The sensitivity of an assessment that an infant <3 months old was toxic varied from 11 to 100% in four studies.[7] This variation may reflect the experience of the clinicians and thus be measuring their clinical acumen. Various researchers have attempted to define and quantify the signs and symptoms for clinical scoring systems to predict the likelihood of serious infection. The Yale Observation Score,[20] the Young Infant Observation Scale,[21] and a Melbourne scoring system[22] have all been evaluated. studies have shown that febrile children who are judged as being toxic are more likely to have SBI, there are problems. Large prospective studies show that scoring systems identify only 33–76% of infants <3 months old with SBI.[7] For older children, clinical scoring systems are even less sensitive,[8] and there is a group of children with high fever and so-called occult bacteremia who are not judged as being

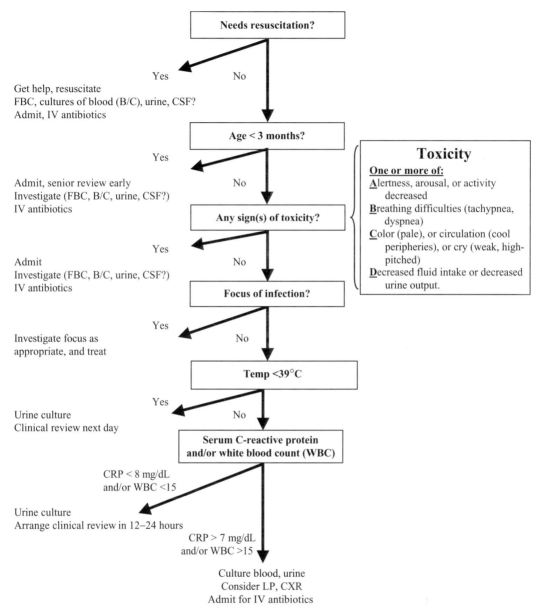

Figure 6.1 Algorithm for management of the febrile child <3 years old. In a population fully immunized with pneumococcal conjugate vaccine, it may not be necessary to measure WBC and serum CRP, but to review these children after 12–24 hours. (Modified from Reference 36.)

toxic by any criteria.[8] Most of these children had occult pneumococcal bacteremia.[8]

If a young febrile child <36 months old is judged as toxic, the risk of their having SBI is increased to the extent that it would seem wise to admit them to hospital for empiric antibiotics, pending the results of cultures. The signs of toxicity described in the infant observation scales[20–22] are one or more of the following: decreased alertness and arousal, altered breathing, blue lips, cold peripheries, weak, high-pitched cry, and decreased fluid intake and/or urine output. These signs are summarized in Box 6.2.

Box 6.2 Signs of toxicity in febrile young children aged 0–36 months.[20–22]

Toxicity: ABCD

The signs of toxicity in infants are:

A = arousal, alertness, and activity (decreased in a toxic child)

B = breathing difficulties (tachypnea or labored breathing)

C = color (pale) and/or circulation (cold peripheries) and/or cry (weak, high pitched)

D = decreased fluid intake (< half normal) and decreased urine output (< 4 wet nappies a day)

· Abnormality of any of these signs places the child at increased risk of serious illness

· The presence of more than one sign increases the risk

· The toxic child may appear drowsy, lethargic or irritable, pale, mottled, and tachycardic

Focus of infection

If there is a clinically apparent focus of infection, this will direct investigations and specific therapy and also alters the likelihood of bacteremia. For example, a child with a high fever who has acute otitis media or acute tonsillopharyngitis is less likely to be bacteremic than a child with no focus of infection.[8] Some children with a focus can be treated with oral antibiotics without further investigation and sent home, e.g., acute otitis media (see Chapter 12). A child who is toxic should be assessed carefully, even if there is a focus of infection, because a child with acute otitis media, for example, may also have systemic sepsis.

6.6   Investigation of febrile child

Not all febrile children need investigations. Indeed, most febrile children are diagnosed as having presumed viral infection and managed safely in the community. The decision as to whether or not to investigate should be made on the basis of an estimate of the risk that the child has SBI. This in turn depends on the criteria already described: age, height of fever, signs of toxicity, and focus of infection.

White blood count

The peripheral blood white blood cell count (WBC) is a relatively poor predictor of SBI in young infants < 3

months old. A review[7] found that the sensitivity of a total WBC > 15,000/mm^3 (15×10^6/L) for SBI was only 31–52% and the specificity 77–96%, although the absolute band count had a better sensitivity of 86–88%. The total WBC is a better predictor of SBI in children aged 3–36 months because most children with pneumococcal infection have a high WBC and, before immunization against *Streptococcus pneumoniae*, pneumococcal infections far outweighed other causes of bacteremia.[8]

In one preimmunization study, 86% of children with pneumococcal bacteremia had a WBC > 15,000/mm^3 (sensitivity 86%), but 23% of non-bacteremic children also had a WBC > 15,000/mm^3 (specificity 77%).[23] In such a population, the WBC can be used to screen highly febrile children with no focus of infection. If the incidence of pneumococcal bacteremia in a population of children aged 3–36 months with fever > 39°C and no focus is 4%,[8] then 40 out of every 1000 highly febrile children will have pneumococcal bacteremia, of whom 34 will have a WBC > 15,000/mm^3, while 960 will not have bacteremia, but 220 will have a WBC > 15. If a cutoff of 20,000/mm^3 is used, then fewer children without bacteremia will be treated, but at the cost of missing more children with pneumococcal bacteremia.[24] The cutoff used determines how many uninfected children are investigated and treated to avoid missing an infected child.

Universal infant immunization with 7-valent pneumococcal conjugate vaccine was introduced in the USA in 2000. Since then, a Kaiser Permanente study[19] found that the incidence of pneumococcal bacteremia in febrile children aged 3–36 months had fallen from 1.3 to 0.2% and the overall incidence of bacteremia from 1.6 to 0.7%. In this population, the sensitivity of a WBC > 15,000/mm^3 was 74% and the specificity 54.5%, which means that the peripheral blood white cell count is a relatively poor predictor of bacteremia in 3–36-month-old children from a population immunized against pneumococcus, only identifying three of four children with bacteremia.

Acute phase reactants

Serum C-reactive protein (CRP) is the most widely used and best studied of the acute phase reactants.[25–31] It is superior to the WBC as a predictor of occult SBI. In one study, a serum CRP > 7 mg/dL had a sensitivity of 79% and a specificity of 91% for predicting occult SBI and a higher likelihood ratio than WCC or absolute neutrophil count.[25] However, these data are from the days before universal pneumococcal immunization, and as for WBC, post-pneumococcal immunization studies may show that there are so few children with occult SBI that using an abnormal serum CRP may lead to treating many children to benefit none or very few.

Other acute phase reactants that are promising but less readily available include serum procalcitonin, IL-6, IL-8, and IL-1 receptor antagonist.[31]

No test has 100% sensitivity for predicting the febrile child with SBI. The use of serum CRP can help identify those children at risk of occult SBI who would benefit from hospitalization and/or systemic antibiotics. The cutoff point for an abnormal CRP can be set to try to obtain the best balance between over- and undertreatment.[25]

Urinalysis and urine culture

Urinary tract infection is the commonest SBI in a febrile child with no clinically apparent focus of infection.[8,32] A completely normal urinalysis makes urinary tract infection extremely unlikely (see Chapter 17), although if there is no focus, urine should be sent for culture. Bag urines should not be used for culture when starting empiric antibiotics because of the high risk of contaminated urine. It is not necessary to send urine for culture if there is another focus, e.g., the child has a respiratory infection, and especially if the urinalysis is also normal.[32]

Cerebrospinal fluid (CSF)

The need for CSF examination depends on the incidence of meningitis, which in turn depends on the age, immunization status (Hib, pneumococcal, meningococcal), and on the clinical examination (see Section 10.1, p. 132). In general, the younger the child, the less reliable is the clinical examination in excluding meningitis and so lower the threshold recommended to perform a lumbar puncture (LP). The arguments for deferring LP in a very sick child are discussed in Chapter 10 (see p. 133 and Table 10.1).

Chest radiograph

Febrile children without respiratory symptoms often have a chest radiograph performed to exclude pneumonia. A systematic review[33] of three observational studies concluded that there is level II evidence that the yield is so low that chest X-ray is not indicated in a febrile child aged <2 years with no respiratory signs or symptoms. One study of febrile children aged 3 months to 15 years found that none of 41 without chest signs had an abnormal chest X-ray.[34] In contrast, 5 of 173 febrile infants aged <3 months without respiratory distress had abnormal chest X-rays.[35] If an abnormal chest X-ray would change practice, in terms of initiating or continuing antibiotics, then it may be indicated in febrile infants <3 months old even in the absence of chest signs.

6.7 Management of the febrile child

An algorithm developed for the management of the febrile child in the era before universal infant pneumococcal immunization,[36] and modified to include serum CRP measurement, is shown in Figure 6.1. We strongly recommend admitting all febrile neonates and treating them with empiric antibiotics. We have recommended also admitting and treating all febrile infants aged 1–3 months, although we acknowledge that it would be reasonable to use the Rochester criteria to identify low-risk infants aged 1–3 months and to manage them as outpatients with or without antibiotics. The data are not yet sufficient to confirm whether or not, in the pneumococcal vaccine era, it is safe to omit measurement of serum CRP and WBC in the well-looking child aged 3–36 months with fever >39°C but no focus of infection.

Antibiotics

The choice of empiric antibiotics for treating a febrile child will depend on the severity of the illness, on the child's and the population's immunization status, and on the epidemiology of local organisms causing sepsis. If the child is severely unwell, see Chapter 15. For the febrile child with no focus of infection, who is well or moderately unwell, has a normal urinalysis, does not have meningitis (normal CSF or old enough for meningitis to be excluded clinically), and for whom antibiotics are indicated, for example, in the algorithm in Figure 6.1, we recommend:

0–3 months old: **amoxi/ampicillin 50 mg/kg IV, 6-hourly** PLUS
gentamicin 7.5 mg/kg IV, daily
4 months to 4 years: **benzylpenicillin 30 mg (50,000 U)/kg IV, 6-hourly** OR

ceftriaxone 50 mg/kg IV or IM, daily OR
Over 4 years: THE COMBINATION OF
**benzylpenicillin 30 mg (50,000 U)/kg (max 1.2 g
or 2 million U) IV, 6-hourly PLUS
di/flucl/oxa/nafcillin 50 mg/kg (max 2 g) IV,
6-hourly** OR, AS A SINGLE AGENT
cefotaxime 50 mg/kg IV, 8-hourly OR
ceftriaxone 50 mg/kg IV or IM, daily

These recommendations are not based on RCTs, but on epidemiologic data on the likely organisms causing infection in industrialized countries.

In babies 0–3 months old, it is necessary to cover for group B streptococcus, meningococcus, *Listeria*, and Gram-negative enteric bacilli, among other organisms.

For children aged 4 months to 4 years with a normal urinalysis, meningococcus and pneumococcus are the major pathogens in industrialized countries, while *Staphylococcus aureus* should also be considered in older children. Benzylpenicillin is acceptable provided meningitis has been excluded and the child is immunized against Hib.

Ceftriaxone 50 mg/kg IM as a daily dose has been widely recommended and often used, especially when hospitalization is not an option or is not preferred. Ceftriaxone is inactive against *Listeria* (which is a rare cause of sepsis aged 1–3 months) and has relatively poor activity against *S. aureus*. These organisms are exceedingly rare in children aged 4 months to 4 years, and IM ceftriaxone is an option for these children. The main disadvantage of giving IM ceftriaxone to children who are being sent home is that the number of children you need to treat to prevent one case of septicemia or meningitis is high (several hundred) and will rise in countries which use universal pneumococcal immunization, and studies have shown that a population of older infants and children can be safely managed as outpatients.

Antipyretics

Antipyretics may be given to reduce fever or to reduce symptoms such as irritability. The most frequently used antipyretics are acetaminophen (which is the same as paracetamol) and ibuprofen.

Question | For febrile children, do antipyretics compared with placebo or other antipyretics reduce fever and irritability?

Literature review | We found 35 RCTs, 2 systematic reviews, and a Cochrane review.[37]

A Cochrane review found only 12 trials that compared the antipyretic effects of paracetamol with placebo or physical methods, and could find no evidence that paracetamol was effective in reducing the overall duration of fever.[37] Although paracetamol did not reduce the duration of fever in one study, children treated with paracetamol were more active and alert, but had no detectable improvement in mood, comfort, appetite, or fluid intake.[38]

A systematic review[39] of 22 articles comparing acetaminophen with ibuprofen found that acetaminophen produced a greater body temperature reduction than ibuprofen 30 minutes after administration. However, ibuprofen provided a longer duration of antipyretic effect than acetaminophen, and the initial temperature decrement lasted longer.[39] A systematic review examined the effect of ibuprofen and acetaminophen on pain and fever in children.[40] Single doses of ibuprofen (4–10 mg/kg) and acetaminophen (7–15 mg/kg) were comparable to analgesics or antipyretics in terms of efficacy and safety for relieving moderate to severe pain.[40] Ibuprofen (5–10 mg/kg) was a more effective antipyretic than acetaminophen (10–15 mg/kg) at 2, 4, and 6 hours post-treatment.[40]

Although there are anecdotal reports of liver toxicity and even hepatic failure with acetaminophen/paracetamol given for fever, such events are rare and usually relate to inadvertent overdose due to persistent administration at high doses, compounded in some cases by infection with a virus that might cause hepatitis.[41] Ibuprofen can be associated with gastrointestinal bleeding, anaphylaxis, and renal failure in adults, although rarely in children.[42] In a study of over 27,000 children randomized to acetaminophen or ibuprofen, 3 children, all in the ibuprofen group, were hospitalized with gastrointestinal bleeding (rate 17 per 100,000 for ibuprofen, not statistically significantly raised).[42] There were no other adverse reactions.

Question | For a febrile child, is giving both acetaminophen (paracetamol) and ibuprofen compared with giving either alone more effective in reducing fever?
Literature review | We found two RCTs of alternating doses of acetaminophen and ibuprofen[43,44] and one RCT comparing giving both at once with either alone.[45]

Two studies suggested that alternating doses of acetaminophen (paracetamol) with doses of ibuprofen on a 4-hourly basis had a greater antipyretic effect than monotherapy with either alone.[43,44] An Israeli study of 464 infants in day care found that the alternating regimen, given for 3 days, was associated with less fever but also with less stress and less absenteeism from day care.[44] While these results are interesting, they are preliminary, and it is unclear whether or not using alternating medications would be confusing and would increase the risk of toxicity. An emergency department-based study found that giving acetaminophen and ibuprofen simultaneously reduced the temperature by less than 0.5°C compared with monotherapy; the authors considered this change insufficient to warrant routine use.[45]

Question | In children with fever, is the response to antipyretics able to distinguish children with bacterial infection from children with viral infection?

Literature review | We found four prospective studies[46–49] and a review.[7]

Children with viral infections respond the same as those with bacterial infection to antipyretics.[7,46–49] It is not possible to differentiate bacterial from viral infection by the response to antipyretics.

Physical methods for reducing fever

A Cochrane review[50] found seven studies (467 children) comparing temperature reduction by physical methods such as tepid sponging with medication or placebo. Tepid sponging had an additive effect on reducing fever when used with an antipyretic. The only adverse effects were shivering and goose pimples.

We give our recommendations on the use of antipyretics and physical methods for managing fever in febrile children in Box 6.3.

6.8 Fever and petechial rash or purpura

Question | When a child presents with fever and petechiae (non-blanching rash), what is the likelihood of meningococcal infection and what of other severe bacterial infections?

Literature review | We found five observational studies (case series) of the incidence of SBI in children presenting with petechiae and fever[51–55] and one case series of non-blanching rash.[56]

Box 6.3 Recommendations on managing fever in children.

- Use antipyretics only if necessary for comfort (child's or parents')
- Try physical methods first, such as tepid sponging
- The recommended dose of acetaminophen/paracetamol is 15 mg/kg (max 600 mg), orally, no more than every 4 h, to a maximum of 4 doses/day (max 2.4 g/day)
- It is not recommended to give acetaminophen/paracetamol for more than 3 days without seeking medical advice
- The recommended dose of ibuprofen is 5–10 mg/kg (max 400 mg), orally, given 6–8-hourly, to a maximum of 4 doses/day
- Ibuprofen is not recommended for babies < 6 mo old

We found five case series of children presenting to hospital with fever and petechial rash, all from industrialized countries.[51–55] The incidence of SBI was much lower in the largest study, from Boston Children's Hospital.[53] The results are summarized in Table 6.1.

In one paper from the USA pre-Hib vaccines, Hib caused 6.2% of cases.[51] In another US study, group A streptococcus was responsible for 10% of cases and viral infections for 14.7%.[52] In the study from Denmark, enterovirus was found in 7% and adenovirus in 4% of cases.[55]

Other causes of fever and petechiae described in these papers, and in case reports and case series, included children with infections with *S. pneumoniae*,[57] *S. aureus*, rickettsial infections including Rocky Mountain spotted fever in North America and Q fever, various viral infections including influenza A, and endocarditis.

In a UK case series of 233 children presenting with non-blanching rash,[56] 26 (11%) had meningococcal disease at a time of relatively high UK incidence of meningococcal infection. Children with meningococcal infection were more likely than children without meningococcal to be assessed as "ill" (not otherwise defined), to be pyrexial (>38.5°C), have purpura, and a capillary refill time <2 seconds. Five of 26 children with meningococcal disease (19.2%) had an axillary temperature below 37.5°C. No child with a rash confined to the distribution of the superior vena cava had meningococcal infection. Investigations were less helpful, although

Table 6.1 Published case series of children with fever and petechial rash.

Study	Country of Study	Number of Children	All SBIs	Meningococcal Infection
Van Nguyen, 1984[51]	USA	129	26 (20.2%)	13 (11.1%)
Baker, 1989[52]	USA	190	32 (16.8%)	13 (6.8%)
Mandl, 1997[53]	USA	411	6 (1.5%)	2 (0.5%)
Brogan, 2000[54]	UK	55	5 (9.9%)	3 (5.5%)
Nielsen, 2001[55]	Denmark	264	45 (17.0%)	40 (15.2%)
Total		**1049**	**104 (10.0%)**	**73 (7.0%)**

children with meningococcal infection were more likely to have an abnormal neutrophil count and a prolonged international normalized ratio. No child with a serum CRP <6 mg/L had meningococcal infection.[56]

Most primary care physicians will never see a child with meningococcal infection in their practice and may or may not have seen infected children during their hospital training. In industrialized countries, about 7% of children presenting to hospital with fever and petechiae have meningococcal infection with a range from 0.5 to 15%.[51–55] Hospital-based series are subject to selection bias. Presumably, children presenting to general practitioners and pediatricians outside hospital with fever and petechial rash are less likely to have meningococcal infection and more likely to have viral infections, although we could not find any case series of the causes of fever and rash in children presenting outside hospital. Children with meningococcal infection are more likely to look ill and have poor perfusion (assessed by capillary refill time), but in one study as many as 19% were afebrile.[56]

Not all children with meningococcal infection have a petechial rash at presentation. In one large case series of 448 children with meningococcal infection, a petechial rash was present in 42% of children <1 year old and 65–70% of older children and adolescents.[58]

The primary care physician and the pediatrician need to decide:

· which children with petechiae and fever need admission to hospital;
· how to identify children with meningococcal infection as early as possible.

The decision on which child with fever and petechiae needs hospital admission will depend on local circumstances, such as the incidence of meningococcal infection, on the experience of the clinician, and on the history and examination, in particular whether the child is well or "toxic" (see below). A survey found substantial differences among North American pediatricians when asked how they would investigate and treat a child with fever and petechial rash who did not appear toxic, with community-based and academic general pediatricians less likely to take blood cultures and admit children to hospital than pediatricians specializing in emergency medicine and infectious diseases.[59]

We will discuss in detail the presentation and clinical management of a child with suspected meningococcal infection in Chapter 15.

6.9 Kawasaki disease (KD)

KD is an acute, self-limited systemic vasculitis, of unknown etiology, which if untreated can lead to coronary artery aneurysms in 25% of cases.[60–63] There is as yet no diagnostic test for KD. Diagnostic criteria have been developed for KD (see Box 6.4). It should be emphasized that these are epidemiologic criteria that were developed more to allow epidemiologic comparisons than to decide which children with KD should be treated.

Some children will not have all the classic diagnostic features of KD, but will nevertheless start to develop coronary artery dilatation and aneurysm formation. Such children are said to have incomplete or atypical KD, and recommendations for the evaluation of children with suspected incomplete KD have been published.[60]

Laboratory tests for KD

Laboratory investigations that can help with the diagnosis of KD are given in Box 6.5. It should be pointed out that only 50–60% of children with KD have a WBC

Box 6.4 Diagnostic criteria for Kawasaki disease.

Fever for 5 or more days
AND
Presence of at least four of:
1 bilateral bulbar conjunctival injection without exudate
2 polymorphous rash
3 oral changes: red, dry, cracked lips, strawberry tongue, oropharyngeal erythema
4 changes in extremities: erythema and/or edema of palms and soles, desquamation
5 cervical lymphadenopathy
AND
Exclusion of other diseases, e.g., measles, group A streptococcal infection, and viral infections
OR
Child with fewer features but who develops coronary artery aneurysms

$>15,000/mm^3$, that 70–90% have raised ESR and/or CRP, that thrombocytosis is unusual at the time of diagnosis, and that abnormalities of liver enzymes and serum albumin are present in less than 50% of children with KD.[60,61] Thus, although laboratory tests can be supportive, KD is primarily a clinical diagnosis and the decision to treat is a clinical one.

Echocardiography in KD

The echocardiogram should not be used as a diagnostic test for KD, and the decision whether or not to start treatment of KD should not depend solely on the echocardiogram findings. Coronary lesions often develop in the convalescent phase, so a normal echocardiogram does not exclude KD. Indeed, the aim of treatment is to prevent the development of coronary lesions.

Box 6.5 Helpful investigations in suspected Kawasaki disease.

Neutrophil leukocytosis: present in the majority of patients, often with toxic changes
Platelet count: thrombocytosis common, but only from second week of illness
Inflammation: raised ESR and serum CRP usual
Liver transaminases raised in up to 40% of patients

Treatment should not be delayed pending an echocardiogram. This is of particular relevance in rural areas where there may be delay in obtaining an echocardiogram. Ideally, however, an echocardiogram should be performed in all patients at or soon after the time of diagnosis, and repeated after 2 and after 6–8 weeks to exclude new lesions, which may rarely develop.[60,61] If coronary lesions are present, more frequent review will be necessary.[60,61]

Management of KD

In reviewing the management of KD, we found 52 guidelines, of which 4 were current and described as evidence-based.[60–63]

Intravenous immunoglobulin (IVIG)

Question | For children with KD, do IVIGs compared with placebo or no IVIG reduce the incidence of coronary artery abnormalities (CAAs)?
Literature review | We found 16 RCTs and a Cochrane review.[64]

The mainstay of the treatment of KD is the use of IVIG. The mechanism of action is uncertain, but there is no doubt about the efficacy of IVIG. A Cochrane meta-analysis of 16 trials of IVIG versus placebo[64] showed a significant decrease in new CAAs in favor of IVIG at 30 days RR = 0.74 (95% CI 0.61–0.90). No statistically significant difference was found thereafter. A sub-group analysis excluding children with CAAs at enrolment also found a reduction of new CAAs in children receiving IVIG: RR = 0.67 (95% CI 0.46–1.00).[64]

Results of dose comparisons showed the number of new CAAs decreased with increased dose. A single dose of 2 g/kg was superior to 400 mg/kg/day for 5 days and showed a statistically significant reduction in CAAs at 30 days (RR = 0.22, 95% CI 0.08–0.65). This comparison also showed a significant reduction in duration of fever with the higher dose.[64]

There was no statistically significant difference noted between different preparations of IVIG.

The authors concluded that children fulfilling the diagnostic criteria for KD should be treated with IVIG (2 g/kg single dose) within 10 days of onset of symptoms.[64]

Aspirin

Question | In children with KD, does high-dose aspirin therapy compared with no aspirin or low-dose aspirin or placebo reduce the incidence of CAAs?

Literature review | We found no studies comparing aspirin with placebo. We found six poor-quality comparative studies. We found a Cochrane review[65] and two non-Cochrane meta-analyses.[66,67]

Before IVIG was studied, aspirin was the mainstay of the treatment of KD. It has never been subjected to a satisfactory RCT. The rationale for aspirin use is either as an anti-inflammatory, when high doses would be better than low, or as an antithrombotic agent, when low dose would be preferred.

The Cochrane review[65] found only one study involving 102 children which was described as randomized, but it was not possible to confirm the method of treatment allocation.[68] The paper compared aspirin alone (30–50 mg/kg/day until defervescence) with aspirin plus IVIG with IVIG alone. The incidence of coronary artery aneurysms was reported as 39–42% with aspirin but 14–21% with IVIG.[68] A non-Cochrane meta-analysis[66] and a sub-sequent retrospective study[69] found no difference in the incidence of coronary artery aneurysms at 30 or 60 days between patients who received high-dose IVIG plus low-dose aspirin (80 mg/kg/day or less) and those who received high-dose IVIG with high-dose aspirin (>80 mg/kg/day). A second non-Cochrane meta-analysis of the role of IVIG and aspirin in KD[67] found the incidence of CAAs was inversely related to dose of IVIG, but independent of dose of aspirin. A paper in which children with KD were not given IVIG compared high-dose aspirin (100 mg/kg/day) with low-dose aspirin (30 mg/kg/day).[70] There was no difference in the rate of coronary aneurysms (17% versus 23%), but the high-dose group developed abnormal liver enzymes. However, the duration of aspirin treatment was longer than is usual.

Finally, a recent study has queried the need for high-dose aspirin. Children diagnosed with KD were given IVIG 2 g/kg but no aspirin initially and 94.4% defervesced within 3 days.[71] The authors concluded that aspirin was unnecessary, but because the study was uncontrolled and there was no aspirin group, it is unsure whether this conclusion is correct.

The current US guidelines[60] are to use aspirin 80–100 mg/kg/day in four divided doses during the acute phase of the illness, while the Australian,[61] UK,[62] and Japanese[63] recommendations are for 30–50 mg/kg/day in three divided doses, to reduce gastrointestinal adverse events.

All authorities[60–63] recommend that as soon as the child defervesces, the dose of aspirin should be dropped to an antithrombotic dose of 3–5 mg/kg once daily. This should be continued, even if the initial echocardiogram is normal, until the follow-up echocardiogram at 6–8 weeks shows no CAA.

We feel that the evidence for using high-dose aspirin in the initial phase of acute KD is weak and that it would be perfectly reasonable to treat with IVIG and only to add high-dose aspirin for children who failed to defervesce. There is no evidence that low-dose aspirin decreases the risk of thrombosis, but this is a relatively benign treatment so that the risks and cost are minimal.

Corticosteroids

Question | In children with KD, do corticosteroids compared with no corticosteroids or placebo improve outcome in KD?

Literature review | We found 10 studies of the use of corticosteroids and a meta-analysis[72] but only 1 RCT.[73]

Corticosteroids were often used in Japan in the early stages of KD treatment. Initial comparisons suggested that corticosteroid-treated children fared worse than children who did not receive corticosteroids. However, the studies were retrospective, non-randomized, and highly subject to confounding by selection bias because the corticosteroid-treated children were almost certainly more severely affected.

There has only been one RCT[73] that compared 21 children given 2 g/kg IVIG plus aspirin with 18 children given 2 g/kg IVIG plus aspirin plus a single dose of 30 mg/kg pulsed IV methylprednisolone. The steroid-treated children had significantly shorter mean duration of fever (1 day versus 2.4 days), shorter mean hospital stay (1.9 days versus 3.3 days), and lower serum acute phase reactants at 6 weeks. There were no differences in coronary artery size.

A meta-analysis[72] of eight studies, of which only one was an RCT, found that corticosteroids, when used in addition to IVIG and aspirin, were associated with a significant reduction in the incidence of coronary artery aneurysms: RR 0.55 (95% CI 0.37–0.80). The data are based on weak studies and have not convinced any authorities to recommend corticosteroids for primary therapy yet. Larger trials are awaited.

Treatment of acute KD should be started as soon as possible after the onset of fever and within 10 days whenever possible.

Recommendation for initial treatment of acute KD:

IVIG 2 g/kg, infused over 8–12 hours
WITH OR WITHOUT
aspirin 30–100 mg/kg orally, 6–8-hourly*

[*Whether or not high-dose aspirin is given initially, we recommend starting or changing to aspirin 3–5 mg/kg orally, daily when the child's fever has resolved.]

About 90–95% of children will respond to this regime with immediate resolution of fever within 36 hours.[60,71]

The above treatment is not indicated if the diagnosis of KD is made retrospectively, e.g., a child who presents with peeling fingers after >2 weeks but who no longer has signs or symptoms of inflammation.

Children with KD resistant to initial treatment

About 5–10% of children diagnosed with KD will have fever and signs of inflammation persisting for >36 hours despite IVIG.[60,71] The possibility of alternate diagnoses should be reconsidered. If the diagnosis of KD seems highly likely, and particularly if the child has coronary artery dilatation, further treatment is indicated.

The children with KD least likely to respond to initial IVIG are also the children most likely to develop coronary artery aneurysms. Risk factors for coronary artery aneurysms include being <1 year old, male, and a biphasic illness with recurrence of fever after initial defervescence.[61–63,74]

There are no good trial data to guide the best treatment for children with persistent KD. Most authorities recommend giving a second dose of IVIG 2 g/kg if fever persists after 48 hours. This was followed by defervescence in 9 of 13 children (69%) in one study, while two more of the 13 resolved after a third dose.[75] Some workers have used 1 g/kg of IVIG for the second dose, but the scanty data suggest that 2 g/kg may be more

effective than 1 g/kg, which resulted in resolution in 18 of 35 children (51%) in one study.[76]

Corticosteroids have been advocated by some for persistent KD. One small RCT[76] randomized 17 patients who had failed to respond to a second dose of IVIG to receive a third dose of IVIG 1 g/kg (8 patients) or 20 mg/kg of methylprednisolone (9 patients). Fever resolved more quickly with corticosteroids (1.4 versus 4.8 days), but perhaps because of low numbers, there was no difference in the incidence of coronary artery aneurysms.

For persistent or recurrent fever after 48 hours, we recommend:

IVIG 2 g/kg infused over 8–12 hours PLUS
aspirin 80–100 mg/kg orally, 6-hourly

If fever continues despite two doses of IVIG 2 g/kg, we recommend:

methylprednisolone 30 mg/kg IV infusion over 2–3 hours for 1–3 days

The evidence for these recommendations is not strong, as already indicated, but they represent our best interpretation of the literature.

6.10 Cat scratch disease

Cat scratch disease is caused by infection with *Bartonella henselae*.[77] *Bartonella* species cause a variety of clinical syndromes in both immunocompetent and immunocompromised hosts. Domestic cats are the natural reservoir and vectors of *B. henselae*. Infection follows a scratch or lick from an infected cat, usually a kitten or sick cat.[77] Asymptomatic *B. henselae* infection is common in early childhood.[77] Cat scratch disease typically produces fever and local lymphadenitis. Mild cases resolve spontaneously, but persistent lymphadenitis may require antibiotics and possibly drainage. Other manifestations of cat scratch disease include granulomatous conjunctivitis with ipsilateral preauricular or sub-mandibular lymphadenopathy (Parinaud oculoglandular syndrome), encephalitis without CSF pleocytosis, endocarditis, hepatitis, osteomyelitis, and fever of unknown origin.[77,78]

If tissue is not available, the diagnosis of cat scratch disease is made serologically using immunofluorescent assays[79] or ELISA,[80] both of which have reasonable sensitivity and specificity. If tissue is available, culture is feasible but PCR is the diagnostic test of choice.[81]

There are no comparative studies of different antibiotics to treat cat scratch disease. Margileth[82] retrospectively reviewed 268 patients with cat scratch disease, measuring outcome by clinical improvement in inflammatory and constitutional symptoms, reduced or resolved lymphadenopathy, and falling ESR. Only 4 of 18 different antimicrobials had apparent demonstrable efficacy: rifampicin in 87% of patients, ciprofloxacin 84%, gentamicin 73%, and trimethoprim-sulfamethoxazole in 58%, but none was compared to placebo.[82] Penicillins, cephalosporins, tetracycline, and erythromycin had minimal or no apparent clinical efficacy.

There is only a single-randomized, double-blind, placebo-controlled study of any antibiotic in cat scratch disease, azithromycin.[83] Patients with lymphadenopathy caused by *B. henselae* received either azithromycin or placebo. Affected lymph nodes reduced in size more quickly in azithromycin recipients, but there were no significant differences after 30 days.

Cat scratch disease is usually self-limiting in immunocompetent children, and most do not require antibiotic therapy. Treatment is recommended for children with systemic disease with organ involvement (e.g., liver, eye), with endocarditis, or with lymphadenopathy which has not resolved after a month, or when the lymphadenopathy is associated with significant morbidity.

For treatment of cat scratch disease, azithromycin is the only antibiotic that has been compared to placebo. We recommend:

azithromycin 10 mg/kg (max 500 mg) orally, on day 1, then 5 mg/kg (max 250 mg) orally, daily for 4 more days

Alternative antibiotics that may be as effective include ciprofloxacin, rifampicin, co-trimoxazole (trimethoprim+sulfamethoxazole), or gentamicin.

Longer duration of treatment is necessary for endocarditis (see p. 19) and for osteomyelitis.

6.11 Lyme disease

Lyme disease is caused by the spirochaete bacterium, *Borrelia burgdorferi*, acquired through a tick bite from the *Ixodes* tick. It was first described in the USA, and is endemic in parts of the USA, Europe, the former Soviet Union, China, Japan, but not Australasia. The clinical manifestations are divided into three stages: early localized, early disseminated, and late disease.

Early localized disease manifests as erythema migrans, a rash that typically begins 7–14 days after a tick bite as a red macule or papule that expands over days or weeks to form a large, red, annular lesion, often with central clearing, with a median diameter of 15 cm. Patients with erythema migrans may also have fever, headache, malaise, myalgia, and arthralgia.[84,85]

Early disseminated disease usually presents as multiple erythema migrans, which are multiple, annular lesions, smaller than the primary lesion, that appear about 4 weeks after the tick bite. They are due to bloodstream spread of the spirochaete. Early disseminated disease may present as facial nerve palsy, other cranial nerve lesions, meningitis, or conjunctivitis, all of which may occur with or without the rash.[84,85] Carditis with heart block can occur in children.

Late disease presents months to years posttick bite, mainly with recurrent pauciarticular arthritis and sometimes with central nervous system (CNS) symptoms.[84,85]

Culture of *B. burgdorferi* is possible from the lesions, but the necessary specialized culture media are not commercially available. Diagnosis is, therefore, made serologically using enzyme immunoassay (EIA) or immunofluorescent antibodies (IFA), with confirmation of equivocal tests by Western blot.[73,74] Serology is complex and should be discussed with the laboratory. The practice of sending *B. burgdorferi* serology on patients with non-specific symptoms such as chronic fatigue is discouraged,[73,74] because any positive results are very likely to be false positives. A systematic review of serology recommended that serology not be sent unless there was a greater than 20% pretest probability (on clinical and epidemiologic criteria) that the patient had Lyme disease.[86] CNS involvement is tested by finding CSF antibodies due to intrathecal synthesis.[84,85]

A systematic review of antibiotics for early Lyme disease found 11 RCTs involving 1213 patients.[87] The review suggested that phenoxymethylpenicillin, amoxicillin, amoxicillin/probenecid, tetracycline, doxycycline, and cefuroxime axetil were equally effective for treating early Lyme disease, although the available studies did not have sufficient power to detect small but potentially clinically relevant differences in efficacy between the individual drugs. Clinical failures with erythromycin, roxithromycin, and azithromycin indicate that macrolides should not be recommended as first line agents. The studies supported the use of treatment courses of 10–21 days for early disease. Based on the systematic review[87] and guidelines based on best available evidence,[84,85] the recommended treatment for early localized disease and early disseminated disease is:

> **doxycycline child >8 years: 2.5 mg/kg (max 100 mg) orally, 12-hourly** OR
> **amoxicillin 25 mg/kg (max 1g) orally, 12-hourly**

It is recommended to use 10–21 days for early localized disease, 21 days for multiple erythema migrans, 21–28 days for isolated facial palsy, and 28 days for arthritis.[84,85]

For persistent or recurrent arthritis (defined as synovitis persisting despite 2 months' antibiotic treatment), carditis, meningitis, or encephalitis, use:

> **ceftriaxone 100 mg/kg (max 2 g) IV, daily** OR
> **benzylpenicillin 60 mg (100,000 U)/kg (max 1.8 g or 3 million U) IV, 4-hourly**

It is recommended to use 14–28 days for persistent or recurrent arthritis or carditis, but 30–60 days for meningitis or encephalitis.[84,85]

6.12 Prolonged fever (fever of unknown origin)

The term pyrexia of unknown origin (PUO) or fever of unknown origin (FUO) is sometimes loosely used to refer to any child with unexplained fever, however long. A traditional definition is an illness with temperature exceeding 38.3°C, evolving over a period of at least 3 weeks, with no diagnosis reached after 1 week of inpatient investigation.[88]

The causes of FUO will vary according to whether or not the child comes from or has visited a developing country, the child's age, referral patterns, and the sophistication of available diagnostic tests. In general, the prognosis of PUO in childhood is better than in adults.

As always, a thorough history and examination is paramount. The history should include travel, animal exposure, and potential exposure to infectious diseases, including from siblings, parents (the parental occupa-

tion may be relevant), household, and other child contacts.

In four case series from USA,[89] Kuwait,[90] Argentina,[91] and Turkey,[92] totaling 536 children with FUO, the cause was an infection in 58% of cases, collagen vascular disease in 10% (but 20% in the USA[89]), malignancy in 6%, and other diagnoses in 11%. No diagnosis was made in 15% of children (ranging from 12% in the USA to 20% in Argentina).

Investigation of the child with prolonged fever

Investigation of the child with prolonged fever should be as selective as possible. Some investigations such as a full blood count, blood film, and cultures of blood and urine are mandatory. Acute phase reactants and sedimentation rate indicate inflammation and are nonspecific, although very high levels may suggest endocarditis or vasculitis. A blood film should be examined for malaria parasites if the child has lived in or traveled to an endemic area (see Section 16.4, p. 257). Most children have serology performed for EBV, CMV, *Mycoplasma pneumoniae*, and any other organisms suggested by history or examination. Antinuclear antibodies and antineutrophil cytoplasmic antibodies should be measured if vasculitis is suspected. A chest X-ray and Mantoux test should usually be performed to exclude tuberculosis. Abdominal ultrasound may be helpful, especially if there is anything to indicate abdominal pathology. The yield is poor from more extensive radiologic or nuclear medicine investigations, such as CT scans, MRI, and bone scans, unless there is a clinical indication. The use of invasive investigations, such as bone marrow or liver biopsy, is dictated by clinical indications or by suggestive laboratory tests.

6.13 Recurrent fever

Most children with recurrent fevers without an apparent focus of infection probably have recurrent viral infections, although it is difficult to prove this. Infectious causes that should be considered and excluded if the child comes from an endemic area include malaria (see Section 16.4, p. 257), brucellosis (see Section 16.2, p. 256), and tuberculosis (see p. 198).

A number of unusual syndromes can cause periodic recurrent bouts of fever, sometimes associated with other symptoms, which have a remitting and relapsing

Table 6.2 Comparative features of some periodic fever syndromes.

Characteristics	PFAPA	FMF	FHF	Hype-IgD Syndrome	Systemic Onset Juvenile Arthritis	Cyclic Neutropenia
Onset < 5 years old	Usual	Uncommon	Rare	Common	Common	Common
Mean length of episodes of fever	4 days	2 days	Days to weeks	4 days	> 30 days	3 days
Interval between episodes	2–8 weeks	4–8 weeks	Not periodic	Not periodic	Hectic quotidian	3–4 weeks
Aphthous ulcers	Usual (two-thirds of cases)	No	No	No	No	Usual
Pharyngitis	Yes	Sometimes	No	No	No	Yes
Cervical adenitis	Tender	No	No	Yes	Yes	No
Abdominal pain	Sometimes	Yes	Rare	Yes	No	No
Joint symptoms	Arthralgia uncommon	Arthralgia	Arthritis	Arthritis or arthralgia	Arthritis	No
Splenomegaly	Sometimes	No	No	Yes	Often	No
Rash	No	Erysipeloid ankle rash	Yes	Yes	Yes	No
Ethnic origin	Not specific	Mediterranean	Irish	Dutch, French, or other European	Not specific	Not specific
Laboratory tests	None	Mutation in pyrin (marenostrin) gene	Mutation in TNF receptor genes	Raised serum IgD	Not specific	Intermittent neutropenia, mutation in ELA2 gene
Complications	None	Amyloidosis	None	None	Polyarthritis	Gingivitis

Adapted from Reference 93, with permission.

course. They can be difficult to diagnose without a high index of clinical suspicion[82] (see Table 6.2).

Familial Mediterranean fever (FMF)

FMF is a disorder of the inflammatory response, causing intermittent widespread serositis. Mutations in the "Mediterranean fever gene" coding for a protein called pyrin or marenostrin can be demonstrated in about 85% of cases. This protein, produced mainly by neutrophils, regulates inflammation by an unknown mechanism, and gene mutations allow recurrent episodes of serositis. The inheritance of FMF is autosomal recessive, but in up to half of patients there is no family history. It characteristically affects people of Italian, Jewish, Turkish, Arabic, or Armenian ancestry, but can also occur in children with no documented Mediterranean background.[83,84]

Symptoms supporting a diagnosis of FMF are:
1 episodes of fever with abdominal and/or chest and/or joint pains;
2 at least three such episodes;
3 a family history of FMF or amyloidosis.

Attacks lasting from hours to 2 or more days comprise high fevers, marked abdominal pain due to peritonitis, pleuritic chest pain, arthritis, and headaches. A characteristic rash around the ankles may also be present. There is a risk of developing amyloidosis later. There are reports of FMF presenting in infancy, but symptoms usually start during childhood, and 80% of patients have their first attack <20 years old. The time between episodes varies. Treatment with colchicine reduces the incidence and the severity of attacks and reduces the risk of amyloid.[94,95]

Hyperimmunoglobulin D (hyper-IgD) syndrome

Hyper-IgD syndrome is a rare familial disorder. Attacks typically occur every 4–8 weeks, causing lymphadenopathy, abdominal pain with diarrhea, hepatosplenomegaly, arthralgia, arthritis, and a vasculitic rash. Acute phase reactants are usually markedly raised during attacks. Serum IgD is characteristically high, both during and between attacks.[96,97]

Familial Hibernian fever (FHF)

A rare but important differential diagnosis, FHF, is caused by a mutation in a tumor necrosis factor (TNF) receptor gene.[98] It is dominantly inherited and affects people of non-Mediterranean background. Abdominal pain is particularly prominent, the attacks tend to occur initially at an older age, and the fever is more prolonged than in FMF. There is no response to colchicine, but steroids are effective.[98]

Cyclic neutropenia

Cyclic neutropenia is a disorder caused by a mutation in the neutrophil elastase gene. It classically results in regular episodes of high fever, often accompanied by mouth ulcers, pharyngitis, or pyogenic infections. The episodes occur every 3–4 weeks. Serial monitoring of white cell counts once weekly for 6–8 weeks shows a cyclical fall in neutrophils, with symptoms corresponding to the nadir. Heterozygous mutations in the ELA2 gene, coding for neutrophil elastase, have been described in the majority of cases of cyclic neutropenia, as well as in most cases of sporadic and autosomal dominant severe congenital neutropenia.[99]

Periodic fever, aphthous stomatitis, pharyngitis, and adenitis (PFAPA syndrome)

The diagnosis of this clinically recognized syndrome is usually made by exclusion.[93,100] The etiology is not yet known. The name documents the symptoms: pharyngitis with negative throat cultures, aphthous mouth ulcers, and tender lymphadenopathy. The mean duration is 4–5 days. The child is healthy between episodes. Cyclic neutropenia needs to be excluded by measuring the white cell count during attacks. The periodicity of attacks in PFAPA syndrome is usually 4 weeks, although sometimes less, sometimes up to 6 weekly, and rarely every 3–4 months. Prednisolone 2 mg/kg daily, given for 1–2 days after onset of symptoms, is characteristically effective in aborting attacks and controlling symptoms. Cimetidine has been tried in refractory cases, with some success. Tonsillectomy is curative in up to 60% of affected children.[100]

Juvenile idiopathic arthritis (JIA)

The systemic presentation of JIA (previously called systemic Still's disease) is often non-specific. The child has high, spiking fevers, usually once or twice a day, continuing for many days. An associated macular, orange-pink, or salmon-colored rash (really the color of smoked salmon) is highly characteristic, but is often evident only at the time of fever. There can be associated splenomegaly and lymphadenopathy. Joint symptoms are not usually prominent, and arthritis may not develop for months to years after the onset of the fever.

References

1 Herzog LW, Coyne LJ. What is fever? Normal temperatures in infants less than three months old. *Clin Pediatr* 1993;32:142–6.

2 Craig JV, Lancaster GA, Williamson PR, Smyth RL. Temperature measured at the axilla compared with rectum in children and young people: systematic review. *BMJ* 2000;320:1174–8.

3 Duce SJ. A systematic review of the literature to determine optimal methods of temperature measurement in neonates, infants and children. Cochrane Library 1996, 1–124. DARE-978207.

4 Craig JV, Lancaster GA, Taylor S, Williamson PR, Smyth RL. Infrared ear thermometry compared with rectal thermometry in children: a systematic review. *Lancet* 2002;360:603–9.

5 El-Radhi AS, Barry W. Thermometry in paediatric practice. *Arch Dis Child* 2006;91:351–6.

6 Dodd SR, Lancaster GA, Craig JV, Smyth RL, Williamson PR. In a systematic review, infrared ear thermometry for fever diagnosis in children finds poor sensitivity. *J Clin Epidemiol* 2006;59:354–7.

7 Neto G. Fever in the young infant. In: Moyer VA (ed.), *Evidence-Based Pediatrics and Child Health*, 2nd edn. London: BMJ Books, 2004:257–66.

8 Bulloch B. Fever without focus in the older infant. In: Moyer VA (ed.), *Evidence-Based Pediatrics and Child Health*, 2nd edn. London: BMJ Books, 2004:267–75.

9 Bonadio W, McElroy K, Smith D. Relationship of fever magnitude to rate of serious bacterial infections in infants aged 4 to 8 weeks. *Clin Pediatr* 1991;30:478–80.

10 Jaffe DM, Fleisher GR. Temperature and total white blood cell count as indicators of bacteremia. *Pediatrics* 1991; 87:670–4.

11 Baker MD, Bell LM. Unpredictability of serious bacterial illness in febrile infants from birth to 1 month of age. *Arch Pediatr Adolesc Med* 1999;153:508–11.

12 Kadish HA, Loveridge B, Tobey J, Bolte RG, Corneli HM. Applying outpatient protocols in febrile infants 1–28 days of age: can the threshold be lowered? *Clin Pediatr (Phila)* 2000;39:81–8.

13 Roberts KB, Borzy MS. Fever in the first eight weeks of life. *Johns Hopkins Med J* 1977;141:9–13.

14 Caspe WB, Chamudes O, Louie B. The evaluation and treatment of the febrile infant. *Pediatr Infect Dis J* 1983;2:131–5.

15 Baraff LJ, Oslund SA, Schriger DL, Stephen ML. Probability of bacterial infection in febrile infants less than three months of age: a meta-analysis. *Pediatr Infect Dis J* 1992;11:257–64.

16 Klassen TP, Rowe PC. Selecting diagnostic tests to identify febrile infants less than 3 months of age as being at low risk for serious bacterial infection: a scientific overview. *J Pediatr* 1992;121:671–6.

17 Dagan R, Powell KR, Hall CB, Mengus MA. Identification of infants unlikely to have serious bacterial infection although hospitalized for suspected sepsis. *J Pediatr* 1985;107:855–60.

18 Dagan R, Sofer S, Philip M, Shachak E. Ambulatory care of febrile infants younger than two months classified as being at low risk for having serious bacterial infections. *J Pediatr* 1988;112:355–60.

19 Herz AM, Greenhow TL, Alcantara J. Changing epidemiology of outpatient bacteremia in 3- to 36-month-old children after the introduction of the heptavalent-conjugated pneumococcal vaccine. *Pediatr Infect Dis J* 2006;25:293–300.

20 McCarthy PL, Sharpe MR, Spiesel SZ et al. Observation scales to identify serious illness in young children. *Pediatrics* 1982;70:802–9.

21 Bonadio WA, Hennes H, Smith D et al. Reliability of observation variables in distinguishing infectious outcome of febrile young infants. *Pediatr Infect Dis J* 1990;12:111–4.

22 Hewson P, Poulakis Z, Jarman F et al. Clinical markers of serious illness in young infants: a multicentre follow-up study. *J Paediatr Child Health* 2000;36:221–5.

23 Lee GM, Harper MB. Risk of bacteremia for febrile young children in the post-*Haemophilus influenzae* type b era. *Arch Pediatr Adolesc Med* 1998;152:624–8.

24 Browne GJ, Ryan JM, McIntyre P. Evaluation of a protocol for selective empiric treatment of fever without localising signs. *Arch Dis Child* 1997;76:129–33.

25 Pulliam PN, Attia MW, Cronan KM. C-reactive protein in febrile children 1 to 36 months of age with clinically undetectable serious bacterial infection. *Pediatrics* 2001;108:1275–9.

26 McCarthy PL, Jekel JF, Dolan TF. Comparison of acute-phase reactants in pediatric patients with fever. *Pediatrics* 1978;62:716–20.

27 Bennish M, Been MO, Ormiste V. C-reactive protein and zeta sedimentation rate as indicators of bacteremia in pediatric patients. *J Pediatr* 1984;104:729–32.

28 Putto A, Ruuskanen O, Meurman O et al. C-reactive protein in the evaluation of febrile illness. *Arch Dis Child* 1986;61:24–9.

29 Peltola H, Jaakkola M. C-reactive protein in early detection of bacteremic versus viral infections in immunocompetent and compromised children. *J Pediatr* 1988;113:641–6.

30 Berger RM, Berger MY, van Steensel-Moll HA, Dzoljic-Danilovic G, Derksen-Lubsen G. A predictive model to estimate the risk of serious bacterial infection in febrile infants. *Eur J Pediatr* 1996;155:468–73.

31 Lacour AG, Gervaix A, Zamora SA et al. Procalcitonin, IL-6, IL-8, IL-1 receptor antagonist and C-reactive protein as identificators of serious bacterial infections in children with fever without localising signs. *Eur J Pediatr* 2001;160:95–100.

32 Moyer VA, Craig J. Acute urinary tract infection. In: Moyer VA (ed), *Evidence-Based Pediatrics and Child Health*, 2nd edn. London: BMJ Books, 2004:429–36.

33 Jadavji T, Law B, Lebel MH, Kennedy WA, Gold R, Wang EE. A practical guide for the diagnosis and treatment of pediatric pneumonia. *CMAJ* 1997;156:S703–11.

34 Leventhal JM. Clinical predictors of pneumonia as a guide to ordering chest roentgenograms. *Clin Pediatr* 1982;21:730–4.

35 Heulitt MJ, Ablow RC, Santos CC, O'Shea TM, Hilfer CL. Febrile infants less than 3 months old: value of chest radiography. *Radiology* 1988;167:135–7.

36 Kilham HA, Isaacs D. *Children's Hospital at Westmead Handbook: Clinical Practice Guidelines for Paediatrics.* Sydney: McGraw-Hill, 2004.

37 Meremikwu M, Oyo-Ita A. Paracetamol for treating fever in children. *The Cochrane Database of Systematic Reviews* 2002;(2):Art No CD003676.

38 Kramer MS, Naimark LE, Roberts-Brauer R, McDougall A, Leduc DG. Risks and benefits of paracetamol antipyresis in young children with fever of presumed viral origin. *Lancet* 1991;337:591–4.

39 Wahba H. The antipyretic effect of ibuprofen and acetaminophen in children. *Pharmacotherapy* 2004;24:280–4.

40 Perrott DA, Piira T, Goodenough B, Champion GD. Efficacy and safety of acetaminophen vs ibuprofen for treating children's pain or fever: a meta-analysis. *Arch Pediatr Adolesc Med* 2004;158:521–6.

41 Mahadevan SBK, McKiernan PJ, Davies P, Kelly DA. Paracetamol induced hepatotoxicity. *Arch Dis Child* 2006;91:598–603.

42 Lesko SM, Mitchell AA. The safety of acetaminophen and ibuprofen among children younger than two years old. *Pediatrics* 1999;104:e39.

43 Nabulsi MM, Tamim H, Mahfoud Z et al. Alternating ibuprofen and acetaminophen in the treatment of febrile children: a pilot study. *BMC Med* 2006;4:4.

44 Sarrell EM, Wielunsky E, Cohen HA. Antipyretic treatment in young children with fever: acetaminophen, ibuprofen, or both alternating in a randomized, double-blind study. *Arch Pediatr Adolesc Med* 2006;160:197–202.

45 Erlewyn-Lajeunesse MD, Coppens K, Hunt LP et al. Randomised controlled trial of combined paracetamol and ibuprofen for fever. *Arch Dis Child* 2006;91:414–6.

46 Torrey S, Heinritig F, Fleisher G. Temperature response to antipyretic therapy in children. Relationship to occult bacteremia. *Am J Emerg Med* 1985;3:190–6.

47 Weisse M, Miller G, Brien J. Fever response to acetaminophen in viral vs bacterial infections. *Pediatr Infect Dis J* 1987;6:1091–5.

48 Yamamoto L, Widger H, Flinger D. Relationship of bacteremia to antipyretic therapy in febrile children. *Pediatr Emerg Care* 1987;3:223–7.

49 Bonadio W, Bellomo T, Brady W, Smith D. Correlating changes in body temperature with infectious outcome in febrile children who receive acetaminophen. *Clin Pediatr* 1993;32:343–6.

50 Meremikwu M, Oyo-Ita A. Physical methods for treating fever in children. *The Cochrane Database of Systematic Reviews* 2003;(2):Art No CD004264.

51 Van Nguyen Q, Nguyen EA, Weiner LB. Incidence of invasive bacterial disease in children with fever and petechiae. *Pediatrics* 1984;74:77–80.

52 Baker RC, Seguin JH, Leslie N, Gilchrist MJ, Myers MG. Fever and petechiae in children. *Pediatrics* 1989;84:1051–5.

53 Mandl KD, Stack AM, Fleisher GR. Incidence of bacteremia in infants and children with fever and petechiae. *J Pediatr* 1997;131:398–404.

54 Brogan PA, Raffles A. The management of fever and petechiae: making sense of rash decisions. *Arch Dis Child* 2000;83:506–7.

55 Nielsen HE, Andersen EA, Andersen J et al. Diagnostic assessment of haemorrhagic rash and fever. *Arch Dis Child* 2001;85:160–5.

56 Wells LC, Smith JC, Weston VC, Collier J, Rutter N. The child with a non-blanching rash: how likely is meningococcal disease? *Arch Dis Child* 2001;85:218–22.

57 Carpenter CT, Kaiser AB. Purpura fulminans in pneumococcal sepsis: case report and review. *Scand J Infect Dis* 1997;29:479–83.

58 Thompson MJ, Ninis N, Perera R et al. Clinical recognition of meningococcal disease in children and adolescents. *Lancet* 2006;367:397–403.

59 Nelson DG, Leake J, Bradley J, Kuppermann N. Evaluation of febrile children with petechial rashes: is there consensus among pediatricians? *Pediatr Infect Dis J* 1998;17:1135–40.

60 Newburger JW, Takahashi M, Gerber MA et al. Diagnosis, treatment, and long-term management of Kawasaki disease: a statement for health professionals from the Committee on Rheumatic Fever, Endocarditis, and Kawasaki Disease, Council on Cardiovascular Disease in the Young, American Heart Association. *Pediatrics* 2004;114:1708–33.

61 Royle J, Burgner D, Curtis N. The diagnosis and management of Kawasaki disease. *J Paediatr Child Health* 2005;41:87–93.

62 Brogan PA, Bose A, Burgner D et al. Kawasaki disease: an evidence based approach to diagnosis, treatment, and proposals for future research. *Arch Dis Child* 2002;86:286–90.

63 Japanese Circulation Society Joint Research Group. Guidelines for diagnosis and management of cardiovascular sequelae in Kawasaki disease. *Pediatr Int* 2005;47:711–32.

64 Oates-Whitehead RM, Baumer JH, Haines L et al. Intravenous immunoglobulin for the treatment of Kawasaki disease in children. *The Cochrane Database of Systematic Reviews* 2003;(4):Art No CD004000.

65 Baumer JH, Love SJL, Gupta A, Haines LC, Maconochie I, Dua JS. Salicylate for the treatment of Kawasaki disease in children. *The Cochrane Database of Systematic Reviews* 2006;(4):Art No CD004175.

66 Durongpisitkul K, Gururaj VJ, Park JM, Martin CF. The prevention of coronary artery aneurysm in Kawasaki disease: a meta-analysis on the efficacy of aspirin and immunoglobulin treatment. *Pediatrics* 1995;96:1057–61.

67 Terai M, Shulman ST. Prevalence of coronary artery abnormalities in Kawasaki disease is highly dependent on gamma globulin dose but independent of salicylate dose. *J Pediatr* 1997;131:888–93.

68 Furusho K, Kamiya T, Nakano H et al. Intravenous gamma-globulin for Kawasaki disease. *Acta Paediatr Jpn* 1991;33:799–804.

69 Saulsbury FT. Comparison of high-dose and low-dose aspirin plus intravenous immunoglobulin in the treatment of Kawasaki syndrome. *Clin Pediatr (Phila)* 2002;41:597–601.

70 Akagi T, Kato H, Inoue O, Sato N. Salicylate treatment in Kawasaki disease: high dose or low dose? *Eur J Pediatr* 1991;150:642–6.

71 Hsieh KS, Weng KP, Lin CC, Huang TC, Lee CL, Huang SM. Treatment of acute Kawasaki disease: aspirin's role in the febrile stage revisited. *Pediatrics* 2004;114:e689–93.

72 Wooditch AC, Aronoff SC. Effect of initial corticosteroid therapy on coronary artery aneurysm formation in Kawasaki disease: a meta-analysis of 862 children. *Pediatrics* 2005;116:989–95.

73 Sundel RP, Baker AL, Fulton DR, Newburger JW. Corticosteroids in the initial treatment of Kawasaki disease: report of a randomized trial. *J Pediatr* 2003;142:611–6.

74 Muta H, Ishii M, Furui J, Nakamura Y, Matsuishi T. Risk factors associated with the need for additional intravenous gamma-globulin therapy for Kawasaki disease. *Acta Paediatr* 2006;95:189–93.

75 Sundel RP, Burns JC, Baker A, Beiser AS, Newburger JW. Gamma globulin re-treatment in Kawasaki disease. *J Pediatr* 1993;123:657–9.

76 Hashino K, Ishii M, Iemura M, Akagi T, Kato H. Risk factors associated with the need for additional intravenous gamma-globulin therapy for Kawasaki disease. *Acta Paediatr* 2006;95:189–93.

77 Massei F, Gori L, Macchia P, Maggiore G. The expanded spectrum of bartonellosis in children. *Infect Dis Clin North Am* 2005;19:691–711.

78 Murakami K, Tsukahara M, Tsuneoka H et al. Cat scratch disease: analysis of 130 seropositive cases. *J Infect Chemother* 2002;8:349–52.

79 Sander A, Berner R, Ruess M. Serodiagnosis of cat scratch disease: response to *Bartonella henselae* in children and a review of diagnostic methods. *Eur J Clin Microbiol Infect Dis* 2001;20:392–401.

80 Not T, Canciani M, Buratti E et al. Serologic response to *Bartonella henselae* in patients with cat scratch disease and in sick and healthy children. *Acta Paediatr* 1999;88:284–9.

81 Hansmann Y, DeMartino S, Piemont Y et al. Diagnosis of cat scratch disease with detection of *Bartonella henselae* by PCR: a study of patients with lymph node enlargement. *J Clin Microbiol* 2005;43:3800–6.

82 Margileth AM. Antibiotic therapy for cat-scratch disease: clinical study of therapeutic outcome in 268 patients and review of the literature. *Pediatr Infect Dis J* 1992;11:474–8.

83 Bass JW, Freitas BC, Freitas AD et al. Prospective randomized double blind placebo-controlled evaluation of azithromycin for treatment of cat-scratch disease. *Pediatr Infect Dis J* 1998;17:447–52.

84 American Academy of Pediatrics. Lyme disease. In: Pickering LK (ed.) *Red Book: 2003 Report of the Committee on Infectious Diseases*, 26th edn. Elk Grove Village, IL: American Academy of Pediatrics, 2003:407–11.

85 American Academy of Pediatrics, Committee on Infectious Diseases. Prevention of Lyme disease. *Pediatrics* 2000;105:142–7.

86 Tugwell P, Dennis DT, Weinstein A et al. Laboratory evaluation in the diagnosis of Lyme disease. Ann Intern Med 1997;127:1109–123.

87 Loewen PS, Marra CA, Marra F. Systematic review of the treatment of early Lyme disease. *Drugs* 1999;57:157–73.

88 Petersdorf RG, Beeson PB. Fever of unexplained origin: report on 100 cases. *Medicine (Baltimore)* 1961;40:1–30.

89 Pizzo PA, Lovejoy FH, Smith DH. Prolonged fever in children: review of 100 cases. *Pediatrics* 1975;55:468–73.

90 Mouaket AE, El-Ghanim EE, Abd-El-Al YK, Al-Quod N. Prolonged unexplained pyrexia: a review of 221 paediatric cases. *Infection* 1990;18:226–9.

91 Chantada G, Casak S, Plata JD, Pociecha J, Bologna R. Children with fever of unknown origin in Argentina: an analysis of 113 cases. *Pediatr Infect Dis J* 1994;13:260–3.

92 Ciftci E, Ince E, Dogru U. Pyrexia of unknown origin in children: a review of 102 patients from Turkey. *Ann Trop Paediatr* 2003;23:259–63.

93 Isaacs D, May M. Recurrent episodes of fever with tonsillitis, mouth ulcers and adenopathy. *J Paediatr Child Health* 2003;39:627–8.

94 El-Shanti H, Majeed HA, El-Khateeb M. Familial mediterranean fever in Arabs. *Lancet* 2006;367:1016–24.

95 Bakkaloglu A. Familial Mediterranean fever. *Pediatr Nephrol* 2003;18:853–9.

96 Drenth JP, Haagsma CJ, van der Meer JW. Hyperimmunoglobulinemia D and periodic fever syndrome. The clinical spectrum in a series of 50 patients. International Hyper-IgD Study Group. *Medicine (Baltimore)* 1994;73:133–44.

97 Oretti C, Barbi E, Marchetti F et al. Diagnostic challenge of hyper-IgD syndrome in four children with inflammatory gastrointestinal complaints. *Scand J Gastroenterol* 2006;41:430–6.

98 Aganna E, Hammond L, Hawkins PN et al. Heterogeneity among patients with tumor necrosis factor receptor-associated periodic syndrome phenotypes. *Arthritis Rheum* 2003;48:2632–44.

99 Ancliff PJ, Gale RE, Linch DC. Neutrophil elastase mutations in congenital neutropenia. *Hematology* 2003;8:165–71.

100 Berlucchi M, Meini A, Plebani A, Bonvini MG, Lombardi D, Nicolai P. Update on treatment of Marshall's syndrome (PFAPA syndrome): report of five cases with review of the literature. *Ann Otol Rhinol Laryngol* 2003;112:365–9.

CHAPTER 7
Gastrointestinal infections

7.1 Acute gastroenteritis

Acute gastroenteritis is a common condition of childhood. It used to cause 5 million deaths a year, almost all being children younger than 5 years old in developing countries, and still causes an estimated 2 million deaths annually worldwide.[1] Gastroenteritis is potentially fatal in any country and causes about 300 deaths a year in the USA.[1] Rotavirus is the most important cause throughout the world, but other intestinal viruses (such as Norwalk), other noroviruses and enteroviruses, bacteria (such as *Salmonella*, *Shigella*), and *Vibrio cholerae*, and protozoa (such as *Cryptosporidium*) are also important causes.

The hallmark of acute gastroenteritis is diarrhea. Diarrhea can be defined as a change in bowel habit for the individual child, resulting in substantially more frequent and/or looser stools.[1,2] The diarrhea may be associated with vomiting: rotavirus gastroenteritis is characterized by 1–2 days of vomiting followed by secretory diarrhea (diarrhea which persists even if the patient takes nothing by mouth).[1]

We offer two important clinical suggestions:

· **Diarrhea and/or vomiting can be non-specific presenting signs in children with systemic sepsis, e.g., meningococcal infection, septicemia, and urinary tract infection. Assess each child carefully.**

· **If a child has vomiting alone, consider the possibility of other diagnoses, e.g., intestinal obstruction (e.g., intussusception), diabetes, or meningitis, rather than assuming vomiting is due to gastroenteritis.**

Features that suggest alternate diagnoses include marked abdominal pain or tenderness, high fever (>38°C for child younger than 3 months old, >39°C for child 3 months or older), pallor, bloody diarrhea, shock, apathy, lethargy, or irritability.[1,2] Having urged caution, the vast majority of children with acute diarrhea, with or without vomiting, do have gastroenteritis.

Evidence-based guidelines have been published on the optimal investigation and management of acute gastroenteritis.[1–3]

Degree of dehydration in acute gastroenteritis

Question | In children with gastroenteritis, can clinical examination predict accurately the degree of dehydration?

Literature review | We found four studies that compared clinical findings with the degree of dehydration.[4–7]

Calculation of the severity of gastroenteritis and of fluid replacement requirements requires assessment of the degree of dehydration. The degree of dehydration is proportional to the weight lost due to fluid lost. Pre-illness weight, if known, provides the most accurate measure of fluid loss. Because the pre-illness weight is not known accurately in most cases, the validity of clinical measures of dehydration has to be assessed retrospectively.

We found four studies in which clinical findings were compared with the degree of dehydration, calculated as the difference between admission weight and post-rehydration weight.[4–7] One study was in Egypt[5] and the other three were in North America[6,7] and Australia.[4] In one study, a clinical score was developed to predict significant dehydration rather than relating clinical findings to weight loss.[7]

The findings of the four studies were very similar. Clinical signs of dehydration became apparent at 3–4% rather than the oft-quoted 5% dehydration. Children could be categorized as having no significant dehydration if they were <3% dehydrated, mild-to-moderate if they were about 5% dehydrated with a range of 3–8%,

Table 7.1 Assessment of degree of dehydration[4–7] and recommended management.

Minimal or No Dehydration	Mild to Moderate Dehydration	Severe Dehydration
< 3% loss in body weight • No signs	3–8% loss in body weight • General appearance abnormal ("looks unwell") • Dry oral mucosa • Absent tears • Sunken eyes • Diminished skin turgor (skin recoil after pinching skin > 2 s) • Capillary return > 2 s	9% or greater loss in body weight • Increasingly marked signs from the mild to moderate group plus: • Deep (acidotic) breathing • Altered neurological status (drowsiness, irritability) • Decreased peripheral perfusion • Circulatory collapse
• Manage at home generally • Normal fluids, continue breast-feeding, normal diet • Admit if very young, diagnosis in doubt, or large losses	• Manage at home or in hospital with oral rehydration solution (ORS) • If ORS not tolerated may require NG tube feeds or IV fluids • Resume normal diet when tolerated	• Measure urea, electrolytes, acid–base balance • Resuscitate with IV bolus if shocked • Rehydrate IV over 2–6 hours with regular clinical and biochemical review

and severely dehydrated if they were 9% dehydrated or greater.

Doctors in industrialized countries tended to overestimate the degree of dehydration clinically. In one study, the overestimate was by a mean of 3.2%, which the authors concluded caused unnecessary hospital admissions and overtreatment with IV fluid.[4]

Signs associated with dehydration in two or more of the four studies are given in Table 7.1, together with advice on management.

A dehydrated child's fluid requirements can be calculated as the volume needed to replace the deficit plus maintenance fluids plus ongoing losses.[8] The volume required for daily maintenance is given in Table 7.2.

For example, if the child weighs 8 kg, the daily maintenance fluid requirements are $(8 \times 100) = 800$ mL. If the child weighs 12 kg, the daily maintenance fluid requirements are $(10 \times 100) + (2 \times 50) = 1100$ mL. If the child weighs 23 kg, daily maintenance is $(10 \times 100) + (10 \times 50) + (3 \times 20) = 1560$ mL.

Examples of calculations of replacement requirements are given in Boxes 7.1 and 7.2.

If the child is **hypernatremic**, there is grave risk of causing cerebral problems by giving fluid too fast.[1–3] It is advised to calculate to replace the deficit over 48 hours rather than 24 hours.[1–3] An RCT showed that rehydration with ORS is safer than IV fluids, with fewer complications from hypernatremia.[9]

A number of studies have shown that hospital doctors in an industrialized country setting tend to overestimate the degree of dehydration, leading to increased hospitalization.[4,10–13] It is more dangerous to overestimate the degree of dehydration if fluids are to be replaced intravenously, because of the danger of fluid overload and serum electrolyte imbalance.

Table 7.2 Daily maintenance fluid requirements.

Weight of Child	Maintenance Fluid Requirements
First 10 kg	100 mL/kg
Second 10 kg	50 mL/kg
Subsequent	20 mL/kg

Route of rehydration for acute gastroenteritis

Question | For children with dehydration from acute gastroenteritis, is oral rehydration as effective and safe as IV rehydration?

Box 7.1 Example of calculation of replacement fluids for child who is 5% dehydrated.

One-year-old child
Estimated clinically as 5% dehydrated
Weight on admission: 10 kg
Maintenance fluids: 100 mL/kg for first 10 kg

Fluid requirements in the first 24 hours

	Replacement: 5% of 10 kg = 500 g (which is the same as 500 mL)	= 500 mL
PLUS	Maintenance fluids (100 mL/kg × 10 kg)	= 1000 mL
PLUS	Ongoing losses, estimated at, say, 180 mL (guesswork)	= 180 mL
TOTAL		1680 mL

Total fluid requirements = 1680 mL in first 24 hours
= 70 mL/h in first 24 hours
Recommended to be given orally using oral rehydration solution (preferably not with nasogastric tube)

Box 7.2 Example of calculation of replacement fluids for child who is 10% dehydrated.[1,2]

One-year old child
Estimated as 10% dehydrated and peripherally shut down
Weight on admission: 9 kg
· Take blood for serum electrolytes, urea and creatinine, blood sugar, and full blood count
· Resuscitate using **intravenous isotonic fluids** : normal saline (0.9% saline) or Hartmann's solution
· Suggest giving rapid bolus of 20 mL/kg = 180 mL
· If still poorly perfused, repeat up to total 40 mL/kg, to restore circulation
· If still shocked, consider sepsis or abdominal crisis (e.g., intussusception, perforation), continue IV infusion, admit to intensive care if possible
When child no longer shocked, and passing urine, calculate requirements for 24 hours (do not subtract resuscitation fluids)
   Because of the dangers of overhydration, it is usual to calculate to replace about 5% of the deficit   and review after 2–4 hours

Fluid requirements in the next 24 hours (after circulation restored)

	Replacement: 5% of 9 kg = 0.45 kg (which is the same as 0.45 L or 450 mL)	= 450 mL
PLUS	Maintenance fluids (100mL/kg × 9kg)	= 900 mL
PLUS	Ongoing losses, estimated at say 300 mL (guesswork)	= 300 mL
TOTAL		= 1650 mL
		= 69 mL/hours

As soon as possible change to oral rehydration solution for ongoing fluids, especially if child is hypernatremic
   Prefer oral fluids, but may need to nasogastric fluids if child not drinking
   If not tolerating enteral fluids, use IV 0.45% saline and 2.5% dextrose (higher dextrose concentration if blood sugar low), and change to oral fluids as soon as tolerated
   Review the child clinically frequently, especially soon after starting and when IV fluids being given

Literature review | We found 18 RCTs, a non-Cochrane meta-analysis,[14] and a Cochrane review[15] comparing oral with IV rehydration.

The first meta-analysis[14] conducted in 11 countries identified 16 trials involving 1545 children. Compared with children treated with IV rehydration, children treated with oral rehydration had significantly fewer major adverse events, including death or seizures (RR 0.36, 95% CI 0.14–0.89), and a significant reduction in length of hospital stay (mean 21 h, 95% CI 8–35 h). There was no significant difference in weight gain between the two groups (mean –26 g, 95% CI –61 to 10 g). The overall failure rate of enteral therapy was 4.0% (95% CI 3.0–5.0%). They concluded that enteral rehydration by the oral or nasogastric route is associated with significantly fewer major adverse events and a shorter hospital stay compared with IV therapy and is successful in most children.[14]

A Cochrane review compared oral rehydration therapy (ORT) with intravenous therapy (IVT) and found 17 trials (1811 participants), all described as being of poor to moderate quality.[15] They found more treatment failures with ORT (relative difference 4%, 95% CI 1–7). There were no significant differences in weight gain, hyponatremia or hypernatremia, duration of diarrhea, or total fluid intake at 6 and 24 hours. The ORT group stayed in hospital for 1.2 days less (95% CI –2.38 to –0.02 days). Phlebitis occurred more often in the IVT group (2%) and paralytic ileus more often in the ORT group (3%). Six deaths occurred in the IVT group and two in the ORT group.[15]

The authors of the Cochrane review concluded that ORT and IVT were equally effective. However, although they found no clinically important differences between ORT and IVT, the ORT group did have a higher risk of paralytic ileus and the IVT group was exposed to the risks of IVT. For every 25 children treated with ORT, one would fail and require IVT.[15]

We conclude that both oral and IV rehydration are safe and effective. In developing countries, where mothers nurse their infants and give frequent oral feeds, oral rehydration is preferred.[13] In industrialized countries, ORT is cheaper and with fewer adverse effects. The choice may depend on the availability of parents or nursing staff to give ORT. They should be encouraged to do so, and informed that if they can give oral

rehydration, the child will avoid an IV line and will get home quicker.

Rapid IV rehydration over 4 hours was advocated in the 1980s by the World Health Organization (WHO) for children in developing countries with moderate to severe dehydration, although there were no RCTs to support this recommendation.[13] In industrialized countries, uncontrolled observational studies have looked at using rapid IVT to rehydrate children with moderate dehydration IV over 1–3 hours and send them home if they can tolerate oral fluids. A recent study concluded this practice was safe and effective,[16] but rapid IVT has not been compared with oral rehydration, may not be safe in all hands, and is unproven in comparison to other therapies for gastroenteritis.[13] The main advantage of rapid IV rehydration is that children recover quicker and can be sent home earlier. The main potential danger of rapid rehydration is causing fluid overload and/or electrolyte disturbances, especially if the child's degree of dehydration is overestimated, which is common.[4,10–13,17] There is also a risk of sending home some children who are in need of hospital care. There seems no reason to recommend rapid IV rehydration if oral rehydration is equally effective and has proven to be safer than IV rehydration in general.[14,15]

Studies have shown that many children who could be rehydrated orally receive unnecessary IV fluids.[10–13,17] Because doctors tend to overestimate the degree of dehydration,[4,10–13] it is particularly important that the risks of treatment are kept to a minimum. The data suggest that oral rehydration is safer than IV fluids for hypernatremic dehydration.[13–15] IV cannulation may be associated with phlebitis and paralytic ileus. The main advantage of ORT is that it is less costly, less traumatic for the child, and results in a shorter hospital stay.

We recommend using oral rehydration for children with mild or moderate dehydration, although it is safe and effective to use IV fluids for children with moderate dehydration, if preferred.

Severe dehydration (9% or greater) is life-threatening and we agree with the consensus view[1–3] and recommend resuscitating severely dehydrated children urgently using IV fluids.

Choice of ORS for oral rehydration in acute gastroenteritis

Since the 1980s, the WHO has recommended a standard ORS with relatively high sodium and glucose content (90 mmol/L sodium, 111mmol/L glucose, total osmolarity 311 mmol/L). The evidence for using this composition has been questioned. A number of studies have now compared the standard WHO ORS with ORS of reduced osmolarity.

Question | For children with dehydration from acute gastroenteritis, is WHO standard ORS as safe and effective as reduced-osmolarity ORS?

Literature review | We found eight RCTs and a Cochrane review[18] comparing standard or reduced ORS for non-cholera diarrhea. We found eight RCTs and a Cochrane review[19] and one later RCT[20] comparing standard or reduced-osmolarity ORS for cholera.

A Cochrane review[18] found 11 studies comparing standard WHO ORS with reduced-osmolarity ORS (defined as total osmolarity 250 mmol/L or less with reduced sodium) and reported the primary outcome, which was unscheduled IV fluid infusion. In a meta-analysis of eight eligible trials, reduced-osmolarity ORS was associated with fewer unscheduled IV fluid infusions than WHO standard ORS (OR 0.59, 95% CI 0.45–0.79), with no evidence for heterogeneity between trials. Stool output was lower and vomiting was less frequent in the reduced-osmolarity ORS group. No additional risk of developing hyponatremia was found with reduced-osmolarity ORS when compared with WHO standard ORS. The meta-analysis clearly favored reduced-osmolarity ORS for non-cholera diarrhea.[18] The WHO now recommends an ORS with a reduced sodium content and osmolarity: see WHO/UNICEF's joint statement—oral rehydration salts (ORS), a new reduced-osmolarity formulation—available on http://www.who.int/medicines/publications/pharmac opoeia/OralRehySalts.pdf (Accessed December 2006).

The situation for cholera is less clear-cut, and will be considered in Section 7.4, p. 83.

> **We recommend using reduced-osmolarity ORS for rehydration of children with mild to moderate non-cholera diarrhea.**

Mode of delivery of oral rehydration: oral feeds or nasogastric tube feeds

Question | For children with dehydration from acute gastroenteritis, are nasogastric tube feeds less likely to lead to treatment failure (need for IV fluids) than oral feeds?

Literature review | We found six observational studies in which at least some children were rehydrated nasogastrically, but no RCTs. We found one study comparing rapid nasogastric rehydration with rapid IV rehydration.[21]

The use of nasogastric tubes to give enteral feeds is increasingly common in some industrialized countries. In a retrospective study from Australia, 166 children were admitted with gastroenteritis: 20 (12%) received IV fluids, 50 (30%) received rehydration fluid orally, and 96 (58%) received rehydration fluid via a nasogastric tube.[22] No patient had to be changed from enteral rehydration therapy to IVT.

A study from the USA compared rapid oral rehydration using nasogastric tube feeds with rapid IV rehydration, both giving 50 mL/kg over 3 hours.[21] There were 96 children aged 3–36 months with moderate dehydration, and four treatment failures. Although the authors conclude that both treatments are safe, effective, and cost-effective, neither has been compared to simple oral feeds.

Pediatric wards in developing countries often supply a large central container of ORS so that mothers can use a ladle to get ORS and then rehydrate their children using a cup and spoon.[13] Children are rehydrated without the need for interventions such as nasogastric tubes.

Nasogastric tube feeds have the advantage of getting fluid in if a child refuses to drink or is vomiting frequently. They are far less invasive, cheaper, and less traumatic then IV fluids. On the other hand, they are more invasive than oral feeds, unpleasant, and have not been shown to have any advantage over oral rehydration.

> **We recommend giving ORT by mouth as the first choice in the treatment of mild to moderate dehydration and that nasogastric fluids be considered if oral intake is insufficient.**

Choice of IV fluids for IV rehydration in acute gastroenteritis

In many industrialized countries, it was tradition, when intravenously rehydrating children with gastroenteritis, to use low-sodium fluids (e.g., N/2 [half normal] or N/4 [quarter normal] saline) made isotonic by adding dextrose. This is because the calculated daily requirements for sodium and other electrolytes suggested that children needed only relatively low amounts of sodium for replacement compared with adults. One problem is that low-sodium fluids made isotonic by adding dextrose rapidly become hypotonic as the dextrose is rapidly metabolized. The use of low-sodium fluids was not subjected to clinical trials, and has recently been questioned, following episodes of catastrophic hyponatremia associated with IV rehydration for gastroenteritis.[23] Hyponatremia is particularly likely to develop in children who concurrently have the syndrome of inappropriate antidiuretic hormone secretion (SIADH). Dehydration, vomiting, and stress are potential causes of SIADH and occur commonly in gastroenteritis.[23–26]

Question | For children with acute gastroenteritis who need IV fluid rehydration, are low-sodium fluids safer or more effective than normal saline?

Literature review | We found a review of cases of severe hospital-acquired hyponatremia,[23] a case-control study of hyponatremia,[24] and one RCT comparing hypotonic with isotonic fluids.[25]

A 10-year review of children with severe hospital-acquired hyponatremia found over 50 reported cases of neurological morbidity and mortality, including 26 deaths, resulting from hospital-acquired hyponatremia in children who were receiving low-sodium parenteral fluids for various indications.[23] These were mainly common childhood conditions requiring parenteral fluids, such as pneumonia and meningitis, dehydration, and the post-operative state. All these conditions are potential non-osmotic stimuli for antidiuretic hormone (ADH) production, which can lead to free water retention and hyponatremia. The authors concluded that the use of isotonic saline for maintenance parenteral fluids is the most important prophylactic measure that can be taken to prevent the development of hyponatremia in children who receive parenteral fluids.[23] It must be remembered, however, that the au-

thors were reporting a highly selected group of children with a predetermined outcome. There was no control group, so the study did not address whether children rehydrated with isotonic fluids might also develop hyponatremia.

A case-control study compared 40 children who developed hyponatremia in hospital over a 3-month period with children whose serum sodium remained normal.[24] The patients who became hyponatremic received significantly more electrolyte-free water and had a higher positive water balance. Two of them had major neurological sequelae and one died.[24]

A prospective observational study looked for evidence of non-osmotic ADH activity in 52 children being rehydrated with 0.45% saline + 2.5% dextrose ("half normal" saline) for gastroenteritis.[26] Serum ADH levels were raised and remained high in both hyponatremic and normonatremic children. Most children had non-osmotic stimuli of ADH secretion and the persistence of the stimulus during IV-fluid administration predisposed to dilutional hyponatremia.

We found only one RCT, in which 102 children with gastroenteritis were randomized to receive either 0.9% saline + 2.5% dextrose (NS) or 0.45% saline + 2.5% dextrose (N/2 saline) at a rate determined by their treating physician according to hospital guidelines and clinical judgment.[25] Hyponatremia was common on admission (36% of patients). No child became hypernatremic after receiving IV fluids, but hyponatremia was more likely to persist or to develop in children given 0.45% saline + 2.5% dextrose than in those given normal saline. Normal saline protected against hyponatremia (no child receiving normal saline became hyponatremic) without causing hypernatremia.

For resuscitation of children with severe gastroenteritis using IV fluids, we recommend using normal saline, with or without added dextrose, to maintain the blood sugar. Hartmann's solution would be an appropriate alternative.

Antibiotics and acute gastroenteritis

Antibiotics are not routinely recommended for acute gastroenteritis. The reasons given are that most episodes of acute gastroenteritis are caused by viruses; that most episodes are self-limiting, including those caused by bacteria; that antibiotic use for gastroenteritis is likely to select for antibiotic resistance; and that antibiotics might increase gastrointestinal motility and cause bacterial overgrowth and thus worsen diarrhea.

Question | For children with acute gastroenteritis, do antibiotics compared with no antibiotics or placebo speed recovery?

Literature review | We found one placebo-controlled RCT of erythromycin[27] and two adult studies of ciprofloxacin for acute gastroenteritis.[28,29]

A small RCT of erythromycin for gastroenteritis in infancy showed no significant clinical benefit.[27] Two RCTs of ciprofloxacin in adults with acute diarrhea did describe modest clinical benefits, but because of the risk of rapid development of quinolone resistance[30] and the risk of adverse effects from quinolones in children, the use of antibiotics in this setting is not justified.[28,29]

We found no evidence to support the routine use of antibiotics for gastroenteritis in children. Traveler's diarrhea (Section 7.10, p. 86) and gastroenteritis due to specific organisms will be considered below.

We do not recommend antibiotics routinely for acute childhood gastroenteritis.

Antiemetics in acute gastroenteritis

A Cochrane review[31] of antiemetics for children with gastroenteritis found two RCTs, with a total of 181 children. Ondansetron and metoclopramide reduced the number of episodes of vomiting due to gastroenteritis in children compared to placebo, but increased the incidence of diarrhea.[32,33] We do not recommend antiemetics in childhood gastroenteritis.

Diet in acute gastroenteritis

Recommendations for maintenance dietary therapy in gastroenteritis depend on the age and diet history of the patient.

Breast-feeding and gastroenteritis

There is widespread consensus that breast-fed babies with dehydration from gastroenteritis should be rehydrated orally (with ORS) or intravenously, but should continue breast-feeding.[1] The reasons are to maintain adequate nutrition and to maintain breast-feeding. There are no RCTs, but this recommendation is an empiric one, which is unlikely to be studied in an RCT.

We recommend that breast-fed infants with acute gastroenteritis should continue breast-feeding on demand.

Lactose-free formula feeds and acute gastroenteritis

Question | For babies with acute gastroenteritis, do lactose-free or lactose-reduced feeds, compared with breast milk or lactose-containing formulas, speed recovery.

Literature review | We found 29 RCTs and a non-Cochrane meta-analysis.[34]

Breast milk contains as much lactose as formula feeds. Despite this, many people advocate low lactose or lactose-free formulas, supposedly because of the risk of lactose intolerance secondary to gastroenteritis. A meta-analysis of 29 RCTs (2215 patients) found no advantage of lactose-free formulas over lactose-containing formulas for the majority of infants, although infants with malnutrition or severe dehydration recovered more quickly when given lactose-free formula.[34]

Lactose intolerance often occurs post-gastroenteritis, due to damage to the mucosa resulting in impaired production of the lactase enzyme used to metabolize lactose, but is usually transient and does not require treatment. Patients with persistent lactose intolerance will have exacerbation of diarrhea when a lactose-containing formula is introduced. The presence of low pH (<6.0) or reducing sub-stances ($>0.5\%$) in the stool is not diagnostic of lactose intolerance in the absence of clinical symptoms.[1]

We recommend that lactose-free or lactose-reduced formulas are not routinely used for acute gastroenteritis and should be given only when there is evidence of lactose intolerance.

Regrading and acute gastroenteritis

Although medical practice has often favored restarting feeds with diluted (e.g., half- or quarter-strength) formula ("regrading feeds"), controlled clinical trials have shown that this practice is not only unnecessary but prolongs symptoms[35] and delays nutritional recovery.[36]

We do not recommend using diluted feeds for children recovering from gastroenteritis.

Soy fiber and acute gastroenteritis

Formulas containing soy fiber have been marketed, particularly to physicians and consumers, in the USA. Added soy fiber has been reported to reduce liquid stools without changing the overall stool output.[37] This cosmetic effect might reduce diaper rash and encourage early resumption of normal diet, but the benefits are probably insufficient to merit its use as a standard of care.[1]

Solids and gastroenteritis

Children receiving semisolid or solid foods should continue to receive their usual diet during episodes of diarrhea. Routinely withholding food for a day or more, which is sometimes advocated, is inappropriate. Early feeding reduces changes in intestinal permeability caused by infection,[38] reduces the duration of illness, and improves nutrition.[39,40] Severe malnutrition can occur after gastroenteritis if prolonged gut rest or clear fluids are prescribed.[41] This is a particular problem in developing communities where children often experience many episodes of gastroenteritis and catch-up growth is not achieved between episodes.

Zinc in diarrheal diseases

Severe zinc deficiency is associated with diarrhea (acrodermatitis enteropathica), which prompted studies on the role of zinc supplementation in preventing and treating acute and chronic diarrhea. In developing countries, prophylactic dietary oral zinc supplementation reduces the incidence and severity of acute diarrheal disease in childhood.[42,43] Furthermore, oral zinc supplements reduce the duration of chronic diarrhea in developing countries.[44,45] A systematic review identified five RCTs of oral zinc supplementation for chronic diarrhea in developing countries.[45] Zinc-supplemented children had a 24% lower probability of continuing diarrhea (95% CI 9–37%) and a 42% lower rate of treatment failure or death (95% CI 10–63%).[45]

For acute diarrhea, a meta-analysis found five RCTs of the use of oral zinc supplements started at the time children presented with acute diarrhea in developing countries. Zinc-supplemented children had a 15% lower probability of continuing diarrhea on a given day (95% CI 5–24%).[45] These benefits were independent of concomitant vitamin A supplementation.[45–50]

Neither zinc nor vitamin A supplementation, however, influenced the duration of acute diarrhea or the rate of readmission with diarrhea in Australian Aboriginal children.[51]

The WHO recommends that oral zinc is given to children in developing countries at the onset of diarrhea.

Vitamin A

The effect of routine dietary vitamin A supplementation on the incidence of diarrheal disease in infants in developing countries is controversial. Large doses of vitamin A have been associated with an increased risk of diarrhea,[52] while other studies showed reduced incidence of diarrhea.[53] A meta-analysis of nine RCTs found that supplemental vitamin A had no consistent benefit on the incidence of diarrhea (RR 1.00, 95% CI 0.94–1.07) and was associated with a slight increase in the incidence of respiratory infections.[54] Vitamin A supplements do not influence the outcome of acute diarrheal illness.[45–50]

We do not recommend vitamin A in acute gastroenteritis.

Probiotics in acute gastroenteritis

Question | For children with acute gastroenteritis, do probiotics compared to no probiotics or placebo shorten the duration of diarrhea?

Literature review | We found a Cochrane review of probiotics in adults and children,[55] a non-Cochrane systematic review of probiotics in children,[56] and a meta-analysis of lactobacilli in children.[57]

Probiotics are live microorganisms in fermented foods or components of microbial cells that have a beneficial effect on the health and well-being of the host.[55] Examples studied in trials include various species of lactobacilli or bifidobacteria and the non-pathogenic yeast *Saccharomyces boulardii*. No serious adverse effects of probiotics have been reported in well people, but infections have been reported in people with impaired immune systems.[55]

One systematic review restricted to placebo-controlled RCTs of probiotics in treating acute diarrhea in infants and children found 8 trials (731 children).[56] Probiotics reduced the risk of diarrhea lasting 3 or more days by 60% and reduced the duration of diarrhea by 18 hours. A meta-analysis restricted to RCTs of lactobacilli in children found 7 studies (675 children).[57] Lactobacilli reduced the duration of diarrhea by 0.7 days. Heterogeneity of results between studies prevented the analysis of the effects of individual strains of lactobacilli. A Cochrane review that included adult and child RCTs found 23 studies (1917 patients).[55] Probiotics reduced the risk of diarrhea at 3 days by 34% and the mean duration of diarrhea by 30.5 hours. There was some heterogeneity.[55]

The CDC advise caution, pointing out that because dietary supplements like probiotics are usually not regulated by the federal government, the potential exists for great variability among them, providing a challenge to the prescribing physician to make an informed recommendation regarding their use.[1] We conclude that further research is needed to determine the optimal type, dosage, and regimen.

We do not recommend routine use of probiotics for prevention or treatment of acute gastroenteritis, but we feel it is likely that their benefit outweighs their harm.

Nitazoxanide in acute gastroenteritis

Nitazoxanide is a thiazolide anti-infective active against protozoan parasites (*Giardia*, *Entamoeba histolytica*, *Cryptosporidium*, *Blastocystis*) and against *Clostridium difficile*. It was studied in rotavirus gastroenteritis in Egypt.[58] In a small RCT, 38 children, aged 5 months to 7 years (median age 11 months), hospitalized for gastroenteritis, with rotavirus as the sole identified cause, were randomly assigned to either 7.5 mg/kg nitazoxanide as an oral suspension or placebo twice a day for 3 days. Nitazoxanide was associated with a significant reduction in time to resolution of illness to 31 hours compared with 75 hours for the placebo group. No significant adverse events were reported. The authors also performed in vitro studies which showed that tizoxanide, a metabolite of nitazoxanide, was potent at inhibiting rotavirus replication.[58] Nitazoxanide may be acting as an antiviral agent or may be treating occult parasitic infection. The study is small and the main author is an employee and stockholder of the company that owns the intellectual property rights for nitazoxanide,[58] and so the results should be interpreted with caution.

Emergency department guidelines on management of acute gastroenteritis

Developing evidence-based guidelines is common. Evaluating the effect of their implementation is far less common. A British group developed guidelines based on best evidence and consensus view and then sought the opinion of the guidelines from a panel of 39 selected medical and nursing staff using a postal Delphi consensus process.[2] When the guidelines were introduced in a pediatric emergency department, oral rehydration was used more appropriately and there was a reduction from 9 to 1% in the proprotion of children receiving unnecessary IV infusions.[59] Management time in the emergency department was reduced from 55 to 40 minutes and documentation improved. The proportion of children investigated with unnecessary blood tests fell from 11 to 4%. Surprisingly, however, the admission rate for diarrhea increased from 27 to 34%.[59] This study shows the importance of evaluating the effect of guidelines, however well-meaning, after they have been introduced to make sure that they are effective and do not have unexpected effects.

7.2 Antibiotic-associated diarrhea

In most cases of antibiotic-associated diarrhea no pathogen is identified, although toxin produced by *C. difficile* is responsible for a minority. Stopping antibiotics usually relieves the problem. Dietary manipulation may help. In a masked, randomized parallel study, older infants and toddlers with diarrhea which developed when receiving antibiotics were fed commercial soy formulas with or without added soy fiber for 10 days.[60] The mean duration of diarrhea was significantly reduced from 51.6 hours for those fed the regular formula to 25.1 hours for children fed the formula with added fiber.

A Cochrane review of nine studies of *C. difficile*-associated diarrhea in adults suggested that mild cases do not need specific treatment, while metronidazole was as effective as vancomycin and other antibiotics in treating severe cases.[61] If it is not possible to stop antibiotics, it is recommended to change to a regimen less likely to cause diarrhea. Amoxicillin, broad-spectrum cephalosporins, quinolones, and some other broad-spectrum antibiotics (e.g., ticarcillin + clavulanate) are the antibiotics most commonly associated with diarrhea.

When *C. difficile* is proven or suspected in symptomatic patients, we recommend:

metronidazole 10 mg/kg (max 400 mg) orally, 8-hourly for 7–10 days

C. difficile or its toxins can occasionally be demonstrated in asymptomatic infants, especially newborns, and some older children. Treatment for asymptomatic carriage is not indicated.

Metronidazole is preferred to vancomycin because of the dangers of selecting for vancomycin-resistant organisms, particularly vancomycin-resistant enterococci, by the use of non-absorbable vancomycin. If, however, the diarrhea does not respond, relapses, or is particularly severe, we recommend:

oral vancomycin 10 mg/kg (max 125 mg) orally, 6-hourly for 7–10 days

Probiotics, given from the start of antibiotic therapy, may be of benefit in preventing antibiotic-associated diarrhea. A meta-analysis found nine RCTs, two in children, in which probiotics were given in combination with antibiotics and the control groups received placebo and antibiotics.[62] Four trials used a yeast (*S. boulardii*), four used lactobacilli, and one used a strain of *Enterococcus* that produced lactic acid. Three trials used a combination of probiotic strains of bacteria. The use of any probiotic was associated with a 61–66% reduction in antibiotic-associated diarrhea.[62]

7.3 Campylobacter enteritis

Question | For children with gastroenteritis due to *Campylobacter*, do antibiotics compared with no antibiotics or placebo speed recovery?

Literature review | We found four placebo-controlled trials of erythromycin for *Campylobacter*.[63–66]

Three studies found that erythromycin shortened excretion of *Campylobacter*, but had no clinical effect on duration of diarrhea.[63–65] One study found that erythromycin hastened the cessation of diarrhea.[66] Campylobacter enteritis is usually self-limited. Antibiotics have relatively little clinical benefit and because of the risk of resistance are not routinely indicated.

Quinolones are effective, but resistance develops rapidly. In one study, Campylobacter with high-level resistance to norfloxacin appeared in three of eight patients within 4–90 days of starting norfloxacin.[30]

Azithromycin was at least as effective as ciprofloxacin for adult travelers with *Campylobacter* infection,[67] but is more expensive than erythromycin, and has not been compared to placebo.

Antibiotic therapy is indicated only when there is high fever or severe illness, suggesting septicemia, usually in infants. If antibiotics are indicated, we recommend:

erythromycin 10 mg/kg (max 500 mg) orally, 6-hourly OR
azithromycin 10 mg/kg (max 500 mg) orally, daily

For proven *Campylobacter* bacteremia, base antibiotics on susceptibility results. For suspected bacteremic disease, we recommend:

gentamicin <10 years: 7.5 mg/kg IV daily, 10 years or older: 6 mg/kg IV daily OR
ciprofloxacin 10 mg/kg (max 400 mg) IV 12-hourly

7.4 Cholera

Rehydration is the basis of cholera treatment and can usually be achieved orally despite massive ongoing losses.[18,19,68,69] A Cochrane review[18] of seven trials (718 participants) found that hyponatremia, defined as serum sodium <130 mmol/L, was more common with reduced-osmolarity ORS than with standard ORS (RR 1.67, CI 1.09–2.57). This did not reach significance for severe hyponatremia, defined as serum Na <125 mmol/L (RR 1.58, CI 0.62–4.04). No trials reported symptomatic hyponatremia or death. No statistically significant difference was found in the need for unscheduled IV infusion. Analyses separating children and adults showed no obvious trends. Two trials (102 participants) examined rice-based ORS. In the reduced-osmolarity group, duration of diarrhea was shorter (weighted mean difference −16.85 h, CI −21.22 to −12.48). A later trial of 176 patients aged 12–60 years with cholera found no difference in serum sodium or risk of hyponatremia, but patients treated with reduced-osmolarity ORS had a significantly lower volume of vomiting and significantly higher urine output than those treated with standard WHO ORS.[19]

A meta-analysis of 13 trials showed that rice-based ORSs significantly reduce the rate of stool output during the first 24 hours by 36% (95% CI 28–44%) in adults with cholera and by 32% (19–45%) in children with cholera.[68] The benefit of rice-based ORS in cholera was confirmed in a Cochrane review of 15 trials[69] and one subsequent RCT.[70] Rice-based ORS is far less effective for non-cholera diarrhea, for which it is not recommended.[68,69]

> **We recommend using standard WHO ORS or rice-based ORS for children with cholera diarrhea.**

Antibiotic therapy reduces the volume and duration of cholera diarrhea.[71,72] Single-dose ciprofloxacin achieves similar or better clinical outcomes than 12-dose erythromycin in children with cholera, but is less effective in eradicating *V. cholerae* from stool.[71] Single-dose azithromycin is as effective as erythromycin and causes less vomiting. We recommend:

> **azithromycin 20 mg/kg orally as a single dose** OR
> **doxycycline child >8 years: 2.5 mg/kg (max 100 mg) orally, 12-hourly for 3 days** OR
> **ciprofloxacin 25 mg/kg (max 1 g) orally as a single dose** OR
> **erythromycin 12.5 mg/kg (max 500 mg) orally, 6-hourly for 3 days**

Antibiotic-resistant strains are now common in some regions, where antibiotics different to those recommended above may be needed.

7.5 Enterohemorrhagic *Escherichia coli* (EHEC) enteritis

Most *E. coli* infections cause self-limiting watery diarrhea which does not require specific therapy. Infection with some EHEC strains, e.g., O157:H7 and O111:H8, can lead to the development of hemolytic uremic syndrome or thrombotic thrombocytopenic purpura.

The use of antibiotics is controversial. A systematic review of *E. coli* O157:H7 infections reported that most isolates are susceptible in vitro to various antibiotics, but that certain antibiotics, especially at sublethal concentrations, increase the release of Shiga-like toxins, which have been associated with the development of hemolytic uremic syndrome/thrombotic thrombocytopenic purpura in humans.[73] Most of the clinical studies involve small numbers of patients. No studies have shown that antibiotics are effective in reducing the duration of *E. coli* O157:H7 infection or the duration of diarrhea or bloody diarrhea. A few studies have supported that some antibiotics, especially quinolones and fosfomycin, may prevent the development of hemolytic uremic syndrome or thrombotic thrombocytopenic purpura. On the other hand, some clinical studies associate antibiotics with a higher risk for hemolytic uremic syndrome and/or longer duration of diarrhea, and even with an increased mortality.[74]

> **We recommend that antibiotics should not be prescribed routinely for children with EHEC infection or hemolytic uremic syndrome.**

7.6 Enteropathogenic *Escherichia coli* (EPEC) enteritis

In a setting where there was a high prevalence of an EPEC (serotype O111:B4), an RCT of infant diarrhea showed a clinical cure on the third day in 79% given mecillinam, 73% trimethoprim-sulfamethoxazole, but only 7% given placebo.[74] This is an uncommon situation. Most EPEC infections occur in developing countries and the organism is never cultured. The main significance is for traveler's diarrhea (see Section 7.10, p. 86).

7.7 Non-typhoid Salmonella enteritis

Question | For children with gastroenteritis due to non-typhoid Salmonella (NTS), do antibiotics compared with no antibiotics or placebo speed recovery?

Literature review | We found 12 RCTs and a Cochrane review[29] comparing the use of antibiotics with placebo for NTS infection.

In industrialized countries, most NTS infections are food-borne, causing acute gastroenteritis alone; extraintestinal complications, such as septicemia, meningitis, and osteomyelitis, are rare.[75] Outbreaks are associated especially with infected food from poultry (meat or eggs), cattle and pigs, and from infections contracted abroad. In contrast, in developing countries, particularly tropical Africa, NTS are an important cause of invasive extraintestinal disease.[76] Rates of *Salmonella* infection appear to be falling in industrialized countries, but this is counterbalanced by an alarming rise in multiresistant strains, which are associated with increased morbidity and mortality.[77]

A Cochrane review[29] of trials of antibiotics for NTS infections found 12 RCTs. There were no significant differences in length of illness, diarrhea, or fever between any antibiotic regimen and placebo. Antibiotic regimens resulted in more negative cultures during the first week of treatment but clinical relapses were more frequent in those receiving antibiotics, and antibiotics prolonged salmonella detection in stools after 3 weeks. Adverse drug reactions were more common in the antibiotic groups. These studies included the newer antibiotics such as quinolones.[29]

> **We recommend that children with uncomplicated NTS infection are not given antibiotics.**

Antibiotics are not indicated for asymptomatic short-term carriers. However, antibiotic therapy is indicated for patients who are proven or suspected to be septicemic. Septicemia is more likely in malnourished infants, infants <3 months old, and immunosuppressed children.[77] If a child with any of these conditions presents with bloody diarrhea and fever and/or has *Salmonella* isolated from feces, antibiotics are recommended, although their value is assumed rather than proven.[77] Antibiotics are also recommended for *Salmonella* infection occurring in association with chronic gastrointestinal disease, malignant neoplasms, hemoglobinopathies, or severe colitis.[78]

The choice of antibiotic to start and to continue treatment should be based on culture results. Amoxicillin is preferred if the organism is susceptible.

For empiric therapy we recommend:

> **ciprofloxacin 10 mg/kg (max 500 mg) orally, 12-hourly** OR
> **azithromycin 20 mg/kg (max 1 g) orally on the first day, then 10 mg/kg (max 500 mg) daily**

The appropriate duration of therapy has not been defined, but 5–7 days is usually effective.

If oral therapy cannot be tolerated until oral antibiotics (as above) can be tolerated, we recommend:

> **ciprofloxacin 10 mg/kg (max 400 mg) IV, 12-hourly** OR
> **ceftriaxone 50 mg/kg (max 2 g) IV daily**

7.8 Typhoid and paratyphoid fevers (enteric fevers)

Typhoid and paratyphoid fevers, due to *Salmonella typhi* and *S. paratyphi*, respectively, are endemic in many developing countries. Almost all infections in industrialized countries are acquired by travelers, although very occasionally cases occur with no history of travel. In these cases, enquiries should be made about contact with travelers, food exposure, and about contact with family members who work in laboratories (laboratory-acquired cases occur and can be transmitted).

Typhoid is a septicemic illness rather than a diarrheal illness, but will be covered in this section. The clinical features in children have been described in a number of studies, each of over 100 children. Typhoid affects children from infancy to adolescence, with a median age of 6–8 years.[79–82] Fewer than 2% of cases are in infants, and they have the highest mortality. The most common clinical features are fever, hepatomegaly, abdominal pain, diarrhea, vomiting, cough, malaise, and headache.[79–82] Hepatomegaly is more common than splenomegaly. Rose spots are rare and children do not have relative bradycardia.[83] Other manifestations of typhoid include febrile convulsions, jaundice, ileus, perforation, and impaired consciousness. Hematologic abnormalities include neutropenia, leucopenia, and thrombocytopenia. The organism can be grown from blood, feces, or urine. Serology can be useful, but more often to make a retrospective diagnosis than in acute diagnosis.

Multidrug resistance is an increasing problem.[84] A Cochrane review[85] of fluoroquinolones for typhoid fever found 33 trials, but study methodology was often poor, and although typhoid mainly affects children, only 3 trials exclusively studied children. The Cochrane review found that quinolones were at least as effective as chloramphenicol, co-trimoxazole, ceftriaxone, cefixime, and azithromycin in adults. In trials of hospitalized children, fluoroquinolones were not statistically significantly different from ceftriaxone or cefixime. Treatment with norfloxacin resulted in clinical failure more often than treatment with other fluoroquinolones. Trials comparing different durations of fluoroquinolone treatment showed no statistically significant differences,[86,87] and two pediatric studies showed 2 days of ofloxacin was safe and highly effective in uncomplicated typhoid in children.[88,89]

Short-course (5 days) oral azithromycin was as effective as ceftriaxone in acute cure,[85] and clinical relapses occurred only with ceftriaxone but not azithromycin.[90,91] In Pakistan, the relapse rate was higher (14%) with 7 days than 14 days of ceftriaxone.[92]

Although in vitro studies suggest that almost all isolates are sensitive to quinolones,[89−92] there are increasing reports of clinical failures when using quinolones to treat infections acquired in the Indian sub-continent and in Vietnam. For the treatment of typhoid and paratyphoid fevers acquired in other areas, we recommend:

ciprofloxacin 15 mg/kg (max 500 mg) orally, 12-hourly for 7–10 days OR
in uncomplicated disease, EITHER
ofloxacin 10 mg/kg (max 400 mg) orally, daily for 2 days OR
azithromycin 20 mg/kg (max 1 g) orally, daily for 5 days

If oral therapy cannot be tolerated, initial therapy, until oral can be tolerated, should be with:

ciprofloxacin 10 mg/kg (max 400 mg) IV, 12-hourly OR
azithromycin 20 mg/kg (max 1 g) IV, daily

Fever often persists for several days with both NTS and typhoid infections, even if using appropriate antityphoid antibiotics, and is less concerning if the child's clinical state is much improved.[89−92] Ibuprofen may be more effective than paracetamol at reducing fever in typhoid fever.[93]

If reduced susceptibility to ciprofloxacin is suspected because of country of acquisition, or is reported by the laboratory (nalidixic acid resistant), or the clinical response is delayed (e.g., child remains unwell or fever >7 days), we recommend:

ceftriaxone 50 mg/kg (max 2 g) IV, daily OR, in uncomplicated disease
azithromycin 20 mg/kg (max 1 g) IV or orally, daily for 5 days

If the organism is sensitive and the child is improving, we recommend oral amoxicillin or oral azithromycin.

7.9 Shigellosis

Antibiotic therapy is recommended for children with shigella dysentery, even if mild, for public health reasons because a very low inoculum causes infection and because antibiotics eliminate the organism. It is stated that antibiotics relieve symptoms, but although we found 34 studies of antibiotics in shigellosis, 16 of them in children, all the studies compared different antibiotics or different doses or duration or different routes of administration. We found no studies that compared antibiotic with placebo or no antibiotics.

Effective antibiotics, if the organism is sensitive, include quinolones,[94,95] ceftriaxone,[94] azithromycin,[96,97] cefixime,[95] and cotrimoxazole.[98] A study in Zimbabwe showed that 3 days of ciprofloxacin was as effective as 5 days in Shigella dysenteriae type 1 infection, and all children had bacteriologic cure without relapse.[95]

The pattern of antibiotic susceptibility of *Shigella* strains varies from country to country, and multidrug-resistant strains are encountered in many regions. Antibiotic therapy should be modified according to the results of culture and susceptibility tests:

ciprofloxacin 15 mg/kg (max 600 mg) orally, 12-hourly for 3 days OR
azithromycin 20 mg/kg (max 1 g) one dose, then 10 mg/kg (max 500 mg) orally, daily for 4 days OR
trimethoprim + sulfamethoxazole 4 + 20 mg/kg (max 160 + 800 mg) orally, 12-hourly for 5 days

7.10 Traveler's diarrhea

Traveler's diarrhea is a common problem, with an attack rate of 20–50% of travelers to high-risk countries. It has been estimated that at least 11 million people annually develop traveler's diarrhea.[99−101]

A working definition is the passage of three or more unformed stools over 24 hours, with symptoms starting during or shortly after a period of foreign travel.[99] The diarrhea is often accompanied by nausea, vomiting, abdominal pain, fever, tenesmus, and blood or mucus in the stools.[99]

Organisms can be isolated from about 50% of episodes of traveler's diarrhea and about 85% of the organisms are bacteria, although the relative importance of different pathogens varies according to the region visited and the season.[99] Worldwide, enterotoxigenic E. coli (ETEC) are the most common bacterial pathogens isolated.[99–102] Two-thirds of ETEC produce a heat-labile toxin similar to cholera toxin which induces secretory diarrhea. Campylobacter jejuni is an ubiquitous pathogen that causes up to 30% of all cases of traveler's diarrhea, particularly in Asia. Salmonellae and shigellae each account for up to 15% of cases, and enteroaggregative E. coli and enteroinvasive E. coli are increasingly recognized as possible causes of traveler's diarrhea.[99]

Prevention of traveler's diarrhea

Prevention can be difficult. "Boil it, cook it, peel it, or forget it" is time-honored advice, but studies do not show that dietary advice is followed or effective.[99]

Contaminated water is probably the major source of traveler's diarrhea. Standard advice to travelers to low-income countries is to avoid drinking the local water.[99] Tap water and ice cubes should be thought of as contaminated. The latter may contain organisms such as Shigella, which have a very low infective dose. Boiling is the most effective way of ensuring that water is safe to drink. Buying bottled water is not totally safe, because empty bottles may be filled with tap water and recycled as if new. Chlorine tablets can be used to purify tap water, which sacrifices palatability for safety: the purified water can be drunk and used to clean teeth. Swimming pool water is also a potential risk, while rivers, standing freshwater, and seawater may be contaminated by sewage. Swimmers are advised to avoid sub-mersion or swallowing water.[99]

Because of the widely varying causes of traveler's diarrhea, the chances of developing an effective vaccine for prophylaxis are limited, although a combination vaccine against ETEC, Campylobacter, and Shigella might be useful in the future. The only combination vaccine currently available is an oral, killed, recombinant B sub-unit, whole-cell vaccine against cholera and ETEC.[102,103] Basic immunization for adults and children comprises two doses of vaccine given at an interval of at least 1 week, and satisfactory protection against cholera and ETEC diarrhea can be expected about 1 week after the second dose.[102,103] There are no efficacy data in children. A study of 615 adult tourists who went to Morocco from Finland showed 52% protection against traveler's diarrhea associated with ETEC strains and 71% protective efficacy against a combination of ETEC and any other pathogen.[102] Another efficacy study of 502 US students traveling to Mexico showed 50% protective efficacy against all ETEC strains, regardless of toxin type.[103] However, ETEC cause only 20–40% of episodes of traveler's diarrhea, so the vaccine will prevent <30% of all cases of traveler's diarrhea. The vaccine is licensed as Dukoral for protection against traveler's diarrhea in only a few countries including Sweden and Canada.[99]

Prophylactic antibiotics are not recommended for healthy travelers and not for children.[68] Antibiotic prophylaxis might be considered for an immunocompromised child traveling for a relatively short time, in which case a fluoroquinolone (ciprofloxacin or norfloxacin) would be the antibiotic of choice.[99]

Treatment of traveler's diarrhea

Question | For children with traveler's diarrhea, does empiric antibiotic therapy compared with no antibiotics or placebo shorten the illness?

Literature review | We found 12 RCTs and a Cochrane review.[104]

A Cochrane review of empiric therapy for traveler's diarrhea found 20 trials (12 placebo-controlled) in which travelers >5 years old with acute non-bloody diarrhea due to unknown organism at allocation were randomly allocated to treatment with antibiotics or placebo.[104] All of the trials reported a significant reduction in duration of diarrhea in participants treated with antibiotics compared with placebo. The trials generally did not report duration of post-treatment diarrhea. Persons taking antibiotics experienced more side effects than those taking placebo. The most effective antibiotics for empiric therapy from trials are quinolones, azithromycin, and rifaximin.[99]

As with other types of diarrhea, all patients should take fluids and electrolytes. Rehydration with ORS is particularly important for young children.

Antimotility drugs, such as loperamide, should be avoided in children, because of the danger of causing paralytic ileus.[105] Mild cases do not usually need antibiotics.[99]

For moderate to severe disease, we recommend:

azithromycin 20 mg/kg (max 1 g) orally, as a single dose OR
ciprofloxacin 20 mg/kg (max 750 mg) orally, as a single dose OR
norfloxacin 20 mg/kg (max 800 mg) orally, as a single dose OR
trimethoprim + sulfamethoxazole 4 + 20 mg/kg (max 160 + 800 mg) orally, 12-hourly for 3 days OR
rifaximin 10 mg/kg orally, 12-hourly for 3 days

If after the above, diarrhea continues or if fever or bloody stools are present, we recommend up to 3 days therapy with:

azithromycin 10 mg/kg (max 500 mg) orally, once daily OR
norfloxacin 10 mg/kg (max 400 mg) orally, 12-hourly OR
ciprofloxacin 10 mg/kg (max 500 mg) orally, 12-hourly

The management of persistent diarrhea in a returned traveler depends on accurate diagnosis of the responsible pathogen(s) or identification of a non-infective cause. Investigations should include stool microscopy and culture. Multiple stool samples may be required to diagnose some parasitic infections. Serology may be helpful in some cases, e.g., amebiasis, schistosomiasis, strongyloidiasis. If no clear diagnosis is identified, empiric therapy for giardiasis should be considered, given the difficulties in diagnosis. If symptoms persist, specialist advice should be sought.

7.11 Protozoal infections

Amebiasis (*Entamoeba histolytica*)

E. histolytica infection can cause non-invasive intestinal infection, which can be asymptomatic or cause amebic dysentery or colitis, ameboma, and/or liver abscess.[106,107] Passage of *Entamoeba* cysts or tropho-zoites in the absence of acute dysenteric illness does not warrant antimicrobial therapy,[106,107] although some authorities recommend a luminal agent (paromomycin, diloxanide furoate, or iodoquinol; see p. 89) for chronic cyst excretors.[108]

Amebic dysentery

Patients with amebic colitis characteristically present with dysenteric symptoms of bloody diarrhea, abdominal pain, and tenderness. Children can have rectal bleeding without diarrhea. The onset can be gradual, with several weeks of symptoms: often multiple, small volume, mucoid stools, but sometimes profuse, watery diarrhea.[106,107] Occasionally, individuals develop fulminant amebic colitis, with profuse bloody diarrhea, fever, pronounced leukocytosis, widespread abdominal pain often with peritoneal signs, and extensive involvement of the colon. Paralytic ileus and concurrent amebic liver abscess may occur. Toxic megacolon complicates amebic colitis in about 0.5% of patients. The main danger is intestinal perforation, which occurs in >75% of individuals with fulminant amebic colitis, with a mortality over 40%.[106,107] Amebomas are localized inflammatory, annular masses of the cecum or ascending colon which can cause obstruction and be confused with carcinomas. Patients on corticosteroids are at particular risk if they develop amebiasis.[106,107]

The diagnosis of amebic colitis rests on the demonstration of *E. histolytica* in the stool or colonic mucosa of patients with diarrhea. Stool microscopy cannot distinguish between *E. histolytica* and *E. dispar*, but is still useful in the correct clinical setting such as a child with bloody diarrhea.[107,108] Commercially available ELISA assays which not only identify *E. histolytica* antigens in stool but distinguish *E. histolytica* from *E. dispar* are more sensitive and less user-dependent than microscopy.[109,110] However, they are not generally used in endemic areas and their reported sensitivity and specificity still need to be confirmed with independent studies. Stool polymerase chain reaction (PCR) may be used in the future.[111] Some patients with acute colitis, especially when amebiasis is suspected on clinical grounds but *E. histolytica* is not initially detected in stools, will benefit from colonoscopy or flexible sigmoidoscopy with examination of scrapings and biopsy samples for amebic trophozoites.[112]

Serum antibodies against amebae are detected by indirect hemagglutination in >70% of patients with symptomatic *E. histolytica* infection[113–116] and are particularly sensitive (>94%) in amebic liver abscess.[107] Serology can be useful when there is diagnostic uncertainty. In some gastroenterology departments, *E. histolytica* serology is performed routinely on all patients with bloody diarrhea, and positive ameba serology has saved more than one child with amebiasis but with a wrong clinical diagnosis of inflammatory bowel disease from a colectomy.[117]

For acute amebic dysentery, the nitroimidazoles (metronidazole, tinidazole, ornidazole) are >90% effective.[105,106] Tinidazole is at least as effective as metronidazole, more effective in some studies,[107] and better tolerated, but is not available in the USA. We recommend:

> **metronidazole 15 mg/kg (max 600 mg) orally, 8-hourly for 7–10 days** OR
> **tinidazole 50 mg/kg (max 2 g) orally, daily for 3 days**

To eradicate cysts and prevent relapse after acute treatment, if available, follow with:

> **paromomycin 10 mg/kg (max 500 mg) orally, 8-hourly for 7 days** OR
> **diloxanide furoate 7 mg/kg (max 500 mg) orally, 8-hourly for 10 days** OR
> **iodonoquil 10 mg/kg (max 650 mg) orally, 8-hourly for 20 days**

Amebic liver abscess

Amebic liver abscess may be diagnosed clinically and radiologically and confirmed serologically.[118] In this case, therapeutic aspiration may be required as an adjunct to specific antiparasitic therapy. Drainage of the abscess should be considered in patients who have no clinical response to drug therapy within 5–7 days or those with a high risk of abscess rupture, as defined by a cavity with a diameter of more than 5 cm or by the presence of lesions in the left lobe.[118] Drainage may also identify the rare child with bacterial coinfection of an amebic liver abscess. Imaging-guided percutaneous treatment (needle aspiration or catheter drainage) has replaced surgical intervention as the procedure of choice for reducing the size of an amebic liver abscess.[118]

For amebic liver abscess, we recommend:

> **metronidazole 15 mg/kg (max 600 mg) orally, 8-hourly for 14 days** OR
> **tinidazole 50 mg/kg (max 2 g) orally, daily for 5 days**

Blastocystis hominis

There is controversy about the pathogenicity of *Blastocystis hominis*, a parasite that can be recovered from 1 to 20% of stool specimens tested for ova, cysts, and parasites. It is generally considered to be a commensal and it is usually recommended to ignore its presence in stools. We found one placebo-controlled RCT of 3 days of nitazoxanide for the treatment of diarrhea and enteritis in children and adults from the Nile delta of Egypt, where *B. hominis* was the sole identified pathogen.[119] Symptoms resolved 4 days after completing therapy in 36 (86%) of 42 patients who received nitazoxanide and 16 (38%) of 42 patients who received placebo (*p* <0.0001). Thirty-six (86%) of 42 patients who received nitazoxanide were free of *B. hominis* organisms in each of three post-treatment stool samples compared with only 5 (12%) of 42 patients who received placebo (*p* < 0.0001). These findings suggest either that *B. hominis* is pathogenic in some patients and can be treated effectively with nitazoxanide or, alternatively, that nitazoxanide is effective in treating other unidentified causes of persistent diarrhea. Other agents that should be active against *Blastocystis* and also against likely occult pathogens such as *Giardia* are metronidazole, tinidazole, albendazole, and furazolidine.

Cryptosporidium

Cryptosporidium parvum infection causes frequent, watery diarrhea, without blood in immunocompetent children.[120] Other prominent symptoms include crampy abdominal pain, fever, and vomiting. Asymptomatic infection is rare. Infections are often waterborne; the cysts are resistant to chlorine, and contaminated water and swimming pools have been the source of large outbreaks.[120] In immunocompetent children, infection usually resolves after 10 days (range 1–20) and requires no specific treatment.[120]

Immunocompromised children can develop severe chronic diarrhea, which may be life-threatening. In patients with HIV infection, highly active antiretroviral therapy often reduces symptoms.

Immunocompetent patients tend to respond better to antiparasitic agents than immunocompromised patients for whom the agents are most needed. Trials have shown conflicting results. Paromomycin showed promise in a small RCT of HIV-infected patients,[121] but a larger multicenter study found it was no better than placebo.[122] In two studies of immunocompetent children with *Cryptosporidium* infection, spiramycin was found to have modest benefits in terms of shortening diarrhea and reducing oocyst excretion in one study,[123] but no benefit in another study.[124] Azithromycin improved symptoms in HIV-positive patients but did not prevent continued oocyst excretion.[125] Nitazoxanide (see p. 82) shows most promise. In immunocompetent children, nitazoxanide reduces the duration of diarrhea and of oocyst excretion.[126,127] In one study of immunocompetent children in Egypt, nitazoxanide reduced mortality (0 of 25 compared with 4 of 22 in the placebo group).[127] The data are less clear-cut in HIV-infected patients, with some studies in adults showing benefit,[128,129] while others, including a pediatric study,[126] showed none.[127,130]

We do not recommend treating immunocompetent children with Cryptosporidium diarrhea routinely, because treatment benefits are marginal at best and the disease self-limiting. In contrast, *Cryptosporidium* infection can be life-threatening in immunocompromised children. We recommend reducing immunosuppression, if possible. To treat *Cryptosporidium* infection in immunocompromised children, we recommend:

> nitazoxanide 1–3 years: 100 mg 12-hourly; 4–11 years: 200 mg 12-hourly; 12 years or older: 500 mg orally 12-hourly, for 3 days

Giardiasis

Giardia lamblia is a flagellate protozoan parasite with a worldwide distribution. Infection is primarily waterborne, and although humans are the main reservoir of infection, animals such as dogs and cats can contaminate water with infectious cysts. Infection can be asymptomatic, can be acute with watery diarrhea and abdominal pain, or protracted with chronic or intermittent foul-smelling stools, abdominal distension, flatulence, and anorexia.[131] Diagnosis is by detecting cysts in stool. Although ELISA tests on stool are slightly more sensitive than direct microscopy for ova and parasites,[132,133] one study suggested that both tests

need to be performed to achieve a sensitivity >90%.[133] Immunofluorescent antibody testing of stool has also been claimed to be more sensitive than microscopy.[134] Sensitivity of any of these tests is <95%, so that diagnosis in difficult cases may require examination of aspirated duodenal fluid.

There are few RCTs of treatment of acute or chronic giardiasis, and the outcome of trials is often reported as parasitologic rather than clinical cure. This is problematic, because most authorities agree that treatment of patients with asymptomatic passage of *Giardia* cysts is unwarranted. The traditional treatment of symptomatic patients is with metronidazole, which is 80–95% effective in clinical cure but has unpleasant adverse effects of nausea and unpleasant taste.[131] In adult studies, tinidazole is at least as effective as metronidazole at curing symptoms and eradicating cysts[135,136] and in one study was superior,[136] and tinidazole has fewer reported adverse events.[135,136] In one RCT in children, single-dose tinidazole was more effective than single-dose metronidazole and only minor adverse events were reported.[137] In two RCTs in children, tinidazole was more effective than albendazole at eradicating cysts.[138,139] Tinidazole is not licensed in the USA because of insufficient safety data in children. Furazolidone was as effective as metronidazole in one RCT.[140] Albendazole was as effective as metronidazole in children in India[141,142] and Turkey,[143] but less effective in children than tinidazole in Indonesia[138] and Chile.[139] Nitazoxanide was as effective as metronidazole in Peruvian children.[143]

For symptomatic patients, we recommend:

> tinidazole 50 mg/kg (max 2 g) orally, as a single dose OR
> metronidazole 5 mg/kg (max 250 mg) orally, 8-hourly for 5 days

Albendazole, furazolidone, and nitazoxanide are alternatives. Treatment failure is more common in immunocompromised children who may require prolonged treatment with one of the above agents or may need combinations of the above drugs. For immunocompetent children who fail therapy, it is usual to repeat the original course while investigating whether reinfection may have occurred from a family member or water source. There is no good evidence on this approach or on prolonging the treatment or increasing the dose.

Isospora belli gastroenteritis

I. belli usually causes gastroenteritis only in HIV-infected and other immunocompromised subjects. The clinical features resemble cryptosporidiosis. We recommend:

> **trimethoprim + sulfamethoxazole 4 + 20 mg/kg (max 160 + 800 mg) orally, 6-hourly for 10 days**

Long-term suppressive therapy with trimethoprim + sulfamethoxazole 4 + 20 mg/kg (max 160 + 800 mg) orally three times per week is generally required to prevent relapse in HIV-infected patients.[144]

Microsporidium

Microsporidia such as *Enterocytozoon bieneusi* and *Encephalitozoon (Septata) intestinalis* can cause chronic diarrhea in immunocompromised patients, particularly HIV-infected patients, and the latter organism can disseminate. Microsporidia can also cause sub-acute diarrheal illness in immunocompetent children.[145] In an RCT, albendazole produced clinical improvement within 48 hours in 95% of immunocompetent children with chronic diarrhea (>10 days) due to Microsporidia.[146]

We recommend:

> **albendazole 10 mg/kg (max 400 mg) orally, 12-hourly for 7 days**

7.12 *Helicobacter pylori* infection

Acute *H. pylori* infection can cause a self-limiting gastritis. Chronic *H. pylori* infection is an important cause of chronic active gastritis and of peptic ulcers in adults, but much less often in children. Children with recurrent abdominal pain and suspected gastritis or peptic ulceration can be screened non-invasively for *H. pylori* infection with a urea breath test. The ^{13}C-urea breath test is a highly useful screening tool which was found in a large multicenter study to have sensitivity 96.2% and specificity 97.3% compared to endoscopically confirmed infection.[147] Although biopsy is often recommended to confirm the diagnosis by culture or histopathology, the urea breath test is so accurate that a case can be made for treating children with a positive urea breath test empirically and only doing a biopsy if they fail treatment.[147]

Treatment is complicated by varying response rates, perhaps due to antibiotic resistance, which varies geographically. The standard triple therapy is a proton pump inhibitor (usually lansoprazole or omeprazole) plus amoxicillin plus clarithromycin for 10 days: this was 74% effective in eradicating the organism, compared to 9% spontaneous recovery in a large placebo-controlled RCT.[148] The benefits of susceptibility testing are debatable, but patients who do not respond to standard triple therapy often respond if metronidazole or tinidazole is used instead of clarithromycin.[149,150] An alternate proposal which improved efficacy to 97% in an RCT[151] is to use 5 days of omeprazole plus amoxicillin followed by 5 days of omeprazole plus clarithromycin plus tinidazole.

7.13 Liver abscess

Liver abscesses in children are rare, particularly in industrialized countries. They are pyogenic, amebic (see p. 89), or hydatid (see p. 257). Pyogenic liver abscesses usually spread from an intra-abdominal source of infection, such as appendicitis. Abscesses can be single or multiple. Polymicrobial infections, with aerobic and anaerobic bowel flora are common, but occasionally an organism of the *Streptococcus anginosus/milleri* group may be found alone. In pediatric series, *Staphylococcus aureus* is a common isolate,[152,153] and so are Gram-negative enteric bacilli including *E. coli*[153] and *Klebsiella pneumoniae*.[154] The latter organism is increasingly cultured from liver abscesses in adults in Asia.[155,156]

Children with pyogenic abscesses usually present with fever, abdominal pain, and an enlarged, tender liver.[152,153] Occasionally children will have fever without other signs or symptoms. Imaging is critical to make the diagnosis and for guided aspiration, which is important therapeutically and to distinguish pyogenic abscesses from abscesses due to ameba or hydatid disease. If aspiration cannot be done or amebic liver abscess or hydatid disease is suspected, we recommend serological testing for *Entamoeba. histolytica* (amoeba) and *Echinococcus granulosus* (hydatid).

For empiric treatment of pyogenic liver abscess, to cover *S. aureus*, anaerobic streptococci, and Gram-negative organisms, we recommend:

> **clindamycin 10 mg/kg (max 450 mg) IV, 8-hourly PLUS**
> **gentamicin <10 years: 7.5 mg/kg IV, daily; 10 years or older: 6 mg/kg IV, daily**

7.14   Hepatitis A

Hepatitis A virus is an RNA virus classified as a picornavirus (from pico = small + RNA). Infection can be asymptomatic. Symptomatic infection develops after an average incubation period of 28 days (range 15–50 days).[157] Onset is typically abrupt with fever, malaise, anorexia, nausea, and abdominal discomfort, followed by dark urine and jaundice. The likelihood of infection causing symptoms is related to age. In children aged <6 years, 70% of infections are asymptomatic, and if illness does occur it is typically not accompanied by jaundice.[158] In older children and adults, infection typically is symptomatic, with jaundice occurring in over 70% of patients.[159] Signs and symptoms typically last up to 2 months, although 10–15% of symptomatic persons have prolonged or relapsing disease lasting up to 6 months.[160] The overall case-fatality ratio in the USA is approximately 0.3–0.6%.[161] There is no specific treatment for hepatitis A virus infection. However, hepatitis A infection can be prevented. Important preventive measures are active immunization with one of the inactivated hepatitis A vaccines or passive protection with human immunoglobulin. Hepatitis A vaccine is routine in some countries and is recommended for travelers to high-risk countries.

Prophylaxis of unimmunized family contacts with normal human immunoglobulin is recommended by public health authorities, and it is stated that normal human immunoglobulin contains enough antibodies against hepatitis A for post-exposure prophylaxis and short-term prophylaxis.[161] What is the evidence?

Question | For persons exposed to hepatitis A infection, does normal human immunoglobulin compared to no treatment or placebo prevent hepatitis A virus infection?

Literature review | We found six RCTs and a non-Cochrane systematic review.[162]

A non-Cochrane systematic review found six studies of variable quality and heterogeneity. Compared with placebo or no treatment, human immunoglobulin was 83% effective in primary prevention (RR 0.17, 95% CI 0.15–0.19) and 69% effective in prevention after exposure (RR 0.31, 95% CI 0.20–0.47).[151] The average duration of passive protection was 3 months.[162] Some of the variability may relate to when prophylaxis was given. Immunoglobulin is most effective in preventing symptomatic hepatitis A infection when administered early in the incubation period, although administration later in the incubation period can reduce the severity of infection.[163] Normal human immunoglobulin is safe and has not transmitted other virus infections, such as hepatitis B or HIV.[161]

The dose recommended for short-term protection (e.g., for an unimmunized traveler who is going to leave the country too soon to be fully immunized) and for post-exposure prophylaxis (for a family member of a person with hepatitis A) is:

normal human immunoglobulin 0.02 mL/kg, IM

Normal human immunoglobulin is no longer routinely recommended to protect travelers, because safe and effective killed vaccines are now readily available.

7.15   Hepatitis B

Hepatitis B virus (HBV) is a DNA virus that causes one of the commonest infections in the world. The most important antigens of HBV are the surface antigen (s), the core antigen (c), and the early antigen (e).

There are over 400 million persons chronically infected with HBV worldwide (carriers).[164,165] Carriers of HBV have large amounts of infectious virus in their serum, as well as in their liver, but little or no antibody. This is referred to as being surface antigen positive or HBsAg positive. Chronic hepatitis B infection can progress to cirrhosis and liver cancer. The virus is responsible for more than 300,000 cases of liver cancer every year and for similar numbers of gastrointestinal hemorrhage and ascites. More than a quarter of all carriers with chronic hepatitis B will die of liver disease, and more than 1 million people with this infection die every year.[164,165]

Prevention of HBV infection

Routine immunization against hepatitis B

Primary immunization of persons at birth or in adolescence with hepatitis B vaccine before exposure to HBV is at least 95% protective against infection.[164–166] In many countries, both developing and industrialized, hepatitis B immunization is part of the primary childhood immunization schedule.

Management of baby born to mother who is an HBV carrier

Children can acquire HBV infection by mother-to-child transmission before or around the time of birth from their carrier mother (sometimes called "vertical infection") or postnatally from exposure to the virus ("horizontal transmission"). In Southeast Asia, the vast majority of carriers are infected vertically (mother-to-child), while in contrast most children in Africa who become carriers acquire HBV horizontally.[164,165]

Perinatal transmission is believed to account for 35–50% of all hepatitis B carriers.[165] If the mother is a chronic carrier (surface antigen positive), and particularly if she is e-antigen positive, which is a marker of infectivity (i.e., HBsAg and HBeAg positive), the risk of mother-to-child transmission is 70–90% without intervention.[166,167] Studies have examined the use of hepatitis B vaccines, containing surface antigen purified from plasma or obtained by recombinant DNA technology, and hepatitis B immunoglobulin (immunoglobulin with a high titer against HBV) to prevent mother-to-child transmission.

Question | For babies born to hepatitis B carrier mothers, does hepatitis B vaccine plus immunoglobulin or vaccine alone or immunoglobulin alone compared with no treatment or placebo vaccine prevent mother-to-child transmission of HBV?

Literature review | We found 29 RCTs and a Cochrane review.[168]

A Cochrane review looked at the safety and efficacy of hepatitis B immunoglobulin and/or hepatitis B vaccine given at birth to the infants of HbsAg-positive mothers to prevent mother-to-child transmission of hepatitis B.[168] The reviewers found 29 RCTs, of which 5 were considered of high quality. Only 3 trials reported inclusion of hepatitis B e-antigen-negative mothers. Compared with placebo or no intervention, hepatitis vaccine reduced hepatitis B transmission by 72% (RR 0.28, 95% CI 0.20–0.40). No significant difference in efficacy was found between recombinant vaccine versus plasma-derived vaccine or between high-dose versus low-dose vaccine. Compared with placebo or no intervention, hepatitis B immunoglobulin reduced hepatitis B transmission by 50% (RR 0.50, 95% CI 0.41–0.60). The combination of vaccine plus hepatitis B immunoglobulin was more effective than either alone. Vaccine plus hepatitis B immunoglobulin reduced hep-

atitis B occurrence by 92% compared with no intervention or placebo (RR 0.08, 95% CI 0.03–0.17, 3 trials).[167]

We recommend giving hepatitis B vaccine plus immunoglobulin at birth to babies born to women who are carriers of hepatitis B.

Mother-to-child transmission could occur transplacentally (intrauterine), peripartum, or post-natally from breast milk (carriers' breast milk is known to contain live virus).[163,164] The fact that most mother-to-child transmission can be interrupted by interventions at birth implies that most transmission occurs peripartum or post-natally rather than in utero. The only proviso is that HBV has a long incubation period (6 wk to 6 mo) and so it is possible that intrauterine infection could be altered by active and passive immunization at birth. Why does the baby not mount an immune response? The most likely explanation is that the baby's immune system views the virus as "self" rather than foreign, and thus becomes "tolerant" of HBV. If they remain tolerant and unable to mount an immune response to the virus, this explains why later antiviral treatment is relatively ineffective at eradicating HBV from children who acquired HBV perinatally (see p. 94).

Even if hepatitis B immunization is part of the primary immunization schedule and the first dose is given at birth, it is still recommended to screen pregnant women for HBV status. This is because if they are HBeAg positive, their babies should be given immunoglobulin as well as vaccine at birth. If HBV vaccine is not in the primary immunization schedule, maternal screening is even more important.

The doses of vaccine and immunoglobulin vary from country to country. Prescribers should consult local guidelines.

Post-exposure prophylaxis

If an unimmunized child is accidentally exposed to hepatitis B or to a situation where there is a risk of hepatitis B, e.g., a needlestick injury, household, or sexual exposure, it is recommended to give hepatitis B immunoglobulin immediately and to start a course of hepatitis B vaccine (at 0, 1, and 6 mo) simultaneously.[161] Because strong immunological memory persists more than 10 years after immunization of infants and adolescents with a primary course of vaccination, it is not considered necessary to give hepatitis B immunoglobulin or booster doses of vaccine following accidental exposure,[169] because evidence suggests that children will mount an anamnestic response and boost their antibody levels.[170]

Treatment of chronic carriers

Carriers may be treated when they are asymptomatic to reduce their long-term risk of progressing to cirrhosis or they may need treatment because they have already started to develop liver disease, either symptomatic or discovered from liver function tests. Treatment of the former aims to induce seroconversion and clear HBV, while in the latter case treatment aims to improve liver function. The treatment of chronic carriers is complex, particularly children.

Adults may occasionally clear surface antigen spontaneously and start producing surface antibody. The proportion of adults seroconverting and clearing the virus can be improved by using antivirals, such as interferon-α or lamivudine.[171] Seroconversion is often associated with a transient rise in transaminases.[163,164] Children who acquired HBV perinatally are far less likely to seroconvert than children who acquired HBV horizontally.[172–175] This is presumably because perinatally infected children remain tolerant of the virus. A number of studies have shown that treatment of carrier children with interferon-α,[172] lamivudine,[173] interferon-α plus lamivudine,[174] or with interferon-α plus steroids[175] can improve liver function (reduced elevated liver enzymes, reduced viral load, and sometimes clearance of e antigen and production of e antibody). However, none of these regimens was associated with an increased rate of eradication of surface antigen; i.e., the children still remained carriers. For this reason, we do not recommend treating carriers who are well and whose liver enzymes are normal or near normal. Chronic carriers should be followed with regular clinical examination and liver function tests (enzymes, viral load, serology). If there is a sustained rise in liver enzymes to greater than twice normal, we recommend discussion with a pediatric gastroenterologist with a view to possible liver biopsy and treatment with antivirals.

7.16 Hepatitis C

More than 170 million people worldwide are chronically infected with hepatitis C virus (HCV), resulting in more than 100,000 cases of liver cancer per year and similar numbers of episodes of gastrointestinal hemorrhage and ascites.[176] The combination of pegylated interferon and ribavirin can eradicate the virus in more than 50% of patients.[177,178] These antiviral treatments reduce liver fibrosis progression and can reverse cirrhosis. Although there are few studies in children, RCTs in children with chronic active hepatitis C show that a sustained response can be achieved in 36% of children treated with interferon-α alone[179] and 46% of children given interferon-α plus ribavirin.[180] Adverse reactions associated with interferon, notably fevers, arthralgia, malaise, and psychiatric problems, are common at any age but particularly in children, and often lead to dose modification or cessation of treatment.[179,180] The treatment of chronic hepatitis C infection in children is specialized, and we recommend that it be undertaken in joint consultation between a pediatric gastroenterologist and a pediatric infectious disease specialist.

There is no vaccine against hepatitis C and human immunoglobulin contains no HCV antibodies, and so mother-to-child transmission of HCV is not preventable currently. The risk of perinatal transmission is about 5–10%, and virtually occurs only if mother is HCV RNA positive at delivery.[176] Co-infection with HIV increases the risk. In a study of HCV-infected children of HCV-positive mothers, babies were tested 3 days after birth using PCR on blood.[179] At least a third and perhaps as many as a half of all children were infected in utero, and this implied that post-partum transmission was rare.[181] Although low-titer HCV RNA can be detected in the breast milk of viremic mothers, there is no demonstrable increased risk of transmission from breast-feeding.[181,182] One study suggested that Caesarean section might reduce transmission,[183] but this has not been confirmed[181] and Caesarean section is not currently recommended, even for viremic mothers.[184]

We recommend to HCV-infected mothers that Caesarean section is not indicated and that it is almost certainly safe to breast-feed. All infants born to infected women should be screened for hepatitis C.

7.17 Worms

Worm infestation impairs growth and possibly intellectual function and there is limited evidence that the treatment of children with helminth infestation improves growth.[185,186] Albendazole, mebendazole, and thiabendazole are not recommended in children <6 months of age because of lack of safety data, but pyrantel is reported to be safe in this age group.

Tapeworm (*Echinococcus granulosus*)

The larval forms of *E. granulosus*, and in adults, *E. multilocularis*, can cause hydatid disease (see p. 257).

Hookworm (*Ancylostoma duodenale* or *Necator americanus*)

Albendazole is superior to mebendazole or pyrantel in the treatment of hookworm,[187,188] although price and availability can be important issues. For the treatment of hookworm we recommend:

> **albendazole 400 mg (child ≤10 kg but not <6 months old: 200 mg) orally, as a single dose** OR
> **mebendazole 100 mg (child ≤10 kg but not <6 months old: 50 mg) orally, 12-hourly for 3 days** OR
> **pyrantel 20 mg/kg (max 750 mg) orally, as a single dose (repeat after 7 days if heavy infection)**

Strongyloidiasis (*Strongyloides stercoralis*)

For the treatment of strongyloidiasis in immunocompetent patients, ivermectin is superior to albendazole.[189] We recommend:

> **ivermectin 200 µg/kg (adult and child >5 years) orally, single dose** OR
> **albendazole 400 mg (child ≤10 kg: 200 mg) orally, daily for 3 days**

Some authorities recommend repeating each course 1–2 weeks later, but an RCT suggested this is unnecessary and increases toxicity.[190] Treatment is not always successful, especially in immunosuppressed patients, and may need to be repeated at monthly intervals or a longer course given.

Pinworm or threadworm (*Enterobius vermicularis*)

Pinworm and threadworm are common names for the same organism, *Enterobius vermicularis*. We found no RCTs of treatment, only observational studies. Drugs that have been shown in observational studies to be effective are:

> **mebendazole 100 mg (child ≤10 kg: 50 mg) orally, as a single dose** OR
> **pyrantel 10 mg/kg (max 750 mg) orally, as a single dose** OR
> **albendazole 400 mg (child ≤10 kg: 200 mg) orally, as a single dose**

Whipworm (*Trichuris trichiura*)

In an RCT of treatment of asymptomatic children with whipworm (trichuriasis), albendazole was more effective than pyrantel for children with heavy infestation, but the opposite was true if infestation was less severe.[184] For the treatment of whipworm, we recommend:

> **mebendazole 100 mg (child ≤10 kg: 50 mg) orally, 12-hourly for 3 days** OR
> **pyrantel 10 mg/kg (max 750 mg) orally, as a single dose** OR
> **albendazole 400 mg (child ≤10 kg: 200 mg) orally, daily for 3 days**

Community worm programs

Age-targeted chemotherapy has been recommended because some overseas studies have found that treatment of helminth worm infestation improves nutrition and growth. A Cochrane review[191] of 30 trials (>1500 children) found that a single dose of any anthelminth was associated with short-term weight gain of a mean of 0.17–0.38 kg. If repeat doses were given, there was a non-significant mean weight gain of 0.12 kg a year later. Results from studies of cognitive performance were mixed and inconclusive. Thus the benefits were marginal.

If it is decided to treat children aged 6 months to 12 years in a community where helminthic infections are endemic, the recommended treatment is:

> **albendazole 400 mg (child ≤10 kg: 200 mg) orally, as a single dose every 4–6 months**

References

1 King CK, Glass R, Bresee JS, Duggan C, for the Centers for Disease Control and Prevention. Managing acute gastroenteritis among children: oral rehydration, maintenance, and nutritional therapy. *MMWR Recomm Rep* 2003;52(RR-16):1–16.

2 Armon K, Stephenson T, MacFaul R et al. An evidence and consensus based guideline for acute diarrhea management. *Arch Dis Child* 2001;85:132–42.

3 American Academy of Pediatrics. Practice parameter: the management of acute gastroenteritis in young children. American Academy of Pediatrics Provisional Committee on Quality Improvement, Sub-committee on Acute Gastroenteritis. *Pediatrics* 1996;97:424–35.

4 Mackenzie A, Barnes G, Shann F. Clinical signs of dehydration in children. *Lancet* 1989;2:605–7.

5 Duggan C, Refat M, Hashem M, Wolff M, Fayad I, Santosham M. How valid are clinical signs of dehydration in infants? *J Pediatr Gastroenterol Nutr* 1996;22:56–61.

6 Gorelick MH, Shaw KN, Murphy KO. Validity and reliability of clinical signs in the diagnosis of dehydration in children. *Pediatrics* 1997;99:E6.

7 Friedman JN, Goldman RD, Srivastava R, Parkin PC. Development of a clinical dehydration scale for use in children between 1 and 36 months of age. *J Pediatr* 2004;145:201–7.

8 Kilham HA, Isaacs D. *Children's Hospital at Westmead Handbook. Clinical Practice Guidelines for Paediatrics.* Sydney: McGraw-Hill, 2004.

9 Sharifi J, Ghavami F, Nowrouzi Z et al. Oral versus intravenous rehydration therapy in severe gastroenteritis. *Arch Dis Child* 1985;60:856–60.

10 Mackenzie A, Barnes GL. Randomised controlled trial comparing oral and intravenous rehydration therapy in children with diarrhea. *BMJ* 1991;303:393–6.

11 O'Loughlin EV, Notaras E, McCullough C et al. Home-based management of children hospitalised with acute gastroenteritis. *J Paediatr Child Health* 1995;31:189–91.

12 Elliott EJ, Backhouse JA, Leach JW. Pre-admission management of acute gastroenteritis. *J Paediatr Child Health* 1996;32:18–21.

13 Brewster DR. Dehydration in acute gastroenteritis. *J Paediatr Child Health* 2002;38:219-22.

14 Fonseca BK, Holdgate A, Craig JC. Enteral vs intravenous rehydration therapy for children with gastroenteritis: a meta-analysis of randomized controlled trials. *Arch Pediatr Adolesc Med* 2004;158:483–90.

15 Hartling L, Bellemare S, Wiebe N, Russell K, Klassen TP, Craig W. Oral versus intravenous rehydration for treating dehydration due to gastroenteritis in children. *The Cochrane Database of Systematic Reviews* 2006;(3): Art No CD004390.

16 Reid SR, Bonadio WA. Outpatient rapid intravenous rehydration to correct dehydration and resolve vomiting in children with acute gastroenteritis. *Ann Emerg Med* 1996;28:318–23.

17 Conway SP, Newport MJ. Are all hospital admissions for acute gastroenteritis necessary? *J Infect* 1994;29:5–8.

18 Hahn S, Kim Y, Garner P. Reduced osmolarity oral rehydration solution for treating dehydration caused by acute diarrhea in children. *The Cochrane Database of Systematic Reviews* 2002;(1):Art No CD002847.

19 Pulungsih SP, Punjabi NH, Rafli K et al. Standard WHO-ORS versus reduced-osmolarity ORS in the management of cholera patients. *J Health Popul Nutr* 2006;24:107–12.

20 Murphy C, Hahn S, Volmink J. Reduced osmolarity oral rehydration solution for treating cholera. *The Cochrane Database of Systematic Reviews* 2004;(4):Art No CD003754.

21 Nager AL, Wang VJ. Comparison of nasogastric and intravenous methods of rehydration in pediatric patients with acute dehydration. *Pediatrics* 2002;109:566–72.

22 Yiu WL, Smith AL, Catto-Smith AG. Nasogastric rehydration in acute gastroenteritis. *J Paediatr Child Health* 2003;39:159–61.

23 Moritz ML, Ayus JC. Prevention of hospital-acquired hyponatremia: a case for using isotonic saline. *Pediatrics* 2003;111:227–30.

24 Hoorn EJ, Geary D, Robb M, Halperin ML, Bohn D. Acute hyponatremia related to intravenous fluid administration in hospitalized children: an observational study. *Pediatrics* 2004;113:1279–84.

25 Neville KA, Verge CF, Rosenberg AR, O'Meara MW, Walker JL. Isotonic is better than hypotonic saline for intravenous rehydration of children with gastroenteritis: a prospective randomised study. *Arch Dis Child* 2006;91:226–32.

26 Neville KA, Verge CF, O'Meara MW, Walker JL. High antidiuretic hormone levels and hyponatremia in children with gastroenteritis. *Pediatrics* 2005;116:1401–7.

27 Robins-Browne RM, Coovadia HM, Bodasing MN, Mackenjee MK. Treatment of acute non-specific gastroenteritis of infants and young children with erythromycin. *Am J Trop Med Hyg* 1983;32:886–90.

28 Pichler H, Diridl G, Wolf D. Ciprofloxacin in the treatment of acute bacterial diarrhea: a double blind study. *Eur J Clin Microbiol* 1986;5:241–3.

29 Dryden MS, Gabb RJ, Wright SK. Empirical treatment of severe acute community-acquired gastroenteritis with ciprofloxacin. *Clin Infect Dis* 1996;22:1019–25.

30 Wretlind B, Stromberg A, Ostlund L, Sjogren E, Kaijser B. Rapid emergence of quinolone resistance in *Campylobacter jejuni* in patients treated with norfloxacin. *Scand J Infect Dis* 1992;24:685–6.

31 Alhashimi D, Alhashimi H, Fedorowicz Z. Antiemetics for reducing vomiting related to acute gastroenteritis in children and adolescents. *The Cochrane Database of Systematic Reviews* 2006;(3):Art No CD005506.

32 Cubeddu LX, Trujillo LM, Talmaciu I et al. Antiemetic activity of ondansetron in acute gastroenteritis. *Aliment Pharmacol Ther* 1997;11:185–91.

33 Ramsook C, Sahagun-Carreon I, Kozinetz CA, Moro-Sutherland D. A randomized clinical trial comparing oral ondansetron with placebo in children with vomiting from acute gastroenteritis. *Ann Emerg Med* 2002;39:397–403.

34 Brown KH, Peerson JM, Fontaine O. Use of non-human milks in the dietary management of young children with acute diarrhea: a meta-analysis of clinical trials. *Pediatrics* 1994;93:17–2.

35 Santosham M, Foster S, Reid R *et al.* Role of soy-based, lactose-free formula during treatment of acute diarrhea. *Pediatrics* 1985;76:292–8.

36 Brown KH, Gastanaduy AS, Saavedra JM et al. Effect of continued oral feeding on clinical and nutritional outcomes

of acute diarrhea in children. *J Pediatr* 1988;112:191–200.

37 Brown KH, Perez F, Peerson J et al. Effect of dietary fiber (soy polysaccharide) on the severity, duration, and nutritional outcome of acute, watery diarrhea in children. *Pediatrics* 1993;92:241–7.

38 Isolauri E, Juntunen M, Wiren S, Vuorinen P, Koivula T. Intestinal permeability changes in acute gastroenteritis: effects of clinical factors and nutritional management. *J Pediatr Gastroenterol Nutr* 1989;8:466–73.

39 Duggan C, Nurko S. "Feeding the gut": the scientific basis for continued enteral nutrition during acute diarrhea. *J Pediatr* 1997;131:801–8.

40 Sandhu BK, for the European Society of Paediatric Gastroenterology, Hepatology, and Nutrition Working Group on Acute Diarrhea. Rationale for early feeding in childhood gastroenteritis. *J Pediatr Gastroenterol Nutr* 2001;33(suppl 2):S13–6.

41 Baker SS, Davis AM. Hypocaloric oral therapy during an episode of diarrhea and vomiting can lead to severe malnutrition. *J Pediatr Gastroenterol Nutr* 1998;27:1–5.

42 Bhutta ZA, Black RE, Brown KH et al., for the Zinc Investigators' Collaborative Group. Prevention of diarrhea and pneumonia by zinc supplementation in children in developing countries: pooled analysis of randomized controlled trials. *J Pediatr* 1999;135:689–97.

43 Bhandari N, Bahl R, Taneja S et al. Substantial reduction in severe diarrheal morbidity by daily zinc supplementation in young north Indian children. *Pediatrics* 2002;109:e86.

44 Penny ME, Peerson JM, Marin RM et al. Randomized, community-based trial of the effect of zinc supplementation, with and without other micronutrients, on the duration of persistent childhood diarrhea in Lima, Peru. *J Pediatr* 1999;135(2, pt 1):208–17.

45 Bhutta ZA, Bird SM, Black RE et al. Therapeutic effects of oral zinc in acute and persistent diarrhea in children in developing countries: pooled analysis of randomized controlled trials. *Am J Clin Nutr* 2000;72:1516–22.

46 Sazawal S, Black RE, Bhan MK, Bhandari N, Sinha A, Jalla S. Zinc supplementation in young children with acute diarrhea in India. *N Engl J Med* 1995;333:839–44.

47 Faruque AS, Mahalanabis D, Haque SS, Fuchs GJ, Habte D. Double-blind, randomized, controlled trial of zinc or vitamin A supplementation in young children with acute diarrhea. *Acta Paediatr* 1999;88:154–60.

48 Baqui AH, Black RE, El Arifeen S et al. Effect of zinc supplementation started during diarrhea on morbidity and mortality in Bangladeshi children: community randomised trial. *BMJ* 2002;325:1059.

49 Strand TA, Chandyo RK, Bahl R et al. Effectiveness and efficacy of zinc for the treatment of acute diarrhea in young children. *Pediatrics* 2002;109:898–903.

50 Bhatnagar S, Bahl R, Sharma PK, Kumar GT, Saxena SK, Bhan MK. Zinc with oral rehydration therapy reduces stool output and duration of diarrhea in hospitalized children: a randomized controlled trial. *J Pediatr Gastroenterol Nutr* 2004;38:34–40.

51 Valery PC, Torzillo PJ, Boyce NC et al. Zinc and vitamin A supplementation in Australian Indigenous children with acute diarrhea: a randomised controlled trial. *Med J Aust* 2005;182:530–5.

52 Andreozzi VL, Bailey TC, Nobre FF et al. Random-effects models in investigating the effect of vitamin A in childhood diarrhea. *Ann Epidemiol* 2006;16:241–7.

53 Stansfield SK, Pierre-Louis M, Lerebours G, Augustin A. Vitamin A supplementation and increased prevalence of childhood diarrhea and acute respiratory infections. *Lancet* 1993;342:578–82.

54 Grotto I, Mimouni M, Gdalevich M, Mimouni D. Vitamin A supplementation and childhood morbidity from diarrhea and respiratory infections: a meta-analysis. *J Pediatr* 2003;142:297–304.

55 Allen SJ, Okoko B, Martinez E, Gregorio G, Dans LF. Probiotics for treating infectious diarrhea. *The Cochrane Database of Systematic Reviews* 2003;(4):Art No CD003048.

56 Szajewska H, Kotowska M, Mrukowicz JZ, Armanska M, Mikolajczyk W. Efficacy of lactobacillus GG in prevention of nosocomial diarrhea in infants. *J Pediatr* 2001;138:361–5.

57 Van Niel CW, Feudtner C, Garrison MM, Christakis DA. Lactobacillus therapy for acute infectious diarrhea in children: a meta-analysis. *Pediatrics* 2002;109:678–84.

58 Rossignol JF, Abu-Zekry M, Hussein A, Santoro MG. Effect of nitazoxanide for treatment of severe rotavirus diarrhea: randomised double-blind placebo-controlled trial. *Lancet* 2006;368:124–9.

59 Armon K, MacFaul R, Hemingway P, Werneke U, Stephenson T. The impact of presenting problem based guidelines for children with medical problems in an accident and emergency department. *Arch Dis Child* 2004;89:159–64.

60 Burks AW, Vanderhoof JA, Mehra S, Ostrom KM, Baggs G. Randomized clinical trial of soy formula with and without added fiber in antibiotic-induced diarrhea. *J Pediatr* 2001;139:578–82.

61 Bricker E, Garg R, Nelson R, Loza A, Novak T, Hansen J. Antibiotic treatment for *Clostridium difficile*-associated diarrhea in adults. *The Cochrane Database of Systematic Reviews* 2005;(1):Art No CD004610.

62 D'Souza AL, Rajkumar C, Cooke J, Bulpitt CJ. Probiotics in prevention of antibiotic associated diarrhea: meta-analysis. *BMJ* 2002;324:1361–6.

63 Anders BJ, Lauer BA, Paisley JW, Reller LB. Double-blind placebo controlled trial of erythromycin for treatment of campylobacter enteritis. *Lancet* 1982;1:131–2.

64 Pai CH, Gillis F, Tuomanen E, Marks MI. Erythromycin in treatment of campylobacter enteritis in children. *Am J Dis Child* 1983;137:286–8.

65 Mandal BK, Ellis ME, Dunbar EM, Whale K. Double-blind placebo-controlled trial of erythromycin in the treatment of clinical campylobacter infection. *J Antimicrob Chemother* 1984;13:619–23.

66 Salazar-Lindo E, Sack RB, Chea-Woo E et al. Early treatment with erythromycin of *Campylobacter jejuni*-associated dysentery in children. *J Pediatr* 1986;109:355–60.

67 Kuschner RA, Trofa AF, Thomas RJ et al. Use of azithromycin for the treatment of campylobacter enteritis in travelers to Thailand, an area where ciprofloxacin resistance is prevalent. *Clin Infect Dis* 1995;21:536–41.

68 Gore SM, Fontaine O, Pierce NF. Impact of rice based oral rehydration solution on stool output and duration of diarrhea: meta-analysis of 13 clinical trials. *BMJ* 1992;304: 287–91.

69 Fontaine O, Gore SM, Pierce NF. Rice-based oral rehydration solution for treating diarrhea. *The Cochrane Database of Systematic Reviews* 2000;(2):Art No CD001264.

70 Zaman K, Yunus M, Rahman A, Chowdhury HR, Sack DA. Efficacy of a packaged rice oral rehydration solution among children with cholera and cholera-like illness. *Acta Paediatr* 2001;90:505–10.

71 Khan WA, Saha D, Rahman A, Salam MA, Bogaerts J, Bennish ML. Comparison of single-dose azithromycin and 12-dose, 3-day erythromycin for childhood cholera: a randomised, double-blind trial. *Lancet* 2002;360:1722–7.

72 Saha D, Khan WA, Karim MM, Chowdhury HR, Salam MA, Bennish ML. Single-dose ciprofloxacin versus 12-dose erythromycin for childhood cholera: a randomised controlled trial. *Lancet* 2005;366:1085–93.

73 Panos GZ, Betsi GI, Falagas ME. Systematic review: are antibiotics detrimental or beneficial for the treatment of patients with *Escherichia coli* O157:H7 infection? *Aliment Pharmacol Ther* 2006;24:731–42.

74 Thoren A, Wolde-Mariam T, Stintzing G, Wadstrom T, Habte D. Antibiotics in the treatment of gastroenteritis caused by enteropathogenic *Escherichia coli*. *J Infect Dis* 1980;141:27–31.

75 Sirinavin S, Garner P. Antibiotics for treating salmonella gut infections. *The Cochrane Database of Systematic Reviews* 1999;(1):Art No CD001167.

76 Weinberger M, Keller N. Recent trends in the epidemiology of non-typhoid Salmonella and antimicrobial resistance: the Israeli experience and worldwide review. *Curr Opin Infect Dis* 2005;18:513–21.

77 Graham SM, Molyneux EM, Walsh AL, Cheesbrough JS, Molyneux ME, Hart CA. Non-typhoidal Salmonella infections of children in tropical Africa. *Pediatr Infect Dis J* 2000;19:1189–96.

78 American Academy of Pediatrics. Salmonella infections. In: Pickering LK (ed.), *Red Book: 2003 Report of the Committee on Infectious Diseases*, 26th edn. Elk Grove Village, IL: American Academy of Pediatrics, 2003:541–7.

79 Laditan AA, Alausa KO. Problems in the clinical diagnosis of typhoid fever in children in the tropics. *Ann Trop Paediatr* 1981;1:191–5.

80 Choo KE, Razif A, Ariffin WA, Sepiah M, Gururaj A. Typhoid fever in hospitalized children in Kelantan, Malaysia. *Ann Trop Paediatr* 1988;8:207–12.

81 Rathore MH, Bux D, Hasan M. Multidrug-resistant *Salmonella typhi* in Pakistani children: clinical features and treatment. *South Med J* 1996;89:235–7.

82 Malik AS, Malik RH. Typhoid fever in Malaysian children. *Med J Malaysia* 2001;56:478–90.

83 Davis TM, Makepeace AE, Dallimore EA, Choo KE. Relative bradycardia is not a feature of enteric fever in children. *Clin Infect Dis* 1999;28:582–6.

84 Rasaily R, Dutta P, Saha MR, Mitra U, Lahiri M, Pal SC. Multi-drug resistant typhoid fever in hospitalised children. Clinical, bacteriological and epidemiological profiles. *Eur J Epidemiol* 1994;10:41–6.

85 Thaver D, Zaidi AK, Critchley J, Madni SA, Bhutta ZA. Fluoroquinolones for treating typhoid and paratyphoid fever (enteric fever). *The Cochrane Database of Systematic Reviews* 2005;(2):Art No CD004530.

86 Cao XT, Kneen R, Nguyen TA, Truong DL, White NJ, Parry CM, for the Dong Nai Pediatric Center Typhoid Study Group. A comparative study of ofloxacin and cefixime for treatment of typhoid fever in children. *Pediatr Infect Dis J* 1999;18:245–8.

87 Huai Y, Zhu Q, Wang X. Ceftriaxone vs. norfloxacin in the treatment of resistant typhoid fever in 60 children. *Zhonghua Er Ke Za Zhi* [Chinese *Journal of Pediatrics*] 2000;38:386–8.

88 Vinh H, Wain J, Vo TN et al. Two or three days of ofloxacin treatment for uncomplicated multidrug-resistant typhoid fever in children. *Antimicrob Agents Chemother* 1996;40:958–61.

89 Vinh H, Duong NM, Phuong le T et al. Comparative trial of short-course ofloxacin for uncomplicated typhoid fever in Vietnamese children. *Ann Trop Paediatr* 2005;25: 17–22.

90 Frenck RW, Jr, Mansour A, Nakhla I et al. Short-course azithromycin for the treatment of uncomplicated typhoid fever in children and adolescents. *Clin Infect Dis* 2004;38:951–7.

91 Frenck RW, Jr, Nakhla I, Sultan Y et al. Azithromycin versus ceftriaxone for the treatment of uncomplicated typhoid fever in children. *Clin Infect Dis* 2000;31:1134–8.

92 Bhutta ZA, Khan IA, Shadmani M. Failure of short-course ceftriaxone chemotherapy for multidrug-resistant typhoid fever in children: a randomized controlled trial in Pakistan. *Antimicrob Agents Chemother* 2000;44:450–2.

93 Vinh H, Parry CM, Hanh VT et al. Double blind comparison of ibuprofen and paracetamol for adjunctive treatment of uncomplicated typhoid fever. *Pediatr Infect Dis J* 2004;23:226–30.

94 Leibovitz E, Janco J, Piglansky L et al. Oral ciprofloxacin vs. intramuscular ceftriaxone as empiric treatment of acute invasive diarrhea in children. *Pediatr Infect Dis J* 2000;19: 1060–7.

95 Zimbabwe, Bangladesh, South Africa (Zimbasa) Dysentery Study Group. Multicenter, randomized, double blind clinical trial of short course versus standard course oral ciprofloxacin for *Shigella dysenteriae* type 1 dysentery in children. *Pediatr Infect Dis J* 2002;21:1136–41.

96 Basualdo W, Arbo A. Randomized comparison of azithromycin versus cefixime for treatment of shigellosis in children. *Pediatr Infect Dis J* 2003;22:374–7.

97 Miron D, Torem M, Merom R, Colodner R. Azithromycin as an alternative to nalidixic acid in the therapy of childhood shigellosis. *Pediatr Infect Dis J* 2004;23:367–8.

98 Ashkenazi S, Amir J, Waisman Y et al. A randomized, double-blind study comparing cefixime and trimethoprim-sulfamethoxazole in the treatment of childhood shigellosis. *J Pediatr* 1993;123:817–21.

99 Al-Abri SS, Beeching NJ, Nye FJ. Traveller's diarrhea. *Lancet Infect Dis* 2005;5:349–60.

100 Steffen R. Epidemiologic studies of travelers' diarrhea, severe gastrointestinal infections, and cholera. *Rev Infect Dis* 1986;8(suppl 2):S122–30.

101 Jiang ZD, Lowe B, Verenkar MP et al. Prevalence of enteric pathogens among international travelers with diarrhea acquired in Kenya (Mombasa), India (Goa), or Jamaica (Montego Bay). *J Infect Dis* 1985;185:497–502.

102 Peltola H, Siitonen A, Kyronseppa H et al. Prevention of travellers' diarrhea by oral B-sub-unit/whole-cell cholera vaccine. *Lancet* 1991;338:1285–9.

103 Scerpella EG, Sanchez JL, Mathewson JJ, III et al. Safety, immunogenicity, and protective efficacy of the whole-cell/recombinant B sub-unit (WC/rBS) oral cholera vaccine against travelers' diarrhea. *J Travel Med* 1995;2:22–7.

104 De Bruyn G, Hahn S, Borwick A. Antibiotic treatment for travellers' diarrhea. *The Cochrane Database of Systematic Reviews* 2000;(3):Art No CD002242.

105 von Muhlendahl KE, Bunjes R, Krienke EG. Loperamide-induced ileus. *Lancet* 1980;1:209.

106 Haque R, Huston CD, Hughes M, Houpt E, Petri WA, Jr. Amebiasis. *N Engl J Med* 2003;348:1565–73.

107 Stanley SL, Jr. Amoebiasis. *Lancet* 2003;361:1025–34.

108 American Academy of Pediatrics. Amebiasis. In: Pickering LK (ed.), *Red Book: 2003 Report of the Committee on Infectious Diseases*, 26th edn. Elk Grove Village, IL: American Academy of Pediatrics, 2003:192–4.

109 Haque R, Mollah NU, Ali IK et al. Diagnosis of amebic liver abscess and intestinal infection with the TechLab *Entamoeba histolytica* II antigen detection and antibody tests. *J Clin Microbiol* 2000;38:3235–9.

110 Pillai DR, Keystone JS, Sheppard DC et al. *Entamoeba histolytica* and *Entamoeba dispar*: epidemiology and comparison of diagnostic methods in a setting of non-endemicity. *Clin Infect Dis* 1999;29:1315–8.

111 Mirelman D, Nuchamowitz Y, Stolarsky T. Comparison of use of enzyme-linked immunosorbent assay-based kits and PCR amplification of rRNA genes for simultaneous detection of *Entamoeba histolytica* and *E. dispar*. *J Clin Microbiol* 1997;35:2405–7.

112 Blumencranz H, Kasen L, Romeu J, Waye JD, LeLeiko NS. The role of endoscopy in suspected amebiasis. *J Gastroenterol* 1983;78:15–8.

113 Krupp IM, Powell SJ. Comparative study of the antibody response in amebiasis: persistence after successful treatment. *Am J Trop Med Hyg* 1971;20:421–4.

114 Krogstad DJ, Spencer HC, Jr, Healy GR, Gleason NN, Sexton DJ, Herron CA. Amebiasis: epidemiologic studies in the United States, 1971–1974. *Ann Intern Med* 1978;88:89–97.

115 Haque R, Ali IKM, Akther S, Petri WA, Jr. Comparison of PCR, isoenzyme analysis, and antigen detection for diagnosis of Entamoeba histolytica infection. *J Clin Microbiol* 1998;36:449–52.

116 Pillai DR, Keystone JS, Sheppard DC, MacLean JD, MacPherson DW, Kain KC. *Entamoeba histolytica* and *Entamoeba dispar*: epidemiology and comparison of diagnostic methods in a setting of non-endemicity. *Clin Infect Dis* 1999;29:1315–8.

117 Patel AS, DeRidder PH. Amebic colitis masquerading as acute inflammatory bowel disease: the role of serology in its diagnosis. *J Clin Gastroenterol* 1989;11:407–10.

118 van Sonnenberg E, Mueller PR, Schiffman HR et al. Intrahepatic amebic abscesses: indications for and results of percutaneous catheter drainage. *Radiology* 1985;156:631–5.

119 Rossignol JF, Kabil SM, Said M, Samir H, Younis AM. Effect of nitazoxanide in persistent diarrhea and enteritis associated with *Blastocystis hominis*. *Clin Gastroenterol Hepatol* 2005;3:987–91.

120 Huang DB, Chappell C, Okhuysen PC. Cryptosporidiosis in children. *Semin Pediatr Infect Dis* 2004;15:253–9.

121 White AC, Jr, Chappell CL, Hayat CS, Kimball KT, Flanigan TP, Goodgame RW. Paromomycin for cryptosporidiosis in AIDS: a prospective, double-blind trial. *J Infect Dis* 1994;170:419–24.

122 Hewitt RG, Yiannoutsos CT, Higgs ES et al, for the AIDS Clinical Trial Group. Paromomycin: no more effective than placebo for treatment of cryptosporidiosis in patients with advanced human immunodeficiency virus infection. *Clin Infect Dis* 2000;31:1084–92.

123 Saez-Llorens X, Odio CM, Umana MA, Morales MV. Spiramycin vs. placebo for treatment of acute diarrhea caused by Cryptosporidium. *Pediatr Infect Dis J* 1989;8:136–40.

124 Wittenberg DF, Miller NM, van den Ende J. Spiramycin is not effective in treating cryptosporidium diarrhea in infants: results of a double-blind randomized trial. *J Infect Dis* 1989;159:131–2.

125 Kadappu KK, Nagaraja MV, Rao PV, Shastry BA. Azithromycin as treatment for cryptosporidiosis in human immunodeficiency virus disease. *J Postgrad Med* 2002;48:179–81.

126 Rossignol JF, Ayoub A, Ayers MS. Treatment of diarrhea caused by *Cryptosporidium parvum*: a prospective randomized, double-blind, placebo-controlled study of nitazoxanide. *J Infect Dis* 2001;184:103–6.

127 Amadi B, Mwiya M, Musuku J et al. Effect of nitazoxanide on morbidity and mortality in Zambian children with cryptosporidiosis: a randomised controlled trial. *Lancet* 2002;360:1375–80.

128 Rossignol JF, Hidalgo H, Feregrino M et al. A double-"blind" placebo-controlled study of nitazoxanide in the treatment of cryptosporidial diarrhea in AIDS patients in Mexico. *Trans R Soc Trop Med Hyg* 1998;92:663–6.

129 Zulu I, Kelly P, Njobvu L et al. Nitazoxanide for persistent diarrhea in Zambian acquired immune deficiency syndrome patients: a randomized-controlled trial. *Aliment Pharmacol Ther* 2005;21:757–63.

130 Doumbo O, Rossignol JF, Pichard E et al. Nitazoxanide in the treatment of cryptosporidial diarrhea and other intestinal

parasitic infections associated with acquired immunodeficiency syndrome in tropical Africa. *Am J Trop Med Hyg* 1997;56:637–9.

131 Ochoa TJ, Salazar-Lindo E, Cleary TG. Management of children with infection-associated persistent diarrhea. *Semin Pediatr Infect Dis* 2004;15:229–36.

132 Scheffler EH, Van Etta LL. Evaluation of rapid commercial enzyme immunoassay for detection of *Giardia lamblia* in formalin-preserved stool specimens. *J Clin Microbiol* 1994;32:1807–8.

133 Hanson KL, Cartwright CP. Use of an enzyme immunoassay does not eliminate the need to analyze multiple stool specimens for sensitive detection of *Giardia lamblia*. *J Clin Microbiol* 2001;39:474–7.

134 Rashid SM, Nagaty IM, Maboud AI, Fouad MA, Shebl A. Comparative study on ELISA, IFA and direct methods in diagnosis of giardiasis. *J Egypt Soc Parasitol* 2002;32:381–9.

135 Kyronseppa H, Pettersson T. Treatment of giardiasis: relative efficacy of metronidazole as compared with tinidazole. *Scand J Infect Dis* 1981;13:311–2.

136 Speelman P. Single-dose tinidazole for the treatment of giardiasis. *Antimicrob Agents Chemother* 1985;27:227–9.

137 Gazder AJ, Banerjee M. Single-dose treatment of giardiasis in children: a comparison of tinidazole and metronidazole. *Curr Med Res Opin* 1977;5:164–8.

138 Pengsaa K, Limkittikul K, Pojjaroen-anant C et al. Single-dose therapy for giardiasis in school-age children. *Southeast Asian J Trop Med Public Health* 2002;33:711–7.

139 Escobedo AA, Nunez FA, Moreira I, Vega E, Pareja A, Almirall P. Comparison of chloroquine, albendazole and tinidazole in the treatment of children with giardiasis. *Ann Trop Med Parasitol* 2003;97:367–71.

140 Quiros-Buelna E. Furazolidone and metronidazole for treatment of giardiasis in children. *Scand J Gastroenterol Suppl* 1989;169:65–9.

141 Dutta AK, Phadke MA, Bagade AC et al. A randomised multicentre study to compare the safety and efficacy of albendazole and metronidazole in the treatment of giardiasis in children. *Indian J Pediatr* 1994;61:689–93.

142 Misra PK, Kumar A, Agarwal V, Jagota SC. A comparative clinical trial of albendazole versus metronidazole in children with giardiasis. *Indian Pediatr* 1995;32:779–82.

143 Yereli K, Balcioglu IC, Ertan P, Limoncu E, Onag A. Albendazole as an alternative therapeutic agent for childhood giardiasis in Turkey. *Clin Microbiol Infect* 2004;10:527–9.

144 Ortiz JJ, Ayoub A, Gargala G, Chegne NL, Favennec L. Randomized clinical study of nitazoxanide compared to metronidazole in the treatment of symptomatic giardiasis in children from Northern Peru. *Aliment Pharmacol Ther* 2001;15:1409–15.

145 Verdier RI, Fitzgerald DW, Johnson WD, Jr, Pape JW. Trimethoprim-sulfamethoxazole compared with ciprofloxacin for treatment and prophylaxis of *Isospora belli* and Cyclospora cayetanensis infection in HIV-infected patients: a randomized, controlled trial. *Ann Intern Med* 2000;132:885–8.

146 Tremoulet AH, Avila-Aguero ML, Paris MM, Canas-Coto A, Ulloa-Gutierrez R, Faingezicht I. Albendazole therapy for Microsporidium diarrhea in immunocompetent Costa Rican children. *Pediatr Infect Dis J* 2004;23:915–8.

147 Megraud F, for the European Paediatric Task Force on Helicobacter pylori. Comparison of non-invasive tests to detect *Helicobacter pylori* infection in children and adolescents: results of a multicenter European study. *J Pediatr* 2005;146:198–203.

148 Gottrand F, Kalach N, Spyckerelle C et al. Omeprazole combined with amoxicillin and clarithromycin in the eradication of *Helicobacter pylori* in children with gastritis: a prospective randomized double-blind trial. *J Pediatr* 2001;139:664–8.

149 Gessner BD, Bruce MG, Parkinson AJ et al. A randomized trial of triple therapy for pediatric *Helicobacter pylori* infection and risk factors for treatment failure in a population with a high prevalence of infection. *Clin Infect Dis* 2005;41:1261–8.

150 Faber J, Bar-Meir M, Rudensky B et al. Treatment regimens for Helicobacter pylori infection in children: is in vitro susceptibility testing helpful? *J Pediatr Gastroenterol Nutr* 2005;40:571–4.

151 Francavilla R, Lionetti E, Castellaneta SP et al. Improved efficacy of 10-Day sequential treatment for *Helicobacter pylori* eradication in children: a randomized trial. *Gastroenterology* 2005;129:1414–9.

152 Wang DS, Chen DS, Wang YZ, Li JS. Bacterial liver abscess in children. *J Singapore Paediatr Soc* 1989;31:75–8.

153 Kumar A, Srinivasan S, Sharma AK. Pyogenic liver abscess in children—South Indian experiences. *J Pediatr Surg* 1998;33:417–21.

154 Tsai CC, Chung JH, Ko SF et al. Liver abscess in children: a single institutional experience in Southern Taiwan. *Acta Paediatr Taiwan* 2003;44:282–6.

155 Lederman ER, Crum NF. Pyogenic liver abscess with a focus on *Klebsiella pneumoniae* as a primary pathogen: an emerging disease with unique clinical characteristics. *Am J Gastroenterol* 2005;100:322–31.

156 Rahimian J, Wilson T, Oram V, Holzman RS. Pyogenic liver abscess: recent trends in etiology and mortality. *Clin Infect Dis* 2004;39:1654–9.

157 Krugman S, Giles JP. Viral hepatitis: new light on an old disease. *JAMA* 1970;212:1019–29.

158 Hadler SC, Webster HM, Erben JJ, Swanson JE, Maynard JE. Hepatitis A in day-care centers: a community-wide assessment. *N Engl J Med* 1980;302:1222–7.

159 Lednar WM, Lemon SM, Kirkpatrick JW, Redfield RR, Fields ML, Kelley PW. Frequency of illness associated with epidemic hepatitis A virus infection in adults. *Am J Epidemiol* 1985;122:226–33.

160 Glikson M, Galun E, Oren R, Tur-Kaspa R, Shouval D. Relapsing hepatitis A: review of 14 cases and literature survey. *Medicine* 1992;71:14–23.

161 Fiore AE, Wasley A, Bell BP, for the Advisory Committee on Immunization Practices (ACIP). Prevention of hepatitis A through active or passive immunization: recommendations

of the Advisory Committee on Immunization Practices (ACIP). *MMWR Recomm Rep* 2006;55(RR-7):1–23.

162 Bianco E, De Masi S, Mele A, Jefferson T. Effectiveness of immune globulins in preventing infectious hepatitis and hepatitis A: a systematic review. *Dig Liver Dis* 2004;36: 834–42.

163 Winokur PL, Stapleton JT. Immunoglobulin prophylaxis for hepatitis A. *Clin Infect Dis* 1992;14:580–6.

164 Lee WM. Hepatitis B infection virus. *N Engl J Med* 1997;337:1733–45.

165 Lai CL, Ratziu V, Yuen M-F et al. Viral hepatitis B. *Lancet* 2003;362:2089–94.

166 Chang MH. Decreasing incidence of hepatocellular carcinoma among children following universal hepatitis B immunization. *Liver Int* 2003;23:309–14.

167 Yao JL. Perinatal transmission of hepatitis B virus infection and vaccination in China. *Gut* 1996;38(suppl 2):S37–8.

168 Lee C, Gong Y, Brok J, Boxall EH, Gluud C. Hepatitis B immunisation for newborn infants of hepatitis B surface antigen-positive mothers. *The Cochrane Database of Systematic Reviews* 2006;(2):Art No CD004790.

169 American Academy of Pediatrics. Hepatitis B. In: Pickering LK (ed.), *Red Book: 2003 Report of the Committee on Infectious Diseases*, 26th edn. Elk Grove Village, IL: American Academy of Pediatrics, 2003:318–36.

170 Zanetti AR, Mariano A, Romano L. Long-term immunogenicity of hepatitis B vaccination and policy for booster: an Italian multicentre study. *Lancet* 2005;366:1379–84.

171 Mellerup MT, Krogsgaard K, Mathurin P, Gluud C, Poynard T. Sequential combination of glucocorticosteroids and alfa interferon versus alfa interferon alone for HBeAg-positive chronic hepatitis B. *The Cochrane Database of Systematic Reviews* 2005;(3):Art No CD000345.

172 Vo Thi Diem H, Bourgois A, Bontems P et al. Chronic hepatitis B infection: long term comparison of children receiving interferon alpha and untreated controls. *J Pediatr Gastroenterol Nutr* 2005;40:141–5.

173 Jonas MM, Mizerski J, Badia IB et al. Clinical trial of lamivudine in children with chronic hepatitis B. *N Engl J Med* 2002;346:1706–13.

174 Dikici B, Bosnak M, Kara IH et al. Lamivudine and interferon-alpha combination treatment of childhood patients with chronic hepatitis B infection. *Pediatr Infect Dis J* 2001;20:988–92.

175 Boxall EH, Sira J, Ballard AL, Davies P, Kelly DA. Long-term follow-up of hepatitis B carrier children treated with interferon and prednisolone. *J Med Virol* 2006;78:888–95.

176 Poynard T, Yuen MF, Ratziu V, Lai CL. Viral hepatitis C. *Lancet* 2003;362:2095–100.

177 Myers RP, Regimbeau C, Thevenot T et al. Interferon for acute hepatitis C. *The Cochrane Database of Systematic Reviews* 2001;(4):Art No CD000369.

178 Brok J, Gluud LL, Gluud C. Ribavirin plus interferon versus interferon for chronic hepatitis C. *The Cochrane Database of Systematic Reviews* 2005;(2):Art No CD005445.

179 Jacobson KR, Murray K, Zellos A, Schwarz KB. An analysis of published trials of interferon monotherapy in children with chronic hepatitis C. *J Pediatr Gastroenterol Nutr* 2002;34: 52–8.

180 Gonzalez-Peralta RP, Kelly DA, Haber B et al. Interferon alfa-2b in combination with ribavirin for the treatment of chronic hepatitis C in children: efficacy, safety, and pharmacokinetics. *Hepatology* 2005;42:1010–8.

181 Mok J, Pembrey L, Tovo PA, Newell ML, for the European Paediatric Hepatitis C Virus Network. When does mother to child transmission of hepatitis C virus occur? *Arch Dis Child Fetal Neonatal Ed* 2005;90:F156–60.

182 Ruiz-Extremera A, Salmeron J, Torres C et al. Follow-up of transmission of hepatitis C to babies of human immunodeficiency virus-negative women: the role of breast-feeding in transmission. *Pediatr Infect Dis J* 2000;19:511–6.

183 Gibb DM, Goodall RL, Dunn DT et al. Mother-to-child transmission of hepatitis C virus: evidence for preventable peripartum transmission. *Lancet* 2000;356:904–7.

184 Pembreya L, Newella ML, Tovo PA, for the EPHN Collaborators. The management of HCV infected pregnant women and their children European paediatric HCV network. *J Hepatol* 2005;43:515–25. [Names misspelt in PubMed: should be Pembrey L, Newell ML]

185 Dickson R, Awasthi S, Demellweek C, Williamson P. Anthelmintic drugs for treating worms in children: effects on growth and cognitive performance. *The Cochrane Database of Systematic Reviews* 2000(2):Art No CD000371.

186 Forrester JE, Bailar JC, III, Esrey SA, Jose MV, Castillejos BT, Ocampo G. Randomised trial of albendazole and pyrantel in symptomless trichuriasis in children. *Lancet* 1998;352: 1103–8.

187 Sacko M, De Clercq D, Behnke JM, Gilbert FS, Dorny P, Vercruysse J. Comparison of the efficacy of mebendazole, albendazole and pyrantel in treatment of human hookworm infections in the southern region of Mali, West Africa. *Trans R Soc Trop Med Hyg* 1999;93:195–203.

188 Rahman WA. Comparative trials using albendazole and mebendazole in the treatment of soil-transmitted helminths in schoolchildren on Penang, Malaysia. *Southeast Asian J Trop Med Public Health* 1996;27:765–7.

189 Marti H, Haji HJ, Savioli L et al. A comparative trial of a single-dose ivermectin versus three days of albendazole for treatment of *Strongyloides stercoralis* and other soil-transmitted helminth infections in children. *Am J Trop Med Hyg* 1996;55:477–81.

190 Gann PH, Neva FA, Gam AA. A randomized trial of single- and two-dose ivermectin versus thiabendazole for treatment of strongyloidiasis. *J Infect Dis* 1994;169:1076–9.

191 Dickson R, Awasthi S, Demellweek C, Williamson P. Anthelmintic drugs for treating worms in children: effects on growth and cognitive performance. *The Cochrane Database of Systematic Reviews* 2000;(2):Art No CD000371.

CHAPTER 8
HIV infection

The management of HIV infection in pregnancy, the management of babies born to HIV-infected mothers, and the management of children with post-natally acquired HIV infection are all highly specialized. There are regularly updated Web sites that provide detailed information on many aspects of the management of HIV infection in adults and children.[1–3] Because of the complexity, we strongly recommend consultation with HIV experts when faced with difficult treatment decisions.

In this chapter, we will discuss the diagnosis of HIV infection, general principles about antiretroviral therapy, the prevention of mother-to-child transmission (MTCT) of HIV infection, and the management of potential needlestick or sexual exposure to HIV.

8.1 Clinical presentation of HIV infection in babies and children

HIV-infected infants and children may develop early acquired immunodeficiency syndrome (AIDS)-defining illness or can remain asymptomatic for years before developing an opportunist infection.[4–10] A bimodal distribution of perinatally infected infants has been described. Babies infected with HIV by MTCT can progress rapidly and present in the first few months of life with failure to thrive or severe malnutrition, diarrhea, persistent or recurrent oral candidiasis, or with *Pneumocystis jiroveci* (previously *P. carinii*) pneumonia (still called PCP).[4–10] The classic presentation of PCP is with non-productive cough, fever, tachypnea, and dyspnea, increasing in severity over a period of 2–3 weeks.[11] Oxygen saturation is often low, but cyanosis is a late sign. Children with PCP sometimes have a more fulminant presentation.[11]

A minority of perinatally HIV-infected children are so-called slow progressors and may remain asymptomatic for years.[4] Slow progressors may present with lymphoid interstitial pneumonitis (LIP), persistent or recurrent oral candidiasis, neurologic signs due to HIV encephalopathy, or with opportunist infections, which are considered to be AIDS-defining illnesses, such as PCP, esophageal candidiasis, chronic or disseminated infections secondary to CMV, HSV, or VZV, tuberculosis (TB), atypical mycobacterial infections, chronic diarrhea due to *Cryptosporidium* or other intestinal parasites, and rarely with cerebral toxoplasmosis or cryptococcosis.[4–10] Children who are perinatally infected despite receiving antiretroviral therapy progress slower than untreated children.[12] Children with LIP may also develop hepatosplenomegaly, generalized lymphadenopathy, bilateral parotitis, and finger clubbing.[7] This presentation can be difficult to distinguish from TB and also from disseminated Kaposi sarcoma, both of which occur in association with childhood HIV infection in Africa.[7,13] Other common presenting features in HIV-infected children in Africa are chronic fever, recurrent pneumonia, and chronic dermatitis.[7] TB, including neonatal TB and miliary TB in older children, is common in HIV-infected children in many developing countries.[4,7,13]

It is relatively rare for HIV-infected children to develop malignancy. Tumors represent about 2% of the AIDS-defining events in children in the USA, most commonly non-Hodgkin lymphoma and smooth muscle tumors, although the incidence of Burkitt lymphoma is also increased in HIV infection.[14,15] In Africa, children may present with dark lesions of the palate, gums, and skin and with lymphadenopathy and hepatosplenomegaly due to Kaposi sarcoma,[15] and this clinical picture may be difficult to distinguish from TB.

HIV-infected persons started on highly active antiretroviral therapy (HAART) may develop exacerbations of preexisting chronic infections as a consequence of restoration of the immune response. These diseases are called immune reconstitution syndrome (IRS) or immune reconstitution inflammatory syndrome or immune restoration diseases. They have been described mainly in adults. In Thailand, 19% of children developed immune reconstitution diseases over a median of 4 weeks (range 2–31) after starting HAART.[16] Mycobacterial infections, due to *Mycobacterium tuberculosis*, BCG, or atypical mycobacterial infection, were the commonest diseases and presented with discharging lymph nodes, skin abscesses, or pulmonary infection.[16,17] Other manifestations of IRS in these children were classic zoster, HSV infections (mostly herpes labialis but one child had HSV encephalitis), and recurrence of cryptococcal meningitis.[16] IRS is being increasingly reported in children in industrialized countries.[1–3]

8.2 Diagnosis of HIV infection in babies and children

There are various tests that are or have been used to diagnose HIV infection (see Table 8.1).

Question | For a baby or child with suspected HIV infection, which tests are sensitive and specific enough to be used to make a reliable diagnosis of HIV infection?
Literature review | We found a non-Cochrane meta-analysis comparing viral culture with antigen detection and clinical examination.[8] We found 32 studies and a non-Cochrane meta-analysis of polymerase chain reaction (PCR) testing in infants and children.[24] We found 5 studies comparing DNA PCR with RNA PCR.

HIV viral antigen

In the early days of testing for HIV infection in babies, HIV antigen detection was used as a rapid diagnostic assay when culture was unavailable or too slow and antibodies were likely to be maternal. The most useful antigen was the viral capsid protein antigen, p24. However, the test is not as sensitive as viral culture and has been superseded by molecular techniques.[8]

Viral culture

In the first 6 months of life, viral culture is more sensitive for detecting HIV infection than physical examination, serum immunoglobulin determination, or HIV p24 antigen determination.[8,18] Viral culture is slow and expensive and PCR techniques have made viral culture less essential. Viral culture is still useful for determining sensitivities to antiretrovirals and for serotyping HIV, so we recommend performing viral culture if virus is detected by PCR.

HIV IgG antibodies

Serum IgG antibodies specific to HIV are present in all HIV-infected persons. The only exceptions are immunocompromised persons who become so hypogammaglobulinemic that they have lost HIV antibodies and acutely infected subjects in the "window period" before they mount an immune response. For a child over 18 months old with suspected HIV infection, an HIV ELISA is the recommended test of choice to screen cheaply for HIV infection.[1–3,8] If the ELISA is positive and there is sufficient serum left, the laboratory will repeat the ELISA and perform a Western blot assay to

Table 8.1 Tests for HIV infection.

Category	Test	Comment
HIV antigen	Serum HIV p24 antigen	No longer used due to low sensitivity[8]
Virus	HIV viral culture	Sensitive, but slow and costly
HIV IgG antibodies	ELISA test, confirmed with Western blot assay	Transplacentally acquired maternal IgG antibody persists for up to 18 months
HIV IgM antibodies	ELISA test	Unreliable and not commercially available[8]
HIV DNA	HIV DNA PCR	Sensitive and specific test for diagnosing HIV infection in child < 18 months old[18–23]
HIV RNA	HIV RNA PCR	Recent papers suggest at least as sensitive as DNA PCR[8]

look for antibodies to different HIV antigens. Transplacentally acquired maternal IgG antibody persists for up to 18 months, and so detecting HIV IgG antibodies in a child <18 months old does not distinguish an HIV-infected from an uninfected child.[1–3,8]

HIV IgM antibodies

Attempts to develop serum IgM assays for HIV have been unsuccessful, and there is no reliable commercial HIV IgM test available.

PCR tests for diagnosis of HIV

A meta-analysis of 32 studies on PCR testing of infants and children[24] found that the median sensitivity for diagnosing HIV infection was 91.6% (range 31–100%) and the median specificity was 100% (range 50–100%). The joint sensitivity and specificity was significantly higher in older infants (98.2%) than in neonates (93.3%). When there was a low risk of perinatal transmission (probability of transmission 8.3%), the positive predictive value for PCR was 55.8% in neonates (so almost half of the positive PCR tests were false positives) and 83.2% in older infants. A negative PCR result reduced the probability of HIV infection to less than 3%.

HIV DNA PCR

DNA PCR identifies 25–45% of HIV-infected babies in the first week of life, rising to over 90% by 14 days of age, and 95–100% by 2 months old.[18–23] The sensitivity is high, 95–100%, although specificity may be decreased by false positives due to contamination.[18–23] HIV DNA is more sensitive than HIV viral culture,[18] as well as easier and cheaper to perform.

HIV RNA PCR

RNA PCR can be used as a qualitative test (detected or not detected) or as a quantitative test (how much RNA is detected). Like DNA PCR, RNA PCR is highly sensitive and specific. The term "quantitative RNA PCR" means the same as "viral load." The sensitivity of RNA PCR for detecting HIV infection is 29–47% in the first week, rising to 78% at 8–28 days, and 95–100% by 2 months old.[20–23,25–27]

We found five studies comparing sensitivity and specificity of DNA PCR and RNA PCR.[21–23,25,26] One study reported no difference,[26] while the others reported marginally better sensitivity in the first week of life for RNA PCR compared with DNA PCR, but no difference thereafter.[21–23,25]

PCR techniques are sensitive and specific, quick, and relatively cheap.[8] Although they are the best available tests for diagnosis of HIV infection in neonates and infants, the results are not definitive and should be interpreted with the aid of careful clinical follow-up examinations.

We recommend using either RNA PCR or DNA PCR to diagnose HIV infection in the first 18 months of life. After 18 months, we recommend HIV antibody testing by ELISA, confirmed by Western blot and PCR.

8.3 Antiretroviral therapy

When to start HAART

HAART has been associated with a significant fall in mortality from HIV infection, in rate of progression to AIDS,[28,29] and in incidence of opportunist infections.[30] There is no controversy that a child with AIDS should be started on HAART if it is available.[1–3] However, there are issues of adherence, adverse effects of HAART, and drug interactions. There is no good evidence that starting all asymptomatic HIV-infected children on HAART improves survival, and there is at least a theoretical risk that starting HAART earlier might increase the risk of selecting for resistant HIV strains.

In a non-Cochrane meta-analysis of 3941 children from Europe and the USA, CD4 T-cell percentage (CD4%) was found to be more reliable than viral load in predicting death or progression to AIDS.[31] CD4% was more reliable than absolute CD4 count in younger children. The risk of death increased sharply when CD4% was less than about 10%. The risk of AIDS increased when CD4 was <15%. The risk of progression increased when viral load exceeded about 10^5 copies/mL, although this association was more gradual compared with CD4%.

In another non-Cochrane meta-analysis, CD4 count was a more reliable predictor of outcome than CD4% or viral load.[32] The estimated risk of disease progression in children older than 4 or 5 years increased sharply when the CD4 cell count fell below 200–300 cells/μL. As with other immunologic markers, CD4 cell count was less prognostic in younger children.[32]

We conclude that for asymptomatic HIV-infected children >4 years old, it is reasonable not to start HAART unless the child develops a significant

opportunist infection or an AIDS-defining illness or until the CD4 count falls rapidly or falls below 300 cells/μL, or CD4% falls below 15%.

Before effective antiretroviral therapy was available, about 20% of infants in industrialized countries developed AIDS and 10% died within the first year of life.[33–36] HAART has been associated with a significant fall in mortality in HIV-infected infants.[37–39] HIV-1 RNA and CD4 count and percentage are poor predictors of disease progression and of death during infancy,[31,32,37] which makes it more difficult to predict outcome for infants. There is some controversy whether or not all asymptomatic perinatally infected infants should be started immediately on antiretroviral therapy, for the same concerns expressed for older asymptomatic children.[37] A French group has reported encephalopathy in untreated but not in treated infants.[38] Treated infants in the French and in an American population-based cohort,[39] but not in the British cohort,[37] were reported to be less likely to progress to AIDS. Currently, most authorities recommend considering starting antiretroviral therapy for all infected children in the first year of life. We feel the evidence is not conclusive and are unable to make a firm recommendation.

Antiretroviral therapy

There are three major classes of antiretrovirals:
· The nucleoside or nucleotide analogue reverse transcriptase inhibitors (NRTIs) contain a molecule such as thymidine that mimics a nucleotide or nucleoside and thus inhibits the activity of the HIV reverse transcriptase enzyme necessary for HIV replication.
· The non-nucleoside reverse transcriptase inhibitors (NNRTIs) act in different ways from NRTIs, but also block reverse transcriptase.
· The protease inhibitors (PIs) act on the protease enzyme of HIV. A boosted PI is one used with a small dose of the PI ritonavir, resulting in a far higher concentration of the active drug.[40–42]
Other active drugs include the fusion inhibitors (FIs) such as enfuvirtide that prevent infection by blocking fusion of HIV to the CD4 T lymphocyte.

Integrase inhibitors are currently in development.

Fixed drug combinations of two antiretroviral drugs in one tablet are increasingly available. Examples are zidovudine+lamivudine, lamivudine+abacavir, and emcitrabine+tenofovir. They may improve adherence, but allow less flexibility in dosing for children.

The antiretroviral drugs commonly used in children are shown in Table 8.2.

The recommended doses of antiretrovirals are sometimes expressed by weight (dose/kg) and sometimes by surface area (dose/m^2). This reflects the sad lack of pharmacokinetic data in children. Because recommendations change frequently, we have not given doses but advise consulting one of the regularly updated Web sites.[1–3] In addition, the Web site should be consulted for adverse drug reactions associated with each drug. We recommend that antiretrovirals should not be started or changed without expert consultation.

Antiretroviral drugs and drug interactions
The PIs and NNRTIs inhibit or induce the cytochrome P450 enzymes and interact with many other drugs. For example, rifampin (rifampicin) should not be used with any of the NNRTIs or PIs except efavirenz.

A comprehensive, up-to-date interaction Web site maintained by the University of Liverpool (UK) can be found at www.hiv-druginteractions.org/.

Antiretroviral combinations

Question | For HIV-infected children being treated with antiretroviral therapy, are three or four antiretroviral drugs more effective than one or two?
Literature review | We found three studies and a Cochrane review.[43]

A Cochrane review compared HIV maintenance regimens using three or four antiretrovirals with regimens using fewer drugs.[43] Four trials were identified including three published studies and one abstract, all in adults. Compared to three- or four-drug maintenance therapy, maintenance therapies including fewer drugs were associated with a higher risk of virologic failure (loss of HIV suppression to non-detectable levels). Combining the results of all four studies yielded an OR for treatment failure of 5.6 (95% CI 3.1–9.8).[41] Maintenance regimens of zidovudine and lamivudine compared to maintenance regimens with zidovudine, lamivudine, and indinavir were associated with significantly higher rates of virologic failure. Similarly, maintenance regimens that discontinued one or more PI after including them in induction therapy were also

Table 8.2 Antiretroviral drugs used in children.

Class of Drug	Examples	Toxicity (Class Effect)
NRTI	Abacavir (ABC)* Didanosine (ddl) Emcitrabine (FTC) Lamivudine (3TC) Stavudine (d4T) Tenofovir (TDF) Zalcitabine (ddC) Zidovudine (AZT, ZDV)	Class effect: lactic acidosis, hepatic steatosis, lipodystrophy
NNRTI	Efavirenz (EFV) Nevirapine (NVP)	Class effect: rash (including Stevens–Johnson syndrome), abnormal liver function, fever
PI	Nelfinavir (NFV)	Class effect: lipodystrophy (abnormal fat accumulation with central obesity, breast enlargement, buffalo hump or lipoatrophy (fat wasting in limbs and face), hyperglycemia, hyperlipidemia, abnormal liver function
Boosted PI	Atazanavir/ritonavir Saquinavir/lopinavir/ritonavir Tipranovir/ritonavir	Class effect: lipodystrophy (abnormal fat accumulation with central obesity, breast enlargement, buffalo hump or lipoatrophy (fat wasting in limbs and face), hyperglycemia, hyperlipidemia, abnormal liver function
FI	Enfuvirtide (T20)	Injection site reactions, hypersensitivity, increased incidence of bacterial pneumonia

*Potentially fatal hypersensitivity reactions develop in first 6 weeks in 5% of children on abacavir: fever, fatigue, malaise, nausea, vomiting, diarrhea, abdominal pain, dyspnea: *stop drug* and *do not reintroduce*.

associated with a significantly higher risk of virologic failure.[43]

The usual combination for initial antiretroviral therapy is:

Two NRTIs plus one NNRTI OR
Two NRTIs plus one boosted PI

The choice of when to start antiretroviral therapy (see p. 104) and which antiretroviral drugs to use is complex and we strongly recommend expert input.

8.4 Prophylaxis against PCP

Co-trimoxazole (trimethoprim-sulfamethoxazole, TMP-SMX) is effective chemoprophylaxis against pneumonia due to *P. jiroveci* (PCP) in immunocompromised persons when given daily[44] or thrice weekly.[45] A Cochrane review[46] found only one RCT of TMP-SMX prophylaxis in HIV-infected children in Zambia.[47] The study showed a 33% reduction in mortality in children given prophylaxis.[47] African adults given co-trimoxazole have similar reductions in mortality.[48] We found no RCTs in industrialized countries.

HIV-infected children who are significantly immunocompromised are at highest risk of PCP, and TMP-SMX prophylaxis is indicated. The current recommendations state that these are children aged 1–5 years old with CD4 counts <500 cells/μL (<500 × 10^9 cells/L) or children >5 years old with CD4 counts <200 cells/μL (<200 × 10^9 cells/L).[49,50] The current US guidelines also recommend giving TMP-SMX to all HIV-exposed babies aged 4 weeks to 4 months and to babies aged 4–12 months with indeterminate status.[49] Because of the very low risk of transmission (<1%) when MTCT prevention measures have been taken (see Section 8.8, p. 108), this policy will expose a large number of children to TMP-SMX for little return.

The sensitivity of PCR tests is so high that we recommend stopping TMP-SMX prophylaxis at 3 months if an exposed baby is well and all tests including PCR tests are consistently negative.

In contrast, breast-fed babies in developing countries are at ongoing risk of catching HIV from breast milk, and the WHO recommends they are given

TMP-SMX prophylaxis from 6 weeks of age while they are still breast-feeding.[51]

> **We recommend giving all perinatally exposed children in developing countries co-trimoxazole (TMP-SMX) prophylaxis until they stop breast-feeding and are documented to be HIV negative.**

8.5 Immunization of HIV-infected children

Children with HIV infection who are immunocompromised will not mount as good an immune response to immunization (reduced T-helper cells leading to reduced cell-mediated immunity and reduced antibody production).[52–54] In addition, they may be at risk of disseminated disease from live viral vaccines, such as measles vaccine, or from live bacterial vaccines, such as BCG. Indeed, there has been a case report of an adult with HIV who died from pneumonitis due to measles vaccine,[55] and rare but potentially fatal cases of disseminated atypical mycobacterial disease (BCGosis) with BCG vaccine.[24,56] Varicella vaccine is safe and immunogenic in HIV-infected children who are not immunocompromised.[57]

Vaccine recommendations vary with the child's immune status and also with the child's country of origin, which determines risk of exposure. Our current recommendations are given in Table 8.3.

8.6 Treating opportunist infections

The treatment of opportunist infections is dealt with in different chapters in this book. Expert recommendations on managing opportunist infections in children are available from Centers for Disease Control and Prevention (CDC)[58] and in guidelines.[1–3]

8.7 Additional management issues for HIV-infected children and adolescents

There are many other management issues, in addition to giving antiretroviral drugs and monitoring for toxicity.[59] These include to:

- counsel the child and the parents about the disease and the treatment;
- screen family members and contacts for infection, after counseling, and as appropriate;
- provide patient support and educational interventions (found by a Cochrane review[39] to improve adherence to antiretroviral therapy);
- deal with ongoing psychosocial issues for the child and family;
- deal with school issues;
- educate adolescents about condom use (found by a Cochrane review[60] to reduce heterosexual transmission of HIV by 80%).

Table 8.3 Recommendations on immunization of HIV-infected children.

Vaccine	Industrialized Country, Asymptomatic	Industrialized Country, Symptomatic	Developing Country
BCG	No	No	Yes, at birth
DTP	Yes	Yes	Yes
Hepatitis A	Yes	Yes	Not usually available
Hepatitis B	Yes	Yes	Yes
Hib	Yes	Yes	Yes, if available
Influenza (inactivated)	Yes	Yes	Yes, but not usually available
Measles or MMR	Yes	Yes, unless severely immunocompromised*	Yes
Meningococcal	Yes	Yes	Yes, if available
Pneumococcal	Yes	Yes	Yes, if available
Polio vaccine	IPV	IPV	OPV
Varicella	Yes[57]	No	Not usually available

*Defined as CD4 count <750 cells/μL if <12 months, <500 aged 1–5 years, <200 aged >5 years.
Modified from References 52–54.

8.8 Prevention of MTCT of HIV infection

The risk of MTCT of HIV infection in the era before the use of antiretrovirals and other interventions to reduce transmission ranged from 13% in Europe[61] to 45% in Africa.[62] With the advent of maternal screening, HAART, bottle feeding, and caesarean section, the rate of transmission has fallen to <1% in industrialized countries.[63,64]

Question | For pregnant women with HIV infection, does giving antiretrovirals to mother and/or baby compared with no treatment reduce MTCT of HIV infection? What is the most effective regimen? For pregnant women with HIV infection, does caesarean section compared to normal vaginal delivery reduce the risk further? For babies born to HIV-infected mothers, does bottle feeding compared to breast-feeding reduce the risk of HIV infection?

Literature review | We found a Cochrane systematic review[65] and a more recent Clinical Evidence review[66] of interventions to reduce MTCT of HIV. We found 15 RCTs on the use of antiretrovirals. We found 1 RCT on caesarean section. We found observational studies on bottle feeding.

Antiretrovirals to prevent MTCT of HIV infection

Early studies before the HAART era showed that monotherapy with zidovudine to treat mother and baby reduced MTCT of HIV infection. The seminal PACTG 076 study[67] showed that treating mother and baby with zidovudine (AZT) compared with placebo reduced the rate of MTCT from 25.5 to 8.3%. Such studies were important to show effectiveness, but the regimens have been superseded. In industrialized countries, more effective regimens using HAART to treat HIV-infected women during pregnancy have reduced the risk of transmitting HIV to the baby to <1%. In developing countries, novel cheap and effective regimens can reduce the transmission rate to <2% (see Combination regimens, below).

Zidovudine monotherapy

Based on four trials (1585 women), any zidovudine regimen giving zidovudine to mother and baby significantly reduces the risk of MTCT compared with no treatment or placebo (OR 0.46, 95% CI 0.35–0.60).[65,66] Zidovudine is also associated with a decreased risk of infant death within the first year (OR 0.57, 95% CI 0.38–0.85) and a decreased risk of maternal death (OR 0.32, 95% CI 0.16–0.66).

Nevirapine

The HIVNET 012 study of 626 women from a predominantly breast-feeding population in Uganda compared zidovudine with nevirapine.[68] Nevirapine, given to mothers as a single oral dose at the onset of labor and to infants as a single dose within 72 hours of birth, significantly reduced the incidence of HIV infection at 14–16 weeks to 15% compared to 26% with oral zidovudine given to women during labor and to their newborns for 7 days after birth (RR 0.58, 95% CI 0.40–0.83).[68]

There are some concerns about maternal hepatotoxicity from nevirapine. A case series from Ireland reported that 8 of 123 women given nevirapine as part of combination antiretroviral therapy during pregnancy developed significant hepatotoxicity, and 2 of them died from fulminant hepatitis.[69] However, large RCTs have not reported increased hepatotoxicity or mortality in mothers and babies taking nevirapine compared with other regimens.[65,70–73]

Zidovudine plus lamivudine

We found one RCT, the Petra study, that compared zidovudine+lamivudine with placebo in 1797 predominantly breast-feeding women in South Africa, Uganda, and Tanzania.[70] Antiretroviral drugs given in the antenatal period (from 36 weeks), intrapartum, and post-partum (to mother and baby for 1 week) significantly reduced the risk of HIV transmission at 6 weeks to 5.7% compared with 15.3% in controls (RR 0.37, 95% CI 0.21–0.65).

Combination regimens

The most impressive results in developing country are from Thailand.[74] In a large RCT of 1844 non-breast-feeding women, a regimen of zidovudine from 28 weeks' gestation plus a single dose of nevirapine to mothers and a single dose of nevirapine at birth followed by 1 week of zidovudine to babies reduced the transmission rate at 6 months to 2%.[74]

Recommendations on antiretrovirals for newborn babies

Recommendations on antiretroviral treatment for babies are complicated and depend on circumstances such as the mother's antiretroviral therapy, her HIV viral load, mode of delivery, and breast- or bottle feeding. Advice is available from Web sites such as the US Department of Human Health and Services Web site[2] (http://aidsinfo.nih.gov/guidelines/) and is regularly updated. If in doubt, consult a specialist.

The US recommendations[2] at the time of writing refer to four clinical scenarios. We have modified these scenarios into situations that we feel clinicians are likely to face in current practice. We have given the doses of antiretrovirals for full-term babies. For preterm babies, see below.

Scenario 1: Pregnant mother, no prior antiretroviral therapy, has detectable virus

We recommend starting the mother on HAART.

The recommendation for the baby will depend on whether or not the mother has detectable virus at delivery (see Scenarios 2 and 3).

Scenario 2: Mother in labor, already on HAART, no detectable virus

A collaborative European and US study of mothers with viral load <1000 copies/mL found that the transmission rate to babies of mothers taking antiretrovirals was 1% compared with 9.8% for mothers not taking antiretroviral treatment.[75] If the mother was treated with antiretrovirals, her newborn usually was, too.[75] For this reason, we recommend treating mothers with no detectable virus and their babies using antiretrovirals. The regimen used is debatable because of lack of data. One of the concerns is toxicity because antiretrovirals given to the mother are sometimes associated with mitochondrial damage in babies.[76] It would not be unreasonable to give three antiretrovirals, as in Scenario 4 below. However, as a balance between risk and benefit, we currently recommend only zidovudine, a drug that has been shown in a meta-analysis to halve the risk of transmission.[65] For the baby, we recommend:

zidovudine (AZT) syrup 4 mg/kg orally, 12-hourly for 6 weeks

The British HIV Association (BHIVA) guidelines,[1] however, recommend giving the baby triple therapy in this situation, based on expert opinion.

Scenario 3: Mother in labor, already on HAART, has detectable virus

This situation suggests probable resistance to antiretrovirals and/or non-adherence and is complex. We recommend seeking expert advice.

Scenario 4: Mother in labor, no prior antiretroviral therapy, has detectable virus

The optimum therapy has not been proven, but because of the high risk to the baby when mother has detectable virus at delivery and the proven efficacy of three-drug regimens,[43] we recommend giving IV zidovudine to the mother followed by treatment of the baby with:

zidovudine (AZT) syrup 4 mg/kg orally 12-hourly for 6 weeks PLUS
lamivudine (3TC) syrup 2 mg/kg orally, 12-hourly for 6 weeks PLUS
nevirapine syrup 2 mg/kg single dose orally at 48–72 hours old

The BHIVA guidelines[1] recommend 4 weeks of antiretrovirals for the baby, based on expert opinion.

Antiretroviral drug doses for preterm babies

For preterm babies >30 weeks gestation at birth (if they can tolerate oral therapy), the dose is:

zidovudine (AZT) syrup 2 mg/kg orally, 12-hourly for 2 weeks, THEN
zidovudine (AZT) syrup 2 mg/kg orally, 8-hourly for 4 weeks

For babies unable to take oral medication, zidovudine (AZT) is the only IV antiretroviral available. Change to the oral dosage as soon as one can tolerate oral feeds. We recommend:

>34 weeks gestation at birth: **zidovudine (AZT) 1.5 mg/kg IV, 6-hourly**
30–34 weeks gestation at birth: **zidovudine (AZT) 1.5 mg/kg IV, 12-hourly for 2 weeks THEN zidovudine (AZT) 1.5 mg/kg IV, 8-hourly, from 2 to 6 weeks of age**
<30 weeks gestation at birth: **zidovudine (AZT) 1.5 mg/kg IV, 12-hourly for 4 weeks THEN zidovudine (AZT) 1.5 mg/kg IV, 8-hourly, from 4 to 6 weeks of age**

There is no dose adjustment of lamivudine (3TC) or nevirapine for preterm infants.

The BHIVA guidelines[1] recommend 4 weeks of antiretrovirals for the baby, based on expert opinion.

Caesarean section

There is only one RCT comparing elective caesarean section with anticipation of vaginal delivery.[77] This European study was in the pre-HAART era and involved 436 participants. Caesarean section significantly reduced the risk of MTCT of HIV infection to 1.8% compared with 10.5% with vaginal delivery (RR 0.17, 95% CI 0.05–0.55).

Two Cochrane systematic reviews found no RCTs of caesarean section since HAART was used. They found, however, that maternal post-partum morbidity was greater with elective caesarean section than with vaginal delivery, although morbidity is greater still with emergency caesarean section.[78,79]

Post-partum morbidity rates for HIV-1-infected women have declined over time,[80] suggesting that the risk of post-partum morbidity with elective caesarean section is decreasing as the medical (antiretroviral therapy) and surgical (peripartum antibiotic prophylaxis) management of HIV-1-infected women improves.

The benefit of elective caesarean section delivery is unclear for HIV-1-infected women with less advanced or well-controlled HIV-1 disease whose risk of MTCT is extremely low (<2%). In such a setting, the short-term risk of the intervention (i.e., morbidity experienced by the mother within the first 6 weeks after delivery) may exceed the rare but important long-term benefit (prevention of HIV-1 transmission to the infant). For women with poorly controlled HIV-1 disease and/or no antiretroviral prophylaxis or treatment, the benefit of elective caesarean section generally outweighs the risk of maternal morbidity.

Obstetric management of HIV-1-infected women with a very low risk of transmission to infants, irrespective of mode of delivery, should be individualized after discussion between the woman and her obstetrician.

Breast-feeding

Most data on the risk of HIV transmission through breast-feeding come from non-randomized observational studies in developing countries. An early meta-analysis estimated that if a baby born to an HIV-infected mother was not infected at birth, there was a 14% additional risk of post-natal transmission from breast-feeding.[81] The risk for babies born to women who developed HIV infection post-partum was higher at 29%, presumably because the latter women were more viremic.[81]

A review found that the cumulative probability of late post-natal transmission was 9.3% by 18 months, and the overall risk of late post-natal transmission was 8.9 transmissions/100 child-years of breast-feeding.[82]

Early mixed bottle- and breast-feeding is associated with a fourfold increased risk of HIV transmission compared with breast-feeding alone.[83] This may be because cow's milk causes mucosal damage.

There has been only one intervention study, an RCT from Kenya in which children born to 425 HIV-infected women were randomized to breast-feeding or replacement feeding.[84,85] The results showed that 44% of infant HIV infections were acquired through breast-feeding and that most infections were acquired during the first few months of life. The cumulative probability of HIV-1 infection at 24 months was 36.7% in the breast-feeding arm and 20.5% in the formula arm ($p = 0.001$), giving an estimated rate of breast milk transmission of 16.2% (95% CI 6.5–25.9%). Most breast milk transmission occurred early, with 75% of the risk difference occurring by 6 months, although transmission continued throughout the duration of exposure. The 2-year mortality rate was similar in both arms (breast-feeding 24.4% versus formula feeding 20.0%, $p = 0.30$). At 2 years, babies in the breast-feeding arm were less likely to be free of HIV infection (58.0%) than babies in the formula feeding arm (70.0%, $p = 0.02$).[84,85] This RCT casts doubt on the WHO recommendation that women in developing countries should breast-feed because bottle feeding is more dangerous.

Although the WHO and others have traditionally recommended that women in developing countries should breast feed, because the risk of diarrheal and other diseases attributable to formula feeding outweighed the risk of contracting HIV, this rule no longer seems to be generally applicable. Current data suggest that in some African countries, the risk of breast-feeding may be greater than the risk of formula feeding.[83–86] An alternative which is being investigated in some countries[87] is to use pasteurized (heat-treated) expressed breast milk to feed babies, but it seems unlikely that this will be practical in resource-poor settings.

In industrialized countries, HIV-infected women should be advised to feed their babies with formula and not to breast feed.

8.9 Post-exposure prophylaxis against HIV infection

Post-exposure prophylaxis against HIV infection should be considered following exposure to a person known to be HIV-infected or when the person may be HIV-infected but their HIV status is unknown. The common routes of exposure are from needlestick injuries in health care or associated with IV drug-using equipment, sexual exposure, or breast milk.

Question | For persons exposed to HIV infection, does antiretroviral therapy compared with no treatment or placebo reduce the risk of acquiring HIV infection?

Literature review | We found a non-Cochrane systematic review of the risk of infection following parenteral exposure to HIV.[88] We found a non-Cochrane systematic review of post-exposure prophylaxis for non-occupational exposure to HIV.[89] We found guidelines on post-exposure prophylaxis for adults[90,91] and children.[89]

A review of post-exposure prophylaxis found no RCTs.[89] A case-control study from the USA and Europe evaluated 33 health-care workers who acquired HIV infection after occupational exposure and 679 controls who did not acquire HIV infection after 6 months follow-up despite occupational exposure.[92] After adjustment for confounding factors, people who had acquired HIV infection were less likely to have taken post-exposure prophylaxis with zidovudine than the controls who had not acquired HIV (adjusted OR 0.19, 95% CI 0.06–0.52, $p = 0.003$).

We found no controlled studies of post-exposure prophylaxis using combinations of antiretrovirals and no studies of the efficacy of post-exposure prophylaxis in the community outside the health-care setting.

Zidovudine prophylaxis is associated with adverse events such as fatigue, nausea, vomiting, and gastrointestinal discomfort in 50–75% of health-care workers and about 30% of them stop taking post-exposure prophylaxis.[92] The frequency of reported adverse ef-

Table 8.4 Estimate risk of HIV infection following single exposure.

Nature of Exposure	Risk of Acquiring HIV
Needlestick from HIV-infected patient[88]	0.23% (95% CI 0–0.46%)
Needlestick injury from discarded needle or syringe from IV drug user[89]	No cases of transmission reported
Sexual: unprotected anal[89]	0.5–3.2%
Sexual: receptive vaginal[89]	0.05–0.15%
Sexual: insertive vaginal[89]	0.03–0.09%
Breast milk[89]	0.001–0.004%

fects (50–90%) is higher in people taking a combination of antiretroviral drugs, so multidrug prophylaxis might reduce adherence to post-exposure prophylaxis.[93] Adverse effects are rarely severe or serious, and even severe adverse events are transient.[93]

Risk of acquiring HIV from exposure

A systematic review of transmission risks quantified the risk of acquiring HIV, which varies according to the nature of the exposure.[89] The results are summarized in Table 8.4.

General principles of post-exposure prophylaxis against HIV

The decision on whether or not to recommend post-exposure prophylaxis will depend on factors such as risk and probable adherence. In the absence of data on efficacy outside of the health-care setting, the decision is best made by experienced clinicians in collaboration with the exposed person and/or parents after a careful discussion of the risks of transmission and the burden and potential complications of antiretroviral therapy.[91]

Some authorities recommend using three drugs for high-risk exposures and fewer for exposures defined as low risk.[94] Others recommend consideration of a two-drug regimen (AZT+3-TC) if it is likely to improve compliance. If it is decided to start prophylaxis, it is recommended to start as soon as possible and continue for 4 weeks.[91,94] Prophylaxis is not usually recommended >72 hours after exposure, unless the risk is very high.[91,94]

Children exposed to HIV may also have been exposed to other blood-borne viruses such as HBV and HCV, in which case they should have prophylaxis against HBV infection (see p. 93) and counseling about risk and follow-up.

If the source is found to be HIV antibody negative, and unlikely to be in the window period between infection and seroconversion, no further follow-up testing is required for the source or child. In all other circumstances, the child should have follow-up HIV antibody testing, usually at 6 weeks, 3 months, and 6 months, together with tests for other blood-borne viruses such as HBV and HCV as indicated.[91,94]

Post-exposure prophylaxis regimen

If it is decided to give post-exposure prophylaxis, we recommend:

lamivudine 4 mg/kg (max 150 mg) AND zidovudine 8 mg/kg (max 300 mg) orally, 12-hourly for 4 weeks or until source shown to be HIV negative PLUS EITHER lopinavir 300 mg/m^2 (max 400 mg) AND ritonavir 75 mg/m^2 (max 100 mg) orally, 12-hourly (Kaletra) for 4 weeks or until source shown to be HIV negative OR nelfinavir <13 years: 55 mg/kg (max 2 g) orally, 12-hourly; >12 years: 1250 mg orally, 12-hourly for 4 weeks or until source shown to be HIV negative

Needlestick exposure to HIV (percutaneous injury)

Needlestick exposure to HIV occurs most commonly from health-care exposure or from discarded IV drug-using equipment. The risks are extremely different.

Exposure to needlestick in health-care setting

A systematic review found 22 studies of needlestick exposure where the source was known to be HIV-infected.[88] The mean risk from contaminated needlestick injury was 0.23% (95% CI 0–0.46%) or 1 in 435 needlestick injuries,[88] although the estimates ranged from 0 to 2.38%.

Exposure to needlestick in community

Needlestick injuries in the community usually occur when a child handles or steps on a needle and syringe in the park or on a beach. The risk is almost certainly far lower than with health-care exposures, but has not been quantified.

HIV is very susceptible to drying. In the laboratory setting, HIV can survive for up to 28 days in syringes containing as little as 20 μL of blood.[95] On the other hand, when HIV is placed on a surface exposed to air, the 50% tissue culture infective dose decreases by about 6 logs in 72 hours (1 log every 9 h).[96]

No HIV proviral DNA could be detected in 28 syringes discarded in public places and 10 syringes from a needle exchange program for injection drug users.[97] We found that over 300 children have been followed up after community needlestick exposures from discarded needles and syringes and none have acquired HIV infection.[98–101] We calculated that the 95% CI for the risk of transmission is 0–1%. There have been no confirmed reports of HIV acquisition from percutaneous injury by a needle found in the community.[89]

Parents are understandably upset after an accidental needlestick exposure, and reassurance about the low risk is paramount. We counsel against post-exposure prophylaxis with antiretrovirals in this setting, although we would be guided by the parents if they wanted prophylaxis despite the low risk. We advise to make sure always that the child is protected against hepatitis B virus infection (see p. 93).

Sexual exposure to HIV

The risks of HIV infection from sexual exposure have been explored in a number of studies[102–107] and are given in Table 8.4. The risk varies according to the nature of the sexual act. HIV infection has been described following oral sex,[108] but the risk from a single episode is unknown and presumably very low. Decisions about whether or not to initiate post-exposure prophylaxis after sexual abuse or rape will need to take into account the risk of HIV infection (see Table 8.4), the potential harms of antiretroviral therapy, and the likelihood of adherence.[89]

Accidental ingestion of breast milk

It is not uncommon that a baby is accidentally given breast milk expressed by another mother. The risk is extremely low, even if the breast milk is from an

HIV-infected woman[89] (see Table 8.4). There are no reports of HIV transmission to a person handling human milk in a nursery from a single episode of exposure to HIV-infected human milk, or to an infant from a single enteral exposure to HIV-infected human milk.[89]

We do not recommend antiretroviral prophylaxis for accidental ingestion of breast milk, but the risks and benefits of antiretrovirals should be considered and discussed with the baby's parents.

8.10 Useful Web sites on HIV infection

British HIV Association (BHIVA) Web site includes guidelines on the management of HIV infection: http://www.bhiva.org/

US Department of Human Health and Services Web site includes guidelines on the management of HIV infection: http://aidsinfo.nih.gov/guidelines/

Australasian Society for HIV Medicine Web site includes guidelines on the management of HIV infection: http://www.ashm.org.au/

References

1 British HIV Association (BHIVA). Guidelines on the management of HIV infection. Available at http://www.bhiva.org/.

2 US Department of Human Health and Services. Guidelines on the management of HIV infection. Available at http://aidsinfo.nih.gov/guidelines/.

3 Australasian Society for HIV Medicine. Guidelines on the management of HIV infection. Available at http://www.ashm.org.au/.

4 Chearskul S, Chotpitayasunondh T, Simonds RJ et al. Survival, disease manifestations, and early predictors of disease progression among children with perinatal human immunodeficiency virus infection in Thailand. *Pediatrics* 2002;110:e25.

5 Morris CR, Araba-Owoyele L, Spector SA, Maldonado YA. Disease patterns and survival after acquired immunodeficiency syndrome diagnosis in human immunodeficiency virus-infected children. *Pediatr Infect Dis J* 1996;15:321–8.

6 Bamji M, Thea DM, Weedon J et al., for the New York City Perinatal HIV Transmission Collaborative Study Group. Prospective study of human immunodeficiency virus 1-related disease among 512 infants born to infected women in New York City. *Pediatr Infect Dis J* 1996;15:891–8.

7 Spira R, Lepage P, Msellati P et al., for Mother-to-Child HIV-1 Transmission Study Group. Natural history of human immunodeficiency virus type 1 infection in children: a five-year prospective study in Rwanda. *Pediatrics* 1999;104:e56.

8 Kline MW, Hollinger FB, Rosenblatt HM, Bohannon B, Kozinetz CA, Shearer WT. Sensitivity, specificity and predictive value of physical examination, culture and other laboratory studies in the diagnosis during early infancy of vertically acquired human immunodeficiency virus infection. *Pediatr Infect Dis J* 1993;12:33–6.

9 Miller TL, Easley KA, Zhang W et al. Maternal and infant factors associated with failure to thrive in children with vertically transmitted human immunodeficiency virus-1 infection: the prospective, P2C2 human immunodeficiency virus multicenter study. *Pediatrics* 2001;108:1287–96.

10 Ciuta ST, Boros S, Napoli PA, Pezzotti P, Rezza G. Predictors of survival in children with acquired immunodeficiency syndrome in Italy, 1983 to 1995. *AIDS Patient Care STDS* 1998;12:629–37.

11 Graham SM. Non-tuberculosis opportunistic infections and other lung diseases in HIV-infected infants and children. *Int J Tuberc Lung Dis* 2005;9:592–602.

12 Berk DR, Falkovitz-Halpern MS, Sullivan B, Ruiz J, Maldonado YA. Disease progression among HIV-infected children who receive perinatal zidovudine prophylaxis. *J Acquir Immune Defic Syndr* 2007;44:106–11.

13 Zar HJ. Pneumonia in HIV-infected and HIV-uninfected children in developing countries: epidemiology, clinical features, and management. *Curr Opin Pulm Med* 2004;10:176–82.

14 Mueller BU. Cancers in children infected with the human immunodeficiency virus. *Oncologist* 1999;4:309–17.

15 Orem J, Otieno MW, Remick SC. AIDS-associated cancer in developing nations. *Curr Opin Oncol* 2004;16:468–76.

16 Puthanakit T, Oberdorfer P, Akarathum N, Wannarit P, Sirisanthana T, Sirisanthana V. Immune reconstitution syndrome after highly active antiretroviral therapy in human immunodeficiency virus-infected Thai children. *Pediatr Infect Dis J* 2006;25:53–8.

17 Puthanakit T, Oberdorfer P, Punjaisee S, Wannarit P, Sirisanthana T, Sirisanthana V. Immune reconstitution syndrome due to bacillus Calmette-Guerin after initiation of antiretroviral therapy in children with HIV infection. *Clin Infect Dis* 2005;41:1049–52.

18 McIntosh K, Pitt J, Brambilla D et al., for the Women and Infants Transmission Study Group. Blood culture in the first 6 months of life for the diagnosis of vertically transmitted human immunodeficiency virus infection. *J Infect Dis* 1994;170:996–1000.

19 Bremer JW, Lew JF, Cooper E et al. Diagnosis of infection with human immunodeficiency virus type 1 by a DNA polymerase chain reaction assay among infants enrolled in the Women and Infants' Transmission Study. *J Pediatr* 1996;129:198–207.

20 Dunn DT, Brandt CD, Krivine A et al. The sensitivity of HIV-1 DNA polymerase chain reaction in the neonatal period and the relative contributions of intra-uterine and intra-partum transmission. *AIDS* 1995;9:F7–11.

21 Kovacs A, Xu J, Rasheed S et al. Comparison of a rapid non-isotopic polymerase chain reaction assay with four commonly used methods for the early diagnosis of human

immunodeficiency virus type 1 infection in neonates and children. *Pediatr Infect Dis J* 1995;14:948–54.

22 Steketee RW, Abrams EJ, Thea DM et al, for the New York City Perinatal HIV Transmission Collaborative Study Group. Early detection of perinatal human immunodeficiency virus (HIV) type 1 infection using HIV RNA amplification and detection. *J Infect Dis* 1997;175:707–11.

23 Cunningham CK, Charbonneau TT, Song K et al. Comparison of human immunodeficiency virus 1 DNA polymerase chain reaction and qualitative and quantitative RNA polymerase chain reaction in human immunodeficiency virus 1-exposed infants. *Pediatr Infect Dis J* 1999;18:30–5.

24 Owens DK, Holodniy M, McDonald TW, Scott J, Sonnad S. A meta-analytic evaluation of the polymerase chain reaction for the diagnosis of HIV infection in infants. *JAMA* 1996;275:1342–8.

25 Young NL, Shaffer N, Chaowanachan T et al. Early diagnosis of HIV-1-infected infants in Thailand using RNA and DNA PCR assays sensitive to non-B sub-types. *J Acquir Immune Defic Syndr* 2000;24:401–7.

26 Nesheim S, Palumbo P, Sullivan K et al. Quantitative RNA testing for diagnosis of HIV-infected infants. *J Acquir Immune Defic Syndr* 2003;32:192–5.

27 Simonds RJ, Brown TM, Thea DM et al., for Perinatal AIDS Collaborative Transmission Study. Sensitivity and specificity of a qualitative RNA detection assay to diagnose HIV infection in young infants. *AIDS* 1998;12:1545–9.

28 Gortmaker SL, Hughes M, Cervia J et al. Effect of combination therapy including protease inhibitors on mortality among children and adolescents infected with HIV-1. *N Engl J Med* 2001;345:1522–8.

29 Gibb DM, Duong T, Tookey PA et al. Decline in mortality, AIDS, and hospital admissions in perinatally HIV-1 infected children in the United Kingdom and Ireland. *BMJ* 2003;327:1019–25.

30 Gona P, Van Dyke RB, Williams PL et al. Incidence of opportunistic and other infections in HIV-infected children in the HAART era. *JAMA* 2006;296:292–300.

31 Dunn D, for the HIV Paediatric Prognostic Markers Collaborative Study Group. Short-term risk of disease progression in HIV-1-infected children receiving no antiretroviral therapy or zidovudine monotherapy: a meta-analysis. *Lancet* 2003;362:1605–11.

32 HIV Paediatric Prognostic Markers Collaborative Study. Predictive value of absolute CD4 cell count for disease progression in untreated HIV-1-infected children. *AIDS* 2006;20:1289–94.

33 Walker AS, Doerholt K, Sharland M, Gibb DM, for the Collaborative HIV Paediatric Study (CHIPS) Steering Committee. Response to highly active antiretroviral therapy varies with age: the UK and Ireland Collaborative HIV Paediatric Study. *AIDS* 2004;18:1915–24.

34 The European Collaborative Study. Natural history of vertically acquired human immunodeficiency virus-1 infection. *Pediatrics* 1994;94:815–9.

35 Blanche S, Newell ML, Mayaux MJ et al., for the French Pediatric HIV Infection Study Group and European Collaborative Study Group. Morbidity and mortality in European children vertically infected by HIV-1. *J Acquir Immune Defic Syndr Hum Retrovirol* 1997;14:442–50.

36 The Italian register for HIV Infection in Children. Rapid disease progression in HIV-1 perinatally infected children born to mothers receiving zidovudine monotherapy during pregnancy. *AIDS* 1999;13:927–33.

37 Doerholt K, Duong T, Tookey P et al. Outcomes for human immunodeficiency virus-1-infected infants in the United kingdom and Republic of Ireland in the era of effective antiretroviral therapy. *Pediatr Infect Dis J* 2006;25:420–6.

38 Faye A, Le Chenadec J, Dollfus C et al. Early versus deferred antiretroviral multidrug therapy in infants infected with HIV type 1. *Clin Infect Dis* 2004;39:1692–8.

39 Berk DR, Falkovitz-Halpern MS, Hill DW et al., for the California Pediatric HIV Study Group. Temporal trends in early clinical manifestations of perinatal HIV infection in a population-based cohort. *JAMA* 2005;11:2221–31.

40 Walmsley S, Bernstein B, King M et al. Lopinavir-ritonavir versus nelfinavir for the initial treatment of HIV infection. *N Engl J Med* 2002;346:2039–46.

41 Cohen C, Nieto-Cisneros L, Zala C et al. Comparison of atazanavir with lopinavir/ritonavir in patients with prior protease inhibitor failure: a randomized multinational trial. *Curr Med Res Opin* 2005;21:1683–92.

42 Ananworanich J, Kosalaraksa P, Hill A et al. Pharmacokinetics and 24-week efficacy/safety of dual boosted saquinavir/lopinavir/ritonavir in nucleoside-pretreated children. *Pediatr Infect Dis J* 2005;24:874–9.

43 Rutherford GW, Sangani PR, Kennedy GE. Three- or four-versus two-drug antiretroviral maintenance regimens for HIV infection. *The Cochrane Database of Systematic Reviews* 2003; (4): Art No CD002037.

44 Hughes WT, Kuhn S, Chaudhary S et al. Successful chemoprophylaxis for *Pneumocystis carinii* pneumonitis. *N Engl J Med* 1977;297:1419–26.

45 Hughes WT, Rivera GK, Schell MJ, Thornton D, Lott L. Successful intermittent chemoprophylaxis for *Pneumocystis carinii* pneumonitis. *N Engl J Med* 1987;316:1627–32.

46 Grimwade K, Swingler GH. Cotrimoxazole prophylaxis for opportunistic infections in children with HIV infection. *The Cochrane Database of Systematic Reviews* 2006; (1):Art No CD003508.

47 Chintu C, Bhat GJ, Walker AS et al. Cotrimoxazole as prophylaxis against opportunistic infections in HIV-infected Zambian children (CHAP): a double-blind randomised placebo-controlled trial. *Lancet* 2004;364:1865–71.

48 Grimwade K, Swingler G. Cotrimoxazole prophylaxis for opportunistic infections in adults with HIV. *The Cochrane Database of Systematic Reviews* 2003; (3):Art No CD003108.

49 Kaplan JE, Masur H, Holmes KK. Guidelines for preventing opportunistic infections among HIV-infected persons—2002. Recommendations of the US Public Health Service and the Infectious Diseases Society of America. *MMWR Recomm Rep* 2002;51(RR-8):1–52.

50 American Academy of Pediatrics. *Pneumocystis jiroveci* infections. In: Pickering LK (ed.), *Red Book: 2003 Report of the*

Committee on Infectious Diseases, 26thedn. Elk Grove Village, IL: American Academy of Pediatrics, 2003:500–5.

51 Gill CJ, Sabin LL, Tham J, Hamer DH. Reconsidering empirical cotrimoxazole prophylaxis for infants exposed to HIV infection. *Bull World Health Organ* 2004;82:290–7.

52 American Academy of Pediatrics. Human immunodeficiency virus infection. In: Pickering LK (ed.), *Red Book: 2003 Report of the Committee on Infectious Diseases*, 26th edn. Elk Grove Village, IL: American Academy of Pediatrics, 2003:360–82.

53 Moss WJ, Clements CJ, Halsey NA. Immunization of children at risk of infection with human immunodeficiency virus. *Bull World Health Organ* 2003;81:61–70.

54 Obaro SK, Pugatch D, Luzuriaga K. Immunogenicity and efficacy of childhood vaccines in HIV-1-infected children. *Lancet Infect Dis* 2004;4:510–8.

55 Centers for Disease Control and Prevention Measles. Pneumonitis following measles-mumps-rubella vaccination of a patient with HIV infection: 1993. *MMWR Morb Mortal Wkly Rep* 1996;45:603–6.

56 Hesseling AC, Rabie H, Marais BJ et al. Bacille Calmette-Guerin vaccine-induced disease in HIV-infected and HIV-uninfected children. *Clin Infect Dis* 2006;42:548–58.

57 Levin MJ, Gershon AA, Weinberg A et al. Administration of livevaricella vaccine to HIV-infected children with current or past significant depression of CD4(+) T cells. *J Infect Dis* 2006;194:247–55.

58 Benson CA, Kaplan JE, Masur H et al. Treating opportunistic infections among HIV-exposed and infected children: recommendations from CDC, the National Institutes of Health, and the Infectious Diseases Society of America. *MMWR Recomm Rep* 2004;53(RR-15):1–112.

59 Rueda S, Park-Wyllie LY, Bayoumi AM et al. Patient support and education for promoting adherence to highly active antiretroviral therapy for HIV/AIDS. *The Cochrane Database of Systematic Reviews* 2006; (3):Art No CD001442.

60 Weller SC, Davis-Beaty K. Condom effectiveness in reducing heterosexual HIV transmission. *The Cochrane Database of Systematic Reviews* 2002; (1):Art No CD003255.

61 European Collaborative Study. Children born to women with HIV-1 infection: natural history and risk of transmission. *Lancet* 1991;337:253–60.

62 The Working Group on Mother-to-Child Transmission of HIV. Rates of mother-to-child transmission of HIV-1 in Africa, America, and Europe: results from 13 perinatal studies. *J Acquir Immune Defic Syndr Hum Retrovirol* 1995;8:506–10.

63 Centers for Disease Control and Prevention (CDC). Achievements in public health. Reduction in perinatal transmission of HIV infection—United States, 1985–2005. *MMWR Morb Mortal Wkly Rep* 2006;55:592–7.

64 Gilling-Smith C, Nicopoullos JD, Semprini AE, Frodsham LC. HIV and reproductive care—a review of current practice. *BJOG* 2006;113:869–78.

65 Brocklehurst P, Volmink J. Antiretrovirals for reducing the risk of mother-to-child transmission of HIV infection. *The Cochrane Database of Systematic Reviews* 2002; (2):Art No CD003510.

66 Volmink J, Mahlati U. HIV mother to child transmission. *Clin Evid* September 1, 2005. Available at: http://www.clinicalevidence.com/ceweb/conditions/hiv/0909/0909_I1.jsp. Accessed December 31, 2006.

67 Connor EM, Sperling RS, Gelber R et al., for the Pediatric AIDS Clinical Trials Group Protocol 076 Study Group. Reduction of maternal-infant transmission of human immunodeficiency virus type 1 with zidovudine treatment. *N Engl J Med* 1994;331:1173–80.

68 Guay L, Musoke P, Fleming T et al. Intrapartum and neonatal single-dose nevirapine compared with zidovudine for prevention of mother-to-child transmission of HIV-1 in Kampala, Uganda: HIVNET 012 randomised trial. *Lancet* 1999;354:795–802.

69 Lyons F, Hopkins S, Kelleher B et al. Maternal hepatotoxicity with nevirapine as part of combination antiretroviral therapy in pregnancy. *HIV Med* 2006;7:255–60.

70 Petra Study Team. Efficacy of three short-course regimens of zidovudine and lamivudine in preventing early and late transmission of HIV-1 from mother to child in Tanzania, South Africa, and Uganda (Petra study): a randomised, double-blind, placebo-controlled trial. *Lancet* 2002;359:1178–86.

71 Moodley D, Moodley J, Coovadia H et al. A multicenter randomized controlled trial of nevirapine versus a combination of zidovudine and lamivudine to reduce intrapartum and early post-partum mother-to-child transmission of human immunodeficiency virus type 1. *J Infect Dis* 2003;187:725–35.

72 Taha TE, Kumwenda NI, Gibbons A et al. Short post-exposure prophylaxis in newborn babies to reduce mother-to-child transmission of HIV-1: NVAZ randomised clinical trial. *Lancet* 2003;362:1171–7.

73 Taha TE, Kumwenda NI, Hoover DR, et al. Nevirapine and zidovudine at birth to reduce perinatal transmission of HIV in an African setting: a randomized controlled trial. *JAMA* 2004;292:202–9.

74 Lallemant M, Jourdain G, Le Coeur S et al. Single-dose perinatal nevirapine plus standard zidovudine to prevent mother-to-child transmission of HIV-1 in Thailand. *N Engl J Med* 2004;351:217–28.

75 Ioannidis JPA, Abrams EJ, Ammann A et al. Perinatal transmission of human immunodeficiency virus type 1 by pregnant women with RNA virus loads <1000 copies/mL. *J Infect Dis* 2001;183:539–45.

76 Poirier MC, Divi RL, Al-Harthi L et al. Long-term mitochondrial toxicity in HIV-uninfected infants born to HIV-infected mothers. *J Acquir Immune Defic Syndr* 2003;33:175–83.

77 The European Mode of Delivery Collaboration. Elective Caesarean-section versus vaginal delivery in prevention of vertical HIV-1 transmission: a randomised clinical trial. *Lancet* 1999;353:1035–9.

78 Read JS, Newell ML. Efficacy and safety of cesarean delivery for prevention of mother-to-child transmission of HIV-1.

The Cochrane Database of Systematic Reviews 2005;(4):Art No CD005479.

79 Brocklehurst P. Interventions for reducing the risk of mother-to-child transmission of HIV infection. *The Cochrane Database of Systematic Reviews* 2002;(1):Art No CD000102.

80 Read JS, Tuomala R, Kpamegan E et al. Mode of delivery and post-partum morbidity among HIV-infected women: the Women and Infants Transmission study. *JAIDS* 2001;26:236–45.

81 Dunn DT, Newell ML, Ades AE, Peckham CS. Risk of human immunodeficiency virus type 1 transmission through breastfeeding. *Lancet* 1992;340:585–8.

82 Coutsoudis A, Dabis F, Fawzi W et al. Late post-natal transmission of HIV-1 in breast-fed children: an individual patient data meta-analysis. *J Infect Dis* 2004;189:2154–66.

83 Iliff PJ, Piwoz EG, Tavengwa NV et al. Early exclusive breastfeeding reduces the risk of post-natal HIV-1 transmission and increases HIV-free survival. *AIDS* 2005;19:699–708.

84 Nduati R, John G, Mbori-Ngacha D et al. Effect of breastfeeding and formula feeding on transmission of HIV-1: a randomized clinical trial. *JAMA* 2000;283:1167–74.

85 Mbori-Ngacha D, Nduati R, John G et al. Morbidity and mortality in breastfed and formula-fed infants of HIV-1-infected women: a randomized clinical trial. *JAMA* 2001;286:2413–20.

86 Coutsoudis A, Pillay K, Spooner E, Coovadia HM, Pembrey L, Newell ML. Morbidity in children born to women infected with human immunodeficiency virus in South Africa: does mode of feeding matter? *Acta Paediatr* 2003;92:890–5.

87 Israel-Ballard KA, Maternowska MC, Abrams BF et al. Acceptability of heat treating breast milk to prevent mother-to-child transmission of human immunodeficiency virus in Zimbabwe: a qualitative study. *J Hum Lact* 2006;22:48–60.

88 Baggaley RF, Boily MC, White RG, Alary M. Risk of HIV-1 transmission for parenteral exposure and blood transfusion: a systematic review and meta-analysis. *AIDS* 2006;20:805–12.

89 Havens PL, for the American Academy of Pediatrics Committee on Pediatric AIDS. Post-exposure prophylaxis in children and adolescents for non-occupational exposure to human immunodeficiency virus. *Pediatrics* 2003;111:1475–89.

90 Smith DK, Grohskopf LA, Black RJ. Antiretroviral post-exposure prophylaxis after sexual, injection-drug use, or other non-occupational exposure to HIV in the United States: recommendations from the U.S. Department of Health and Human Services. *MMWR Recomm Rep* 2005;54(RR-2): 1–20.

91 Talbot MD. HIV infection. Post-exposure prophylaxis in health care workers. *Clin Evid* April 1, 2006. Available at http://www.clinicalevidence.com/ceweb/conditions/hiv/09 02/0902_I3.jsp. Accessed December 31, 2006.

92 Cardo DM, Culver DH, Ciesielski CA et al., for the Centers for Disease Control and Prevention Needlestick Surveillance Group. A case-control study of HIV seroconversion in health care workers after percutaneous exposure. *N Engl J Med* 1997;337:1485–90.

93 Wang SA, Panlilio AL, Doi PA, White AD, Stek M, Jr, Saah A. Experience of healthcare workers taking post-exposure prophylaxis after occupational HIV exposures: findings of the HIV Post-exposure Prophylaxis Registry. *Infect Control Hosp Epidemiol* 2000;21:780–5.

94 Therapeutic Guidelines Ltd. Prophylaxis: medical. In: *Therapeutic Guidelines: Antibiotic*, 13th edn. Melbourne: Therapeutic Guidelines Ltd, 2006:176–87.

95 Abdala N, Stephens PC, Griffith BP, Heimer R. Survival of HIV-1 in syringes. *J Acquir Immune Defic Syndr Hum Retrovirol* 1999;20:73–80.

96 Resnick L, Veren K, Salahuddin SZ, Tondreau S, Markham PD. Stability and inactivation of HTLV-III/LAV under clinical and laboratory environments. *JAMA* 1986;255: 1887–91.

97 Zamora AB, Rivera MO, Garcia-Algar O, Cayla Buqueras J, Vall Combelles O, Garcia-Saiz A. Detection of infectious human immunodeficiency type 1 virus in discarded syringes of intravenous drug users. *Pediatr Infect Dis J* 1998;17: 655–7.

98 Walsh SS, Pierce AM, Hart CA. Drug abuse: a new problem. *BMJ (Clin Res Ed)* 1987;295:526–7.

99 Montella F, DiSora F, Recchia O. Can HIV-1 infection be transmitted by a "discarded" syringe? *J Acquir Immune Defic Syndr* 1992;5:1274–5.

100 Aragon Pena AJ, Arrazola Martinez MP, Garcia de Codes A, Davila Alvarez FM, de Juanes Pardo JR. [Hepatitis B prevention and risk of HIV infection in children injured by discarded needles and/or syringes]. *Aten Primaria* 1996;17:138–40.

101 Nourse CB, Charles CA, McKay M, Keenan P, Butler KM. Childhood needlestick injuries in the Dublin metropolitan area. *Ir Med J* 1997;90:66–9.

102 Katz MH, Gerberding JL. The care of persons with recent sexual exposure to HIV. *Ann Intern Med* 1998;128: 306–12.

103 Mastro TD, de Vincenzi I. Probabilities of sexual HIV-1 transmission. *AIDS* 1996;10:S75–82.

104 DeGruttola V, Seage GR, III, Mayer KH, Horsburgh CR, Jr. Infectiousness of HIV between male homosexual partners. *J Clin Epidemiol* 1989;42:849–56.

105 Wiley JA, Herschkorn SJ, Padian NS. Heterogeneity in the probability of HIV transmission per sexual contact: the case of male-to-female transmission in penile-vaginal intercourse. *Stat Med* 1989;8:93–102.

106 Peterman TA, Stoneburner RL, Allen JR, Jaffe HW, Curran JW. Risk of human immunodeficiency virus transmission from heterosexual adults with transfusion-associated infections. *JAMA* 1988;259:55–8.

107 Downs AM, DeVincenzi I. Probability of heterosexual transmission of HIV: relationship to the number of unprotected sexual contacts. *J Acquir Immune Defic Syndr Hum Retrovirol* 1996;11:388–95.

108 Keet IP, Albrecht van Lent N, Sandfort TG, Coutinho RA, van Griensven GJ. Orogenital sex and the transmission of HIV among homosexual men. *AIDS* 1992;6: 223–6.

CHAPTER 9
Immune deficiency

9.1 Febrile neutropenia

Definition of febrile neutropenia

A working definition of febrile neutropenia is fever, defined as a single oral temperature of $\geq 38.3°C$ (101°F) or a temperature of $\geq 38.0°C$ (100.4°F) for ≥ 1 hour, together with neutropenia, defined as neutrophils <500 cells/mm^3 (0.5 × 10^9 cells/L), or <1000 cells/mm^3(1 × 10^{9}cells/L) with a predicted decline to <500 cells/mm^3 (0.5 × 10^{9}cells/L).[1] In patients with febrile neutropenia, the risk of overwhelming septicemia is sufficiently high, at 20–30%,[1–3] that urgent empiric IV therapy with broad-spectrum antimicrobials is a universally accepted principle.[1–3]

Clinical features in children

A meta-analysis comparing 759 children and 2321 adults with febrile neutropenia enrolled in treatment trials looked at differences in presentation and outcome.[2] Children were more likely than adults to have acute lymphoblastic leukemia (ALL) or solid tumors undergoing intensive myelosuppressive therapy, but were less likely to have acute myeloid leukemia (AML). Children were less likely to have a defined site of infection, and had more upper respiratory tract infections but fewer lung infections than adults. There was a similar low incidence of shock at presentation in the two groups but the children's median neutrophil count was lower, and their median duration of granulocytopenia before the trial was shorter. The incidence of bacteremia was similar, but clinically documented infection was less frequent and fever of unknown origin more common in children.[2]

In general, the prognosis is better for children. In the review, the mortality from infection was only 1% in children compared with 4% in adults ($p = 0.001$), and time to defervescence was shorter in children.[2] In the younger age group, high temperature, prolonged neutropenia before the trial, and shock were prognostic

indicators for bacteremia. Solid tumor patients were significantly less likely to have bacteremia.[2]

Organisms causing febrile neutropenia in children

There has been a well-documented shift since the 1980s, when Gram-negative bacilli were the major cause of bacteremia in adult febrile neutropenic patients, to a predominance of Gram-positive organisms.[3] In a meta-analysis, published in 1997, children developed more streptococcal bacteremias and fewer staphylococcal bacteremias than adults ($p = 0.003$) but the relative incidence of Gram-negative bacillary infections was similar.[2] We found seven studies published from 2001 to 2005 that reported bloodstream isolates.[4–10] Overall, Gram-positive cocci were isolated from 65% of episodes; half of these episodes were due to staphylococci, with coagulase negative staphylococci more frequently reported than *Staphylococcus aureus*, and half were due to streptococci, mostly of the viridans group. Gram-negative bacilli were grown in 22% of episodes and fungi in 5%. Bacteremia due to *Pseudomonas aeruginosa* is relatively rare, but because mortality is high, empiric regimens usually cover this organism. These data are very similar to the data on adult patients in the USA with nosocomial bloodstream infections associated with neutropenia.[11]

The responsible organisms depend on the degree of immunosuppression, the likelihood of infection, and contamination of indwelling intravascular catheters. The organisms grown and the outcome of infections determine what empiric antimicrobial therapy we should consider. Local data on organisms and their sensitivities often influence antibiotic choices.

Laboratory markers of infection in children with febrile neutropenia

Studies have shown that serum acute phase reactants, such as C-reactive protein, IL-6, IL-8, and procalcitonin, are sensitive and specific indicators of infection in febrile neutropenic children.[12,13] Procalcitonin appears to be the best, with a sensitivity >90% and specificity of 90%, but none of the markers has 100% sensitivity.[12,13] Because febrile neutropenic children, like neonates, can deteriorate rapidly and unpredictably, and because the risk of bacteremia is as high as 20–30%, it is considered mandatory to treat with empiric antibiotics pending the results of cultures.[1–3] In this case, measurement of acute phase reactants will not guide decisions about starting therapy.

Empiric antibiotic treatment of febrile neutropenia in children

Question | For children with febrile neutropenia, does combination therapy using a beta-lactam and an aminoglycoside compared with monotherapy with a beta-lactam reduce mortality or treatment failures? Is combination therapy more likely than monotherapy to select for resistant organisms?

Literature review | We found 46 RCTs, only 5 of them in children,[14–18] a Cochrane systematic review,[19] and a non-Cochrane meta-analysis[20] comparing a beta-lactam plus an aminoglycoside with monotherapy.

Most of the data on antibiotics come from studies in adults. The Cochrane review[19] included RCTs comparing any beta-lactam antibiotic monotherapy with any combination of a beta-lactam and an aminoglycoside antibiotic, for the initial, empiric treatment of febrile neutropenic cancer patients. It identified 46 trials (7642 patients) but only 5 trials (431 children) were pediatric.[14–18]

When all 46 studies were combined, there was no significant difference between monotherapy and combination therapy in all-cause mortality (RR 0.85, 95% CI 0.72–1.02).[19] When we analyzed the pediatric studies alone, there were no conclusive results.

When treatment failure was the outcome, there was no significant difference between studies that compared one beta-lactam with the same beta-lactam plus an aminoglycoside, but a significant advantage to monotherapy for studies comparing different beta-lactams (RR 0.86, 95% CI 0.80–0.93). Bacterial and fungal superinfections developed with similar frequencies in the monotherapy and combination treatment groups. Adverse events were significantly more common in the combination treatment group (RR 0.83,

95% CI 0.72–0.97). These included events associated with significant morbidity, primarily renal toxicity.[19]

The authors conclude that the meta-analysis showed an advantage to broad-spectrum beta-lactam monotherapy over beta-lactam/aminoglycoside combination therapy for febrile neutropenia (in adults). The advantages were (1) a similar, if not better, survival, (2) a significantly lower treatment failure rate, (3) comparable probability for secondary infections, and (4) most importantly, a lower rate of adverse events associated with significant morbidity. They conclude that monotherapy should be regarded as the standard of care for febrile neutropenic patients. While their data are primarily in adults, the pediatric data are not inconsistent with their conclusions. The non-Cochrane review of 29 studies (4795 episodes) found that monotherapy was better than combination therapy in terms of mortality and treatment failures.[20]

A separate meta-analysis of eight RCTs compared the effects of the two different regimens on resistance.[21] Beta-lactam monotherapy was associated with significantly fewer superinfections (OR 0.62, 95% CI 0.42–0.93) and fewer treatment failures (OR 0.62, 95% CI 0.38–1.01) than the aminoglycoside/beta-lactam combination, and there was a trend for monotherapy to be associated with a lower emergence of resistant organisms (OR 0.90, 95% CI 0.56–1.47).[21]

> **For children with febrile neutropenia, we recommend using monotherapy with a beta-lactam antibiotic with activity against *Pseudomonas*.**

Question | For children with febrile neutropenia, does the addition of an antibiotic with enhanced activity against Gram-positive organisms such as vancomycin or teicoplanin compared with the standard empiric antibiotic regimen reduce mortality or treatment failures?

Literature review | We found 13 RCTs and a Cochrane review[22] comparing the addition of an antibiotic with enhanced Gram-positive activity to a standard regimen. None were in children. We found 2 RCTs in children which compared two different regimens, 1 of which included vancomycin.[23,24]

A Cochrane review included RCTs where only one antibiotic regimen for the treatment of febrile neutropenic cancer patients was compared to the same regimen with the addition of an antibiotic active against Gram-positive organisms (usually vancomycin or teicoplanin).[22] It included 13 trials and 2392 patients. Empiric anti-Gram-positive antibiotics were given at the onset of treatment in 11 studies and for persistent fever in 2 studies. The addition of an antibiotic with Gram-positive activity did not decrease mortality or treatment failures. The authors conclude that the use of vancomycin or teicoplanin as empiric therapy or added later without proof of a Gram-positive infection does not improve outcome.[22] The two studies in children showed that regimens that included vancomycin conferred no added advantage over standard regimens without vancomycin.[23,24]

We do not recommend empiric use of vancomycin or teicoplanin for children with febrile neutropenia.

Question | For children with febrile neutropenia, does one regimen compared with other regimens reduce mortality or treatment failures or antibiotic resistance?

Literature review | We found 33 RCTs and a non-Cochrane systematic review[25] comparing different beta-lactams used with or without vancomycin. Five of these studies were in children.[26–30] We found 8 RCTs and a non-Cochrane meta-analysis comparing ceftriaxone with an antipseudomonal beta-lactam.[31]

Monotherapy using a beta-lactam antibiotic with activity against *Pseudomonas* is an accepted regimen for febrile neutropenia,[1–3] and is supported by the evidence.[14–20] Although a meta-analysis of eight trials found no difference between ceftriaxone, an antibiotic with no useful antipseudomonal activity, and beta-lactam antibiotics with activity against *Pseudomonas*,[31] the studies were done at a time when *Pseudomonas* infection was very uncommon and most authorities would not recommend ceftriaxone monotherapy for febrile neutropenia.

A non-Cochrane systematic review and meta-analysis of RCTs compared different antipseudomonal beta-lactams, given with or without vancomycin.[25] Thirty-three trials fulfilled inclusion criteria, of which five were in children.[26–30] Cefepime was associated with higher all-cause mortality at 30 days than other beta-lactams (RR 1.44, 95% CI 1.06–1.94, 3123 participants). Carbapenems (imipenem or meropenem) were associated with fewer treatment modifications, including addition of glycopeptides, than ceftazidime or other comparators. Adverse events were significantly more frequent with carbapenems, specifically pseudomembranous colitis (RR 1.94, 95% CI 1.24–3.04). All-cause mortality was unaltered. Piperacillin/tazobactam was compared only with cefepime and carbapenems in six trials. No significant differences were demonstrated, but there was insufficient data to be certain about all-cause mortality.

The increased mortality associated with cefepime is unexplained. For the three pediatric studies (263 children)[26,28,30] there was a trend toward higher mortality with cefepime when compared with ceftazidime (RR 2.28, 95% CI 0.53–9.79) and no difference in the one study that compared cefepime with meropenem.[29] Empiric use of carbapenems was associated with an increased rate of pseudomembranous colitis. The use of quinolones, such as ciprofloxacin, although effective either as monotherapy or in combination, is discouraged because of the rapid emergence of resistance.[32]

Ceftazidime, piperacillin/tazobactam, imipenem/cilastatin, and meropenem appear to be suitable agents for monotherapy. We prefer to keep carbapenems in reserve for multiresistant organisms.

For the empiric treatment of children with fever and neutropenia, unless there are local factors such as organisms resistant to these antibiotics, we recommend:

ceftazidime 50 mg/kg (max 2 g) IV, 8-hourly OR piperacillin/tazobactam 100 + 12.5 mg/kg (max 4 + 0.5 g) IV, 8-hourly

Question | For children with cancer or other causes of severe immune compromise being treated with aminoglycosides, is once-daily compared with multiple-daily dosing safe and effective?

Literature review | We found six RCTs in febrile neutropenic children comparing once-daily with multiple-daily dosing of aminoglycosides.[33–38]

Studies in febrile neutropenic children have shown that once-daily aminoglycoside treatment is less nephrotoxic and at least as effective as multiple-daily dosing.[33–38] All but one of the studies, however, included other antibiotics such as beta-lactams, which made interpretation of the data uncertain. As a result, once-daily therapy has not yet been recommended routinely when using aminoglycosides to treat children with fever and neutropenia.[1] Subsequent to the 2002

US guidelines,[1] a study of tobramycin monotherapy in febrile neutropenic children undergoing stem cell transplantation found once-daily tobramycin was less nephrotoxic and more efficacious than thrice daily.[38]

The evidence appears to be accumulating that once-daily dosing of aminoglycosides is safer than multiple-daily dosing and at least as effective. Because immune compromised children vary in their degree of immune compromise and their renal function, studies may be needed in a number of different settings.

We believe the evidence favors once-daily dosing of aminoglycosides for the majority of children with cancer or immune compromise.

Outpatient management of febrile neutropenia

It is possible to identify a group of febrile neutropenic children at low risk for bacteremia, who might be considered for outpatient management. In an observational study,[39] children were defined as low risk if they were outpatients at the time of presentation with febrile neutropenia, had an anticipated duration of neutropenia <7 days, and no significant comorbidity. They were compared with febrile neutropenic children not meeting the low-risk criteria, who were defined as high risk. The low-risk children had fewer episodes of bacteremia, other documented infection, and serious medical complications compared to the high-risk group, and shorter duration of neutropenia and hospital stay, but no shorter duration of fever. Overall, the rate of any adverse event was 4% in the low-risk group compared with 41% in the high-risk group. Thus, it is possible to identify a low-risk group, using simple readily available criteria. There are obvious dangers in trying to manage even low-risk children with febrile neutropenia as outpatients, but an economic analysis favored the use of home-based care for low-risk children.[40]

Duration of treatment

In several studies, the time it takes for febrile neutropenic patients with cancer who receive different antibiotic regimens to defervesce is 2–7 days (median 5 days).[1] The median time to defervescence for low-risk patients is 2 days, compared with 5–7 days for high-risk patients.[1]

If no organism is grown, the child becomes afebrile and remains afebrile, and the neutrophil count recovers to >500 cells/mm^3 (500×10^9 cells/L) in less than 7 days, a number of studies have shown that antibiotics can be stopped safely.[41–44] However, the IDSA guidelines recommend continuing with oral cefixime to a total of 7 days, citing a lack of good evidence for stopping earlier.[1]

If an organism is grown, therapy should be changed to the most appropriate regimen to treat that organism. The optimum duration of therapy for proven infection is unknown, but the IDSA recommends at least 7 days.[1]

Persistent fever and neutropenia

If fever and neutropenia persist, but cultures are negative, there are a number of options.

Question | For a child with febrile neutropenia that persists after 3–5 days with negative blood cultures, does stopping antibiotics compared with continuing the same empiric antibiotics compared with adding vancomycin or teicoplanin compared with adding one or more antifungals decrease morbidity or increase treatment failures or mortality?

Literature review | We found 1 RCT comparing stopping antibiotics with continuing antibiotics and with adding amphotericin.[45] We found 2 studies comparing adding vancomycin or teicoplanin with continuing antibiotics.[46,47] We found 31 studies and a Cochrane review[48] of antifungals.

Continuing antibiotic treatment for prolonged fever and neutropenia

In an early study, 50 child, adolescent, and adult patients with persistent fever and neutropenia despite 7 days of antibiotics (cephalothin, gentamicin, and carbenicillin) were randomized to discontinue antibiotics (Group 1), to continue antibiotics (Group 2), or to continue antibiotics and add empiric amphotericin B (Group 3).[45] The duration of neutropenia was comparable in the three groups (median 24 days, range 8–51 days). Clinically or microbiologically demonstrable infections occurred in 9 of 16 patients who discontinued antibiotics (Group 1) (6 also experienced shock, $p < 0.01$), in 6 of 16 who continued antibiotics (Group 2) (fungal infection developed in 5), and in 2 of 18 who continued antibiotics plus amphotericin B (Group 3).

The incidence of infections was lower for patients receiving antibiotics plus amphotericin B (Group 3) than for patients in Group 1 who discontinued antibiotics ($p = 0.013$).[45]

There has only been one RCT exclusively in children of stopping antibiotics despite persistent fever and neutropenia.[44] In this study from Chile, about a third of all children with febrile neutropenia could be defined on admission as low risk for bacterial infection and had negative blood cultures on day 3. The 68 low-risk children (75 episodes) were randomized to continue or to stop antibiotics. There were few infections and no deaths.[44]

Because patients with persistent fever and neutropenia have a high rate of subsequent infection with bacteria or fungi[45] and because of the high mortality from such infections, it is not recommended to stop all antimicrobial therapy and observe children with persistent fever and neutropenia.[1]

The use of antifungals for persistent fever in febrile neutropenia was examined in a Cochrane review.[48] The review included 31 RCTs of different antifungals compared with placebo or no treatment in 4155 cancer patients with neutropenia. Unfortunately, the review combines studies of antifungal prophylaxis with studies of antifungals given empirically for persistent fever. The incidence of invasive fungal infection decreased significantly with administration of amphotericin B (RR 0.39, 95% CI 0.20–0.76), fluconazole (RR 0.39, 95% CI 0.27–0.57), and itraconazole (RR 0.53, 95% CI 0.29–0.97), but not with miconazole or ketoconazole.

Prophylactic or empiric treatment with antifungals as a group had no statistically significant effect on mortality (RR 0.96, 95% CI 0.83–1.11). Amphotericin B showed a trend toward reduced mortality (RR 0.73, 95% CI 0.52–1.03), but fluconazole, ketoconazole, miconazole, and itraconazole did not reduce mortality.

We recommend starting antifungal therapy for children with fever and neutropenia that persists for more than 5 days.

Empiric use of antifungals for persistent fever and neutropenia

There are four classes of antifungals used for invasive fungal infections: polyenes (amphotericin B and lipid formulations of amphotericin), azoles (fluconazole, itraconazole, voriconazole, and posaconazole), echinocandins (caspofungin), and nucleoside analogues (flucytosine). The polyenes and azoles target ergosterol in the fungal cell membrane, echinocandins interfere with cell wall biosynthesis, and nucleoside analogues interfere with nucleotide synthesis.

Question | For children with persistent fever and neutropenia, is one antifungal regimen compared with other regimens safe and effective and cost-effective?

Literature review | We found 1 RCT[49] and a Cochrane review[50] comparing liposomal amphotericin with voriconazole. We found 4 RCTs[51–54] and a Cochrane review[55] comparing fluconazole with conventional amphotericin B. We found 1 RCT comparing itraconazole with conventional amphotericin B.[56] We found 1 RCT comparing liposomal amphotericin with caspofungin.[57] We found 12 RCTs and a Cochrane review[58] comparing lipid soluble formulations of amphotericin B with conventional amphotericin B.

Liposomal amphotericin versus voriconazole for persistent fever and neutropenia

We found one RCT[49] comparing liposomal amphotericin with voriconazole in 849 patients >12 years old with fever >96 hours. The trial was sponsored by the pharmaceutical company marketing voriconazole. The study authors claimed no difference in mortality, but a significant reduction in the number of breakthrough fungal infections with voriconazole.[49] The study was considered in a Cochrane review.[50] The Cochrane reviewers felt voriconazole was significantly inferior to liposomal amphotericin B according to the authors' prespecified criteria. More patients died in the voriconazole group (RR 1.37, 95% CI 0.96–1.96, $p = 0.10$), and the claimed significant reduction in the number of breakthrough fungal infections disappeared when patients arbitrarily excluded from analysis by the authors were included.[50]

Fluconazole versus conventional amphotericin B for persistent fever and neutropenia

We found four RCTs, none of them in children,[51–54] and a Cochrane review[55] comparing fluconazole with conventional amphotericin B for fluconazole-naïve cancer patients with persistent fever and neutropenia. Fluconazole was at least as effective as conventional amphotericin B and less toxic.

Itraconazole versus conventional amphotericin B for persistent fever and neutropenia

A single RCT found that itraconazole (IV, then oral) was equivalent to conventional amphotericin B in efficacy and less toxic in patients with persistent fever and neutropenia.[56]

Liposomal amphotericin versus caspofungin for persistent fever and neutropenia

A large RCT found that caspofungin had comparable efficacy to liposomal amphotericin, and was associated with less nephrotoxicity and fewer infusion-related events.[57] At present, the price of caspofungin exceeds that of all other antifungals considerably. We do not recommend its use unless it is shown to be cost-effective compared with other antifungals.

Liposomal amphotericin versus conventional amphotericin B for persistent fever and neutropenia

A Cochrane review[58] found 12 RCTs comparing lipid-soluble formulations of amphotericin B with conventional amphotericin B for the treatment or prophylaxis of neutropenic cancer patients. Only two studies were in children. Lipid-based amphotericin B was not more effective than conventional amphotericin B for mortality (RR 0.83, 95% CI 0.62–1.12), but decreased invasive fungal infection (RR 0.65, 95% CI 0.44–0.97), nephrotoxicity, defined as a 100% increase in serum creatinine (RR 0.45, 95% CI 0.37–0.54), and number of treatment dropouts (RR 0.78, 95% CI 0.62–0.97).

For liposomal amphotericin (AmBisome), the drug used in most patients, a meta-analysis of three trials (1149 patients) found no significant difference in mortality (RR 0.74, 95% CI 0.52–1.07) whereas it tended to be more effective than conventional amphotericin B for invasive fungal infection (RR 0.63, 95% CI 0.39–1.01, $p = 0.053$).[58]

AmBisome, amphotericin B in Intralipid (six trials, 379 patients), amphotericin B colloidal dispersion (ABCD) (two trials, 262 patients), and amphotericin B lipid complex (ABLC) (one trial, 105 patients) all decreased the occurrence of nephrotoxicity, but conventional amphotericin B was rarely administered under optimal circumstances.[58]

A pharmacoeconomic analysis compared the additional cost of liposomal amphotericin against the costs of toxicity from conventional amphotericin B for adult patients.[59] The analysis favored conventional amphotericin B, but was very sensitive to the cost of the drugs. Because of the risk of cumulative nephrotoxicity, most authorities prefer liposomal amphotericin to conventional amphotericin B, provided it can be afforded and its use does not divert funds from other more effective treatments.

Continuous infusion of conventional amphotericin B for persistent fever and neutropenia

An RCT of 80 mostly neutropenic patients with refractory fever and suspected or proved invasive fungal infections compared 1 mg/kg conventional amphotericin B given either by continuous infusion over 24 hours or by rapid infusion over 4 hours.[60] Patients in the continuous infusion group had fewer side effects and significantly reduced nephrotoxicity than those in the rapid infusion group. The overall mortality was significantly lower during treatment and after 3 months' follow-up in the continuous infusion group.[60]

The study was small and did not include bone marrow transplant patients or patients on cyclosporine, so the results should not be generalized without further studies. Despite the success of this study, there have been no further RCTs comparing continuous infusion of conventional amphotericin B with the newer, far more expensive drugs, such as liposomal amphotericin, voriconazole, and caspofungin. It is difficult not to be cynical about the reason for the dearth of studies. Such studies would be extremely welcome.

Recommended empiric antifungal therapy for prolonged fever and neutropenia

We define patients at high risk of nephrotoxicity as:
· hematopoietic stem cell recipients;
· children with underlying renal insufficiency;
· children receiving two or more nephrotoxic drugs;
· children who develop nephrotoxicity on conventional amphotericin B.

The rest are low risk. For patients at low risk of nephrotoxicity who have prolonged fever with neutropenia >5 days, we recommend:

amphotericin 1 mg/kg IV, daily OR (if fluconazole-naïve)
fluconazole 6 mg/kg IV, daily (not if *Aspergillus* infection likely)

The risk of nephrotoxicity with conventional amphotericin B can be reduced by prior hydration and of infusion-related adverse events by premedication with corticosteroids or acetaminophen.[50] We recommend changing patients to liposomal amphotericin if they develop nephrotoxicity while taking conventional amphotericin, defined as a doubling or rapid rise in serum creatinine.[50]

For high-risk patients who have prolonged fever with neutropenia >5 days, we recommend:

liposomal amphotericin 1 mg/kg IV, daily OR
*voriconazole 6 mg/kg IV, 12-hourly for two doses, then 4 mg/kg IV, 12-hourly

Although it is tempting to recommend continuous infusion of amphotericin, the data are not yet sufficiently robust.

Recommended antifungal therapy for candidemia or invasive candidosis

In non-neutropenic patients, a non-Cochrane meta-analysis found that fluconazole was as effective as conventional amphotericin B and less toxic.[61] No other RCTs have shown that any other antifungal is superior to fluconazole or conventional amphotericin B for invasive candidiasis, although caspofungin was shown to be at least as effective as conventional amphotericin B.[62] Prior fluconazole therapy is a risk factor for fluconazole-resistant candidiasis,[63] so amphotericin B is preferred for children who have previously received fluconazole.

For fluconazole-naïve children, we recommend:

fluconazole 6 mg/kg IV, daily

For children with fluconazole-resistant *Candida* and children who have already received fluconazole, if they are at low risk for renal impairment, we recommend:

amphotericin 1 mg/kg IV, daily

For children with fluconazole-resistant *Candida* and children who have already received fluconazole who have preexisting renal impairment or are at high risk of developing it, we recommend:

liposomal amphotericin 3 mg/kg IV, daily OR
*voriconazole 6 mg/kg IV, 12-hourly for two doses, then 4 mg/kg IV, 12-hourly

Recommended antifungal therapy for invasive aspergillosis

An RCT compared voriconazole with conventional amphotericin B for confirmed and presumed invasive *Aspergillus* infections in 391 patients 12 years or older with mainly hematologic malignancies or stem cell transplants.[64] The trial was sponsored by the pharmaceutical company marketing voriconazole. The study authors reported that voriconazole had significant benefit at 12 weeks, in terms of response to therapy and mortality.[64] A Cochrane review commented, however, that conventional amphotericin B was used without adequate attention to reducing its adverse effects by premedication and hydration.[50] This resulted in a marked difference in the duration of treatment on trial drugs (77 days with voriconazole versus 10 days with amphotericin B), and they felt precluded meaningful comparisons of the benefits and harms of the two drugs.[50]

Liposomal preparations of amphotericin are less toxic but have not been shown to be more effective than conventional amphotericin B for invasive aspergillosis. An RCT found that ABCD was almost identical to conventional amphotericin B in terms of response and mortality, was less nephrotoxic, but costs far more.[65] We recommend:

*voriconazole 6 mg/kg IV 12-hourly for two doses, then 4 mg/kg IV 12-hourly for at least 7 days, then 4 mg/kg (max 200 mg) orally 12-hourly OR
liposomal amphotericin 3–5 mg/kg IV, daily OR
amphotericin B desoxycholate 1 mg/kg IV, daily

[*It is recommended that voriconazole levels be monitored.]

Empiric use of glycopeptide antibiotic for persistent fever and neutropenia

Two RCTs compared the addition of glycopeptides, vancomycin,[43] or teicoplanin,[44] with continuing therapy in patients with fever that persisted for 72–96 hours. They found no benefit, and concluded that a glycopeptide such as vancomycin should not be started empirically unless there is evidence of infection with a vancomycin-susceptible organism, such as MRSA. A Cochrane review came to the same conclusion.[22]

We do not recommend adding vancomycin or teicoplanin for persistent fever and neutropenia routinely, unless positive blood cultures are positive for a sensitive organism.

Preventive therapy for children with febrile neutropenia

Prophylactic antibiotics in afebrile neutropenic patients

Question | For neutropenic children who are afebrile but at risk of bacterial infection, do prophylactic antibiotics compared with no antibiotics or placebo reduce the incidence of bacterial infection and do they increase antibiotic resistance?

Literature review | We found 101 trials and a Cochrane review.[66]

A Cochrane review of RCTs or quasi-RCTs compared different types of antibiotic prophylaxis with placebo or no intervention or another antibiotic to prevent bacterial infections in afebrile neutropenic patients.[66] They included 101 trials (12,599 patients) performed between the years 1973 and 2005. Antibiotic prophylaxis significantly decreased the risk for death when compared with placebo or no intervention (RR 0.66, 95% CI 0.55–0.79). The authors estimated that 50 patients needed to be treated to prevent one death from all causes. Prophylaxis resulted in a significant decrease in the risk of infection-related death (RR 0.59, 95% CI 0.47–0.75) and in the occurrence of fever (RR 0.77, 95% CI 0.74–0.81). A reduction in mortality was also evident when the more recently conducted quinolone trials were analyzed separately. Quinolone prophylaxis reduced the risk for all-cause mortality (RR 0.52, 95% CI 0.37–0.74).

Although the authors recommend that antibiotic prophylaxis should be considered, particularly with a quinolone,[66] current recommendations do not favor prophylaxis, because of the risk of resistance.[1,2]

We do not recommend prophylactic antibiotics to prevent bacterial infections in afebrile neutropenic patients, except trimethoprim-sulfamethoxazole to prevent PCP (see Section 9.4, p. 126).

Prophylactic antifungals in febrile neutropenia

Question | For neutropenic children who are afebrile but at risk of fungal infection, do prophylactic antifungals compared with no antifungals or placebo reduce the incidence of fungal infection and do they increase antifungal resistance?

Literature review | We found 31 RCTs and a Cochrane review of prophylactic antifungals for neutropenic patients.[48] We found 12 RCTs and a Cochrane review of antifungal prophylaxis in non-neutropenic, critically ill adult patients.[67]

As previously stated (see p. 121), a Cochrane review of randomized trials of antifungals in cancer patients with neutropenia did not separate prophylaxis from treatment.[48] This review found that antifungals reduced the incidence of fungal infections but not the mortality.

A Cochrane review of antifungal prophylaxis in non-neutropenic, critically ill adult patients found 12 trials (8 fluconazole and 4 ketoconazole) involving 1606 randomized patients.[67] When combined, fluconazole or ketoconazole reduced total mortality by about 25% (RR 0.76, 95% CI 0.59–0.97) and invasive fungal infections by about 50% (RR 0.46, 95% CI 0.31–0.68). Prophylactic antifungals were not associated with a detectable increase in the incidence of infection or colonization with the azole-resistant fungal pathogens *Candida glabrata* or *C. krusei*, although the confidence intervals were wide and trials were not powered to exclude such an effect. Adverse effects were not more common among patients receiving prophylaxis.

We recommend that antifungal prophylaxis with fluconazole should be considered for patients at increased risk of invasive fungal infections.

Colony-stimulating factors to prevent febrile neutropenia

A Cochrane review found six studies (332 participants) of the use of colony-stimulating factors to prevent febrile neutropenia in children with ALL.[68] The use of colony stimulating factors significantly reduced the number of episodes of febrile neutropenia, the length of hospitalization, and the number of infectious disease episodes, but did not influence the length of episodes of neutropenia. There were insufficient data to assess the effect on survival. There was substantial heterogeneity between included trials.[68] The role of cerebrospinal fluid for preventing febrile neutropenia episodes is still uncertain.

9.2 Immunization and leukemia

Children with acute leukemia and other malignancies who have been previously immunized often lose antibodies to vaccine antigens. It is not clear whether this means they have become susceptible to those diseases and so whether or not they need booster doses of vaccine. When the vaccines are live vaccines such as measles or VZV vaccines that are contraindicated for immunodeficient children, it is not clear whether or not the children need passive protection if they are exposed to wild-type disease.

A non-Cochrane systematic review[69] found eight studies published since 1980 on vaccination of children with ALL. The number of children who had preserved defined protective titers of antibodies after treatment for ALL ranged from 17 to 98% for diphtheria, from 27 to 82% for *Bordetella pertussis*, from 20 to 98% for tetanus, from 62 to 100% for poliomyelitis, from 35 to 100% for *Haemophilus influenzae* type b (Hib), from 29 to 92% for mumps, from 29 to 60% for measles, and from 72 to 92% for rubella. Most patients, however, responded to revaccination, demonstrating immunological recovery. Although the designs and results of the included studies varied widely, it can be concluded that chemotherapy for ALL in children results in a temporary reduction of specific antibody levels. Memory is preserved but revaccination may be warranted.

9.3 Prevention of sepsis due to asplenia or splenectomy

Children with functional or anatomic asplenia are at increased risk from infections with encapsulated organisms, particularly pneumococci.[70] Asplenic patients present with high fever and rapidly develop shock or purpura fulminans. In a paper reporting 26 episodes of pneumococcal sepsis in 22 asplenic patients, 7 had shock, 7 had petechiae or purpura, 5 had disseminated intravascular coagulation, and 5 had respiratory distress Six died (27%).[71]

Guidelines on the management of children with functional or anatomical asplenia have been published.[72–74]

The most common problem concerning asplenia in children is functional asplenia due to sickle cell disease.[75] Before the use of penicillin prophylaxis, pneumococcal polysaccharide vaccines, and neonatal screening for hemoglobinopathies, rates of invasive pneumococcal disease in children with sickle cell disease were 20- to 100-fold higher than those in healthy children, with the greatest risk in children <5 years old.[75] Children with sickle cell hemoglobinopathy and certain other sickle cell hemoglobinopathies (including thalassemias) have lower rates of infection than children with SS hemoglobinopathy, but their rates are much higher than those of other children, and deaths attributable to fulminant pneumococcal infection have been reported in these children as well.[76] Despite the use of pneumococcal polysaccharide vaccines and penicillin prophylaxis, high rates of invasive pneumococcal infection have continued to be observed in some groups of children with sickle cell disease.[77,78]

The risk of post-splenectomy sepsis was examined in a non-Cochrane meta-analysis of 19,680 adults and children followed for a mean of 6.9 years. The incidence of infection was 3.3% for children and 3.2% for adults, and the mortality was 1.7% for children and 1.3% for adults.[79] The incidence of sepsis was even higher in 200 children splenectomized as part of their staging for Hodgkin lymphoma: there were 20 episodes in 18 children, and 8 died (4% overall mortality).[80]

The risk of sepsis in children with congenital asplenia, usually associated with congenital heart disease, is extremely high. In a review, 59 children with congenital asplenia (7 with isolated asplenia and 52 with complex congenital heart disease) were compared with a control group of eusplenic children with comparable cardiac lesions.[81] Sixteen (27%) of the asplenic children had documented sepsis. In children <6 months of age, the organism was usually a Gram-negative bacillus (*Escherichia coli* or Klebsiella), but from 6 months on was usually *Streptococcus pneumoniae* or *H. influenzae*. Children with asplenia syndrome who survived the first month of life were at greater risk of dying from sepsis than from their heart disease.[81] The data support giving prophylactic antibiotics to children with congenital asplenia. For children with congenital asplenia, consideration should be given to using amoxicillin-clavulanic acid or ciprofloxacin in the first 6 months because of the risk of Gram-negative sepsis and to switching to amoxicillin at 6 months.

Antibiotic prophylaxis for patients with anatomical or functional asplenia

Antibiotic prophylaxis is recommended for all children with sickle cell disease beginning at 2 months of age or earlier, as well as children with congenital asplenia or surgical splenectomy.[70-74] These recommendations are based on demonstrated efficacy against invasive pneumococcal infection in children with sickle cell disease.[82,83] In a prospective multicenter, double-blind RCT of prophylactic penicillin administration (125 mg of penicillin V potassium, administered orally twice daily to 3 years of age, and 250 mg twice daily thereafter), the antibiotic prophylaxis group had an 84% decrease in the incidence of pneumococcal infection.[82] In another prospective RCT, infants given monthly IM benzathine penicillin injections at home were compared with infants receiving a 14-valent pneumococcal polysaccharide vaccine.[83] No episodes of pneumococcal infection occurred among the infants with sickle cell disease receiving benzathine penicillin compared with 10 cases in concurrently followed infants who were immunized but not given monthly injections of penicillin.[83]

A multicenter RCT of children with sickle cell disease examined the safety of stopping penicillin prophylaxis after 5 years of age.[84] Children with sickle cell disease or thalassemia who had received at least 2 years of penicillin prophylaxis and one dose of pneumococcal polysaccharide vaccine before their fifth birthday were randomized to receive continued prophylaxis or placebo. There was no difference in the rate of invasive pneumococcal infection among the children receiving penicillin prophylaxis, four cases (2%), and those receiving placebo, two cases (1%).[843]

Pneumococcal immunization does not prevent all cases of pneumococcal sepsis.[77,78] It used to be thought that the risk from post-splenectomy sepsis was mostly within the first few years, but in one large series, most cases of post-splenectomy sepsis occurred after 10–30 years and only 11% within 4 years of splenectomy.[85] In contrast, a retrospective study of 318 patients aged 10–26 years and followed for up to 17 years found that overwhelming post-splenectomy infection (OPSI) occurred in 18 patients (5.7%), 56% within the first 6 months.[79] The rate in patients on regular and irregular prophylactic oral penicillin was 2.7% and 10%, respectively ($p < 0.01$). The incidence of OPSI also decreased from 7.3 to 3.2% after routine administra-

tion of pneumococcal vaccine ($p < 0.05$).[86] Antibiotic prophylaxis may be beneficial after 5 years of age, but there are scanty data to support it.

Currently the USA[72] and Canada[73] recommend stopping antibiotic prophylaxis at 5 years or 1 year after splenectomy,[72] provided the child is immunized against pneumococcus, whereas the British recommend that lifelong prophylactic antibiotics should be offered in all cases of asplenia, especially in the first 2 years after splenectomy, for all up to age 16 and when there is underlying impaired immune function.[74]

Immunizations for patients with anatomic or functional asplenia

Patients with anatomic or functional asplenia can safely be given both live attenuated and killed vaccines.[72-74] As these patients are at high risk for developing life-threatening infection due to all encapsulated bacteria, additional immunizations against *S. pneumoniae*, *H. influenzae* type b, and *Neisseria meningitidis* are recommended.[72-74,87,88]

In patients having elective splenectomy, it is recommended to complete immunizations at least 2 weeks prior to the date of surgery because this improves the immune response.[72-74]

In case of emergency splenectomy, the patient should be immunized post-splenectomy. Acceptable antibody levels have been demonstrated after vaccination with 23-valent polysaccharide pneumococcal vaccine when the vaccine was given as early as the first day post-operatively.[89] However, patients receiving the vaccination within 14 days post-operatively are more likely to require revaccination and the antibody levels achieved in adult, post-splenectomy patients, although protective, are lower than the levels attained by healthy adult subjects.[90] It is recommended to immunize patients undergoing emergency splenectomy for trauma 14 days or more after surgery.[91,92]

A summary of our recommendations, based on the evidence in Section 9.3 (p. 125), is given in Table 9.1.

9.4 Prophylaxis against PCP

Trimethoprim-sulfamethoxazole (TMP-SMX; co-trimoxazole) reduces the risk of *P. jiroveci* (previously *P. carinii*) pneumonia (still called PCP) in children with impaired T-cell function at increased risk of PCP

Table 9.1 Recommendations to reduce risk of infections in children with anatomical or functional asplenia.[72–74,87,88]

Intervention	Under 24 mo	2–5 yr	Over 5 yr
Antibiotic prophylaxis	Penicillin V 125 mg, orally, daily or amoxicillin 10 mg/kg orally, 12-hourly	Penicillin V 125 mg, orally, 12-hourly or amoxicillin 10 mg/kg orally, 12-hourly	Not recommended, but should wear Medi-Alert bracelet and review fevers early in hospital
Pneumococcal vaccines (pneumococcal conjugate, e.g., Prevenar 7-valent, and pneumococcal polysaccharide, e.g., Pneumovax)	Give pneumococcal *conjugate* vaccine: primary course and booster dose at 12 months plus dose of pneumococcal polysaccharide vaccine at 2 year of age	Two doses of conjugate vaccine 2 months apart, and then single dose of pneumococcal polysaccharide vaccine at least 1 month later (if not previously immunized)	Two doses of conjugate vaccine 2 months apart, and then single dose of pneumococcal polysaccharide vaccine at least 1 month later (if not previously immunized)
Hib conjugate vaccine	As per routine childhood schedule	Single dose	Single dose
Meningococcal vaccines (meningococcal conjugate Group C or Groups A and C vaccine and meningococcal polysaccharide vaccine A, C, W-135,Y)	Give conjugate vaccine at 2, 4, 6 months. Give single dose if over 1 year of age	Give single dose of conjugate vaccine, and then single dose of polysaccharide vaccine at least 1 month later	Give single dose of conjugate vaccine, then single dose of polysaccharide vaccine at least 1 month later

including cancer patients in developed countries[93] and HIV-infected children in developing countries.[94,95]. It is effective when given thrice weekly.[96] Toxicity to TMP-SMX is much less common in children than in adults.[97] Alternatives in the event of severe rash or other toxicity to TMP-SMX are dapsone[98] and IV or aerosolized pentamidine.[99]

For children with impaired T-cell function, we recommend:

trimethoprim+sulfamethoxazole (trimethoprim 150 mg/m^2+ sulfamethoxazole 750 mg/m^2) orally, as a single dose, thrice weekly on consecutive days, e.g., Monday–Tuesday–Wednesday OR **trimethoprim+sulfamethoxazole 4 + 20 mg/kg (max 80 + 400 mg) orally, as a single dose, thrice weekly on consecutive days, e.g., Monday–Tuesday–Wednesday** OR **dapsone 2 mg/kg (max 100 mg) orally, daily or 4 mg/kg (max 200 mg), once a week** OR **pentamidine 4 mg/kg (max 300 mg) IV or aerosolized every 4 weeks**

References

1 Hughes WT, Armstrong D, Bodey GP et al. 2002 guidelines for the use of antimicrobial agents in neutropenic patients with cancer. *Clin Infect Dis* 2002;34:730–51.

2 Hann I, Viscoli C, Paesmans M, Gaya H, Glauser M, for the International Antimicrobial Therapy Cooperative Group (IATCG) of the European Organization for Research and Treatment of Cancer (EORTC). A comparison of outcome from febrile neutropenic episodes in children compared with adults: results from four EORTC studies. *Br J Haematol* 1997;99:580–8.

3 Viscoli C, Varnier O, Machetti M. Infections in patients with febrile neutropenia: epidemiology, microbiology, and risk stratification. *Clin Infect Dis* 2005;40(suppl 4): S240–5.

4 Hemsworth S, Nunn AJ, Selwood K, Osborne C, Jones A, Pizer B. Once-daily netilmicin for neutropenic pyrexia in pediatric oncology. *Acta Paediatr* 2005;94:268–74.

5 Muller J, Garami M, Constantin T, Schmidt M, Fekete G, Kovacs G. Meropenem in the treatment of febrile neutropenic children. *Pediatr Hematol Oncol* 2005;22:277–84.

6 Aksoylar S, Cetingul N, Kantar M, Karapinar D, Kavakli K, Kansoy S. Meropenem plus amikacin versus piperacillin-tazobactam plus netilmicin as empiric therapy for high-risk febrile neutropenia in children. *Pediatr Hematol Oncol* 2004;21:115–23.

7 Ammann RA, Hirt A, Luthy AR, Aebi C. Predicting bacteremia in children with fever and chemotherapy-induced neutropenia. *Pediatr Infect Dis J* 2004;23:61–7.

8 Santolaya ME, Alvarez AM, Aviles CL et al. Prospective evaluation of a model of prediction of invasive bacterial infection risk among children with cancer, fever, and neutropenia. *Clin Infect Dis* 2002;35:678–83.

9 Fleischhack G, Schmidt-Niemann M et al. Piperacillin, beta-lactam inhibitor plus gentamicin as empirical therapy of a sequential regimen in febrile neutropenia of pediatric cancer patients. *Support Care Cancer* 2001;9:372–9.

10 Haupt R, Romanengo M, Fears T, Viscoli C, Castagnola E. Incidence of septicaemias and invasive mycoses in children undergoing treatment for solid tumours: a 12-year experience at a single Italian institution. *Eur J Cancer* 2001;37: 2413–9.

11 Wisplinghoff H, Seifert H, Wenzel RP, Edmond MB. Current trends in the epidemiology of nosocomial bloodstream infections in patients with hematological malignancies and solid neoplasms in hospitals in the United States. *Clin Infect Dis* 2003;36:1103–10.

12 Fleischhack G, Kambeck I, Cipic D, Hasan C, Bode U. Procalcitonin in pediatric cancer patients: its diagnostic relevance is superior to that of C-reactive protein, interleukin 6, interleukin 8, soluble interleukin 2 receptor and soluble tumour necrosis factor receptor II. *Br J Haematol* 2000;111:1093–102.

13 Stryjewski GR, Nylen ES, Bell MJ et al. Interleukin-6, interleukin-8, and a rapid and sensitive assay for calcitonin precursors for the determination of bacterial sepsis in febrile neutropenic children. *Pediatr Crit Care Med* 2005;6:129–35.

14 Agaoglu L, Devecioglu O, Anak S et al. Cost-effectiveness of cefepime+netilmicin or ceftazidime+amikacin or meropenem monotherapy in febrile neutropenic children with malignancy in Turkey. *J Chemother* 2001;13:281–7.

15 Duzova A, Kutluk T, Kanra G et al. Monotherapy with meropenem versus combination therapy with piperacillin plus amikacin as empiric therapy for neutropenic fever in children with lymphoma and solid tumors. *Turk J Pediatr* 2001;43:105–9.

16 Jacobs RF, Vats TS, Pappa KA, Chaudhary S, Kletzel M, Becton DL. Ceftazidime versus ceftazidime plus tobramycin in febrile neutropenic children. *Infection* 1993;21:223–8.

17 Morgan G, Duerden BI, Lilleyman JS. Ceftazidime as a single agent in the management of children with fever and neutropenia. *J Antimicrob Chemother* 1983;12(suppl A):347–51.

18 Smith L, Will AM, Williams RF, Stevens RF. Ceftriaxone vs. azlocillin and netilmicin in the treatment of febrile neutropenic children. *J Infect* 1990;20:201–6.

19 Paul M, Soares-Weiser K, Grozinsky S, Leibovici L. Beta-lactam versus beta-lactam-aminoglycoside combination therapy in cancer patients with neutropenia. *The Cochrane Database of Systematic Reviews* 2003; (3):Art No CD003038.

20 Furno P, Bucaneve G, Del Favero A. Monotherapy or aminoglycoside-containing combinations for empirical antibiotic treatment of febrile neutropenic patients: a meta-analysis. *Lancet Infect Dis* 2002;2:231–42.

21 Bliziotis IA, Samonis G, Vardakas KZ, Chrysanthopoulou S, Falagas ME. Effect of aminoglycoside and beta-lactam combination therapy versus beta-lactam monotherapy on the emergence of antimicrobial resistance: a meta-analysis of randomized, controlled trials. *Clin Infect Dis* 2005;41: 149–58.

22 Paul M, Borok S, Fraser A, Vidal L, Cohen M, Leibovici L. Additional anti-Gram-positive antibiotic treatment for febrile neutropenic cancer patients. *The Cochrane Database of Systematic Reviews* 2005;(3):Art No CD003914.

23 Granowetter L, Wells H, Lange BJ. Ceftazidime with or without vancomycin vs. cephalothin, carbenicillin and gentamicin as the initial therapy of the febrile neutropenic pediatric cancer patient. *Pediatr Infect Dis J* 1988;7:165–70.

24 Viscoli C, Moroni C, Boni L et al. Ceftazidime plus amikacin versus ceftazidime plus vancomycin as empiric therapy in febrile neutropenic children with cancer. *Rev Infect Dis* 1991;13:397–404.

25 Paul M, Borok S, Fraser A, Vidal L, Leibovici L. Empirical antibiotics against Gram-positive infections for febrile neutropenia: systematic review and meta-analysis of randomized controlled trials. *J Antimicrob Chemother* 2005;55:436–44.

26 Chuang YY, Hung IJ, Yang CP et al. Cefepime versus ceftazidime as empiric monotherapy for fever and neutropenia in children with cancer. *Pediatr Infect Dis J* 2002;21:203–9.

27 Fleischhack G, Hartmann C, Simon A et al. Meropenem versus ceftazidime as empirical monotherapy in febrile neutropenia of pediatric patients with cancer. *J Antimicrob Chemother* 2001;47:841–53.

28 Kebudi R, Gorgun O, Ayan I et al. Randomized comparison of cefepime versus ceftazidime monotherapy for fever and neutropenia in children with solid tumors. *Med Pediatr Oncol* 2001;36:434–41.

29 Kutluk T, Kurne O, Akyuz C et al. Cefepime vs. meropenem as empirical therapy for neutropenic fever in children with lymphoma and solid tumours. *Pediatr Blood Cancer* 2004;42: 284–6.

30 Mustafa MM, Carlson L, Tkaczewski I et al. Comparative study of cefepime versus ceftazidime in the empiric treatment of pediatric cancer patients with fever and neutropenia. *Pediatr Infect Dis J* 2001;20:362–9.

31 Furno P, Dionisi MS, Bucaneve G, Menichetti F, Del Favero A. Ceftriaxone versus beta-lactams with antipseudomonal activity for empirical, combined antibiotic therapy in febrile neutropenia: a meta-analysis. *Support Care Cancer* 2000;8:293–301.

32 Bliziotis IA, Michalopoulos A, Kasiakou SK et al. Ciprofloxacin vs an aminoglycoside in combination with a beta-lactam for the treatment of febrile neutropenia: a meta-analysis of randomized controlled trials. *Mayo Clin Proc* 2005;80:1146–56.

33 Charnas R, Luthi AR, Ruch W, for the Writing Committee for the International Collaboration on Antimicrobial Treatment of Febrile Neutropenia in Children. Once daily ceftriaxone plus amikacin vs. three times daily ceftazidime plus amikacin for treatment of febrile neutropenic children with cancer. *Pediatr Infect Dis J* 1997;16:346–53.

34 Ariffin H, Arasu A, Mahfuzah M, Ariffin WA, Chan LL, Lin HP. Single-daily ceftriaxone plus amikacin versus thrice-daily ceftazidime plus amikacin as empirical treatment of febrile neutropenia in children with cancer. *J Paediatr Child Health* 2001;37:38–43.

35 Postovsky S, Ben Arush MW, Kassis E, Elhasid R, Krivoy N. Pharmacokinetic analysis of gentamicin thrice and single daily dosage in pediatric cancer patients. *Pediatr Hematol Oncol* 1997;14:547–54.

36 The International Antimicrobial Therapy Cooperative Group of the European Organization for Research and Treatment of Cancer. Efficacy and toxicity of single daily doses of amikacin and ceftriaxone versus multiple daily doses of amikacin and ceftazidime for infection in patients with cancer and granulocytopenia. *Ann Intern Med* 1993;119:584–93.

37 Rubinstein E, Lode H, Grassi C, for the Antibiotic Study Group. Ceftazidime monotherapy vs. ceftriaxone/tobramycin for serious hospital-acquired Gram-negative infections. *Clin Infect Dis* 1995;20:1217–28.

38 Sung L, Dupuis LL, Bliss B et al. Randomized controlled trial of once- versus thrice-daily tobramycin in febrile neutropenic children undergoing stem cell transplantation. *J Natl Cancer Inst* 2003;95:1869–77.

39 Alexander SW, Wade KC, Hibberd PL, Parsons SK. Evaluation of risk prediction criteria for episodes of febrile neutropenia in children with cancer. *J Pediatr Hematol Oncol* 2002;24:38–42.

40 Raisch DW, Holdsworth MT, Winter SS, Hutter JJ, Graham ML. Economic comparison of home-care-based versus hospital-based treatment of chemotherapy-induced febrile neutropenia in children. *Value Health* 2003;6:158–66.

41 Mullen CA, Buchanan GR. Early hospital discharge of children with cancer treated for fever and neutropenia: identification and management of the low-risk patient. *J Clin Oncol* 1990;8:1998–2004.

42 Griffin TC, Buchanan GR. Hematologic predictors of bone marrow recovery in neutropenic patients hospitalized for fever: implications for discontinuation of antibiotics and early discharge from the hospital. *J Pediatr* 1992;121:28–33.

43 Jones GR, Konsler GK, Dunaway RP et al. Risk factors for recurrent fever after the discontinuation of empiric antibiotic therapy for fever and neutropenia in pediatric patients with a malignancy or hematologic condition. *J Pediatr* 1994;124:703–8.

44 Santolaya ME, Villarroel M, Avendano LF, Cofre J. Discontinuation of antimicrobial therapy for febrile, neutropenic children with cancer: a prospective study. *Clin Infect Dis* 1997;25:92–7.

45 Pizzo PA, Robichaud KJ, Gill FA, Witebsky FG. Empiric antibiotic and antifungal therapy for cancer patients with prolonged fever and granulocytopenia. *Am J Med* 1982;72:101–11.

46 Cometta A, Kern WV, De Bock R et al. Vancomycin versus placebo for treating persistent fever in patients with neutropenic cancer receiving piperacillin-tazobactam monotherapy. *Clin Infect Dis* 2003;37:382–9.

47 Erjavec Z, de Vries-Hospers HG, Laseur M, Halie RM, Daenen S. A prospective, randomized, double-blinded, placebo-controlled trial of empirical teicoplanin in febrile neutropenia with persistent fever after imipenem monotherapy. *J Antimicrob Chemother* 2000;45:843–9.

48 Gøtzsche PC, Johansen HK. Routine versus selective antifungal administration for control of fungal infections in patients with cancer. *The Cochrane Database of Systematic Reviews* 2002;(2):Art No CD000026.

49 Walsh TJ, Pappas P, Winston DJ et al. Voriconazole compared with liposomal amphotericin B for empirical antifungal therapy in patients with neutropenia and persistent fever. *N Engl J Med* 2002;346:225–34.

50 Jørgensen KJ, Gøtzsche PC, Johansen HK. Voriconazole versus amphotericin B in cancer patients with neutropenia. *The Cochrane Database of Systematic Reviews* 2006;(1):Art No CD004707.

51 Malik IA, Moid I, Aziz Z, Khan S, Suleman M. A randomized comparison of fluconazole with amphotericin B as empiric anti-fungal agents in cancer patients with prolonged fever and neutropenia. *Am J Med* 1998;105:478–83.

52 Silling-Engelhardt G, Fegeler W, Roos N, Schomaker R, Essink M, Büchner T. Early empiric antifungal treatment of infections in neutropenic patients comparing fluconazole with amphotericin B/5-flucytosine. *Blood* 1994;10(suppl 1):306a.

53 Viscoli C, Castagnola E, Van Lint MT et al. Fluconazole versus amphotericin B as empirical antifungal therapy of unexplained fever in granulocytopenic cancer patients: a pragmatic, multicentre, prospective and randomised clinical trial. *Eur J Cancer* 1996;32A:814–20.

54 Winston DJ, Hathorn JW, Schuster MG, Schiller GJ, Territo MC. A multicenter, randomized trial of fluconazole versus amphotericin B for empiric antifungal therapy of febrile neutropenic patients with cancer. *Am J Med* 2000;108:282–9.

55 Johansen HK, Gøtzsche PC. Amphotericin B versus fluconazole for controlling fungal infections in neutropenic cancer patients. *The Cochrane Database of Systematic Reviews* 2002;(2):Art No CD000239.

56 Boogaerts M, Winston DJ, Bow EJ et al. Intravenous and oral itraconazole versus intravenous amphotericin B deoxycholate as empirical antifungal therapy for persistent fever in neutropenic patients with cancer who are receiving broad-spectrum antibacterial therapy. *Ann Intern Med* 2001;135:412–22.

57 Walsh TJ, Teppler H, Donowitz GR et al. Caspofungin versus liposomal amphotericin for empirical antifungal therapy in patients with persistent fever and neutropenia. *N Engl J Med* 2004;351:1391–402.

58 Johansen HK, Gøtzsche PC. Amphotericin B lipid soluble formulations versus amphotericin B in cancer patients with neutropenia. *The Cochrane Database of Systematic Reviews* 2000;(3):Art No CD000969.

59 Cagnoni PJ, Walsh TJ, Prendergast MM et al. Pharmacoeconomic analysis of liposomal amphotericin B versus conventional amphotericin B in the empirical treatment

of persistently febrile neutropenic patients. *J Clin Oncol* 2000;18:2476–83.

60 Eriksson U, Seifert zB, Schaffner A. Comparison of effects of amphotericin B deoxycholate infused over 4 or 24 hours: randomized, controlled trial. *BMJ* 2001;322:1–6.

61 Kontoyiannis DP, Bodey GP, Mantzoros CS. Fluconazole vs. amphotericin B for the management of candidaemia in adults: a meta-analysis. *Mycoses* 2001;44:125–35.

62 Mora-Duarte J, Betts R, Rotstein C et al. Comparison of caspofungin and amphotericin B for invasive candidiasis. *N Engl J Med* 2002;347:2020–9.

63 Nguyen MH, Peacock JE, Jr, Morris AJ et al. The changing face of candidemia: emergence of non-*Candida albicans* species and antifungal resistance. *Am J Med* 1996;100: 617–23.

64 Herbrecht R, Denning DW, Patterson TF et al. Voriconazole versus amphotericin B for primary therapy of invasive aspergillosis. *N Engl J Med* 2002;347:408–15.

65 Bowden R, Chandrasekar P, White MH et al. A double-blind, randomized, controlled trial of amphotericin B colloidal dispersion versus amphotericin B for treatment of invasive aspergillosis in immunocompromised patients. *Clin Infect Dis* 2002;35:359–66.

66 Gafter-Gvili A, Fraser A, Paul M, van de Wetering M, Kremer L, Leibovici L. Antibiotic prophylaxis for bacterial infections in afebrile neutropenic patients following chemotherapy. *The Cochrane Database of Systematic Reviews* 2005;(4):Art No CD004386.

67 Playford EG, Webster AC, Sorrell TC, Craig JC. Antifungal agents for preventing fungal infections in non-neutropenic critically ill patients. *The Cochrane Database of Systematic Reviews* 2006;(1):Art No CD004920.

68 Sasse EC, Sasse AD, Brandalise S, Clark OA, Richards S. Colony stimulating factors for prevention of myelosupressive therapy induced febrile neutropenia in children with acute lymphoblastic leukaemia. *The Cochrane Database of Systematic Reviews* 2005;(3):Art No CD004139.

69 van Tilburg CM, Sanders EA, Rovers MM, Wolfs TF, Bierings MB. Loss of antibodies and response to (re-) vaccination in children after treatment for acute lymphocytic leukemia: a systematic review. *Leukemia* 2006;20:1717–22.

70 Overturf GD, for the American Academy of Pediatrics Committee on Infectious Diseases. Technical report: prevention of pneumococcal infections, including the use of pneumococcal conjugate and polysaccharide vaccines and antibiotic prophylaxis. *Pediatrics* 2000;106:367–76.

71 Schutze GE, Mason EO, Jr, Barson WJ et al. Invasive pneumococcal infections in children with asplenia. *Pediatr Infect Dis J* 2002;21:278–82.

72 American Academy of Pediatrics Committee on Infectious Diseases. Policy statement: Recommendations for the prevention of pneumococcal infections, including the use of pneumococcal conjugate vaccine (Prevnar), pneumococcal polysaccharide vaccine, and antibiotic prophylaxis. *Pediatrics* 2000;106:362–6.

73 Infectious Diseases and Immunization Committee, Canadian Pediatric Society. Prevention and therapy of bacterial infec-tions for children with asplenia or hyposplenia. *Paediatr Child Health* 1999;4:417–21.

74 British Committee for Standards in Haematology. Davies JM, Barnes R, Milligan D, for the Working Party of the Haematology/Oncology Task Force. Update of guidelines for the prevention and treatment of infection in patients with an absent or dysfunctional spleen. *Clin Med* 2002;2:440–3.

75 Overturf GD, Powars D, Baraff LJ. Bacterial meningitis and septicemia in sickle cell disease. *Am J Dis Child* 1977;131: 784–7.

76 Lane PA, Rogers ZR, Woods GM. Fatal pneumococcal septicemia in hemoglobin SC disease. *J Pediatr* 1994;124: 859–62.

77 Zarkowsky HS, Gallagher D, Gill FM. Bacteremia in sickle hemoglobinopathies. *J Pediatr* 1986;109:579–85.

78 Overturf GD. Infections and immunizations of children with sickle cell disease. *Adv Pediatr Infect Dis* 1999;14:191–218.

79 Bisharat N, Omari H, Lavi I, Raz R. Risk of infection and death among post-splenectomy patients. *J Infect* 2001;43: 182–6.

80 Chilcote RR, Baehner RL, Hammond D et al. Septicemia and meningitis in children splenectomized for Hodgkin's disease. *N Engl J Med* 1976;295:798–800.

81 Waldman JD, Rosenthal A, Smith AL, Shurin S, Nadas AS. Sepsis and congenital asplenia. *J Pediatr* 1977;90:555–9.

82 Gaston MH, Verter JI, Woods G et al. Prophylaxis with oral penicillin in children with sickle cell anemia: a randomized trial. *N Engl J Med* 1986;314:1593–9.

83 John AB, Ramlal A, Jackson H, Maude GH, Sharma AW, Serjeant GR. Prevention of pneumococcal infection in children with homozygous sickle cell disease. *BMJ* 1984;288: 1567–70.

84 Falleta JM, Woods GM, Verter JI et al. Discontinuing penicillin prophylaxis in children with sickle cell anemia: Prophylactic Penicillin Study II. *J Pediatr* 1995;127:685–90.

85 Waghorn DJ. Overwhelming infection in asplenic patients: current best practice preventive measures are not being followed. *J Pathol* 2001;54:214–8.

86 El-Alfy MS, El-Sayed MH. Overwhelming post-splenectomy infection: is quality of patient knowledge enough for prevention? *Hematol J* 2004;5:77–80.

87 American Academy of Pediatrics. Pneumococcal infections. In: Pickering LK (ed.), *Red Book: 2003 Report of the Committee on Infectious Diseases,* 26th edn. Elk Grove Village, IL: American Academy of Pediatrics, 2003:490–500.

88 NHMRC. *Australian Immunisation Handbook,* 9th edn. Canberra: Government Publishing Services, 2007.

89 Shatz DV, Schinsky MF, Pais LB et al. Immune responses of splenectomized trauma patients to the 23-valent pneumococcal polysaccharide vaccine at 1 versus 7 versus 14 days after splenectomy. *J Trauma* 1998;44:760–5.

90 Konradsen HB, Rasmussen C, Ejstrud P et al. Antibody levels against *Streptococcus pneumoniae* and *Haemophilus influenzae* type B in a population of splenectomized individuals with varying vaccination status. *Epidemiol Infect* 1997;119: 167–74.

91 Shatz DV, Romero-Steiner S, Elie CM et al. Antibody responses in post-splenectomy trauma patients receiving the 23-valent pneumococcal polysaccharide vaccine at 14 versus 28 days post-operatively. *J Trauma* 2002;53:1037–42.

92 Advisory committee on Immunisation Practices (ACIP). Prevention of pneumococcal disease. *MMWR Morb Mortal Wkly Rep* 1997;46(RR-8):1–24.

93 Hughes WT, Kuhn S, Chaudhary S et al. Successful chemoprophylaxis for *Pneumocystis carinii* pneumonitis. *N Engl J Med* 1977;297:1419–26.

94 Grimwade K, Swingler GH. Cotrimoxazole prophylaxis for opportunistic infections in children with HIV infection. *The Cochrane Database of Systematic Reviews* 2006;(1):Art No CD003508.

95 Chintu C, Bhat GJ, Walker AS et al. Cotrimoxazole as prophylaxis against opportunistic infections in HIV-infected Zambian children (CHAP): a double-blind randomised placebo-controlled trial. *Lancet* 2004;364:1865–71.

96 Hughes WT, Rivera GK, Schell MJ, Thornton D, Lott L. Successful intermittent chemoprophylaxis for *Pneumocystis carinii* pneumonitis. *N Engl J Med* 1987;316:1627–32.

97 Karpman E, Kurzrock EA. Adverse reactions of nitrofurantoin, trimethoprim and sulfamethoxazole in children. *J Urol* 2004;172:448–53.

98 McIntosh K, Cooper E, Xu J et al, for the ACTG 179 Study Team. AIDS Clinical Trials Group. Toxicity and efficacy of daily vs. weekly dapsone for prevention of *Pneumocystis carinii* pneumonia in children infected with human immunodeficiency virus. *Pediatr Infect Dis J* 1999;18:432–9.

99 Principi N, Marchisio P, Onorato J et al, for the Italian Pediatric Collaborative Study Group on Pentamidine. Long-term administration of aerosolized pentamidine as primary prophylaxis against *Pneumocystis carinii* pneumonia in infants and children with symptomatic human immunodeficiency virus infection. *J Acquir Immune Defic Syndr Hum Retrovirol* 1996;12:158–63.

CHAPTER 10

Meningitis and central nervous system infections

10.1 Bacterial meningitis

The organisms causing bacterial meningitis vary according to the age of the child. Neonates and babies in the post-neonatal period (up to about 3 mo old) are susceptible to organisms from the maternal genital tract, including group B streptococcus, *Streptococcus faecalis*, *Escherichia coli*, other Gram-negative bacilli, and *Listeria*.[1–4]

The main organisms causing bacterial meningitis in the post-neonatal period are organisms acquired through the respiratory route, *S. pneumoniae* (pneumococcus), *Neisseria meningitidis* (meningococcus), *Haemophilus influenzae* type b (Hib), and, in some countries, *Salmonella*.[1]

Clinical diagnosis of bacterial meningitis

The classical clinical presentation of bacterial meningitis is with fever, headache, and neck stiffness.[1] Similar signs are found in viral meningitis, but children with bacterial meningitis are usually sicker than children with viral meningitis. For example, one study of children with meningeal signs found that a shorter presenting illness, vomiting, signs of meningeal irritation, cyanosis, petechiae and disturbed consciousness were independent clinical predictors of bacterial meningitis.[5] The only independent predictor from subsequent laboratory tests was the serum C-reactive protein (CRP) concentration.[5] In a developing country, clinical predictors of bacterial meningitis were appearing sick, being lethargic or unconscious, poor feeding, stiff neck, and bulging fontanelle.[6]

While clinical signs can suggest a diagnosis of bacterial as opposed to viral meningitis, lumbar puncture is necessary to make the definitive diagnosis for an individual child, to direct antibiotic and other therapy, and to help advise on prognosis (see below).

Laboratory diagnosis of bacterial meningitis

Lumbar puncture (LP)
Which child should have an LP?
The LP is a form of biopsy. Gram stain and cell count are rapidly available after LP, and may suggest which organism is present, may point to an alternate diagnosis (viral meningitis, tuberculous meningitis, subarachnoid hemorrhage, etc.), or may exclude meningitis altogether. Rapid assays on cerebrospinal fluid (CSF) may reveal the organism causing bacterial meningitis even if culture does not, and a positive CSF culture gives antibiotic susceptibility. These are potent reasons for doing an LP when meningitis is suspected. Yet many young doctors are reluctant to perform LP nowadays.

In some situations, it may be unsafe to perform an immediate LP because of the risk of provoking cerebral herniation ("coning"). The signs of impending cerebral herniation are deterioration in level of consciousness, rising blood pressure, falling heart rate, cranial nerve signs, decorticate or decerebrate post-uring.[7–10] All children with bacterial meningitis have raised intracranial pressure,[7,8] and cerebral herniation can occur without LP. Cerebral herniation is reported to occur in 4–6% of children with bacterial meningitis, with or without LP.[8–10] In some children, the onset of signs of cerebral herniation coincided with LP, but it is unclear whether or not LP caused the cerebral herniation.[8–10]

In adults with suspected meningitis, it is common to perform a computerized tomographic (CT) scan of the brain before doing an LP.[11] This is because space-occupying lesions are common in adults, either tumors mimicking meningitis or intracranial suppurative complications of meningitis. In one study, 24% of adults had abnormal CT scans and 5% had a lesion with a mass effect.[11] However, the value of routine LP in adults has been disputed by a consensus group of Canadian neurologists.[12]

Question | In children with suspected meningitis, is CT scan of the brain a reliable predictor of raised intracranial pressure or impending cerebral herniation?

Literature review | We found five observational studies[13–17] and two reviews[18,19] of CT in childhood bacterial meningitis.

A prospective study of 41 children who had routine CT scans for bacterial meningitis found that CT scan showed sub-dural effusions in 8, focal cerebral infarcts in 5, and basal cistern pus in 1.[13] Clinical management was not influenced by the CT findings, which failed to reveal any clinically significant abnormalities that were not suspected on neurologic examination.[13]

In another study, 5 of 14 children with imminent herniation had a normal CT scan.[10] In a retrospective study of 30 children, CT was normal in 10, of whom 6 had clinical evidence of raised intracranial pressure (ICP).[14]

CT is useful in deciding which children with neurologic disease and suspected intracranial complications need surgery.[13–17] CT scan does not exclude raised intracranial pressure and even imminent herniation,[10,13,14] and most children with abnormal CT scans have neurologic signs which would contraindicate LP.[18,19] Furthermore, there are growing concerns that CT scans of the brain may lead to long-term risk of malignancy[20,21]: the estimated lifetime cancer mortality risk attributable to the radiation exposure from a CT scan of the brain in a 1-year-old is 0.07% or 1 in 1430.[20] CT scans are useful in assessing children with suspected intracranial pathology, but only after treatment. Routine use of CT scans before LP looking for raised intracranial pressure or impending herniation or to exclude space-occupying lesions is contrary to the evidence and potentially harmful.

We recommend not using routine CT scans before LP for children with suspected meningitis.

Delayed LP

Concern has been expressed that it is increasingly common to treat children with suspected meningitis with empiric antibiotics without doing an immediate LP.[22,23] Delaying LP risks making the wrong diagnosis and giving the wrong treatment.

Box 10.1 Contraindications to immediate lumbar puncture

· focal neurologic signs
· papilledema
· rapidly deteriorating consciousness or obtundation (Glasgow Coma Score < 8)
· signs of raised intracranial pressure (falling pulse, rising BP, dilated or poorly reacting pupil[s])
· continuous seizure activity
· bleeding diathesis
[NB: LP should be delayed but performed as soon as the child is clinically stable]

Our recommended contraindications to immediate LP are given in Box 10.1. There is general consensus that LP should be delayed if the child is considered to have a high risk of cerebral herniation,[1,9,10,24] and most of the contraindications reflect clinical findings associated with cerebral herniation.[8–10] Some authors have quoted a modified Glasgow Coma Score (GCS) <13 as a contraindication to LP, a figure which was also used in the Advanced Paediatric Life Support Manual produced by the RCPCH advisory committee.[22,23] This cutoff figure for GCS may derive from an adult study, which defined GCS <13 as one of a number of features associated with an abnormal CT scan, but did not comment on its predictive value.[11] We could find no evidence to support using a cutoff GCS of 13 in children with suspected meningitis, and its use would contraindicate LP in most children with suspected meningitis.[23] The rationale for using a GCS <8 as the cutoff comes from a retrospective study,[25] which found that children with GCS <8 were more likely to die from coning than were those with GCS 8 or above (RR 4.6, 95% CI 1.1–35.8).

If it is decided to treat empirically with antibiotics without immediate LP, the LP should be performed as soon as the child is clinically stable, preferably within 2–3 days. Abnormal CSF white count, sugar, and protein usually persist this long in bacterial meningitis,[1] and rapid bacterial tests (e.g., polymerase chain reaction [PCR] for *N. meningitidis*, and antigen detection for pneumoccus and Hib) may still be positive.

CSF examination
Organisms
A Gram's iodine stain of CSF (Gram stain) demonstrates bacteria in 60–90% of patients with bacterial meningitis who have not received prior antibiotics, and has a specificity >97%.[26–28]

CSF white count and differential
It is not safe to rely on total or differential CSF white count to distinguish bacterial meningitis from viral meningitis for management decisions. In untreated bacterial meningitis, the CSF white cell count is usually in the range of 1000–5000 cells/mm^3 (1000–5000 × 10^6 cells/L), although the range is <100 to >10,000 and rarely no white cells are found in the CSF.[26–29] The total CSF white count in viral meningitis is lower on average, but there is considerable overlap.[26–29] There is usually a neutrophil predominance in bacterial meningitis, but a neutrophil predominance is found in more than half of all cases of viral meningitis in the first 24 hours, and often persists.[29] More concerning for decisions about withholding antibiotics, the CSF may show a lymphocyte predominance in Listeria meningitis and in partially treated bacterial meningitis.[1,28] Treatment decisions based on the CSF white cell count and differential should be guarded.

CSF glucose and CSF/serum glucose ratio
The CSF glucose is usually low in bacterial meningitis, but the ratio of CSF and blood glucose is more sensitive and specific than absolute CSF glucose levels.[26–30] A CSF/serum glucose ratio of 0.4 or less is 80% sensitive and 98% specific for bacterial meningitis in children >2 months old.[26–30]

CSF protein
The CSF protein is usually, but not always, >6 mg/dL (0.6 g/L) in bacterial meningitis.[26–30] Very high CSF protein levels should raise suspicion of tuberculous meningitis.[1]

CSF lactate
CSF lactate level has been reported to be more sensitive and specific for bacterial meningitis than other CSF parameters.[31–33] As with other parameters, however, the CSF lactate may be normal in bacterial meningitis. CSF lactate was also reported as being marginally more accurate than CSF/serum glucose ratio in patients with suspected bacterial meningitis post-neurosurgery.[34]

Rapid bacterial assays on CSF
PCR has been used to amplify nucleic acid from N. meningitidis, S. pneumoniae, Hib, S. agalactiae (GBS), and Listeria monocytogenes. The sensitivity and specificity of the different tests are in the range 90–98%. These tests can be used when the patient has received prior antibiotics and with infection with relatively fastidious organisms such as meningococcus.[24,35,36] Latex agglutination tests are simpler and cheaper, but less sensitive[37] and their routine use is not recommended.[1,24] As with PCR, the main use is probably for pretreated patients.

Acute phase reactants
Serum and CSF CRP are often raised in bacterial meningitis. A meta-analysis of 21 studies of CSF CRP and 10 studies of serum CRP found a wide range in sensitivity (69–99%) and specificity (28–99%) of serum CRP to predict bacterial meningitis.[38] The tests were most useful if they were negative, having >97% negative predictive value, but less useful to make a firm diagnosis of bacterial meningitis.

In a small study, plasma procalcitonin distinguished children with bacterial meningitis from viral meningitis.[39]

Treatment of bacterial meningitis
An algorithm for the assessment and early management of a child with suspected meningitis is given in Figure 10.1.

Antibiotics for bacterial meningitis
Neonates and infants under 3 months
For neonates and infants under 3 months, the likely organisms are the neonatal organisms, S. agalactiae, E. coli, other enteric Gram-negative rods, or Listeria, plus the organisms which cause meningitis in older children. The Gram stain will often help decide which antibiotic(s) to start (see Table 10.1), but for empiric therapy when the organism is unknown, we recommend:

amoxi/ampicillin 50 mg/kg IV, 6-hourly PLUS
cefotaxime 50 mg/kg IV, 6-hourly PLUS
vancomycin 15 mg/kg IV, 6-hourly (not needed for early onset neonatal meningitis)

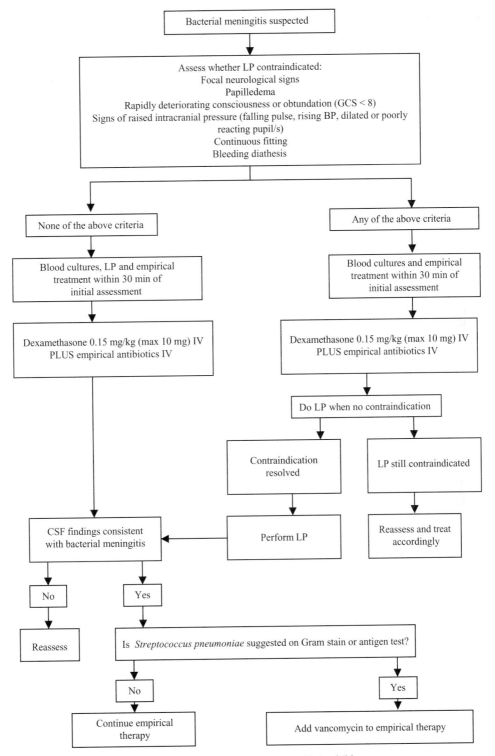

Figure 10.1 Algorithm for management of suspected bacterial meningitis in children.

Table 10.1 Specific antibiotic therapy for neonates and babies <3 months old, according to CSF Gram stain.

Gram Stain	Likely Organism	Suggested Antibiotic Therapy
Gram-positive cocci	Group B streptococcus, *Streptococcus faecalis*, *Streptococcus. pneumoniae*	Cefotaxime 50 mg/kg IV, 6-hourly PLUS vancomycin 15 mg/kg IV, 6-hourly
Gram-negative bacilli	*Escherichia coli*, *Salmonella*, other Gram-negative bacilli	Cefotaxime 50 mg/kg IV, 6-hourly OR cefepime 50 mg/kg IV, 8-hourly
Gram-negative cocci	*Neisseria meningitidis*	Benzylpenicillin 45 mg/kg IV, 4-hourly
Gram-positive bacilli	*Listeria monocytogenes*	Amoxi/ampicillin 50 mg/kg IV, 6-hourly

The third-generation cephalosporins are recommended because of excellent CSF penetration, rapid CSF sterilization, and because of activity against Gram-negative bacilli as well as some Gram-positive organisms.[40] Ceftriaxone is not recommended for neonates because it can displace bilirubin from albumin and because it can cause biliary sludging. Ampicillin or amoxicillin is added to the third-generation cephalosporins because the latter have no activity against Listeria or enterococci.

Cefotaxime has no activity against *Pseudomonas*. If Pseudomonas is suspected to be the cause of meningitis, e.g., because of prior colonization, cefepime (or ceftazidime or meropenem) is recommended.

Vancomycin is used because of the increasing number of cases of infection with *S. pneumoniae* which are relatively insensitive to penicillin.[41–44] The recommendation to use vancomycin is based on convincing clinical descriptions of children with meningitis due to penicillin-insensitive pneumococci who do not improve until vancomycin is started.[41–44] There are no prospective studies comparing vancomycin with other treatments in this situation, but in one retrospective study children with penicillin-insensitive pneumococcal meningitis given vancomycin required shorter duration of treatment than those not given vancomycin.[41]

Children 3 months and older

For children >3 months old, the likely organisms and the recommended treatment are shown in Table 10.2. The frequency of organisms depends on local epidemiology and on immunization practices. *Listeria* meningitis is rare outside the neonatal period, but, if it does occur, is usually in immunodeficient children.

For empiric therapy, when the organism is unknown, we recommend:

vancomycin 15 mg/kg (max 500 mg) IV, 6-hourly PLUS EITHER
cefotaxime 50 mg/kg (max 2 g) IV, 6-hourly OR
ceftriaxone 50 mg/kg (max 2 g) IV, daily

We recommend stopping the vancomycin if a penicillin-susceptible pneumococcus (minimum inhibitory concentration [MIC] <0.125 mg/L) or another organism likely to be susceptible to ceftriaxone/cefotaxime is grown.

Table 10.2 Specific antibiotic therapy for children 3 months old and older, according to CSF Gram stain.

Gram Stain	Likely Organism	Suggested Antibiotic Therapy
Gram-positive cocci	*Streptococcus pneumoniae*	Cefotaxime 50 mg/kg (max 2 g) IV, 6-hourly PLUS vancomycin 15 mg/kg (max 600 mg) IV, 6-hourly
Gram-negative bacilli	*Haemophilus influenzae*	Cefotaxime 50 mg/kg (max 2 g) IV, 6-hourly OR ceftriaxone 50 mg/kg (max 2 g) IV, daily
Gram-negative cocci	*Neisseria meningitidis*	Benzylpenicillin 45 mg/kg (max 1.8 g) IV, 4-hourly
Gram-positive bacilli	*Listeria monocytogenes*	Amoxi/ampicillin 50 mg/kg (max 2 g) IV, 6-hourly

For patients with anaphylactic penicillin or cephalosporin allergy, we recommend:

vancomycin 15 mg/kg (max 500 mg) IV, 6-hourly
PLUS EITHER
ciprofloxacin 15 mg/kg (max 600 mg) IV, 12-hourly OR
moxifloxacin 10 mg/kg (max 400 mg) IV, daily

Subsequent therapy is guided by cultures and other tests.

If meningococcal meningitis and/or septicemia is suspected, e.g., because of a purpuric rash, emergency treatment with parenteral benzylpenicillin before hospital admission is recommended (see p. 249).

Corticosteroids for bacterial meningitis

Question | In children with bacterial meningitis, does adjunctive therapy with corticosteroids compared with no corticosteroids or placebo reduce morbidity or mortality?

Literature review | We found 21 RCTs and a Cochrane review of corticosteroids and bacterial meningitis.[45]

The Cochrane review found 18 RCTs (1853 adults and children) of corticosteroid therapy and bacterial meningitis.[45] Overall, adjuvant corticosteroids were associated with lower case fatality (RR 0.76, 95% CI 0.59–0.98) and lower rates of both severe hearing loss (RR 0.36, 95% CI 0.22–0.60) and long-term neurologic sequelae (RR 0.66, 95% CI 0.44–0.99). However, the meta-analysis was dependent mainly on *H. influenzae* meningitis, which used to be the commonest cause of childhood meningitis but has virtually disappeared post-immunization.[1]

Corticosteroids reduced severe hearing loss in children with *H. influenzae* meningitis (RR 0.31, 95% CI 0.15–0.62) and in meningitis caused by bacteria other than *H. influenzae* (RR 0.42, 95% CI 0.20–0.89). For meningitis caused by bacteria other than *H. influenzae*, 20 children would need to be treated with corticosteroids to prevent one case of hearing loss.[45] The numbers of cases were insufficient to say that corticosteroids reduced hearing loss for any particular organism, except *H. influenzae*.

There was no demonstrated reduction in mortality for pneumococcal meningitis, although a subsequent, retrospective Australian study[46] found that use of corticosteroids before or with parenteral antibiotics was associated with reduced chance of death or severe morbidity from pneumococcal meningitis (adjusted OR 0.21, 95% CI 0.05–0.77). A study from Malawi found no benefit from dexamethasone in children with bacterial meningitis, suggesting that corticosteroids are not beneficial in a developing country setting, where HIV coinfection is likely to be important.[47]

In a subsequent adult study,[48] treatment with dexamethasone was associated with a reduction in mortality (RR 0.48, 95% CI 0.24–0.96) and a halving of poor neurologic outcome from 52 to 26% of cases (RR 0.50, 95% CI 0.30–0.83).

The two major concerns about corticosteroid therapy are whether it is associated with an increased risk of gastrointestinal bleeding and whether corticosteroid therapy might delay sterilization of the CSF, particularly for penicillin-insensitive pneumococci. The Cochrane meta-analysis[45] and subsequent adult study[48] found no increase in gastrointestinal bleeding in association with corticosteroids. There are insufficient data on whether or not dexamethasone therapy delays CSF sterilization in meningitis due to penicillin-insensitive pneumococci.[44]

We believe the evidence favors early treatment with dexamethasone, given before or with the first dose of antibiotic, for children with haemophilus or pneumococcal meningitis. We feel there are insufficient data on corticosteroids for meningococcal meningitis to recommend their routine use (see p. 250), although there is no evidence to suggest they are harmful either. For children with presumed meningitis who are treated empirically without an immediate LP and for children with CSF pleocytosis but no organism seen, we recommend corticosteroids. Data suggest there is no benefit in commencing corticosteroids after the first dose of antibiotic.

We recommend giving dexamethasone just before or with the first dose of antibiotic for children with proven or presumed meningitis (other than meningococcal meningitis).

We recommend:

dexamethasone 0.15 mg/kg (max 10 mg) IV, before or with the first dose of antibiotic, then 6-hourly for 4 days.

If dexamethasone is unavailable, we recommend using hydrocortisone 4 mg/kg (max 200 mg) IV for the initial dose.

Intravenous fluids for bacterial meningitis

Question | In children with bacterial meningitis, does fluid restriction compared with no fluid restriction improve outcome?

Literature review | We found six studies of which three were retrospective and three were RCTs, and a Cochrane review of fluid therapy for bacterial meningitis.[49]

The serum sodium is often low and urine output decreased in bacterial meningitis. For a long time, this was thought to be due to the syndrome of inappropriate antidiuretic hormone secretion, and fluid restriction was recommended for children with bacterial meningitis. This belief has been questioned, and biochemical evidence has been presented that the low urine output and low sodium are due to fluid depletion.[50] Some have even suggested that hyponatremia in treated children is due to the "syndrome of inappropriate fluids."

A Cochrane review found three RCTs from the USA, India, and Papua New Guinea (PNG) which compared maintenance fluids (normal fluid replacement) with fluid restriction.[49] Mortality was high in the PNG study, which was the largest of the three. The meta-analysis found no significant difference between the maintenance-fluid and restricted-fluid groups in number of deaths (RR 0.82, 95% CI 0.53–1.27), acute severe neurologic sequelae (RR 0.67, 95% CI 0.41–1.08), or in mild to moderate sequelae (RR 1.24, 95% CI 0.58–2.65). However, children given maintenance fluids were less likely to develop spasticity (RR 0.50, 95% CI 0.27–0.93), to have seizures at both 72 hours (RR 0.59, 95% CI 0.42–0.83) and 14 days (RR 0.19, 95% CI 0.04–0.88), and to have chronic severe neurologic sequelae at 3-months follow-up (RR 0.42, 95% CI 0.20–0.89).[49]

> **We do not recommend fluid restriction for children with bacterial meningitis.**

Duration of antibiotics for bacterial meningitis

The duration of therapy for bacterial meningitis is dictated more by custom than by evidence.[51,52] The numbers of days of antibiotics given in studies tend to be

Table 10.3 Recommended duration of parenteral antibiotics for uncomplicated meningitis in children.

Organism	Duration of Antibiotics (Days)
Neisseria meningitidis	5
Haemophilus influenzae	7
Streptococcus pneumoniae	10
Group B streptococcus	14–21
Gram-negative bacilli	21
Listeria monocytogenes	21

multiples of "magical numbers," the number of fingers on a hand (5) or days in a week (7).[51]

It has been known for over 30 years that meningococci are extremely sensitive to antibiotics and meningococcal meningitis can be cured with a single dose of long-acting penicillin[53] or chloramphenicol.[54] Treatment of bacterial meningitis, from whatever organism, was, nevertheless, traditionally for at least 10–14 days, and longer if fever persisted or for neonatal meningitis. It was then shown that for children >3 months old who were making an uncomplicated recovery, 7 days treatment with ceftriaxone was as good as 10 days.[55] A study in Chile showed that 4 days of ceftriaxone was equivalent to 7 days for selected children who were improving rapidly[56] (the choice of 4 rather than 5 days contradicted the magical numbers theory).

Our recommendations for antibiotic duration are based on the current Infectious Disease Society of America consensus recommendations[11] and are shown in Table 10.3. The evidence base is poor, and any individual child may need to be treated longer if fever persists. We do not recommend using oral antibiotics for any of the course, because oral antibiotics are unlikely to achieve adequate CSF levels to sterilize the CSF.

Chemoprophylaxis in bacterial meningitis

The secondary attack rate in household contacts is increased to 4.2 per 1000 for meningococcal disease[57] and to 5.2 per 1000 for Hib.[58] Antibiotic prophylaxis is recommended to prevent secondary cases of bacterial meningitis in household contacts of patients with meningitis due to *N. meningitidis* (see p. 251) or Hib. How strong is the evidence?

Question | For household contacts of patients with bacterial meningitis due to meningococcus or Hib, do prophylactic antibiotics compared with no antibiotics or placebo prevent secondary cases?

Literature review | We found a non-Cochrane systematic review[59] and a Cochrane review of prophylactic antibiotics in meningococcal infection[60] and a case-control study in Hib infection.[58]

A non-Cochrane systematic review of the effectiveness of prophylactic antibiotics in meningococcal infection[59] found no high-quality prospective studies, but four retrospective observational studies and one small trial comparing children who did or did not receive chemoprophylaxis. The outcome was secondary cases of meningococcal infection occurring 1–30 days after the index case. Chemoprophylaxis reduced the risk of meningococcal infection for household contacts by an impressive 89%: the risk ratio was 0.11 (95% CI 0.02–0.58) and 218 contacts had to take prophylactic antibiotics to prevent one case of meningococcal infection. In contrast, the data in day-care settings were insufficient to judge whether or not chemoprophylaxis is indicated.

A Cochrane review of chemoprophylaxis[60] found no RCTs and no secondary cases, so could not comment on the effectiveness of chemoprophylaxis. It found that ciprofloxacin, minocycline, and rifamp(ic)in were effective at eradicating nasal carriage of meningococcus at 1 week, but only rifampin (RR 0.20, 95% CI 0.14–0.29) and ciprofloxacin (RR 0.03, 95% CI 0.00–0.42) still proved effective at 1–2 weeks. Rifampin continued to be effective compared to placebo for up to 4 weeks after treatment but resistant isolates were seen following prophylactic treatment. No trials evaluated ceftriaxone against placebo but ceftriaxone was more effective than rifampin after 1–2 weeks of follow-up (RR 5.93, 95% CI 1.22–28.68).

Because there were no cases of meningococcal disease during follow-up in any of the trials, effectiveness regarding prevention of future disease cannot be directly assessed.

We recommend *N. meningitidis* (meningococcus) prophylaxis for household contacts using:

rifamp(ic)in: neonate <1 month 5 mg/kg; child 10 mg/kg (max 600 mg), adult 600 mg, orally, 12-hourly for 2 days (preferred option for children) OR

ciprofloxacin (adult and child ≥12 years) 500 mg orally, child 12.5 mg/kg (max 500 mg) as a single dose OR

ceftriaxone 250 mg (child: 125 mg) IM as a single dose (preferred option during pregnancy).

Rifamp(ic)in is associated with multiple drug interactions, stains contact lenses orange, and is not recommended for persons with severe liver disease. Because they cause cartilage damage in laboratory animals, there are theoretical concerns about quinolones causing skeletal problems in children, although data do not suggest this is a real clinical problem.[61]

A case-control study showed that chemoprophylaxis of household contacts not only reduces carriage of Hib, but appears to prevent secondary cases of Hib disease.[58] Hib disease is rare in countries that routinely use Hib conjugate vaccines. If a case of Hib disease occurs in a well-immunized population, chemoprophylaxis is indicated only if there is an unimmunized or partially immunized child in the household, i.e., any baby 6 months of age or less or else a child <5 years old who is not fully immunized. In that case and in unimmunized populations, prophylaxis should be given to the whole family to reduce the risk of transmission. We recommend:

rifamp(ic)in: neonate <1 month 10 mg/kg; child 20 mg/kg (max 600 mg), adult 600 mg orally, daily for 4 days

Skull fracture and bacterial meningitis

Skull fractures, particularly fractures of the base of the skull, predispose to bacterial meningitis if the dura mater adjacent to the fracture site is torn, placing the central nervous system (CNS) in contact with bacteria from the paranasal sinuses, nasopharynx, or middle ear. A greater associated risk has been reported when CSF leakage occurs, particularly if it persists for more than 7 days.[62]

Question | In patients with post-traumatic CSF leak, do prophylactic antibiotics compared with no antibiotics reduce the risk of bacterial meningitis?

Literature review | We found five RCTs, two non-Cochrane meta-analyses,[63,64] and a Cochrane review.[65]

In one non-Cochrane meta-analysis of patients with post-traumatic CSF leak, the risk of bacterial meningitis was 2.5% if they received antibiotics and 10% if they did not, and the difference was significant.[63] Another non-Cochrane meta-analysis and a Cochrane review, however, found the incidence of meningitis with or without antibiotics was 6–7%, with no demonstrable benefit from prophylactic antibiotics.[64,65]

We do not recommend prophylactic antibiotics for children with post-traumatic CSF leak.

Recurrent bacterial meningitis

For children with recurrent bacterial meningitis, the major causes are anatomic or immunologic abnormalities. Anatomic abnormalities include an occult dural lesion such as a dermal sinus tract, basal encephalocele, or neurenteric cyst, and so physical examination should include a careful search along the craniospinal axis, proceeding to diagnostic imaging (MRI or CT) if there is any suspicion.[66,67] Abnormalities of the inner ear, such as Mondini dysplasia, are usually associated with CSF leak which can be occult.[68] The diagnosis is made by performing thin-cut computed tomography of the temporal bones.[68] Basal skull fractures, usually post-traumatic and associated with CSF leak, should also be considered (see p. 139).

Immunologic abnormalities that should be considered include humoral defects (measure total serum immunoglobulins and consider measuring functional antibody levels to immunizations, such as Hib or pneumococcus) and complement defects. Terminal complement defects are associated with recurrent meningococcal infection.[66,67] Asplenia predisposes to infection with capsulated organisms (see Section 9.3, p. 125) but is an unusual cause of recurrent meningitis.[66,67]

The organism responsible for the recurrent bacterial meningitis may be significant. Pneumococcus or Haemophilus suggests cranial dural defects, *E. coli* or other Gram-negative bacilli suggest spinal dural defects, and meningococci suggest complement deficiency or IgM deficiency.

Recurrence of acute bacterial meningitis due to persistence and recrudescence of the causative organism is more common in neonates than in older children,[2] and may or may not be due to an intracranial collection, such as brain abscess.[66,67] Antibiotic-induced meningitis (usually due to penicillin or trimethoprim-sulfamethoxazole or intrathecal antibiotics) is a rare cause of recurrent aseptic meningitis.[69] Finally, if

there are puzzling aspects of the recurrent meningitis, such as different organisms or failure to respond to apparently adequate treatment, the possibility of Munchausen syndrome by proxy may need to be considered.[70]

Cochlear implants and bacterial meningitis

Cochlear implants are medical devices that electronically stimulate the auditory nerves in the cochlea (inner ear), allowing persons with severe hearing loss to perceive sound.[71] In 2002, a cluster of cases of bacterial meningitis was identified among European cochlear implant recipients.[72,73] Although there was initial suspicion that this was related to one manufacturer and one device, subsequent epidemiologic studies have revealed that the risk of bacterial meningitis for cochlear transplant recipients is increased. In particular, the risk of pneumococcal meningitis is more than 30 times the expected incidence for age in the USA.[74] The risk is also increased in Canada.[75] Although the largest increase by far is for pneumococcal meningitis, there have also been anecdotal reports of meningitis with *H. influenzae* (both type b and untypeable), *N. meningitidis*, *Enterococcus*, *Acinetobacter baumanii*, and *E. coli*.[74–76] Almost all cochlear implant devices are associated with an increased risk of pneumococcal meningitis, although the presence of an extra piece called a "positioner," which holds the electrode in place, greatly increases the risk.[72–75]

In countries with universal infant pneumococcal immunization, it is sufficient to ensure that all children who receive cochlear implants are routinely immunized and are monitored and treated promptly for any bacterial infections after receiving the implant. In countries without universal infant pneumococcal immunization, children with cochlear implants should be immunized as for children with asplenia (see p. 126).

CNS shunt infections

Ventricular shunts are used frequently to treat congenital or post-hemorrhagic hydrocephalus in newborns and to treat various causes of hydrocephalus in older children. The reported incidence of shunt infection varies widely from 1.5 to 39%, although more recently rates of 10–15% have been reported.[76–78] In a retrospective review of patients undergoing CSF shunt operations between 1996 and 1999, three perioperative variables were significantly associated with an increased risk of shunt infection: prematurity, the presence of a post-operative CSF leak, and inadvertent exposure to breached surgical gloves.[78]

The most common pathogens are coagulase-negative staphylococci (50–90%), followed by *Staphylococcus aureus* (13–27%), and a miscellany of other organisms, including aerobic Gram-negative bacilli (10–20%), streptococci (8–10%), and *Propionibacterium* spp.[76–78] Coagulase-negative staphylococci are known to produce a glycocalyx (slime layer), which allows them to survive on the surface of synthetic materials as in shunts and makes it hard to sterilize the shunt with antibiotics.[79]

Babies and older children with CSF shunt infections may present with the acute signs and symptoms of meningitis. More commonly, however, they present more indolently with fever and irritability. The diagnosis is made by obtaining CSF for microscopy and culture. In one study, the serum CRP was elevated in 97.1% of children with CSF shunt infections, with a specificity of 73.5%.[80] CRP may help identify which children are unlikely to be infected, but for optimum management there is no substitute for obtaining CSF.

The options for managing patients with shunt infections[76–78] include:

(A) removal of the entire colonized shunt, external CSF drainage, either by implantation of an external ventricular drain or by regularly tapping the ventricles, administration of antibiotics systemically, intraventricularly, or both, and shunt replacement when the CSF is sterile;

(B) removal of the entire colonized shunt and immediate replacement with a new shunt, followed by a course of antibiotics (either systemic, intraventricular, or both);

(C) antibiotic therapy alone, administered either systemically, intraventricularly, or by both routes.

Variations on these options, with exteriorization of the distal shunt catheter and the administration of systemic and intraventricular antibiotics for between 2 and 4 weeks, followed by revision of either the distal catheter alone or the entire shunt system, have also been described.[78]

A single, small RCT compared patients who received each of options A, B, or C above.[81] All 10 patients in Group A and 9 of 10 in Group B were treated successfully. In contrast, only 3 of 10 in Group C responded to antibiotic treatment without shunt removal.[81] A recent observational paper reports that some adult patients with CSF shunts have been treated successfully with antibiotics alone.[77] In general, however, the evidence suggests most infections in neonates and older children will not resolve without shunt removal.

There is debate on the relative merits of the intravenous and intraventricular routes of antibiotic administration, but few data. An RCT comparing vancomycin treatment of drain-associated staphylococcal ventriculitis in adults found that much higher CSF vancomycin levels were obtained using intraventricular than using intravenous treatment.[82] Intravenous treatment, however, cleared infection as well as intraventricular treatment. Intraventricular treatment also carries the risk of causing CNS damage through direct toxicity or through inflammatory changes consequent on endotoxin-induced cytokine release.[83] A neonatal RCT found that neonates who received intraventricular gentamicin in addition to intravenous antibiotics compared to those receiving intravenous antibiotics alone had no shorter duration of positive cultures and had increased mortality (RR 3.43, 95% CI 1.09–10.74).[84,85] We do not recommend giving intraventricular antibiotics unless the CSF cannot be sterilized using shunt removal, external drainage, and intravenous antibiotics.

Treatment should be based on CSF microscopy and culture. If for some reason cultures cannot be obtained or are delayed, we recommend the following empiric regimen, aimed at staphylococcal and *Pseudomonas* infection. The regimen should be modified, if necessary, as soon as Gram stain and culture results are available.

vancomycin 15 mg/kg (max 500 mg) IV, 6-hourly
PLUS EITHER
ceftazidime 50 mg/kg (max 2 g) IV, 8-hourly OR
meropenem 40 mg/kg (max 2 g) IV, 8-hourly

Meropenem is preferred to imipenem-cilastatin due to the lower risk of seizures.[86]

There is interest in the use of antibiotic-impregnated shunt materials to reduce the risk of infection, but as yet insufficient data to recommend them.[87]

141

10.2 Subdural empyema

Subdural empyema in children usually occurs as a complication of meningitis, sinusitis, or mastoiditis.[88–90] The incidence is biphasic in immunocompetent children, with cases either occurring in children <2 years mainly as a complication of bacterial meningitis, or in children >7 years mainly as a complication of sinusitis.[88–90] The most frequent organism isolated from sinusitis-associated sub-dural empyema is *S. anginosus* (*milleri*), but polymicrobial infection with *S. pneumoniae*, *S. aureus*, Gram-negative bacilli, and anaerobes is common.[88–90] A distinction is sometimes drawn between sub-dural empyema and intracranial epidural abscess,[91] but is not always easy to make in practice.

Although there are anecdotal reports of medical treatment of sub-dural empyema with antibiotics alone, neurosurgical exploration is strongly advised, both for treatment and to identify the causative organisms.

For empiric antibiotic treatment, we recommend:

benzylpenicillin 60 mg (100,000 U)/kg (max 3.6 g or 6 million U) IV, 4-hourly PLUS
metronidazole 12.5 mg/kg (max 500 mg) IV, 8-hourly PLUS
cefotaxime 50 mg/kg (max 2 g) IV, 6-hourly

10.3 Brain abscess

The term *brain abscess* refers to an abscess within the brain parenchyma, as opposed to a sub-dural empyema or an intracranial epidural abscess, which are both extra parenchymal.

We found no RCTs on the treatment of brain abscess in children, but we found observational studies on treatment and outcome,[88–93] and a review on the management of brain abscess in children.[94]

Almost 25% of all brain abscesses occur in children <15 years, with a peak at 4–7 years. The most common predisposing conditions are cyanotic congenital heart disease (hematogenous spread) and direct spread from a contiguous site (middle ear, sinuses, teeth).[94] Brain abscesses are uncommon complications of bacterial meningitis or head trauma (usually with a significant delay from the time of injury). Although conditions such as cystic fibrosis, bronchiectasis, and brain surgery predispose to brain abscess,

no predisposing factor can be identified in up to 30% of children.[94]

Aerobic and anaerobic streptococci, including *S. anginosus* (*milleri*) are grown from 50 to 70% of brain abscesses in children.[94] However, where the likely site of origin is the ear, enteric Gram-negative bacilli are commonly involved (10–25% of all abscesses), while after trauma or surgery, staphylococci predominate (10–30% of total).[88–94] Polymicrobial infection, often involving anaerobic organisms, is found in up to 30% of children.[94] In neonates, Gram-negative enteric bacilli are most common.[95] Immunocompromised hosts can develop brain abscesses caused by *Nocardia*, by fungi such as *Aspergillus* or *Scedosporium*, or by *Mycobacterium tuberculosis*. *Toxoplasma gondii*, a common cause of parasitic brain abscess in adults with AIDS, is rarely encountered in children.[94]

The clinical presentation of brain abscess in infants and children varies depending on the location of the abscess or abscesses, the virulence of the organism and the child's immune status. Headache, fever, and vomiting each occur in 60–70%. Seizures, altered mental status, and focal neurologic signs occur in 25–50%. Meningeal signs occur in <25% and the classic triad of fever, headache, and focal deficits occurs in <30% of children.[94] Thus the clinical features are often nonspecific and a high index of suspicion is required.

Routine laboratory tests are often unhelpful. The CSF may show a pleocytosis, but no organisms are seen and culture is sterile.[94] Other CSF parameters do not distinguish brain abscess from bacterial or aseptic meningitis.[94] Positive blood cultures are found in about 10% of cases. If brain abscess is suspected clinically, imaging with CT and/or MRI (magnetic resonance imaging) is indicated. If imaging studies indicate a brain abscess, LP is generally not indicated because of the low yield.[94]

CT and MRI are the most important diagnostic tools.[94] MRI is superior to CT because of greater sensitivity and better soft tissue details.[94] CT scan with contrast may show a hypodense, ring-enhancing lesion. Because the CT appearances develop slowly and may lag behind the clinical presentation, a normal CT scan does not exclude a brain abscess.[94]

Aspiration or biopsy can guide antimicrobial therapy and is often important for treatment, because antibiotics penetrate relatively poorly into the brain tissue.

For brain abscess associated with sinusitis, mastoiditis, otitis, or cyanotic congenital heart disease, we recommend:

> **metronidazole 12.5 mg/kg (max 500 mg) IV, 8-hourly** PLUS EITHER
> **cefotaxime 50 mg/kg (max 2 g) IV, 6-hourly** OR
> **ceftriaxone 100 mg/kg (max 4 g) IV, daily**

For post-neurosurgical brain abscess, penetrating head trauma, ventriculoperitoneal shunts, or endocarditis where the risk of *S. aureus*, MRSA, and coagulase negative staphylococcal infection is much greater, and for abscesses associated with meningitis, to cover penicillin-insensitive *S. pneumoniae*, we recommend:

> **vancomycin 15 mg/kg (max 500 mg) IV, 6-hourly** PLUS EITHER
> **cefotaxime 50 mg/kg (max 2 g) IV, 6-hourly** OR
> **ceftriaxone 100 mg/kg (max 4 g) IV, daily**

If microscopy and/or culture indicates the need to cover for *Pseudomonas aeruginosa*,[89–94] we recommend using instead of cefotaxime or ceftriaxone:

> **ceftazidime 50 mg/kg (max 2 g) IV, 8-hourly** OR
> **meropenem 40 mg/kg (max 2 g) IV, 8-hourly**

In neonatal brain abscess, where *L. monocytogenes* is possible, ampicillin should be used with cefotaxime, as on p. 134.

For empiric therapy, if aspiration cannot be performed, we recommend:

> **benzylpenicillin 60 mg (100,000 U)/kg (max 3.6 g or 6 million U) IV, 4-hourly** PLUS
> **metronidazole 12.5 mg/kg (max 500 mg) IV, 8-hourly** PLUS EITHER
> **ceftriaxone 100 mg/kg (max 4 g) IV, daily** OR
> **cefotaxime 50 mg/kg (max 2 g) IV, 6-hourly**

Therapy should be modified on the basis of Gram stain and culture results. The optimum duration of treatment is unknown and should be individualized, based on clinical response and radiologic evidence of resolution. Intravenous antibiotics generally should be continued for 4–6 weeks, although a 3–4-week course may be adequate for those who underwent surgical excision. After this time, small residual abscesses may remain but clinical data suggest they are sterile. Some authorities recommend an additional 2–3 months of oral antibiotics, but the benefit is doubtful. Corticosteroids may decrease intracranial pressure but are not routinely recommended because of concerns that they can also decrease antibiotic penetration across the blood–brain barrier and impair clearance of pathogens.[94]

10.4 Spinal epidural abscess

Spinal epidural abscess presents with fever, back pain, diminished movement in the legs (paraplegia or paraparesis), and sometimes urinary retention.[96] Spinal epidural abscesses are frequently associated with adjacent vertebral osteomyelitis or disc infection, and are most likely to be caused by *S. aureus*.[96] The major differential diagnosis is transverse myelitis (see Section 10.13, p. 149).

Spinal epidural abscess is a surgical emergency, especially if associated with neurologic deficit. Immediate radiologic assessment is a priority, because of the risk of progressive neurologic damage with epidural abscess. Magnetic resonance imaging is the best and only reliable non-invasive method for assessing the epidural space and spinal cord. T1-gadolinium sequences will show an epidural mass with peripheral enhancement.[96]

If radiology suggests an epidural abscess, emergency surgical assessment with a view to drainage of the epidural collection is essential. A retrospective study of adults with spinal epidural abscess, mainly lumbar, reported that the outcome was the same in patients treated with surgery plus antibiotics, CT-guided aspiration plus antibiotics, or antibiotics alone.[97] Most authorities advocate surgical or radiologic drainage because of the risk of cord compression leading to irreversible neurologic damage,[96] although a severity grading system might allow conservative medical management of patients at low risk for neurologic damage.[98] Antibiotic treatment should be based on the Gram stain and culture results of operative material, but for empiric therapy prior to surgery, we recommend:

> **di/flucl/oxa/nafcillin 50 mg/kg (max 2 g) IV, 6-hourly** PLUS
> **gentamicin <10 years: 7.5 mg/kg; ≥10 years: 6 mg/kg IV, daily**

Where MRSA infection is likely, because of ethnicity (community-acquired MRSA) or previous colonization or prolonged hospital exposure (hospital-acquired

MRSA), and for patients with anaphylactic penicillin or flucloxacillin allergy, we recommend:

vancomycin 12.5 mg/kg (max 500 mg) IV, 6-hourly PLUS
gentamicin <10 years: 7.5 mg/kg; ≥10 years: 6 mg/kg IV, daily

Clindamycin is a possible alternative to vancomycin when community-acquired MRSA infection is suspected. The duration of therapy is empiric, but we suggest at least 3 weeks, as for osteomyelitis.

Aseptic meningitis

There are a number of reasons that the CSF might be sterile despite evidence of inflammation from raised CSF white cells (CSF pleocytosis). Some examples are given in Box 10.2.

Box 10.2 Causes of CSF pleocytosis with sterile CSF.

· Bacterial meningitis, but no growth
· Partially treated meningitis (prior antibiotics)
· Parameningeal infections, i.e., infection next to meninges (e.g., brain abscess, sub-dural empyema)
· Viral meningitis
· Viral encephalitis, including HSV encephalitis
· Mycoplasma meningoencephalitis
· Acute disseminated encephalomyelitis
· Lyme meningitis
· Tuberculous meningitis
· Fungal meningitis
· Bacterial endocarditis
· Inflammatory , e.g., SLE
· Malignancy
· Drugs, including parenteral and intrathecal antibiotics

10.5   Viral meningitis

Clinical features of viral meningitis

Because of the treatment implications, the major diagnoses to consider in a child with suspected viral meningitis are bacterial meningitis and herpes simplex virus (HSV) encephalitis. Other conditions in Box 10.2 may warrant consideration depending on the clinical situation.

Children with viral meningitis are usually but not always less sick than children with bacterial meningitis, but for any individual child the clinical examination is neither sensitive nor specific enough to determine the need for LP or to suggest it is safe to withhold therapy.[5,6]

HSV can either cause a benign viral meningitis or the much more sinister HSV encephalitis, which will be considered separately in Section 10.7 (p. 145). Children with HSV meningitis may have neck stiffness, headache, and fever, but no significant alteration in level of consciousness and no focal neurologic signs.[99] In contrast, children with HSV encephalitis usually present with one or more of focal or generalized seizures, which often become intractable, decreased level of consciousness, aphasia or neurobehavioral changes, cranial nerve palsies, visual field defects or weakness, which may be hemiplegic or generalized.[99]

A macular or maculopapular rash may occur in enterovirus infections, but children with meningococcal infection can also present with an identical rash,[100] and so the presence of a rash in a child with meningism does not mean it is necessarily safe to withhold antibiotics.

CSF microscopy and biochemistry in viral meningitis

The CSF total white count, neutrophil count, and glucose, protein, lactate, or CRP levels may strongly suggest viral rather than bacterial meningitis, but, as discussed on p. 134, have insufficient sensitivity to withhold antibiotics from a child with meningism and CSF pleocytosis.[26–33] Models based on CSF parameters have been developed which differentiate bacterial meningitis from viral meningitis accurately, but still miss occasional cases of bacterial meningitis.[101,102] It is potentially dangerous to withhold antibiotics on the basis of such a model.

CSF PCR testing in viral meningitis

The use of rapid viral tests, such as PCR on CSF, can help with decisions about treatment, particularly the decision whether it is safe to cease antimicrobial therapy for a child with aseptic meningitis, if PCR results are available in a timely fashion. A review found that enterovirus PCR has >90% sensitivity compared with virus isolation for detecting the enteroviruses: Coxsackie, echo, and polioviruses.[103] The same review also reported that HSV PCR has >90% sensitivity.[103] Mumps is the commonest cause of viral meningitis in unimmunized populations, and outbreaks of mumps are even described despite widespread immunization. Mumps PCR also has a specificity >90%.[103]

Whenever possible when managing a child with suspected viral meningitis, we recommend culturing CSF for viruses (enteroviruses, HSV, and mumps) and sending CSF for PCR to detect enteroviruses and HSV.

Viral culture in viral meningitis

Viral culture of CSF has largely been superseded by PCR in many laboratories, because PCR for enteroviruses and HSV is >90% sensitive and is quicker. When PCR is unavailable, viral culture can still provide valuable information and although enteroviruses grow slowly, HSV cultures may be positive after 2–3 days.[99,104]

Serology in viral meningitis

Serology is rarely helpful for enteroviral infections: children do not mount a detectable antibody response and the tests have poor sensitivity compared with PCR or culture. In one study of children with enteroviral meningitis diagnosed by CSF PCR, 34% had serum IgM to enteroviruses and only 20% had a positive complement fixation test.[105]

Serology may be informative in HSV meningitis or meningoencephalitis, but mainly for making a retrospective diagnosis rather than helping with acute management.[99,104]

Treatment of viral meningitis

The treatment of viral meningitis is primarily supportive, with the exception of HSV encephalitis (see Section 10.7, p. 145). Pleconaril is an antiviral with in vitro activity against enteroviruses, it has some therapeutic efficacy in enteroviral respiratory infections in adults, and there are anecdotal reports of its use in severe enteroviral infections, including meningitis.[106] A double-blind placebo-controlled trial of pleconaril in 20 infants with enteroviral meningitis found no benefit in terms of viral shedding or any clinical outcomes, despite adequate drug levels.[107] Furthermore, there was evidence of drug accumulation and the treatment group had twice as many adverse events.[107]

10.6 Viral encephalitis

The incidence of acute viral encephalitis in childhood is about 10 per 100,000 and up to 30 per 100,000 infants <1 year old.[108–110] It is possible to identify an agent in 40–75% of cases: enteroviruses, *Mycoplasma pneumoniae*, HSV, and influenza are the commonest in recent studies, but arthropod-borne viruses such as West Nile virus and Japanese encephalitis virus are important in some regions.[108–110]

If a child presents with signs and symptoms suggestive of encephalitis, the main priority after resuscitation is to investigate for HSV encephalitis and to treat with acyclovir if there is any doubt. Many experts recommend empiric treatment with acyclovir of all children with acute encephalitis pending further results.[111]

We recommend starting acyclovir for a child with acute encephalitis and continuing until HSV infection has been excluded.

10.7 HSV encephalitis

The annual incidence of HSV encephalitis in the USA is about 20–50 per 100,000 neonates and 3 per 100,000 older children.[108–111] The diagnosis is clinical, supported by laboratory criteria and by imaging. PCR on CSF for HSV nucleic acid is >90% sensitive and specific compared with brain biopsy, and brain biopsy is almost never performed nowadays.[108–111] In neonates, CSF PCR has lower reported sensitivity, at 74–93%.[61] Serology is mostly unhelpful in the acute phase, but serum should be sent to look for specific IgM and IgG to HSV-1 and HSV-2.[102] Support for a diagnosis of HSV encephalitis can be provided by finding focal changes on the EEG or by cerebral imaging using CT scan or MRI scan, all of which characteristically show temporal lobe damage.[99,104] Temporal lobe involvement is sensitive, suggestive MRI changes being found in 90% of patients,[99] but is nonspecific since similar changes can occur in enteroviral encephalitis.[110]

For the treatment of HSV encephalitis in neonates, the recommended treatment[104] is:

acyclovir 20 mg/kg IV, 8-hourly for 21 days

For the treatment of HSV encephalitis in older infants and children, we recommend:

acyclovir 10 mg/kg IV, 8-hourly for 14–21 days

10.8 Mycoplasma meningoencephalitis

M. pneumoniae is a respiratory pathogen that can cause multisystem disease, including the CNS. CNS manifestations include meningoencephalitis, transverse myelitis, stroke, and radiculopathy.[110–113]

The clinical presentation was described in a review of 58 children with *M. pneumoniae* encephalitis, of whom 76% had prior flu-like or respiratory symptoms and 40% had pulmonary infiltrates.[112] Only 57% made a full recovery. Minor to major neurologic sequelae persisted in 34% and 5 patients (9%) died. Poor outcome was associated with higher CSF white count and protein and older age.[112]

Diagnosis is problematic. Serology is the mainstay, but the serum IgM level can remain elevated for many weeks after acute infection, and false-positive IgM tests are well recognized.[110–113] PCR is more reliable on respiratory secretions than CSF: in one study, *M. pneumoniae* was diagnosed in 50 (31%) of 159 children with encephalitis, but CSF PCR was positive in only 11 of them.[110] The diagnosis was confirmed by serology or throat swab PCR in the rest.

The pathogenesis of mycoplasma encephalitis is unknown and the optimum treatment unclear. Various therapies have been used, including antibiotics, corticosteroids, intravenous immunoglobulin (IVIG), and plasmapharesis, but none has been studied in an RCT[110–113]: There is little evidence of active infection in the brain, and some patients recover completely without antibiotics.[110–113] The role of corticosteroids is uncertain. A recent case report described a 17-year-old whose neurologic symptoms resolved while receiving corticosteroid therapy, relapsed after they were stopped, and resolved again when they were restarted.[114] A literature review found that 11 of 14 children (78%) treated with corticosteroids had a near or complete recovery.[114] In a previous study, 56% of children not treated with corticosteroids recovered but the rest died or had severe neurologic sequelae.[115] This sort of comparison with a historic control group provides only weak evidence for steroids.

10.9 Acute disseminated encephalomyelitis (ADEM)

ADEM was first described in the eighteenth century as a post-infectious encephalopathy, usually following measles, chicken pox, or smallpox.[116] A paper published in 1931 described three forms of ADEM: post-infectious cases, cases occurring post-vaccination, and spontaneous cases with no apparent cause.[117] The prognosis was poor for the post-infectious cases, but good for the rest.

Nowadays, ADEM is described as a monophasic, demyelinating disease of the CNS, which is rare (0.8 per 100,000 children per annum) and affects mainly young children and adolescents.[118,119]

ADEM is thought to be a post-infectious phenomenon. In a review of ADEM, 50–75% of patients had fever and often respiratory symptoms in the preceding 4 weeks.[118] An agent is identified in up to 75% of cases,[118] although in one pediatric series only 1 of 18 children had a firm etiologic diagnosis.[118] Cases have been described post-immunization (e.g., with measles or MMR vaccine), although at a far lower rate than with wild-type measles.[116] A wide range of pathogens has been described in association with ADEM, including measles, rubella, varicella, influenza, EBV, CMV, coxsackievirus, HIV, HSV, group A streptococcus, *Mycoplasma, Bartonella henselae, Chlamydia*, and leptospirosis.[118]

Two main pathogenetic mechanisms are postulated. The first is the inflammatory cascade concept in which direct CNS infection results in tissue damage and release of antigens into the systemic circulation, which elicit an immune response. The second is the molecular mimicry concept in which there is some degree of homology between the pathogen and the myelin proteins. A pathogen-initiated immune response can then, theoretically, be reactivated against "self" tissue.[118]

The main clinical features of ADEM are fever, headaches, ataxia, and altered level of consciousness. Focal motor and sensory deficits are more common with increased age.[118]

CSF pleocytosis is usual, although not invariable. Oligoclonal bands may be present. The most characteristic findings on MRI scan of the brain are multifocal white matter lesions, most clearly defined on T2-weighted and FLAIR images, and consistent with widespread CNS demyelination, although these changes are non-specific.[118] ADEM remains a diagnosis based on a poorly defined combination of clinical, laboratory, and radiologic criteria.[118,119]

There are no trials of therapy in the management of ADEM. Intravenous corticosteroids (high-dose methylprednisolone) are the accepted first-line treatment, based on empirical observational studies and expert opinion.[118–120] IVIG and plasmapharesis have been tried in individual cases with variable success.[118–120] The current recommendations are for a 5–7-day course of intravenous corticosteroids followed by a prolonged course (3–6 weeks) of oral steroids.[118,119]

The acute mortality of ADEM is 5–10%. Most patients who survive improve in a few months and 70–90% of patients suffer no residual neurologic symptoms at 18 months.[118–120]

10.10   Lyme meningitis

Children with Lyme meningitis have a more prolonged presentation, on average, than children with viral meningitis, and are more likely to have cranial nerve signs including facial nerve palsy, papilledema, or erythema migrans.[121–123]

The CSF in Lyme meningitis shows a lymphocyte or mononuclear cell predominance. In Lyme meningitis, the proportion of neutrophils is generally lower than in viral meningitis, and a CSF neutrophil count >10% of the total CSF white count makes Lyme meningitis unlikely.[121–123] The CSF protein is higher in Lyme meningitis than in viral meningitis: in one study[122] the respective mean CSF protein was 1.1 and 0.4 g/L. Specific antibodies to *Borrelia burgdorferi* can be demonstrated in the CSF in 25–92% of children with Lyme meningitis, but the sensitivity of PCR on CSF is only 5%.[124]

An RCT of 21 patients with painful Lyme neuroborreliosis radiculitis and neuroborreliosis meningitis found no difference between 10 days' treatment with either penicillin G or cefotaxime.[125]

The American Academy of Pediatrics[126,127] recommends treating Lyme meningitis for 30–60 days, but the Infectious Disease Society of America recommends 14–28 days.[128] We could find no RCTs on duration of treatment, which should be individualized. We recommend:

ceftriaxone 75–100 mg/kg (max 4 g) IV, daily OR
cefotaxime 25 mg/kg (max 1 g) IV, 6-hourly OR
benzylpenicillin 30 mg (50,000 U)/kg (max 1.2 g or 2 million U) IV, 4-hourly

10.11   Tuberculous meningitis (TBM)

Clinical presentation of TBM

TBM usually presents in an indolent fashion, over several days, with non-specific symptoms such as fever, anorexia, intermittent headache, or vomiting, and often with no definite neurologic manifestations. There may be intermittent drowsiness and even fluctuation in level of consciousness.[127,128] TBM has traditionally been classified into three stages,[129] and subsequent studies have shown that the staging has prognostic significance[130]:

Stage I: Non-specific symptoms such as fever, anorexia, intermittent headache, or vomiting, with no definite neurologic manifestations.

Stage II: Drowsiness and disorientation and with signs of meningeal irritation and/or evidence of increased intracranial pressure.

Stage III: Usually unconscious, with paralysis and signs indicating severe intracranial hypertension.

A study in Egypt compared 134 children with culture-proven TBM with 709 children with bacterial meningitis due to pyogenic bacteria.[130] The clinical features that predicted TBM were headache and length of clinical history >5 days.

A retrospective review of 214 children with TBM from Turkey reported a mean age of onset of 4.1 years, with most children (56%) in Stage II.[131]

Diagnosis of TBM

The diagnosis of TBM is based on a combination of one or more of:

· clinical presentation;
· family history of TB;
· tuberculin skin test;
· chest radiographic changes;
· cerebral imaging;
· acid-fast bacilli in sputum or CSF;
· CSF changes: lymphocytosis, high CSF protein, low CSF glucose;
· PCR on CSF;
· culture of TB from CSF or sputum (takes weeks).

Each of the above has a variable incidence in different studies and none was reported to be present in all patients. In the Turkish study, a family history was found in 66%, 30% of children with TBM had a positive tuberculin skin test, and 87% had suggestive radiologic features of hilar adenopathy, miliary TB, infiltrates, or rarely (1%) pleural effusion.[130] Cerebral imaging showed hydrocephalus in 80%, parenchymal cerebral changes in 26%, basal meningitis in 15%, and tuberculomas in 2%. Only 13% of children had acid-fast bacilli seen on Ziehl–Nielsen stain of CSF.[130] In the Egyptian study, the patients with TBM were significantly more likely to have a CSF white cell count <1000 cells/mm^3 (1000×10^6cells/L), CSF lymphocyte count >30% of total, and CSF protein >100 mg/dL (1.0 g/L).[131]

A meta-analysis of commercially available nucleic acid amplification tests (PCR) on CSF for *M. tuberculosis*[132] found a sensitivity of only 56% and specificity of 98%. A positive PCR on CSF is, therefore, likely to be true, but a negative PCR certainly does not exclude TBM. Quantification of CSF interferon-gamma is under investigation.[133]

Treatment of TBM

Antituberculous drugs

Because no combination of the above tests is sufficiently sensitive to be able to confidently exclude TBM and because of the poor prognosis if treatment is delayed, it is not unusual to commence empiric antituberculous therapy on suspicion. If so, the evidence for continuing therapy should be reevaluated regularly.

There is only one RCT of antituberculous antimicrobials in children with TBM, who received isoniazid plus streptomycin plus either rifampin (36 patients) or ethambutol (35 patients).[134] There was no difference in outcome. Streptomycin is rarely used nowadays because it has to be given by IM injection and is toxic. Current recommendations are usually for four antituberculous antimicrobials, but there is no evidence that this is superior to using three.

For the daily regimen, we recommend:

isoniazid 10 mg/kg (max 300 mg) orally, daily for 12 months PLUS
rifamp(ic)in 10 mg/kg (max 600 mg) orally, daily for 12 months PLUS

*ethambutol 15 mg/kg (child $\geq$6 years) orally, daily for 2 months PLUS
pyrazinamide 25 mg/kg (max 2 g) orally, daily for 2 months

For the three-times-weekly regimen, we recommend:

isoniazid 15 mg/kg (max 600 mg) orally, three times weekly for 12 months PLUS
rifampicin 15 mg/kg (max 600 mg) orally, three times weekly for 12 months PLUS
*ethambutol 30 mg/kg (child $\geq$6 years) orally, three times weekly for 2 months PLUS
pyrazinamide 50 mg/kg (max 3 g) orally, three times weekly for 2 months

[*Ethambutol should not be used in young children <6 years old, due to difficulties in assessing optic neuritis. For children <6 years old, we recommend using isoniazid, rifampicin, and pyrazinamide.]

We recommend discontinuing ethambutol once the organism is known to be sensitive to isoniazid and rifampicin, even if this is prior to 2 months; but continuing ethambutol if susceptibility results are not available at 2 months.

[NB: Because of the risk of isoniazid-induced pyridoxine deficiency, it is recommended to give pyridoxine 5 mg orally to breast-fed babies with each dose of isoniazid (you may need to crush a 25 mg tablet, dissolve in 5 mL of water, and give 1 mL).]

Corticosteroids in TBM

Corticosteroid adjunctive therapy improves outcome in TBM.[135–137] One placebo-controlled RCT of prednisolone 2–4 mg/kg/day for 1 month in children with TBM showed corticosteroids improved mortality and intellectual outcome,[135] and this and another RCT[136] both showed that steroid-treated children had more rapid resolution of tuberculomas. Both studies used 4 mg/kg of prednisolone instead of the usual dose of 2 mg/kg for theoretical reasons.

A Cochrane meta-analysis of corticosteroids for TBM showed benefit, but was unable to comment on dose of corticosteroids or to separate adults from children.[137]

In a large placebo-controlled RCT in 545 adults and adolescents with TBM, treatment with dexamethasone was associated with a reduced risk of death (RR 0.69, 95% CI 0.52–0.92), but not with improved morbidity.[138] The dexamethasone regime was a complicated one, not easily extrapolated to children.

We do not feel that the evidence justifies using 4 mg/kg of prednisolone rather than the usual 2 mg/kg. We recommend adjunctive therapy, using:

prednisolone 2 mg/kg (max 80 mg) orally, daily for at least 4 weeks

Thalidomide in TBM

There has been interest in the use of thalidomide as adjunctive therapy in TBM, because of its anti-inflammatory action. An RCT of high-dose thalidomide in children with TBM was terminated early because of a high incidence of adverse events, and possibly increased mortality in the treatment group.[139] Thalidomide is not recommended.

10.12 Cryptococcal meningitis

Cryptococcal meningitis, previously known as torulosis, is caused either by *Cryptococcus neoformans* (particularly in immunocompromised patients, such as HIV infection) or *C. gattii* (previously known as *C. neoformans* var. *gattii*). The diagnosis is made by seeing encapsulated yeast cells on Indian ink or other stain of CSF and by growing the yeast. The management of children with cryptococcal meningitis is complicated and we strongly recommend a pediatric infectious disease consultation.

Because of its rarity, there are no studies of antifungal therapy of immunocompetent patients. Studies of HIV patients have shown that combination therapy with amphotericin B plus flucytosine is superior to amphotericin B alone,[140,141] or to amphotericin B plus fluconazole,[141] or to amphotericin B plus flucytosine plus fluconazole.[141] Liposomal amphotericin sterilizes the CSF more quickly than amphotericin B alone and is less nephrotoxic, but does not improve prognosis and is far more expensive.[142]

The standard recommended treatment[140,141] for cryptococcal meningitis is:

amphotericin B desoxycholate 0.7 mg/kg IV, daily for 6–10 weeks PLUS
flucytosine 25 mg/kg IV or orally, 6-hourly for 6–10 weeks

If amphotericin B causes unacceptable renal or systemic toxicity, liposomal amphotericin B 4 mg/kg IV daily should be used.[142] Patients infected with *C. gattii* may respond slowly and require longer treatment. Alternatively, if the CSF is culture negative after 2 weeks of therapy, it would be reasonable to stop the amphotericin B desoxycholate and flucytosine and commence:

fluconazole 12 mg/kg (max 800 mg) orally or IV for the first dose, then 6 mg/kg (max 400 mg) orally, daily for at least 10 weeks

Itraconazole has been successfully used when fluconazole cannot be used.

In HIV-infected patients, the above regimen has been shown to be successful, without the need for culture negativity at 2 weeks.

Long-term suppressive therapy may be required for immunocompromised patients. If the patient has responded well to 10 weeks of fluconazole at the above dose, secondary prophylaxis is recommended at a reduced dose:

fluconazole 3 mg/kg (max 200 mg) orally, daily, continued while immunosuppressed

10.13 Transverse myelitis

Acute transverse myelitis (ATM) is a rare disease in childhood and adolescence, with an incidence of 1–4 per million new cases annually, and peaks at 10–19 years and 30–39 years.[143] Transverse myelitis is due to inflammation of the spinal cord, usually secondary to infection with enteroviruses,[144] arboviruses, other viruses or *M. pneumoniae*.[145] It has been described in many conditions, including Lyme disease[146] and in cysticercosis. It has occasionally been described in association with immunization with various live and inert vaccines including influenza, MMR, and oral polio vaccines,[147,148] although there is insufficient evidence to say whether immunizations can cause transverse myelitis or whether paralysis from another cause merely occurs coincidentally following immunization.[149]

The clinical presentation of transverse myelitis is characterized by paraplegia, with or without sensory symptoms, and bladder dysfunction. It typically manifests itself over a period of hours to 1 week. The major differential diagnosis is a pyogenic epidural abscess, which requires urgent drainage (see Section 10.4, p. 143). For this reason, radiologic investigation with

MRI or CT scan is a priority. An expert working group has proposed diagnostic criteria.[143]

We found no trials of the use of corticosteroids in ATM, which is hardly surprising given its rarity. A retrospective review of 50 Japanese children with ATM found that younger children and those with neurologic features of paraplegia did worse, and that corticosteroid therapy did not appear to improve outcome.[150] Intravenous corticosteroids (high-dose methylprednisolone as for ADEM; see Section 10.9, p. 146) are often used empirically. ATM often leads to long-term bladder and/or bowel dysfunction.[151]

10.14 Guillain-Barré syndrome

Guillain–Barré syndrome is an acute peripheral neuropathy which causes ascending paralysis due to multifocal inflammation of the spinal roots and peripheral nerves, especially their myelin sheaths. In severe cases the axons are also damaged.[152] In the commonest form of GBS in Europe and North America, the underlying pathologic process is an acute inflammatory demyelinating polyradiculoneuropathy.

In all series, about two-thirds of patients have had an infection within the previous 6 weeks, most commonly a flu-like illness but also gastroenteritis. About a quarter of patients with Guillain–Barré syndrome have had a recent *Campylobacter jejuni* infection, and they are particularly likely to have an axonal neuropathy.[152] Observational and case-control studies implicate a range of bacteria (including *M. pneumoniae*) and viruses such as EBV and CMV as possible triggers for the syndrome. There is also an association with immunization with rabies vaccine[153] (incidence 1 in 1000 doses) and previously but not currently with inactivated influenza vaccine in the USA[154] (1 in 1,000,000 doses).

The pathogenesis is thought to be an autoimmune response directed against antigens in the peripheral nerves that is triggered by a preceding infection. Antibodies or T cells stimulated by antigens on the infecting microbe may cross-react with neural antigens.[152]

Guillain–Barré causes the development of weakness and usually numbness of the limbs and often the facial, swallowing, and breathing muscles. The weakness reaches its nadir within a few days or up to 4 weeks. In 25% of patients it is sufficiently severe to require the use of artificial ventilation, and 3.5–12% of patients die of complications.[152] Recovery takes several weeks or months.

The diagnosis is made clinically and confirmed by neurophysiologic studies.[152] CSF protein is raised in about 80% of cases and there are no white cells in the CSF (the presence of CSF pleocytosis indicates another diagnosis).[152]

A Cochrane review found six studies (649 patients) that compared plasma exchange with supportive therapy and found that plasma exchange hastened motor recovery.[155]

A separate Cochrane review compared IVIG with plasma exchange.[156] There were five eligible RCTs (536 patients). In severe disease, IVIG started within 2 weeks from onset hastened recovery as much as plasma exchange, and was significantly more likely to be completed than plasma exchange. Giving IVIG after plasma exchange did not confer significant extra benefit. There was only one study exclusively in children which found that a total dose of 2 g/kg of IVIG hastened recovery compared with supportive care alone, whether it was given in divided doses over 2 or 5 days.[157]

A Cochrane review of six trials (587 participants) of corticosteroids found limited evidence that oral corticosteroids significantly slow recovery from Guillain–Barré syndrome.[158] Intravenous methylprednisolone alone was not found to produce significant benefit or harm.

We recommend:

IVIG 1 g/kg, infused IV over 8–12 hours, once daily for 2 days

10.15 PANDAS

Pediatric autoimmune neuropsychiatric disorders or PANDAS is a group of disorders which some have suggested are associated with streptococcal infections, possibly analogous to Sydenham's chorea. Patients have prepubertal onset of obsessive-compulsive disorder and tic disorders, and exacerbations may be associated with group A beta-hemolytic streptococcal (GABHS) infections. In one descriptive study of 50 children, the clinical course was characterized by a relapsing–remitting symptom pattern with significant psychiatric comorbidity accompanying the exacerbations of emotional lability, separation anxiety, nighttime fears, bedtime rituals, cognitive deficits, oppositional behavior, and hyperactivity. Symptom onset was reported to be triggered by proven or possible group A streptococcal infection in about 70% of episodes.[159]

There is doubt whether the condition is a real entity. In a controlled study of unselected patients with Tourette syndrome and/or obsessive-compulsive disorder, there was no clear relationship between new GABHS infections and symptom exacerbations.[160] We could find only two controlled treatment studies. In one placebo-controlled study, penicillin prophylaxis did not reduce the number of exacerbations of PANDAS, but nor did it reduce the number of infections.[161] Another study found that children on either penicillin or azithromycin had fewer infections and fewer exacerbations than the previous year, but the results are not helpful as the study did not include a placebo group.[162]

References

1 Chavez-Bueno S, McCracken GH, Jr. Bacterial meningitis in children. *Pediatr Clin North Am* 2005;52:795–810.

2 Isaacs D, Moxon ER. *Handbook of Neonatal Infections: A Practical Guide.* London: WB Saunders, 1999.

3 Kimberlin DW. Meningitis in the neonate. *Curr Treat Options Neurol* 2002;4:239–48.

4 Vergnano S, Sharland M, Kazembe P, Mwansambo C, Heath PT. Neonatal sepsis: an international perspective. *Arch Dis Child Fetal Neonatal Ed* 2005;90:F220–4.

5 Oostenbrink R, Moons KG, Donders AR, Grobbee DE, Moll HA. Prediction of bacterial meningitis in children with meningeal signs: reduction of lumbar punctures. *Acta Paediatr* 2001;90:611–7.

6 Weber MW, Herman J, Jaffar S et al. Clinical predictors of bacterial meningitis in infants and young children in The Gambia. *Trop Med Int Health* 2002;7:722–31.

7 Minns RA, Engleman HM, Stirling H. Cerebrospinal fluid pressure in pyogenic meningitis. *Arch Dis Child* 1989; 64:814–20.

8 Dodge PR, Swartz MN. Bacterial meningitis: review of selected aspects. II. Special neurologic problems, postmeningitic complications and clinicopathological correlations. *N Engl J Med* 1965;272:954–60.

9 Horowitz SJ, Boxerbaum B, O'Bell J. Cerebral herniation in bacterial meningitis in childhood. *Ann Neurol* 1980;7: 524–8.

10 Rennick G, Shann F, de Campo J. Cerebral herniation during bacterial meningitis in children. *BMJ* 1993;306:953–5.

11 Hasbun R, Abrahams J, Jekel J, Quagliarello VJ. Computed tomography of the head before lumbar puncture in adults with suspected meningitis. *N Engl J Med* 2001;345: 1727–33.

12 Archer BD. Computed tomography before lumbar puncture in acute meningitis: a review of the risks and benefits. *CMAJ* 1993;148:961–5.

13 Cabral DA, Flodmark O, Farrell K et al. Prospective study of computed tomography in acute bacterial meningitis. *J Pediatr* 1987;111:201–5.

14 Heyderman RS, Robb SA, Kendall BE, Levin M. Diffusion-weighted imaging in acute bacterial meningitis in infancy. *Neuroradiology* 2003;45:634–9.

15 Bodino J, Lylyk P, del Valle M et al. Computed tomography in purulent meningitis. *Am J Dis Child* 1982;136: 495–501.

16 Packer RJ, Bilaniuk LT, Zimmerman RA. CT parenchymal abnormalities in bacterial meningitis: clinical significance. *J Comput Assist Tomogr* 1982;6:1064–8.

17 Cockrill HH, Jr, Dreisbach J, Lowe B, Yamauchi T. Computed tomography in leptomeningeal infections. *AJR* 1978; 130:511–5.

18 Haslam RHA. Role of computed tomography in the early management of bacterial meningitis. *J Pediatr* 1991;119: 157–9.

19 Oliver WJ, Shope TC, Kuhns LR. Fatal lumbar puncture: fact versus fiction—an approach to a clinical dilemma. *Pediatrics* 2003;112:e174–6.

20 Brenner DJ, Elliston CD, Hall EJ et al. Estimated risks of radiation-induced fatal cancer from pediatric CT. *AJR* 2001;176:289–96.

21 Hall EJ. Lessons we have learned from our children: cancer risks from diagnostic radiology. *Pediatr Radiol* 2002;32: 700–6.

22 Kneen R, Solomon T, Appleton R. The role of lumbar puncture in suspected CNS infection—a disappearing skill? *Arch Dis Child* 2002;87:181–3.

23 Isaacs D, Kneen R, Solomon T, Appleton R. LP and Glasgow coma score. *Arch Dis Child* 2003;88:177.

24 Tunkel AR, Hartman BJ, Kaplan SL et al. Practice guidelines for the management of bacterial meningitis. *Clin Infect Dis* 2004;39:1267–84.

25 Benjamin CM, Newton RW, Clarke MA. Risk factors for death from meningitis. *BMJ* 1988;296:20–1.

26 Bonadio WA. The cerebrospinal fluid: physiologic aspects and alterations associated with bacterial meningitis. *Pediatr Infect Dis J* 1992;11:423–32.

27 Baty V, Viel JF, Schuhmacher H, Jaeger F, Canton P, Hoen B. Prospective validation of a diagnosis model as an aid to therapeutic decision-making in acute meningitis. *Eur J Clin Microbiol Infect Dis* 2000;19:422–6.

28 Feigin RD, McCracken GH, Jr, Klein JO. Diagnosis and management of meningitis. *Pediatr Infect Dis J* 1992;11:785–814.

29 Negrini B, Kelleher KJ, Wald ER. Cerebrospinal fluid findings in aseptic versus bacterial meningitis. *Pediatrics* 2000;105:316–9.

30 Chavanet P, Schaller C, Levy C et al. Performance of a predictive rule to distinguish bacterial and viral meningitis. *J Infect* 2007;54:328–36.

31 Berg B, Gardsell P, Skansberg P. Cerebrospinal fluid lactate in the diagnosis of meningitis: diagnostic value compared

to standard biochemical methods. *Scand J Infect Dis* 1982;14:111–5.

32 Nelson N, Eeg-Olofsson O, Larsson L, Ohman S. The diagnostic and predictive value of cerebrospinal fluid lactate in children with meningitis: its relation to current diagnostic methods. *Acta Paediatr Scand* 1986;75:52–7.

33 Lindquist L, Linne T, Hansson LO, Kalin M, Axelsson G. Value of cerebrospinal fluid analysis in the differential diagnosis of meningitis: a study in 710 patients with suspected central nervous system infection. *Eur J Clin Microbiol Infect Dis* 1988;7:374–80.

34 Leib SL, Boscacci R, Gratzl O, Zimmerli W. Predictive value of cerebrospinal fluid (CSF) lactate level versus CSF/blood glucose ratio for the diagnosis of bacterial meningitis following neurosurgery. *Clin Infect Dis* 1999;29:69–74.

35 Poppert S, Essig A, Stoehr B et al. Rapid diagnosis of bacterial meningitis by real-time PCR and fluorescence in situ hybridization. *J Clin Microbiol* 2005;43:3390–7.

36 Deutch S, Pedersen LN, Podenphant L et al. Broad-range real time PCR and DNA sequencing for the diagnosis of bacterial meningitis. *Scand J Infect Dis* 2006;38:27–35.

37 Maxson S, Lewno MJ, Schutze GE. Clinical usefulness of cerebrospinal fluid bacterial antigen studies. *J Pediatr* 1994;125:235–8.

38 Gerdes LU, Jorgensen PE, Nexo E, Wang P. C-reactive protein and bacterial meningitis: a meta-analysis. *Scand J Clin Lab Invest* 1998;58:383–93.

39 Gendrel D, Raymond J, Assicot M et al. Measurement of procalcitonin levels in children with bacterial or viral meningitis. *Clin Infect Dis* 1997;24:1240–2.

40 Prasad K, Singhal T, Jain N, Gupta PK. Third generation cephalosporins versus conventional antibiotics for treating acute bacterial meningitis. *The Cochrane Database of Systematic Reviews* 2004;(2):Art No CD001832.

41 Kellner JD, Scheifele D, Halperin SA et al. Outcome of penicillin-non-susceptible *Streptococcus pneumoniae* meningitis: a nested case-control study. *Pediatr Infect Dis J* 2002; 21:903–9.

42 Buckingham SC, McCullers JA, Lujan-Zilbermann J, Knapp KM, Orman KL, English BK. Pneumococcal meningitis in children: relationship of antibiotic resistance to clinical characteristics and outcomes. *Pediatr Infect Dis J* 2001;20:837–43.

43 McMaster P, McIntyre P, Gilmour R, Gilbert L, Kakakios A, Mellis C. The emergence of resistant pneumococcal meningitis—implications for empiric therapy. *Arch Dis Child* 2002;87:207–10.

44 McIntyre P. Meningitis. In: Moyer VA (ed.), *Evidence-based pediatrics and child health*, 2nd edn. London: BMJ Books, 2004:285–91.

45 van de Beek D, de Gans J, McIntyre P, Prasad K. Corticosteroids for acute bacterial meningitis. *The Cochrane Database of Systematic Reviews* 2003;(3):Art No CD004405.

46 McIntyre PB, Macintyre CR, Gilmour R, Wang H. A population based study of the impact of corticosteroid therapy and delayed diagnosis on the outcome of childhood pneumococcal meningitis. *Arch Dis Child* 2005;90: 391–6.

47 Molyneux EM, Walsh AL, Forsyth H et al. Dexamethasone treatment in childhood bacterial meningitis in Malawi: a randomised controlled trial. *Lancet* 2002;360:211–8.

48 de Gans J, van de Beek D, for the European Dexamethasone in Adulthood Bacterial Meningitis Study Investigators. Dexamethasone in adults with bacterial meningitis. *N Engl J Med* 2002;347:1549–56.

49 Oates-Whitehead RM, Maconochie I, Baumer H, Stewart MER. Fluid therapy for acute bacterial meningitis. *The Cochrane Database of Systematic Reviews* 2005;(3):Art No CD004786.

50 Powell KR, Sugarman LI, Eskenazi AE et al. Normalization of plasma arginine vasopressin concentrations when children with meningitis are given maintenance plus replacement fluid therapy. *J Pediatr* 1990;117:515–22.

51 Radetsky M. Duration of treatment in bacterial meningitis: a historical inquiry. *Pediatr Infect Dis J* 1990;9:2–9.

52 O'Neill P. How long to treat bacterial meningitis. *Lancet* 1993;341:530.

53 MacFarlane JT, Anjorin FI, Cleland PG et al. Single injection treatment of meningococcal meningitis. 1: Long-acting penicillin. *Trans R Soc Trop Med Hyg* 1979;73:693–7.

54 Wali SS, Macfarlane JT, Weir WR et al. Single injection treatment of meningococcal meningitis. 1: Long-acting chloramphenicol. *Trans R Soc Trop Med Hyg* 1979;73: 698–702.

55 Lin TY, Chrane SF, Nelson JD et al. Seven days of ceftriaxone therapy is as effective as ten days' treatment for bacterial meningitis. *JAMA* 1985;253:3559–63.

56 Roine I, Ledermann W, Foncea LM, Banfi A, Cohen J, Peltola H. Randomized trial of four vs. seven days of ceftriaxone treatment for bacterial meningitis in children with rapid initial recovery. *Pediatr Infect Dis J* 2000;19:219–22.

57 Meningococcal Disease Surveillance Group. Analysis of endemic meningococcal disease by serogroup and evaluation of chemoprophylaxis. *J Infect Dis* 1976;134:201–4.

58 Band JD, Fraser DW, Ajello G. Prevention of *Hemophilus influenzae* type b disease. *JAMA* 1984;251:2381–6.

59 Purcell B, Samuelsson S, Hahne SJM et al. Effectiveness of antibiotics in preventing meningococcal disease after a case: systematic review. *BMJ* 2004;328:1339.

60 Fraser A, Gafter-Gvili A, Paul M, Leibovici L. Antibiotics for preventing meningococcal infections. *The Cochrane Database of Systematic Reviews* 2005;(1):Art No CD004785.

61 Schaad UB. Fluoroquinolone antibiotics in infants and children. *Infect Dis Clin North Am* 2005;19:617–28.

62 Leech PJ, Paterson A. Conservative and operative management of cerebrospinal fluid leakage after closed head injury. *Lancet* 1973;1:1013–5.

63 Villalobos T, Arango C, Kubilis P, Rathore M. Antibiotic prophylaxis after basilar skull fractures: a meta-analysis. *Clin Infect Dis* 1998;27:364–9.

64 Brodie HA. Prophylactic antibiotics for post-traumatic cerebrospinal fluid fistulae: a meta-analysis. *Arch Otolaryngol Head Neck Surg* 1997;123:749–52.

65 Ratilal B, Costa J, Sampaio C. Antibiotic prophylaxis for preventing meningitis in patients with basilar skull fractures.

The Cochrane Database of Systematic Reviews 2006;(1): Art No CD004884.

66 Kline MW. Review of recurrent bacterial meningitis. Pediatr Infect Dis J 1989;8:630–4.

67 Wang HS, Kuo MF, Huang SC. Diagnostic approach to recurrent bacterial meningitis in children. Chang Gung Med J 2005;28:441–52.

68 Ohlms LA, Edwards MS, Mason EO, Igarashi M, Alford BR, Smith RJ. Recurrent meningitis and Mondini dysplasia. Arch Otolaryngol Head Neck Surg 1990;116:608–12.

69 River Y, Averbuch-Heller L, Weinberger M et al. Antibiotic induced meningitis. J Neurol Neurosurg Psychiatry 1994;57:705–8.

70 Mra Z, MacCormick JA, Poje CP. Persistent cerebrospinal fluid otorrhea: a case of Munchausen's syndrome by proxy. Int J Pediatr Otorhinolaryngol 1997;41:59–63.

71 Hannoverschen Cochlear Implant-Gesellschaft e.V. Meeting on post cochlear implantation meningitis. Schiphol Airport, Amsterdam, the Netherlands, July 5, 2002 [Minutes; German]. Available at http://www.hcig.de.

72 French Public Health Agency for Health Product Safety. Recall of Clarion cochlear implants with a positioner made by Advanced Bionics Corporation following cases of meningitis, July 23, 2002 [French]. Available at http://agmed.sante.gouv.fr/htm/alertes/filalert/dm020706.htm.

73 Reefhuis J, Honein MA, Whitney CG et al. Risk of bacterial meningitis in children with cochlear implants. N Engl J Med 2003;349:435–45.

74 Wilson-Clark SD, Squires S, Deeks S, for the Centers for Disease Control and Prevention (CDC). Bacterial meningitis among cochlear implant recipients—Canada, 2002. MMWR Morb Mortal Wkly Rep 2006;55(suppl 1):20–4.

75 Whitney CG. Cochlear implants and meningitis in children. Pediatr Infect Dis J 2004;23:767–8.

76 Venes JL. Infections of CSF shunt and intracranial pressure monitoring devices. Infect Dis Clin North Am 1989;3:289–99.

77 Brown EM, Edwards RJ, Pople IK. Conservative management of patients with cerebrospinal fluid shunt infections. Neurosurgery 2006;58:657–65.

78 Kulkarni AV, Drake JM, Lamberti-Pasculli M. Cerebrospinal fluid shunt infection: a prospective study of risk factors. J Neurosurg 2001;94:195–201.

79 Schuhmann MU, Ostrowski KR, Draper EJ et al. The value of C-reactive protein in the management of shunt infections. J Neurosurg 2005;103(3, suppl):223–30.

80 Ishak MA, Groschel DH, Mandell GL, Wenzel RP. Association of slime with pathogenicity of coagulase-negative staphylococci causing nosocomial septicemia. J Clin Microbiol 1985;22:1025–9.

81 James HE, Walsh JW, Wilson HD, Connor JD, Bean JR, Tibbs PA. Prospective randomized study of therapy in cerebrospinal fluid shunt infection. Neurosurgery 1980;7:459–63.

82 Pfausler B, Spiss H, Beer R et al. Treatment of staphylococcal ventriculitis associated with external cerebrospinal fluid drains: a prospective randomized trial of intravenous compared with intraventricular vancomycin therapy. J Neurosurg 2003;98:1040–4.

83 Mustafa MM, Mertsola J, Ramilo O, Saez-Llorens X, Risser RC, McCracken GH. Increased endotoxin and interleukin1-beta concentrations in cerebrospinal fluid of infants with coliform meningitis and ventriculitis associated with intraventricular gentamicin therapy. J Infect Dis 1989;160:891–5.

84 McCracken GH, Mize SG, Threlkeld N. Intraventricular gentamicin therapy in Gram-negative bacillary meningitis of infancy. Lancet 1980;1:787–91.

85 Shah S, Ohlsson A, Shah V. Intraventricular antibiotics for bacterial meningitis in neonates. The Cochrane Database of Systematic Reviews 2004;(4):Art No CD004496.

86 Schranz J. Comparisons of seizure incidence and adverse experiences between imipenem and meropenem. Crit Care Med 1998;26:1464–6.

87 Govender ST, Nathoo N, van Dellen JR. Evaluation of an antibiotic-impregnated shunt system for the treatment of hydrocephalus. J Neurosurg 2003;99:831–9.

88 Adame N, Hedlund G, Byington CL. Sinogenic intracranial empyema in children. Pediatrics 2005;116:e461–7.

89 Leotta N, Chaseling R, Duncan G, Isaacs D. Intracranial suppuration. J Paediatr Child Health 2005;41:508–12.

90 Tsai YD, Chang WN, Shen CC et al. Intracranial suppuration: a clinical comparison of sub-dural empyemas and epidural abscesses. Surg Neurol 2003;59:191–6.

91 Le Moal G, Landron C, Grollier G et al. Characteristics of brain abscess with isolation of anaerobic bacteria. Scand J Infect Dis 2003;35:318–21.

92 Kao PT, Tseng HK, Liu CP, Su SC, Lee CM. Brain abscess: clinical analysis of 53 cases. J Microbiol Immunol Infect 2003;36:129–36.

93 Jansson AK, Enblad P, Sjolin J. Efficacy and safety of cefotaxime in combination with metronidazole for empirical treatment of brain abscess in clinical practice: a retrospective study of 66 consecutive cases. Eur J Clin Microbiol Infect Dis 2004;23:7–14.

94 Yogev R, Bar-Meir M. Management of brain abscesses in children. Pediatr Infect Dis J 2004;23:157–9.

95 Renier D, Flandin C, Hirsch E, Hirsch JF. Brain abscesses in neonates: a study of 30 cases. J Neurosurg 1988;69:877–82.

96 An HS, Seldomridge JA. Spinal infections: diagnostic tests and imaging studies. Clin Orthop 2006;444:27–33.

97 Siddiq F, Chowfin A, Tight R, Sahmoun AE, Smego RA, Jr. Medical vs surgical management of spinal epidural abscess. Arch Intern Med 2004;164:2409–12.

98 Khanna RK, Malik GM, Rock JP, Rosenblum ML. Spinal epidural abscess: evaluation of factors influencing outcome. Neurosurgery 1996;39:958–64.

99 Tyler KL. Herpes simplex virus infections of the central nervous system: encephalitis and meningitis, including Mollaret's. Herpes 2004;11(suppl 2):57A–64A.

100 Marzouk O, Thomson AP, Sills JA, Hart CA, Harris F. Features and outcome in meningococcal disease presenting with maculopapular rash. Arch Dis Child 1991;66:485–7.

101 Nigrovic LE, Kuppermann N, Malley R. Development and validation of a multivariable predictive model to distinguish

bacterial from aseptic meningitis in children in the post-*Haemophilus influenzae* era. *Pediatrics* 2002;110:712–9.

102 Bonsu BK, Harper MB. Differentiating acute bacterial meningitis from acute viral meningitis among children with cerebrospinal fluid pleocytosis: a multivariable regression model. *Pediatr Infect Dis J* 2004;23:511–7.

103 Cinque P, Bossolasco S, Lundkvist A. Molecular analysis of cerebrospinal fluid in viral diseases of the central nervous system. *J Clin Virol* 2003;26:1–28.

104 Kimberlin D. Herpes simplex virus meningitis and encephalitis in neonates. *Herpes* 2004;11(suppl 2):65A–76A.

105 Terletskaia-Ladwig E, Metzger C, Schalasta G, Enders G. Evaluation of enterovirus serological tests IgM-EIA and complement fixation in patients with meningitis, confirmed by detection of enteroviral RNA by RT-PCR in cerebrospinal fluid. *J Med Virol* 2000;61:221–7.

106 Hayden FG, Herrington DT, Coats TL et al. Efficacy and safety of oral pleconaril for treatment of colds due to picornaviruses in adults: results of 2 double-blind, randomized, placebo-controlled trials. *Clin Infect Dis* 2003;36:1523–32.

107 Abzug MJ, Cloud G, Bradley J et al. Double blind placebo-controlled trial of pleconaril in infants with enterovirus meningitis. *Pediatr Infect Dis J* 2003;22:335–41.

108 Koskiniemi M, Rautonen J, Lehtokoski-Lehtiniemi E, Vaheri A. Epidemiology of encephalitis in children: a 20-year survey. *Ann Neurol* 1991;29:492–7.

109 Kolski H, Ford-Jones EL, Richardson S et al. Etiology of acute childhood encephalitis at the Hospital for Sick Children, Toronto, 1994–1995. *Clin Infect Dis* 1998;26:398–409.

110 Bitnun A, Ford-Jones EL, Petric M et al. Acute childhood encephalitis and *Mycoplasma pneumoniae*. *Clin Infect Dis* 2001;32:1674–84.

111 Lewis P, Glaser CA. Encephalitis. *Pediatr Rev* 2005;26:353–63.

112 Daxboeck F, Blacky A, Seidl R, Krause R, Assadian O. Diagnosis, treatment, and prognosis of *Mycoplasma pneumoniae* childhood encephalitis: systematic review of 58 cases. *J Child Neurol* 2004;19:865–71.

113 Tsiodras S, Kelesidis I, Kelesidis T, Stamboulis E, Giamarellou H. Central nervous system manifestations of *Mycoplasma pneumoniae* infections. *J Infect* 2005;51:343–54.

114 Carpenter T. Corticosteroids in the treatment of severe mycoplasma encephalitis in children. *Crit Care Med* 2002;30:925–7.

115 Lehtokoski-Lehtiniemi E, Koskiniemi ML. *Mycoplasma pneumoniae* encephalitis: a severe entity in children. *Pediatr Infect Dis J* 1989;8:651–3.

116 Lucas J. An account of uncommon symptoms succeeding the measles with additional remarks on the infection of measles and smallpox. *Lond Med J* 1790;11:325–31.

117 McAlpine D. Acute disseminated encephalomyelitis: its sequelay and its relationship to disseminated sclerosis. *Lancet* 1931;846–52.

118 Menge T, Hemmer B, Nessler S et al. Acute disseminated encephalomyelitis. *Arch Neurol* 2005;62:1673–80.

119 Murthy SN, Faden HS, Cohen ME, Bakshi R. Acute disseminated encephalomyelitis in children. *Pediatrics* 2002;110:e21.

120 Shahar E, Andraus J, Savitzki D, Pilar G, Zelnik N. Outcome of severe encephalomyelitis in children: effect of high-dose methylprednisolone and immunoglobulins. *J Child Neurol* 2002;17:810–4.

121 Shah SS, Zaoutis TE, Turnquist J, Hodinka RL, Coffin SE. Early differentiation of Lyme from enteroviral meningitis. *Pediatr Infect Dis J* 2005;24:542–5.

122 Tuerlinckx D, Bodart E, Garrino MG, de Bilderling G. Clinical data and cerebrospinal fluid findings in Lyme meningitis versus aseptic meningitis. *Eur J Pediatr* 2003;162:150–3.

123 Avery RA, Frank G, Glutting JJ, Eppes SC. Prediction of Lyme meningitis in children from a Lyme disease-endemic region: a logistic-regression model using history, physical, and laboratory findings. *Pediatrics* 2006;117:e1–7.

124 Avery RA, Frank G, Eppes SC. Diagnostic utility of *Borrelia burgdorferi* cerebrospinal fluid polymerase chain reaction in children with Lyme meningitis. *Pediatr Infect Dis J* 2005;24:705–8.

125 Pfister HW, Preac-Mursic V, Wilske B, Einhaupl KM. Cefotaxime vs penicillin G for acute neurologic manifestations in Lyme borreliosis: a prospective randomized study. *Arch Neurol* 1989;46:1190–4.

126 American Academy of Pediatrics. Lyme disease. In: Pickering LK (ed.), *Red Book: 2003 Report of the Committee on Infectious Diseases*, 26th edn. Elk Grove Village, IL: American Academy of Pediatrics, 2003:407–11

127 American Academy of Pediatrics, Committee on Infectious Diseases. Prevention of Lyme disease. *Pediatrics* 2000;105:142–7.

128 Wormser GP, Nadelman RB, Dattwyler RJ et al, for the Infectious Disease Society of America. Practice guidelines for the treatment of Lyme disease. *Clin Infect Dis* 2000;31 (suppl 1):1–14.

129 Lincoln EM, Sordillo VR, Davies PA. Tuberculous meningitis in children: a review of 167 untreated and 74 treated patients with special reference to early diagnosis. *J Pediatr* 1960;57:807–23.

130 Yaramis A, Gurkan F, Elevli M et al. Central nervous system tuberculosis in children: a review of 214 cases. *Pediatrics* 1998;102:e49.

131 Youssef FG, Afifi SA, Azab AM et al. Differentiation of tuberculous meningitis from acute bacterial meningitis using simple clinical and laboratory parameters. *Diagn Microbiol Infect Dis* 2006;55:257–8.

132 Pai M, Flores LL, Pai N, Hubbard A, Riley LW, Colford JM, Jr. Diagnostic accuracy of nucleic acid amplification tests for tuberculous meningitis: a systematic review and meta-analysis. *Lancet Infect Dis* 2003;3:633–43.

133 Juan RS, Sanchez-Suarez C, Rebollo MJ et al. Interferon gamma quantification in cerebrospinal fluid compared with PCR for the diagnosis of tuberculous meningitis. *J Neurol* 2006;253:1323–30.

134 Girgis NI, Yassin MW, Laughlin LW, Edman DC, Farid Z, Watten RH. Rifampicin in the treatment of tuberculous meningitis. *Am J Trop Med Hyg* 1978;81:246–7.

135 Schoeman JF, Van Zyl LE, Laubscher JA, Donald PR. Effect of corticosteroids on intracranial pressure, computed tomographic findings, and clinical outcome in young children with tuberculous meningitis. *Pediatrics* 1997;99:226–31.

136 Karak B, Garg RK. Corticosteroids in tuberculous meningitis. *Indian Pediatr* 1998;35:193–4.

137 Prasad K, Volmink J, Menon GR. Steroids for treating tuberculous meningitis. *The Cochrane Database of Systematic Reviews* 2006;(1):Art No CD002244.

138 Thwaites GE, Nguyen DB, Nguyen HD et al. Dexamethasone for the treatment of tuberculous meningitis in adolescents and adults. *N Engl J Med* 2004;351:1741–51.

139 Schoeman JF, Springer P, van Rensburg AJ et al. Adjunctive thalidomide therapy for childhood tuberculous meningitis: results of a randomized study. *J Child Neurol* 2004;19:250–7.

140 van der Horst CM, Saag MS, Cloud GA et al, for the National Institute of Allergy and Infectious Diseases Mycoses Study Group and AIDS Clinical Trials Group. Treatment of cryptococcal meningitis associated with the acquired immunodeficiency syndrome. *N Engl J Med* 1997;337:15–21.

141 Brouwer AE, Rajanuwong A, Chierakul W et al. Combination antifungal therapies for HIV-associated cryptococcal meningitis: a randomised trial. *Lancet* 2004;363:1764–7.

142 Leenders AC, Reiss P, Portegies P et al. Liposomal amphotericin B (AmBisome) compared with amphotericin B both followed by oral fluconazole in the treatment of AIDS-associated cryptococcal meningitis. *AIDS* 1997;11:1463–71.

143 Transverse Myelitis Consortium Working Group. Proposed diagnostic criteria and nosology of acute transverse myelitis. *Neurology* 2002;59:499–505.

144 Kelly H, Brussen KA, Lawrence A, Elliot E, Pearn J, Thorley B. Polioviruses and other enteroviruses isolated from faecal samples of patients with acute flaccid paralysis in Australia, 1996–2004. *J Paediatr Child Health* 2006;42:370–6.

145 Tsiodras S, Kelesidis T, Kelesidis I, Voumbourakis K, Giamarellou H. *Mycoplasma pneumoniae*-associated myelitis: a comprehensive review. *Eur J Neurol* 2006;13:112–24.

146 Meurs L, Labeye D, Declercq I, Pieret F, Gille M. Acute transverse myelitis as a main manifestation of early stage II: neuroborreliosis in two patients. *Eur Neurol* 2004;52:186–8.

147 Kelly H. Evidence for a causal association between oral polio vaccine and transverse myelitis: a case history and review of the Literature. *J Paediatr Child Health* 2006;42:155–9.

148 Lim S, Park SM, Choi HS et al. Transverse myelitis after measles and rubella vaccination. *J Paediatr Child Health* 2004;40:583–4.

149 Stratton KR, Howe CJ, Johnston RB. Adverse events associated with childhood vaccines other than pertussis and rubella: Summary of a report from the Institute of Medicine. *JAMA* 1994;271:1602–5.

150 Miyazawa R, Ikeuchi Y, Tomomasa T, Ushiku H, Ogawa T, Morikawa A. Determinants of prognosis of acute transverse myelitis in children. *Pediatr Int* 2003;45:512–6.

151 Tanaka ST, Stone AR, Kurzrock EA. Transverse myelitis in children: long-term urological outcomes. *J Urol* 2006;175:1865–8.

152 Raphaël JC, Chevret S, Hughes RAC, Annane D. Plasma exchange for Guillain–Barré syndrome. *The Cochrane Database of Systematic Reviews* 2002;(2):Art No CD001798.

153 Hughes RA, Cornblath DR. Guillain–Barre syndrome. *Lancet* 2005;366:1653–66.

154 Hemachudha T, Griffin DE, Chen WW, Johnson RT. Immunologic studies of rabies vaccination-induced GBS. *Neurology* 1988;38:375–8.

155 Lasky T, Terracciano GJ, Magder L et al. The Guillain–Barré syndrome and the 1992–1993 and 1993–1994 influenza vaccines. *N Engl J Med* 1998;339:1797–802.

156 Hughes RAC, Raphaël J-C, Swan AV, van Doorn PA. Intravenous immunoglobulin for Guillain–Barré syndrome. *The Cochrane Database of Systematic Reviews* 2006;(1):Art No CD002063.

157 Korinthenberg R, Schessl J, Kirschner J, Monting JS. Intravenous immunoglobulin in the treatment of childhood Guillain–Barre syndrome: a randomized trial. *Pediatrics* 2005;116:8–14.

158 Hughes RAC, Swan AV, van Koningsveld R, van Doorn PA. Corticosteroids for Guillain–Barré syndrome. *The Cochrane Database of Systematic Reviews* 2006;(2):Art No CD001446.

159 Swedo SE, Leonard HL, Garvey M et al. Pediatric autoimmune neuropsychiatric disorders associated with streptococcal infections: clinical description of the first 50 cases. *Am J Psychiatry* 1998;155:264–71.

160 Luo F, Leckman JF, Katsovich L et al. Prospective longitudinal study of children with tic disorders and/or obsessive-compulsive disorder: relationship of symptom exacerbations to newly acquired streptococcal infections. *Pediatrics* 2004;113:e578–85.

161 Garvey MA, Perlmutter SJ, Allen AJ et al. A pilot study of penicillin prophylaxis for neuropsychiatric exacerbations triggered by streptococcal infections. *Biol Psychiatry* 1999;45:1564–71.

162 Snider LA, Lougee L, Slattery M, Grant P, Swedo SE. Antibiotic prophylaxis with azithromycin or penicillin for childhood-onset neuropsychiatric disorders. *Biol Psychiatry* 2005;57:788–92.

CHAPTER 11
Osteomyelitis and septic arthritis

11.1 Acute osteomyelitis

Acute osteomyelitis is rare in infants and children, with an annual incidence in children of 1 in 5,000 to 1 in 10,000 per annum.[1–4] Infection is usually hematogenous, although organisms can be introduced by trauma or iatrogenically or can spread from contiguous structures such as joints. About a third of children with acute osteomyelitis give a history of recent minor trauma,[1–4] but such a history would probably be equally common in young children without osteomyelitis.

Boys are twice as likely to be affected as girls and half of the children are <5 years old. Infection of the long bones (femur, tibia, humerus) is more common in children than infection elsewhere, such as the spine or pelvis, whereas involvement of the axial skeleton is more likely in adults.[1–4] A single site of infection is most common, but 5–20% of children have multifocal pyogenic osteomyelitis.[1–4]

Diagnosis of acute osteomyelitis
Osteomyelitis can be misdiagnosed as cellulitis, which also presents with fever, tenderness, and swelling. Conditions that can mimic osteomyelitis include fractures and tumors.

Clinical features of acute osteomyelitis
The cardinal clinical features of acute osteomyelitis in children are fever, pain, limitation of movement of the limb, and exquisite sensitivity to local pressure ("point tenderness").[1–3] This is because an abscess forms under the periosteum. In a series of 100 children with extremity pain, 61 had bone scans suggestive of osteomyelitis.[5] Although usually acute, infection can sometimes be indolent.

The antibiotics and doses recommended in this chapter are based on those in *Therapeutic Guidelines: Antibiotic*, 13th edn, Therapeutic Guidelines Ltd, Melbourne, 2006.

In newborns and young infants, the periosteum is thin and pus can rupture through into the soft tissues, so they tend to present with local swelling, resembling cellulitis, or skin abscess, but with less local tenderness.[6,7] In addition, babies are more likely to have septic arthritis as well as osteomyelitis, probably because pus ruptures from the bone into the joint.[6,7]

Laboratory tests in acute osteomyelitis
The ESR and acute phase reactants such as CRP (C-reactive protein) are raised in at least 90% of children with acute osteomyelitis.[1–4] Normal values make osteomyelitis less likely but do not exclude it, while raised values are non-specific. The peripheral blood white cell count is often normal and is less useful than ESR and CRP.[1–4]

Blood cultures may be positive in up to 60% of patients,[8] although the proportion with positive blood cultures is usually much lower.[1–4] The diagnostic yield can be increased substantially, to 50–80%, by using needle aspiration or surgical biopsy to obtain bone, soft tissue, or joint fluid. The needle aspiration can be ultrasound guided to improve the yield in difficult cases.[9]

Imaging in acute osteomyelitis
Plain radiographs are of little use in the early diagnosis of pediatric osteomyelitis, except occasionally in neonatal osteomyelitis. In older children, the X-ray may show non-specific soft-tissue swelling in the first 3 days, but typical changes of osteopenia or osteolysis do not appear until after 7 days, periosteal elevation from 10 to 20 days, and osteosclerosis not before 30 days.[10]

Ultrasound scans can be useful in localizing collections such as sub-periosteal abscesses, in distinguishing infection from other diagnoses, and in directing fine needle aspiration.[9] Ultrasound is non-invasive, cheap, and less subject to movement artifact than magnetic resonance imaging (MRI) or computed tomography

(CT) (so does not require a general anesthetic in young children).[9] In a prospective study of imaging of 65 children with suspected osteomyelitis, ultrasound influenced treatment in 30% of cases, second only to MRI (45%) and better than CT scan.[11]

Bone scan in acute osteomyelitis

The technetium radionuclide bone scan involves IV injection of radioactive technetium-99m (^{99m}Tc). This is carried in the bloodstream to areas of maximum perfusion, so a scan within an hour of injection will show increased uptake (a "hot spot") in areas of hyperemia including both cellulitis and osteomyelitis. After a few hours, however, the ^{99m}Tc is preferentially taken up by osteoblasts.[12] Delayed bone scans will, therefore, show increased uptake in areas of increased new bone formation. Technetium bone scan has a sensitivity of 80–100% in diagnosing acute osteomyelitis in children of all ages,[12–16] including neonates.[7,17]

The main diagnostic pitfalls are that the bone scan may be normal early in the infection[18] and that the scan may show areas of decreased uptake of isotope due to impaired bone perfusion causing bony necrosis in children with more aggressive osteomyelitis.[16,19]

Nuclear medicine is particularly useful in identifying multifocal pyogenic osteomyelitis, which is more common in children than adults.[12–16] In this case, bone scan may demonstrate multiple "hot spots," which may or may not be associated with signs or symptoms. Multifocal pyogenic osteomyelitis is different from chronic multifocal osteomyelitis, which is non-infective (see Section 11.4, p. 160).

Other radionuclide scans

Gallium scanning using the radioactive isotope ^{67}Ga depends on gallium being taken up preferentially by iron-metabolizing cells, including neutrophils. It is most useful in spinal osteomyelitis.[20] Intense uptake of gallium in two adjacent vertebrae with loss of the disc space is highly suggestive of spinal osteomyelitis.[20,21]

Indium-labeled white cell scanning using ^{111}In is no more accurate than ^{99m}Tc scanning,[22] takes longer and is more difficult, and is rarely necessary in pediatric osteomyelitis.

MRI and CT scans in acute osteomyelitis

MRI with enhancement has a sensitivity of 88–100% for diagnosing acute osteomyelitis,[23–26] can reveal sub-periosteal and epiphyseal involvement not seen otherwise, and is more sensitive than CT.[11] Although the specificity is usually quoted[23–26] as >90%, MRI scans may incorrectly identify healing fractures, infarcted bone and healing infection as acute osteomyelitis,[23,24] and are not usually necessary in uncomplicated cases.[11]

CT scans are most useful for guided interventional procedures (e.g., aspiration or drainage) and for evaluation of sinus tracts in chronic infections.[27]

Organisms in acute osteomyelitis

Staphylococcus aureus causes >80% of childhood osteomyelitis,[1–4,28–31] including developing countries.[28] To date, MRSA osteomyelitis, either community-acquired (cMRSA) or nosocomially acquired, is responsible for <10% of cases in most countries worldwide, although there may be regional variation.[1–4,28–31] In the USA, in contrast, cMRSA is responsible for an increasing proportion of cases, over 50% in recent series.[32–36]

Other organisms are relatively uncommon causes of acute osteomyelitis, but should be strongly considered in certain settings:
- Group B streptococcus is an important cause of neonatal osteomyelitis, and MRSA should also be considered.[6,7]
- *Streptococcus pneumoniae* and *Salmonella* are important causes in sickle cell disease.[37]
- *Kingella kingae* is increasingly recognized as a cause of osteoarticular infections in children <5 years old.[38]
- Penetrating injuries to the sole of the foot ("sneaker osteomyelitis") are strongly associated with *Pseudomonas* infection.[3,39]
- *Haemophilus influenzae* type b (Hib), which was an important cause of osteoarticular infections in children <5 years old, is scarcely reported in well-immunized populations, but should be considered in unimmunized children.[1–4,28–31]
- *Bartonella henselae* (cat scratch) can cause acute or chronic vertebral osteomyelitis.[40]
- Children with chronic granulomatous disease are susceptible to fungal osteomyelitis, particularly with *Aspergillus*,[41] as of course are highly immunocompromised children.

Other organisms that can cause osteomyelitis include group A streptococcus (often in association with chicken pox[42]), anaerobes,[43] *Salmonella* (in association with food poisoning), other Gram-negative organisms (in developing countries[28] and in association with surgery), and coagulase negative staphylococci (virtually always in association with surgery).

Antibiotic therapy of acute osteomyelitis

Treatment should be based on cultures from bone, soft tissue, joint fluid, and of course blood cultures, whenever possible. We could find only 1 RCT comparing different antibiotics for acute pediatric osteomyelitis[44] (we excluded 1 RCT that had only nine children with osteomyelitis[45]). This small study, before cMRSA was reported, found no difference between IV clindamycin and IV methicillin or nafcillin.[44] We found observational studies indicating that several different regimens were effective. We found a non-Cochrane systematic review that found no difference in outcome of acute osteomyelitis between beta-lactam and macrolide antibiotics, although only 1 of 12 studies included was an RCT.[46]

Antibiotic therapy of acute osteomyelitis
For **empiric therapy**, in the absence of any other indications, we recommend:

> **di/flucl/oxa/nafcillin 50 mg/kg (max 2 g) IV, 6-hourly** OR
> **cephalothin 50 mg/kg (max 2 g) IV, 6-hourly** OR
> **cephazolin 50 mg/kg (max 2 g) IV, 8-hourly**

followed as soon as possible (see p. 159) by:

> **di/flucloxacillin 25 mg/kg (max 1 g) orally, 6-hourly** OR
> **cephalexin 25 mg/kg (max 1 g) orally, 8-hourly**

When **cMRSA** infection is suspected, because of local prevalence and/or ethnicity,[47] or clindamycin-sensitive cMRSA is grown, we recommend:

> **clindamycin 10 mg/kg (max 450 mg) IV, 8-hourly** THEN (if susceptible)
> **clindamycin 10 mg/kg (max 450 mg) orally, 8-hourly**

Clindamycin is rapidly and almost completely absorbed after oral administration, and is effective.[47] We recommend to change to oral therapy once the patient is responding to IV treatment.

For patients with anaphylactic penicillin allergy, we recommend:

> **vancomycin <12 years: 30 mg/kg (max 1 g) IV, 12-hourly; 12 years and older: 25 mg/kg (max 1 g) IV, 12-hourly** OR
> **clindamycin 10 mg/kg (max 450 mg) IV, 8-hourly** THEN (if susceptible)
> **clindamycin 10 mg/kg (max 450 mg) orally, 8-hourly**

If *S. aureus* is grown and is resistant to macrolides, and the patient is allergic to penicillin, we recommend basing oral therapy following vancomycin on proven susceptibility. Suitable oral options may be trimethoprim+sulfamethoxazole or doxycycline.

For patients with probable or proven **hospital-acquired MRSA**, we recommend:

> **vancomycin <12 years: 30 mg/kg (max 1 g) IV, 12-hourly; 12 years and older: 25 mg/kg (max 1 g) IV, 12-hourly** THEN (if susceptible)
> **rifamp(ic)in 10 mg/kg (max 600 mg) orally, daily** PLUS EITHER
> **fusidate sodium tablets 12 mg/kg (max 500 mg) orally, 12-hourly** OR
> **fusidic acid suspension 18 mg/kg (max 750 mg) orally, 12-hourly**

If **Gram-negative infection** (other than *Pseudomonas*) is suspected, and for children <5 years not immunized against Hib, we recommend:

> **cefotaxime 50 mg/kg (max 2 g) IV, 8-hourly** OR
> THE COMBINATION OF
> **ceftriaxone 50 mg/kg (max 2 g) IV, daily** PLUS
> **di/flucl/oxa/nafcillin 50 mg/kg (max 2 g) IV, 6-hourly**
> THEN (if susceptible)
> **amoxicillin+clavulanate 22.5 + 3.2 mg/kg (max 875 + 125 mg) orally, 8-hourly**

For suspected *Pseudomonas* osteomyelitis (penetrating wound to foot through sneaker), we recommend:

> **ceftazidime 50 mg/kg (max 2 g) IV, 8-hourly** OR
> **ciprofloxacin 10 mg/kg (max 400 mg) IV, 12-hourly** OR
> **piperacillin 100 mg/kg (max 4 g) IV, 8-hourly** OR
> **ticarcillin 50 mg/kg (max 3 g) IV, 6-hourly**

We recommend changing antibiotics if indicated by culture and sensitivity results. If the clinical response is good and the culture results are negative or if sensitive *S. aureus* is cultured, continue with the appropriate regimen mentioned above.

Antibiotics for acute osteomyelitis due to other organisms

For directed therapy of osteomyelitis due to other organisms, we recommend advice from an infectious diseases physician or clinical microbiologist. We recommend not using aminoglycosides for longer than a week, because of the risk of cumulative toxicity (see Appendix 2)

Mode of delivery of antibiotics for acute osteomyelitis

Question | For children with osteomyelitis, does changing from parenteral to oral antibiotics after less than a week compared with longer parenteral therapy result in increased morbidity?

Literature review | We found 1 RCT, 12 observational studies, and a non-Cochrane systematic review of antibiotic duration.[46] We found 1 observational study on adverse effects of prolonged IV therapy.[48]

A systematic review compared the outcome at 6 months in children aged 3 months to 16 years with acute osteomyelitis treated with 3–6 days of IV antibiotics followed by oral antibiotics, and in children treated with 7 or more days of IV antibiotics followed by oral antibiotics.[46] Most of the cases were due to *S. aureus*. The overall cure rate at 6 months for the short course of IV therapy was not significantly different from the longer course: 95.2% (95% CI 90.4–97.7) and 98.8% (95% CI 93.6–99.8), respectively.[46]

Prolonged IV therapy is not without risks. An observational study reported that 41% of 75 children given IV antibiotics by central venous catheter had one or more catheter-associated complication.[48]

> **To treat acute osteomyelitis in children 3 months or older, we recommend changing from IV antibiotics to oral antibiotics after 3–6 days if the child is afebrile and improving clinically.**
> **To treat newborns and infants <3 months old, whose absorption and intake of oral medications is unreliable, therapy should be given intravenously for the entire duration.**

Duration of antibiotics for acute osteomyelitis

We could find no RCTs on overall duration of antibiotics for acute osteomyelitis. A systematic review of short-course IV therapy[46] identified two old studies, each including over 100 children, in which antibiotics were given for <3 weeks, and the success rates were only 82 and 81%.[1,49] For this reason, it is recommended to treat with a total of at least 3 weeks of antibiotics (IV plus oral). There is, however, wide variation between studies regarding failure rates according to treatment duration. A series of smaller studies quoting 1–52 days of parenteral antimicrobial therapy reported success rates from 81 to 100%.[46] There is no evidence that giving antibiotics for longer than 3 weeks improves the success rate.

Serum CRP levels falls quicker than ESR in children recovering from acute osteomyelitis. Studies that measured serial CRP and ESR found that children with raised CRP levels were more likely to have symptoms or extensive radiographic abnormalities.[50,51] This does not mean that a raised CRP after 3 weeks of antibiotics would be an indication to continue treatment if the child was asymptomatic, but it might be an indication to examine the child carefully and to perform imaging.

> **We recommend treating children with acute osteomyelitis with antibiotics for a total of at least 3 weeks.**

11.2 Acute diskitis (discitis)

Childhood diskitis is probably a continuum of spinal infections, from infection of the intervertebral disk alone to vertebral osteomyelitis with soft-tissue abscess. It has been recognized for decades in the pediatric population, with controversy about the etiology and optimal treatment.[52–54] Diskitis is now generally accepted as a bacterial infection involving the disk space and adjacent vertebral end plates.[52,53]

Childhood diskitis can occur in the thoracic, lumbar, or sacral spine and can affect children of all ages, but lumbar diskitis in children <5 years is commonest.[52–54] The presentation of diskitis varies with age. Classically, the child refuses to walk, crawl, or stand, and may have back pain or pain on changing diapers. Nighttime crying can be a feature in toddlers,[54] and limp with irritability in older children. Fever is often low grade or absent, and acute phase reactants are less likely to be elevated than in acute osteomyelitis.[53,54]

CT-guided biopsy yields an organism in only 37–60% of cases,[54] probably due to confounding factors such as low numbers of organisms, previous antibiotics and technique, rather than absence of infection. This yield is compatible with biopsy results in pediatric acute osteomyelitis and septic arthritis.[54] Biopsy is not considered necessary for children with a classic clinical presentation, but is indicated for those whose symptoms do not resolve rapidly with treatment or who have an atypical presentation.[53,54] The diagnosis is usually made clinically and confirmed by changes in the plain radiograph, bone scan, or MRI scan. Blood cultures may be positive.[54]

The most common organism identified is S. aureus,[52–54] but other organisms including Salmonella,[55] K. kingae,[38] and anaerobes[56] have been described.

Most children improve rapidly with antibiotics. We recommend using the same antibiotics as for acute osteomyelitis (see p. 158). There are no RCTs for treatment of diskitis, and the optimum duration of therapy is unknown.[54] Pain often persists and the course can be indolent. There is no evidence and little reason to continue IV antibiotics once the child is afebrile and mobile, usually after about a week. A recent review suggested that oral antibiotics should be continued for about 4–6 weeks, depending on resolution of symptoms.[54] Diskitis often behaves more like chronic than acute osteomyelitis, so extending the duration of oral antibiotics seems reasonable.

Rest and immobilization with a lumbosacral corset or thoracolumbosacral orthosis are sometimes recommended in conjunction with antibiotics, particularly if imaging studies show sagittal or coronal deformity of the spine, or extensive bony destruction and soft-tissue involvement.[54]

Young children do not like rest, corsets, and orthoses, and there is no good evidence that they improve outcome. Children generally recover without them.

There is little value in repeating radiographs or MRI scans frequently in follow-up, because these are slow to resolve and do not equate with cure.[54] Imaging is necessary only if there are problems, and possibly at 12–18 months to show regrowth of the disk space.[54] The duration of oral antibiotics can be determined by clinical response, and the return of acute phase reactants to normal may be useful in this setting.[50,51]

11.3 Chronic osteomyelitis

Chronic osteomyelitis has been defined as bone infection requiring more than one episode of treatment and/or a persistent infection lasting more than 6 weeks.[57] The diagnosis is usually made clinically and confirmed by plain X-ray and/or scan followed by biopsy. A systematic review of diagnostic techniques in chronic osteomyelitis occurring at all ages, including cases associated with metal implants, found that positron emission tomography was most sensitive (96%), compared with MRI (84%) and bone scan (82%).[58]

In chronic infections, sinus cultures are often misleading, because the sinus tract becomes secondarily infected with water-loving Gram-negative bacilli.[59–61] Deep bone biopsy is recommended, whenever possible, although may be negative because of prior antibiotics and low organism load. Chronic osteomyelitis or arthritis associated with prosthetic material rarely recovers unless the prosthetic material is removed.[62] Chronic osteomyelitis of the mandible should rouse suspicion of actinomycosis.[63]

There is no evidence for or against the practice of using probenecid to increase antibiotic levels, but probenecid is often poorly tolerated and so may impair compliance. Nor is there evidence about the use of antibiotic-impregnated beads in chronic infection, usually containing gentamicin,[64,65] but more recently ceftriaxone,[66] although there are concerns that this could induce antibiotic resistance.

We found no good studies, not even observational ones, on duration of treatment for chronic infectious osteomyelitis. Most authorities recommend at least 6 months of oral antibiotics, but the duration of IV therapy is unknown, and even whether IV antibiotics are needed at all, provided adequate bone levels can be achieved with oral therapy. Unless there is evidence to suggest otherwise, we recommend that the antibiotic regimen includes an antibiotic against S. aureus.

11.4 Chronic recurrent multifocal osteomyelitis

Chronic recurrent multifocal osteomyelitis (CRMO) is a rare condition characterized by multifocal recurrent lesions with no infectious agents detectable in the bone lesion.[67,68] The lesions are often lytic. The lesion is a sterile inflammation of bone, of unknown etiology, although it has been post-ulated that patients may have a spondyloarthropathy.[67,68]

CRMO is thought to be a non-infective condition, distinct from acute multifocal osteomyelitis caused by *S. aureus* and other pyogenic organisms, and distinct from chronic pyogenic osteomyelitis (see Section 11.3, p. 160).

Some patients can present with a single non-infectious lesion that recurs in the same site, with the same clinical, radiological, and histological features as CRMO. This condition, sometimes called chronic recurrent unifocal osteomyelitis, is probably the same disease as CRMO.[67,68]

CRMO can be associated with SAPHO (synovitis, acne, pustulosis, hyperostosis, osteitis) syndrome,[69] although few patients presenting with CRMO have all the features of the syndrome.[67,68] If CRMO is suspected, the patient should be asked about and examined for palmar or plantar pustulosis, for psoriasis, and for joint involvement (including sacroiliac joints). Enthesitis (inflammation at the point of attachment of skeletal muscles to bone) may be present or may develop later.[68] Inflammatory bowel disease is also described in association with CRMO.[67,68]

CRMO mimics bacterial osteomyelitis clinically and histologically, and the diagnosis at first presentation is almost inevitably acute or chronic osteomyelitis. The recurrence of lesions despite adequate antibiotic treatment should alert the clinician to a possible diagnosis of CRMO. The median time to diagnosis was 8 months in one study.[68]

The condition is too rare for RCTs of treatment, but the consensus view is that non-steroidal anti-inflammatory drugs relieve symptoms, while antibiotics make no difference.[68]

11.5 Septic arthritis

Septic arthritis can occur as a result of hematogenous spread of organisms, with or without accompanying osteomyelitis, as a result of contiguous spread from osteomyelitis (e.g., in neonates, when pus is more likely to rupture through the periosteum) or following penetrating trauma. Arthritis may be monoarticular or occasionally polyarticular.

The major pathogen worldwide is *S. aureus*, and cMRSA is being reported from the USA,[69] Europe,[70] Taiwan,[71] and Australia.[72] The organisms causing septic arthritis are similar to those causing osteomyelitis (see p. 157), and include *S. pneumoniae*, group A (and in neonates, group B) streptococcus, *K. kingae*, and *Salmonella* species.[69–72] In unimmunized populations, Hib is a major cause. There are, however, some organisms that are sometimes isolated from joints but virtually never from bone. These include *Neisseria meningitidis*, *N. gonorrhoeae*, and *Enterobacter* species.[69–72]

Children with septic arthritis present with pain, swelling, redness, and reluctance to move the joint. The diagnosis is primarily clinical,[73] although a high fever (>38.5°C orally) and a high serum CRP[74] can help distinguish septic arthritis of the hip from irritable hip.[75] Diagnostic specimens, including a joint aspirate and blood cultures, should be taken before starting therapy, although the yield from Gram stain in one study[76] was only 45%. The yield from synovial fluid culture is also lower, at 38–58%, than for bone cultures, presumably due to the antibacterial properties of synovial fluid.[70–73] Because there may be minimal osteoblastic activity in septic arthritis, bone scan is less sensitive diagnostically than for osteomyelitis. Ultrasound can be useful in determining whether or not there is an effusion in a swollen joint and in aiding percutaneous drainage.

Drainage of infected joints is important for therapeutic as well as diagnostic reasons. Pus in the joint can cause permanent damage and impairs the action of antibiotics. Drainage may be achieved percutaneously, but open or arthroscopic surgery, often leaving a drain in situ, is usually needed for adequate drainage. Inflammation sometimes settles initially but recurs. This is an indication that further exploration and drainage is needed.[70–73]

If possible, antibiotic therapy should be based on Gram stain of joint fluid. If not, empiric therapy should be as for osteomyelitis (see p. 158).

Gonococcal arthritis should be treated with cefotaxime or ceftriaxone until susceptibility tests are known. Treatment should continue for a total of 7 days. Joint washouts are usually unnecessary.

Tuberculous arthritis usually presents with a chronic monoarthritis, with no fever, and little or no inflammation. If tuberculous arthritis is suspected or proven, see p. 201 for treatment.

The optimal duration of antibiotic therapy is unknown, but in line with treatment of osteomyelitis, we recommend IV therapy until there is an initial sustained clinical response (usually 3–7 days) followed by oral antibiotics to a total of at least 3 weeks, depending on clinical response.

A placebo-controlled RCT examined the use of 4 days of IV dexamethasone in 123 children with acute septic arthritis.[77] Dexamethasone significantly shortened the duration of symptoms during the acute phase and reduced residual dysfunction at the end of therapy, after 6 months and after 12 months. We recommend, for proven acute septic arthritis, in addition to antibiotics:

> **dexamethasone 0.2 mg/kg/dose IV, 8-hourly for 4 days**

An evaluation of the implementation of clinical guidelines for the management of possible septic arthritis of the hip in children showed excellent results compared to historic controls.[78] The patients treated using the guideline were more likely to have CRP measured before and after treatment, and had a significantly lower rate of initial bone scanning (13% versus 40%) and of presumptive drainage (13% versus 47%), greater compliance with recommended antibiotic therapy (93% versus 7%), faster change to oral antibiotics (3.9 days versus 6.9 days), and shorter hospital stay (4.8 days versus 8.3 days).[78] Because there are great advantages to all in reducing the time on IV antibiotics, we recommend the application of evidence-based guidelines for treating septic arthritis and osteomyelitis.

11.6 Arthritis associated with other infections

Arthritis can be associated with many different infections. Infections include viral arthritis, e.g., rubella or parvovirus B19 infection (see Chapter 18), mycoplasma infections, and arthritis associated with bacterial infections. With bacterial infections the arthritis may be due to direct invasion, i.e., septic arthritis, or may occur as part of an immunological reaction to infection, as with *Brucella* (see Section 16.2, p. 256) or *Yersinia* infection. In some infections, such as meningococcal or Hib infections, it is not always clear whether the arthritis is due to direct invasion or due to a post-infectious inflammatory response. Post-infectious arthritis and rheumatic fever (see p. 25) are well-recognized with group A streptococcal infection.

11.7 Open fractures

A Cochrane review of seven studies (913 participants) of antibiotics for open fractures found that prophylactic antibiotics were associated with a reduction in the risk of infection (RR 0.41, 95% CI 0.27–0.63).[79] The absolute risk reduction was 8% and 13 children had to be given antibiotics to prevent one infection. (95% CI 8–25).[79] Although the Cochrane review did not compare different regimens, the data show that the antibiotic should have antistaphylococcal activity.

We recommend:

> **di/flucl/oxa/nafcillin 50 mg/kg (max 2 g) IV, 6-hourly for 1–3 days OR**
> **cephalothin 50 mg/kg (max 2 g) IV, 6-hourly OR**
> **cephazolin 25 mg/kg (max 1 g) IV, 8-hourly**

For patients with anaphylactic penicillin allergy, we recommend:

> **clindamycin 10 mg/kg (max 450 mg) IV or orally, 8-hourly**

The duration of prophylaxis should be longer (5–7 days) if presentation is delayed for 8 hours or longer. If bone infection is established, treat as for osteomyelitis (see p. 158).

If wound soiling or tissue damage is severe and/or devitalized tissue is present, we recommend:

> **piperacillin+tazobactam 100 + 12.5 mg/kg (max 4 + 0.5 g) IV, 8-hourly OR**
> **ticarcillin+clavulanate 50 + 1.7 mg/kg (max 3 + 0.1 g) IV, 6-hourly FOLLOWED BY**
> **amoxicillin+clavulanate 22.5 + 3.2 mg/kg (max 875 + 125 mg) orally, 12-hourly**

If there has been significant fresh- or saltwater exposure, we recommend:

> **ciprofloxacin 10 mg/kg (max 400 mg) IV, 12-hourly OR**
> **ciprofloxacin 15 mg/kg (max 750 mg) orally, 12-hourly PLUS**
> **clindamycin 10 mg/kg (max 450 mg) IV or orally, 8-hourly**

References

1 Dich VQ, Nelson JD, Haltalin KC. Osteomyelitis in infants and children: a review of 163 cases. *Am J Dis Child* 1975;129: 1273–8.

2 Scott RJ, Christofersen MR, Robertson WW, Jr, Davidson RS, Rankin L, Drummond DS. Acute osteomyelitis in children: a review of 116 cases. *J Pediatr Orthop* 1990;10: 649–52.

3 Faden H, Grossi M. Acute osteomyelitis in children. Reassessment of etiologic agents and their clinical characteristics. *Am J Dis Child* 1991;145:65–9.

4 Dahl LB, Hoyland AL, Dramsdahl H, Kaaresen PI. Acute osteomyelitis in children: a population-based retrospective study 1965 to 1994. *Scand J Infect Dis* 1998;30:573–7.

5 Park HM, Rothschild PA, Kernek CB. Scintigraphic evaluation of extremity pain in children: its efficacy and pitfalls. *AJR Am J Roentgenol* 1985;145:1079–84.

6 Isaacs D, Moxon ER. *Handbook of Neonatal Infections. A Practical Guide.* London: WB Saunders, 1999.

7 Wong M, Isaacs D, Howman-Giles R, Uren R. Clinical and diagnostic features of osteomyelitis occurring in the first three months of life. *Pediatr Infect Dis J* 1995;14:1047–53.

8 Howard CB, Einhorn M, Dagan R, Yagupski P, Porat S. Fine-needle bone biopsy to diagnose osteomyelitis. *J Bone Joint Surg Br* 1994;76:311–4.

9 Robben SG. Ultrasonography of musculoskeletal infections in children. *Eur Radiol* 2004;14(suppl 4):L65–77.

10 Capitanio MA, Kirkpatrick JA. Early roentgen observations in acute osteomyelitis. *Am J Roentgenol Radium Ther Nucl Med* 1970;108:488–96.

11 Kaiser S, Jorulf H, Hirsch G. Clinical value of imaging techniques in childhood osteomyelitis. *Acta Radiol* 1998;39: 523–31.

12 Kim EE, Haynie TP, Podoloff DA, Lowry PA, Harle TS. Radionuclide imaging in the evaluation of osteomyelitis and septic arthritis. *Crit Rev Diagn Imaging* 1989;29:257–305.

13 Sullivan DC, Rosenfield NS, Ogden J, Gottschalk A. Problems in the scintigraphic detection of osteomyelitis in children. *Radiology* 1980;135:731–6.

14 Howie DW, Savage JP, Wilson TG, Paterson D. The technetium phosphate bone scan in the diagnosis of osteomyelitis in childhood. *J Bone Joint Surg Am* 1983;65:431–7.

15 Hamdan J, Asha M, Mallouh A, Usta H, Talab Y, Ahmad M. Technetium bone scintigraphy in the diagnosis of osteomyelitis in children. *Pediatr Infect Dis J* 1987;6:529–32.

16 Tuson CE, Hoffman EB, Mann MD. Isotope bone scanning for acute osteomyelitis and septic arthritis in children. *J Bone Joint Surg Br* 1994;76:306–10.

17 Bressler EL, Conway JJ, Weiss SC. Neonatal osteomyelitis examined by bone scintigraphy. *Radiology* 1984;152:685–8.

18 Wald ER, Mirro R, Gartner JC. Pitfalls on the diagnosis of acute osteomyelitis by bone scan. *Clin Pediatr (Phila)* 1980;19:597–601.

19 Pennington WT, Mott MP, Thometz JG, Sty JR, Metz D. Photopenic bone scan osteomyelitis: a clinical perspective. *J Pediatr Orthop* 1999;19:695–8.

20 Love C, Patel M, Lonner BS, Tomas MB, Palestro CJ. Diagnosing spinal osteomyelitis: a comparison of bone and Ga-67 scintigraphy and magnetic resonance imaging. *Clin Nucl Med* 2000;25:963–77.

21 Palestro CJ, Torres MA. Radionuclide imaging in orthopedic infections. *Semin Nucl Med* 1997;27:334–45.

22 Flivik G, Sloth M, Rydholm U, Herrlin K, Lidgren L. Technetium-99m-nanocolloid scintigraphy in orthopedic infections: a comparison with indium-111-labeled leukocytes. *J Nucl Med* 1993;34:1646–50.

23 Unger E, Moldofsky P, Gatenby R, Hartz W, Broder G. Diagnosis of osteomyelitis by MR imaging. *AJR Am J Roentgenol* 1988;150:605–10.

24 Erdman WA, Tamburro F, Jayson HT, Weatherall PT, Ferry KB, Peshock RM. Osteomyelitis: characteristics and pitfalls of diagnosis with MR imaging. *Radiology* 1991;180:533–9.

25 Morrison WB, Schweitzer ME, Bock GW et al. Diagnosis of osteomyelitis: utility of fat-suppressed contrast-enhanced MR imaging. *Radiology* 1993;189:251–7.

26 Mazur JM, Ross G, Cummings J, Hahn GA, Jr, McCluskey WP. Usefulness of magnetic resonance imaging for the diagnosis of acute musculoskeletal infections in children. *J Pediatr Orthop* 1995;15:144–7.

27 Restrepo S, Vargas D, Riascos R, Cuellar H. Musculoskeletal infection imaging: past, present, and future. *Curr Infect Dis Rep* 2005;7:365–72.

28 Lauschke FH, Frey CT. Hematogenous osteomyelitis in infants and children in the northwestern region of Namibia. Management and two-year results. *J Bone Joint Surg Am* 1994;76:502–10.

29 Bonhoeffer J, Haeberle B, Schaad UB, Heininger U. Diagnosis of acute haematogenous osteomyelitis and septic arthritis: 20 years experience at the University Children's Hospital Basel. *Swiss Med Wkly* 2001;131:575–81.

30 Kao HC, Huang YC, Chiu CH et al. Acute hematogenous osteomyelitis and septic arthritis in children. *J Microbiol Immunol Infect* 2003;36:260–5.

31 Goergens ED, McEvoy A, Watson M, Barrett IR. Acute osteomyelitis and septic arthritis in children. *J Paediatr Child Health* 2005;41:59–62.

32 Frank AL, Marcinak JF, Mangat PD, Schreckenberger PC. Community-acquired and clindamycin-susceptible methicillin-resistant *Staphylococcus aureus* in children. *Pediatr Infect Dis J* 1999;18:993–1000.

33 Sattler CA, Mason EO, Jr, Kaplan SL. Prospective comparison of risk factors and demographic and clinical characteristics of community-acquired, methicillin-resistant versus methicillin-susceptible *Staphylococcus aureus* infection in children. *Pediatr Infect Dis J* 2002;21:910–7.

34 Martinez-Aguilar G, Avalos-Mishaan A, Hulten K, Hammerman W, Mason EO, Jr, Kaplan SL. Community-acquired, methicillin-resistant and methicillin-susceptible *Staphylococcus aureus* musculoskeletal infections in children. *Pediatr Infect Dis J* 2004;23:701–6.

35 Kaplan SL, Hulten KG, Gonzalez BE et al. Three-year surveillance of community-acquired *Staphylococcus aureus* infections in children. *Clin Infect Dis* 2005;40:1785–91.

36 Bocchini CE, Hulten KG, Mason EO, Jr, Gonzalez BE, Hammerman WA, Kaplan SL. Panton-Valentine leukocidin genes are associated with enhanced inflammatory response and local disease in acute hematogenous *Staphylococcus aureus* osteomyelitis in children. *Pediatrics* 2006;117:433–40.

37 Almeida A, Roberts I. Bone involvement in sickle cell disease. *Br J Haematol* 2005;129:482–90.

38 Kiang KM, Ogunmodede F, Juni BA et al. Outbreak of osteomyelitis/septic arthritis caused by *Kingella kingae* among child care center attendees. *Pediatrics* 2005;116:e206–13.

39 Elliott SJ, Aronoff SC. Clinical presentation and management of *Pseudomonas* osteomyelitis. *Clin Pediatr (Phila)* 1985;24:566–70.

40 Abdel-Haq N, Abuhammour W, Al-Tatari H, Asmar B. Disseminated cat scratch disease with vertebral osteomyelitis and epidural abscess. *South Med J* 2005;98:1142–5.

41 Dotis J, Roilides E. Osteomyelitis due to *Aspergillus* spp. in patients with chronic granulomatous disease: comparison of *Aspergillus nidulans* and *Aspergillus fumigatus*. *Int J Infect Dis* 2004;8:103–10.

42 Ibia EO, Imoisili M, Pikis A. Group A beta-hemolytic streptococcal osteomyelitis in children. *Pediatrics* 2003;112: e22–6.

43 Brook I. Joint and bone infections due to anaerobic bacteria in children. *Pediatr Rehabil* 2002;5:11–9.

44 Kaplan SL, Mason EO, Jr, Feigin RD. Clindamycin versus nafcillin or methicillin in the treatment of *Staphylococcus aureus* osteomyelitis in children. *South Med J* 1982;75:138–42.

45 Kulhanjian J, Dunphy MG, Hamstra S et al. Randomized comparative study of ampicillin/sulbactam vs. ceftriaxone for treatment of soft tissue and skeletal infections in children. *Pediatr Infect Dis J* 1989;8:605–10.

46 Le Saux N, Howard A, Barrowman NJ, Gaboury I, Sampson M, Moher D. Shorter courses of parenteral antibiotic therapy do not appear to influence response rates for children with acute hematogenous osteomyelitis: a systematic review. *BMC Infect Dis* 2002;2:16.

47 Martinez-Aguilar G, Hammerman WA, Mason EO, Jr, Kaplan SL. Clindamycin treatment of invasive infections caused by community-acquired, methicillin-resistant and methicillin-susceptible *Staphylococcus aureus* in children. *Pediatr Infect Dis J* 2003;22:593–8.

48 Blockey NJ, Watson JT. Acute osteomyelitis in children. *J Bone Joint Surg Br* 1970;52B:77–87.

49 Ring D, Johnston CE, II, Wenger DR. Pyogenic infectious spondylitis in children: the convergence of discitis and vertebral osteomyelitis. *J Pediatr Orthop* 1995;15:652–60.

50 Unkila-Kallio L, Kallio MJ, Eskola J, Peltola H. Serum C-reactive protein, erythrocyte sedimentation rate, and white blood cell count in acute hematogenous osteomyelitis of children. *Pediatrics* 1994;93:59–62.

51 Roine I, Faingezicht I, Arguedas A, Herrera JF, Rodriguez F. Serial serum C-reactive protein to monitor recovery from acute hematogenous osteomyelitis in children. *Pediatr Infect Dis J* 1995;14:40–4.

52 Early SD, Kay RM, Tolo VT. Childhood diskitis. *J Am Acad Orthop Surg* 2003;11:413–20.

53 Karabouta Z, Bisbinas I, Davidson A, Goldsworthy LL. Discitis in toddlers: a case series and review. *Acta Paediatr* 2005;94:1516–8.

54 Barkai G, Leibovitz E, Smolnikov A, Tal A, Cohen E. *Salmonella* diskitis in a 2-year old immunocompetent child. *Scand J Infect Dis* 2005;37:232–5.

55 Brook I. Two cases of diskitis attributable to anaerobic bacteria in children. *Pediatrics* 2001;107:E26.

56 Schauwecker DS. Osteomyelitis: diagnosis with In-111-labeled leukocytes. *Radiology* 1989;171:141–6.

57 Termaat MF, Raijmakers PG, Scholten HJ, Bakker FC, Patka P, Haarman HJ. The accuracy of diagnostic imaging for the assessment of chronic osteomyelitis: a systematic review and meta-analysis. *J Bone Joint Surg Am* 2005;87:2464–71.

58 Mackowiak PA, Jones SR, Smith JW. Diagnostic value of sinus tract cultures in chronic osteomyelitis. *JAMA* 1978;239: 2772–5.

59 Perry CR, Pearson RL, Miller GA. Accuracy of cultures of material from swabbing of the superficial aspect of the wound and needle biopsy in the preoperative assessment of osteomyelitis. *J Bone Joint Surg* 1991;73(A):745–9.

60 Patzakis MJ, Wilkins J, Kumar J, Holtom P, Greenbaum B, Ressler R. Comparison of the results of bacterial cultures from multiple sites in chronic osteomyelitis of long bones: a prospective study. *J Bone Joint Surg Am* 1994;76:664–6.

61 Zimmerli W, Trampuz A, Ochsner PE. Prosthetic-joint infections. *N Engl J Med* 2004;351:1645–54.

62 Robinson JL, Vaudry WL, Dobrovolsky W. Actinomycosis presenting as osteomyelitis in the pediatric population. *Pediatr Infect Dis J* 2005;24:365–9.

63 Hedstrom SA, Lidgren L, Torholm C, Onnerfalt R. Antibiotic containing bone cement beads in the treatment of deep muscle and skeletal infections. *Acta Orthop Scand* 1980;51:863–9.

64 Walenkamp GH, Kleijn LL, de Leeuw M. Osteomyelitis treated with gentamicin-PMMA beads: 100 patients followed for 1–12 years. *Acta Orthop Scand* 1998;69:518–22.

65 Alonge TO, Ogunlade SO, Omololu AB, Fashina AN, Oluwatosin A. Management of chronic osteomyelitis in a developing country using ceftriaxone-PMMA beads: an initial study. *Int J Clin Pract* 2002;56:181–3.

66 Huber AM, Lam PY, Duffy CM et al. Chronic recurrent multifocal osteomyelitis: clinical outcomes after more than five years of follow-up. *J Pediatr* 2002;141:198–203.

67 Girschick HJ, Raab P, Surbaum S et al. Chronic non-bacterial osteomyelitis in children. *Ann Rheum Dis* 2005;64:279–85.

68 Beretta-Piccoli BC, Sauvain MJ, Gal I et al. Synovitis, acne, pustulosis, hyperostosis, osteitis (SAPHO) syndrome in childhood: a report of ten cases and review of the literature. *Eur J Pediatr* 2000;159:594–601.

69 Luhmann JD, Luhmann SJ. Etiology of septic arthritis in children: an update for the 1990s. *Pediatr Emerg Care* 1999;15: 40–2.

70 Caksen H, Ozturk MK, Uzum K, Yuksel S, Ustunbas HB, Per H. Septic arthritis in childhood. *Pediatr Int* 2000;42:534–40.

71 Wang CL, Wang SM, Yang YJ, Tsai CH, Liu CC. Septic arthritis in children: relationship of causative pathogens, complications, and outcome. *J Microbiol Immunol Infect* 2003;36:41–6.

72 Goergens ED, McEvoy A, Watson M, Barrett IR. Acute os-teomyelitis and septic arthritis in children. *J Paediatr Child Health* 2005;41:59–62.

73 Kunnamo I, Kallio P, Pelkonen P, Hovi T. Clinical signs and laboratory tests in the differential diagnosis of arthritis in children. *Am J Dis Child* 1987;141:34–40.

74 Levine MJ, McGuire KJ, McGowan KL, Flynn JM. Assessment of the test characteristics of C-reactive protein for septic arthritis in children. *J Pediatr Orthop* 2003;23: 373–7.

75 Caird MS, Flynn JM, Leung YL, Millman JE, D'Italia JG, Dormans JP. Factors distinguishing septic arthritis from transient synovitis of the hip in children: a prospective study. *J Bone Joint Surg Am* 2006;88:1251–7.

76 Faraj AA, Omonbude OD, Godwin P. Gram staining in the diagnosis of acute septic arthritis. *Acta Orthop Belg* 2002;68: 388–91.

77 Odio CM, Ramirez T, Arias G et al. Double blind, randomized, placebo-controlled study of dexamethasone therapy for hematogenous septic arthritis in children. *Pediatr Infect Dis J* 2003;22:883–8.

78 Kocher MS, Mandiga R, Murphy JM et al. A clinical practice guideline for treatment of septic arthritis in children: efficacy in improving process of care and effect on outcome of septic arthritis of the hip. *J Bone Joint Surg Am* 2003;85-A:994–9.

79 Gosselin RA, Roberts I, Gillespie WJ. Antibiotics for preventing infection in open limb fractures. *The Cochrane Database of Systematic Reviews* 2004;(1):Art No CD003764.

CHAPTER 12
Respiratory infections

12.1 Upper respiratory tract infections

Acute otitis media

Acute otitis media (AOM) is an acute infection of the middle ear, characterized by pain, fever, irritability, poor feeding, redness, and bulging of the tympanic membrane.[1] AOM is one of the most frequent diseases in early infancy and childhood. Approximately 10% of children have an episode of AOM by 3 months of age. The peak age-specific incidence is between 6 and 15 months. AOM is common in infancy and in preschool years, is less common in school-age children, and is uncommon in healthy adults.[1]

Children with defective humoral immunity, with low levels of IgG, IgG sub-class deficiency, or with poorly functioning IgG, often have recurrent AOM, implying that antibodies are an important host protection against otitis media. The main anatomic defects predisposing to recurrent AOM involve the palate and thus obstruct Eustachian tube drainage. Environmental factors include exposure to tobacco smoke. There is a group of "otitis-prone" children who get recurrent AOM, but have no identifiable immunologic or anatomic defect.[1]

Diagnosis

Children with colds or viral upper respiratory tract infections (URTI) often have eardrums that look dull and move poorly using pneumatic otoscopy. If tympanocentesis is performed in children with colds or URTI, no middle ear fluid is obtained.[3–7] In contrast, children with AOM usually have middle ear fluid, and if tympanocentesis is performed, bacteria can be isolated from 70 to 90% of middle ear cultures.[3–9] Children with

AOM have acute inflammation, with either erythema of the tympanic membrane or otalgia.[3–9] AOM is different from otitis media with effusion (OME),[10] which is a chronic condition characterized by middle ear effusion without acute inflammation.[3–9] (see p. 169).

Tympanocentesis is commonly performed in the diagnosis and management of AOM in Scandinavian countries, sometimes in North America, and virtually never in the rest of Europe or Australia, because of concerns about pain and efficacy. Tympanocentesis has not been compared to antibiotics without tympanocentesis or to no treatment in RCTs. When AOM is diagnosed by otoscopy and tympanometry, tympanocentesis yields fluid in 85% of cases.[8,9]

Tympanometry has 65–97% sensitivity in diagnosing AOM when compared to tympanocentesis.[2–10] If the diagnosis of AOM is made on the otoscopic appearance, the single most important clinical finding associated with finding a middle ear pathogen in one study, with a sensitivity of 74%, is fullness or bulging of the tympanic membrane.[11] Erythema of the eardrum is less helpful, but when cultures are negative, the drum is usually shiny, dull, or white.[11] Pneumatic otoscopy is recommended in preference to simple otoscopy in order to detect effusions.[1]

Organisms

Bacteria are found in 50–90% of children with AOM with or without otorrhea,[1,12–14] viruses are found in 20–49% of cases, and coinfection with bacteria and viruses in 18–27%.[15,16] The major bacterial pathogens in AOM are *Streptococcus pneumoniae*, untypeable *Haemophilus influenzae*, *Moraxella catarrhalis*, and in children >5 years, *Streptococcus pyogenes*. Although the proportions vary with age and geographic location, these organisms are consistently found.[1,12–14] In places like North America, where pneumococcal conjugate vaccine is routinely given to infants, a shift in the proportion of the major AOM pathogens has been

---

The antibiotics and doses recommended in this chapter are based on those in *Therapeutic Guidelines: Antibiotic*, 13th edn, Therapeutic Guidelines Ltd, Melbourne, 2006.

described so that *H. influenzae* now predominates.[17] A study examined the correlation between nasopharyngeal bacteria and the bacteria obtained by tympanocentesis from children with AOM.[18] The sensitivity and specificity were both 99% for pneumococci but not clinically useful for other bacteria.[18]

Treatment of AOM
Antibiotics for AOM: yes or no?

Question | For children with AOM, do antibiotics compared with no antibiotics or placebo result in more rapid resolution of symptoms?
Literature review | We found 80 studies, 10 high-quality RCTs, a non-Cochrane meta-analysis,[19] and a Cochrane systematic review.[20]

A Cochrane review[20] found 10 RCTs but only 8 high-quality trials (2287 children) that reported clinically relevant data. The trials showed no reduction in pain at 24 hours, but a 30% relative reduction (95% CI 19–40%) in pain after 2–7 days. Since approximately 80% of patients will have settled spontaneously in this time, this means an absolute reduction of 7% or that about 15 children must be treated with antibiotics to prevent one child having some pain after 2 days.[20] The conclusion of the authors was that antibiotics provide a small benefit for AOM in children, and because about 80% cases will resolve spontaneously (the so-called Polyanna phenomenon, from an American book about a girl with a very optimistic approach that things always get better), the benefit from antibiotics must be weighed against the possible adverse reactions from antibiotics and risks of resistance.

A more inclusive meta-analysis that included 80 studies found very similar results.[19] Children with AOM not treated with antibiotics experienced a 1–7-day clinical failure rate of 19% (95% CI 10–28%) and few suppurative complications. When patients were treated with amoxicillin, the 2–7-day clinical failure rate was reduced to 7%, a 12% reduction (95% CI 4–20%). There was no evidence to support any particular antibiotic regimens as more effective at relieving symptoms. Adverse effects, primarily gastrointestinal, were more common among children on cefixime than among those on ampicillin or amoxicillin, and more common among children on amoxicillin-clavulanate than among those on azithromycin.

Suppurative complications such as mastoiditis, which used to be common, are now rare, even without antibiotic treatment.[19,20] A review of trials from 1966 to 1999 estimated the incidence of mastoiditis as 1 in 1000 children with untreated otitis media.[20] In some countries, such as the Netherlands, only about 30% of children with AOM are treated with antibiotics and the rest with close observation.[1]

Antibiotics for AOM: delayed versus immediate prescription

Question | For children with AOM, do delayed antibiotic prescriptions compared with immediate antibiotics reduce antibiotic use and do they result in increased morbidity?
Literature review | We found one high-quality RCT of delayed antibiotic prescription for AOM[21] and a Cochrane review of delayed antibiotic prescription for various respiratory disorders in children.[22]

Because of the emergence of antibiotic-resistant organisms and overuse of antibiotics for self-limiting viral URTIs, there have been a number of studies of delayed antibiotic prescriptions. Parents are given a prescription for antibiotics but advised to fill the prescription only if symptoms persist after 2–3 days.

We found one RCT in which children aged 6 months to 10 years with AOM seen in a UK general practice were randomized to immediate or delayed antibiotics.[21] The delayed antibiotic group was instructed to collect an antibiotic prescription at the parents' discretion after 72 hours if the child was not improving. On average, symptoms resolved after 3 days. Children prescribed antibiotics immediately improved more quickly. On average, their illness lasted 1 day less, they had a reduction in night disturbance of 0.7 of a night, and the paracetamol consumption was half a spoon a day less. There was no difference in school absence or pain or distress scores, since benefits of antibiotics occurred mainly after the first 24 hours when distress was less severe. Parents of 36/150 (24%) of the children given delayed prescriptions used antibiotics. Fewer children in the delayed group had diarrhea (9% versus 19%). The authors concluded that for children who are not very unwell systemically, a wait–and–see approach seems feasible and acceptable to parents and could substantially reduce the use of antibiotics for AOM.[21]

167

The Cochrane review found seven studies, four of sore throat, two of viral respiratory tract infections, and the one of otitis media.[22] For most outcomes there was no difference between immediate and delayed antibiotic groups, but patients in the delayed antibiotic group in three of the studies had significantly more fever.

Duration of antibiotic treatment for AOM

Question | For children with AOM, is treatment with antibiotics for 5 days as effective as treatment with antibiotics for longer?

Literature review | We found 33 RCTs, a non-Cochrane meta-analysis,[23] and a Cochrane review.[24]

A meta-analysis comparing fewer than 7 days of antibiotics with 7 or more days found that 44 children would need to be treated with the longer course of antibiotics to avoid one treatment failure.[23] A Cochrane review of 33 studies (1524 children) by the same authors[24] found a worse treatment outcome at 8–19 days in children treated with antibiotics for 5 days compared with 8–10 days (OR 1.52, 95% CI 1.17–1.98). By 20–30 days, however, outcomes were comparable. The absolute difference in treatment failure at 20–30 days suggests that at least 17 children would need to be treated with the long course of antibiotics to avoid one treatment failure. The authors concluded that 5 days of short-acting antibiotic use is effective treatment for uncomplicated AOM in children.[23,24]

Recommendations for antibiotic therapy for AOM

No antibiotics or delayed prescription

Older children who do not have systemic features (vomiting and fever) are likely to have a good outcome, so the need for immediate antibiotics can be assessed on an individual basis. We recommend the following:

· For children aged 6 months and older with no systemic features, symptomatic treatment (analgesics for pain relief and antipyretics for high fever and irritability[1]) for 2 days is an option. If symptoms persist after 2 days, we recommend reevaluating the patient and reconsidering antibiotic treatment (see below).

· An alternative for children aged 6 months and older without systemic symptoms is to give a delayed prescription for antibiotics with instructions on filling it after 48–72 hours if symptoms persist or returning for reevaluation if they get worse (it is wise to give an expiry date on the prescription to avoid use at a much later date).

· For children aged 6 months to 2 years managed as above, we recommend ensuring contact (visit or telephone) after 24 hours, at which time further observation or antibiotics should be considered.

Immediate antibiotics

· For children aged less than 6 months, we recommend treating with antibiotics immediately. This is because diagnosis can be difficult in this age group and because there is a greater risk of suppurative complications if treatment is delayed.

· For children with systemic features, such as vomiting and fever, immediate antibiotic therapy is indicated.

High-dose amoxicillin is recommended when the incidence of penicillin-insensitive pneumococci is high. We recommend:

amoxicillin 40–50 mg/kg (max 1 g) orally, 12-hourly for 5 days

If the incidence of penicillin-insensitive pneumococci is low, we recommend:

amoxicillin 15 mg/kg (max 500 mg) orally, 8-hourly for 5 days
OR (if compliance is likely to be a problem)
amoxicillin 30 mg/kg (max 1 g) orally, 12-hourly for 5 days

If the patient is allergic to penicillin, we recommend:

cefdinir 7 mg/kg (max 300 mg) orally, 12-hourly for 5 days OR
cefpodoxime 5 mg/kg (max 200 mg) orally, 12-hourly for 5 days OR
cefuroxime 15 mg/kg (max 500 mg) orally, 12-hourly for 5 days

Children who fail to respond to amoxicillin alone are likely to be infected with a beta-lactamase-producing organism, *H. influenzae* or *M. catarrhalis*. Amoxicillin-clavulanate contains clavulanic acid which inhibits beta-lactamase enzymes. Recommended treatment is:

Amoxicillin+clavulanate 22.5 + 3.2 mg/kg (max 875 + 125 mg) orally, 12-hourly for 5 days

If the patient still fails to respond to therapy, we recommend seeking expert advice.

Decongestants and antihistamines

Question | For children with AOM, do decongestants and/or antihistamines compared with no treatment or placebo reduce symptoms and speed recovery?

Literature review | We found 15 RCTs and a Cochrane review.[25]

A Cochrane review of 15 studies of decongestants and antihistamines for AOM found that decongestants or antihistamines alone had no benefit.[25] Combined decongestant-antihistamine use was associated with a decreased incidence of persistent otitis media at 2 weeks, but no benefit for early cure rates, symptom resolution, prevention of surgery, or other complications. There was a five- to eightfold increased risk of side effects for those receiving an intervention, which reached statistical significance for all decongestant groupings. The authors concluded that the clinical significance was minimal, that study design may have biased the results, and that routine use of decongestants or antihistamines could not be recommended.[25]

Recurrent AOM

Possible underlying causes of recurrent AOM and risk factors should be considered. These include immune deficiency (usually humoral), passive smoke exposure (tobacco, wood fires), child care, allergic rhinitis, adenoid disease, and structural anomalies such as cleft palate.[26]

Question | For children with recurrent AOM, does tympanostomy tube insertion (grommets) or adenoidectomy or prophylactic antibiotics compared with no treatment reduce the frequency of episodes of AOM?

Literature review | We found four RCTs of tympanostomy tube insertion,[27–30] four RCTs of adenoidectomy,[31–34] and nine RCTs and a non-Cochrane meta-analysis[35] of prophylactic antibiotics in which a placebo group was included.

Early small studies suggested that tympanostomy tubes were effective in reducing the number of episodes in children with recurrent AOM. The largest study of 264 children, however, found that tympanostomy tubes did not reduce the frequency of AOM compared with placebo, and 3.9% of children who received tubes developed persistent tympanic membrane perforations.[30] The authors also pointed out that the incidence of AOM was far lower than predicted in the placebo group, so any intervention should be viewed in this light.

Early studies suggested some benefit from adenoidectomy,[31,32] but recent studies have found none, irrespective of whether adenoidectomy was performed alone[33] or with tympanostomy tube insertion.[34]

A non-Cochrane meta-analysis of nine studies (958 subjects) found that antibiotic prophylaxis of recurrent otitis media reduced the incidence of AOM by 89% (95% CI 81–97%).[35] Two studies found that antibiotic chemoprophylaxis with amoxicillin reduced the frequency of episodes of AOM,[30,36] but the benefits must be weighed against the dangers of inducing resistance and the natural history of resolution. Early studies found co-trimoxazole chemoprophylaxis to be effective, but more recent studies did not confirm this finding.[33,37]

We do not recommend tympanostomy tubes or adenoidectomy for children with recurrent AOM. Prophylactic amoxicillin is likely to be effective, but the benefits should be weighed against the risks of selecting for resistant organisms and of other adverse events.

Chronic OME ("glue ear")

Chronic OME is the persistence of middle ear effusion for more than 3 months. OME is very common in children, especially between the ages of 1 and 3 years with a prevalence of 10–30% and a cumulative incidence of 80% at the age of 4 years.[38] The usual presentation is with symptoms attributable to hearing loss or pain.

Although many different interventions have been tried to improve short- and long-term hearing in children with chronic OME because of fears of the effect on language development, a meta-analysis of 38 studies found very little evidence that OME impairs later language development.[38] Recommendations about interventions, particularly invasive procedures, should reflect the relatively benign outcome.

Diagnosis of OME

A systematic review of eight methods of diagnosing OME, including pneumatic otoscopy, tympanometry, and acoustic reflectometry, examined 52 studies.[38]

Pneumatic otoscopy performed best with a sensitivity of 94% (95% CI 92–96%) and a specificity of 80% (95% CI 75–86%). However, examiner qualifications were reported inconsistently, and training was not specified. The authors concluded that the finding that pneumatic otoscopy can do as well as or better than tympanometry and acoustic reflectometry has significant practical implications. For the typical clinician, pneumatic otoscopy should be easier to use than other diagnostic methods. The important question may be what degree of training will be needed for the clinician to be as effective with pneumatic otoscopy as were the examiners in the studies reviewed in this report.[38] A practice guideline made a strong recommendation that clinicians use pneumatic otoscopy as the primary diagnostic method to distinguish OME from AOM.[39]

Antibiotics for chronic OME

Question | For children with chronic OME, do antibiotics compared with no antibiotics or placebo speed resolution of effusion?

Literature review | We found 20 RCTs and 3 non-Cochrane meta-analyses.[35,40,41]

Bacteria can be cultured from about 20 to 30% of chronic middle ear effusions. All the three meta-analyses found that antibiotics hasten short-term resolution of chronic OME,[35,40,41] although a meta-analysis of eight studies found that they have no effect on long-term outcome.[35] Because the aim is to speed short-term resolution without invasive intervention, a short course of antibiotics is a sensible first-line treatment option. Recommended treatment is:

> **amoxicillin 40–50 mg/kg (max 1 g) orally, 12-hourly for 10–30 days**

If penicillin-insensitive pneumococci are rare, we recommend:

> **amoxicillin 15 mg/kg (max 500 mg) orally, 8-hourly for 10–30 days**
> OR (if compliance is likely to be a problem)
> **amoxicillin 30 mg/kg (max 1 g) orally, 12-hourly for 10–30 days**

If the patient is allergic to penicillin, we recommend:

> **cefdinir 7 mg/kg (max 300 mg) orally, 12-hourly for 10–30 days** OR

> **cefpodoxime 5 mg/kg (max 200 mg) orally, 12-hourly for 10–30 days** OR
> **cefuroxime 15 mg/kg (max 500 mg) orally, 12-hourly for 10–30 days**

If the children fail to respond to amoxicillin, it may be that they are infected with a beta-lactamase-producing organism or that they would benefit from corticosteroids (see below). We recommend giving amoxicillin-clavulanate, with or without oral corticosteroids:

> **amoxicillin+clavulanate 22.5 + 3.2 mg/kg (max 875 + 125 mg) orally, 12-hourly for 10–30 days**

Corticosteroids for chronic OME

Question | For children with chronic OME, do oral corticosteroids compared with no corticosteroids or placebo speed resolution of effusion?

Literature review | We found RCTs and a Cochrane review[42] of oral corticosteroids.

Inflammation may contribute to persistent OME. Short, 7–14-day courses of oral corticosteroids have been used alone or in combination with antibiotics. A Cochrane systematic review found the OR for OME persisting after short-term follow-up in children treated with oral steroids compared with control was 0.22 (95% CI 0.08–0.63); i.e., there was a 78% reduction. The OR for OME persisting after short-term follow-up for children treated with oral steroids plus antibiotic compared with control plus antibiotic was 0.37 (95% CI 0.25–0.56).[42] As with antibiotics, there was no evidence of long-term benefit.

We recommend that if a child has persistent OME despite a course of antibiotics, the option of giving oral corticosteroids with a second course of amoxicillin or amoxicillin-clavulanate should be strongly considered, and certainly before proceeding to surgery. We recommend:

> **prednisolone 1 mg/kg orally, daily for 7–14 days**

Ventilation tubes (grommets) for chronic OME

Question | For children with chronic OME, do ventilation tubes compared with no tubes reduce the short-term and long-term incidence of effusion and the incidence of hearing loss?

Literature review | We found 21 RCTs and a Cochrane review.[43]

The insertion of ventilation tubes or grommets is the operation most frequently performed on children in North America, Europe, and Australia. Despite its immense popularity, there is increasing evidence that this invasive operation has only very modest benefit. Children treated with grommets spend 32% less time with effusion in the next year, and their hearing levels improved by about 9 dB during the first 6 months and 6 dB at 12 months.[43] The benefit is lost thereafter, and early insertion of grommets has no measurable effect on language development or cognitive function.[43] There may be sub-groups who would benefit more from grommets, notably children with cleft palate or perhaps those attending day care,[44] but there is no good evidence that this is the case. Furthermore, grommets are associated with significant adverse effects, including tympanosclerosis, tympanic membrane atrophy, and chronic ear discharge.[43] In general, we recommend that conservative management with antibiotics and topical or systemic corticosteroids should be tried first, and even if unsuccessful, there is little evidence that the short-term benefits of grommets are outweighed by the risks.

Antihistamines and decongestants for chronic OME

Question | For children with chronic OME, do antihistamines and/or decongestants compared with no treatment or placebo result in more rapid resolution of effusion?

Literature review | We found 18 RCTs and a Cochrane review.[45]

A Cochrane review of 18 studies of antihistamines, decongestants, or antihistamine-decongestant combinations found no statistical or clinical benefit, and 11% of those who received active treatment reported adverse events.[45] We recommend that these agents should not be used.

Recommendations for specialist referral for OME

We recommend specialist ENT referral in the following situations:

· Persistent effusion for >3 months, not responding to antibiotics with or without steroids, in a child with speech or educational delay;
· Persistent effusion for >3 months, not responding to antibiotics with or without steroids, in a child with bilateral hearing loss;
· Structural damage to the tympanic membrane (significant retraction, concern about possible cholesteatoma).

Chronic suppurative otitis media (CSOM)

Question | For children with CSOM, does aural toilet compared with no aural toilet reduce the duration of ear discharge?

Literature review | We found four reasonable quality RCTs of aural toilet, and the use of aural toilet was analyzed as part of a larger Cochrane review of interventions for CSOM.[46]

CSOM is primarily a disease of developing countries and of indigenous children living in Australia, North America, Northern Europe, and New Zealand.[47] CSOM is due to an underlying eardrum perforation and needs to be distinguished from otitis externa (see p. 173) because both can result in purulent exudate in the external ear canal. In children with CSOM, regular aural toilet has been shown to be effective[46,48] and is recommended prior to any topical treatment. Dry mopping with rolled tissue spears or an equivalent (repeated 6–12-hourly until the ear canal is dry) can be taught to family members. Suction kits for use under direct vision are very useful if training and equipment are available. Resolution may take some weeks.

Question | For children with CSOM, do topical antibiotics compared with no topical antibiotics reduce the duration of ear discharge?

Literature review | We found 14 RCTs and a Cochrane review.[49]

The use of topical antibiotics has been shown to speed resolution of CSOM.[49] Topical quinolone antibiotics clear aural discharge better than no drug treatment,[49] better than topical antiseptics,[49] and better than oral antibiotics.[50] Topical quinolones have not been shown to be superior to non-quinolone topical antibiotics.[49] There are theoretical concerns about possible ototoxicity with the use of topical aminoglycosides, such as gentamicin or framycetin. Evidence suggests that short-term use is safe, even in the presence of a non-intact tympanic membrane (including grommets).[49] Use of topical aminoglycosides for more than 7 days in children with tympanic perforations is not advised.

The addition of steroids to topical antibiotics has not been studied well. In one small RCT of Australian Aboriginal children, topical ciprofloxacin was superior to topical framycetin plus dexamethasone in terms of resolution of otorrhea, although follow-up was short.[51]

The use of topical quinolones may select for resistant bacteria,[52] but this risk has to be balanced against the theoretical risk of ototoxicity of topical aminoglycosides. A systematic review of topical antibiotics and resistance found no good evidence that topical antibiotics induce resistance, but the development of resistance has not been well studied, and the evidence that they do not induce resistance was weak.[53] Topical quinolones should be used if there has been no response to first-line therapy after 7 days. Recommended treatment is:

regular ear toilet (as above) AND EITHER ciprofloxacin 0.3% ear drops, five drops into the affected ear, 12-hourly for up to 9 days OR dexamethasone 0.05% + framycetin 0.5% + gramicidin 0.005% ear drops, three drops into the ear 6-hourly for not longer than a total of 7 days

Persistent discharge may require more prolonged courses of preparations not containing aminoglycosides. Topical quinolones should be used if there has been no response to dexamethasone plus framycetin after 7 days.

Although systemic antibiotics offer no advantage over topical antibiotics for CSOM,[49,50] if aural discharge is from a recent perforation (i.e., within the last 6 weeks), we recommend oral antibiotics to treat AOM (see p. 168) as well as topical treatment.

In severe persistent cases, referral to an ENT specialist is recommended for more detailed examination and to exclude cholesteatoma or chronic mastoiditis (see p. below).

Mastoiditis

Mastoiditis is an infection of the air cells within the mastoid bone. It is a complication of otitis media and occurs because the mucoperiosteal lining of the mastoid is continuous with that of the middle ear.[54] Mastoiditis may be acute or chronic.

Acute mastoiditis

Acute mastoiditis is now rare in industrialized countries. A systematic review estimated the incidence of mastoiditis as 1 in 1000 children with untreated otitis media.[20] The diagnosis of acute mastoiditis is clinical. Children presented with redness or swelling behind the ear, which is pushed forward, and associated with redness and bulging of the tympanic membrane.[55] Other features include pain, fever, and irritability. Complications include CNS (central nervous system) involvement with meningitis or lateral sinus thrombosis, and lower motor neurone facial palsy.[55–59]

Because of its rarity, immune deficiency, particularly humoral (antibody production), should be strongly considered in a young child with acute mastoiditis in an industrialized country. Initial investigations should at least include a blood count and serum immunoglobulin and IgG sub-class levels, while B- and T-cell subsets may also be indicated if there is a suggestion that defective antibody production is secondary to a T-cell defect.

The organisms isolated from the middle ear of children with acute mastoiditis are not quite the same as for AOM. The commonest in order of frequency are *S. pneumoniae*, *S. pyogenes*, and *Staphlococcus aureus*.[55–59] Less common isolates are *H. influenzae*, Gram-negative bacilli, enterococci, anaerobes, and even *Mycobacterium tuberculosis*.[55–59]

The recommended management is surgical drainage of the middle ear, usually involving tympanocentesis followed by myringotomy or tympanostomy tubes (grommets), plus antibiotics. We recommend:

cefotaxime 25 mg/kg (max 1 g) IV, 8-hourly PLUS di/flucl/oxa/nafcillin 50 mg/kg (max 2 g) IV, 6-hourly

For children with CNS involvement, particularly when meningitis is suspected and LP contraindicated, to cover penicillin-resistant pneumococci we recommend:

cefotaxime 25 mg/kg (max 1 g) IV, 8-hourly PLUS vancomycin 15 mg/kg (max 500 mg) IV, 6-hourly

Chronic mastoiditis

Chronic mastoiditis is associated with CSOM (see p. 171). There is chronic infection of the mastoid air cells, which may result in sub-periosteal abscess, chronic osteomyelitis, cholesteatoma, and intracranial suppuration. The diagnosis should be suspected in any child with chronic suppurative ear discharge. The diagnosis can be confirmed and extent of damage delineated by computed tomography and magnetic resonance imaging scan.[60]

The organisms most commonly isolated are different from acute mastoiditis. Gram-negative bacilli, including *Pseudomonas*, are the most frequent, followed by *S. aureus* and anaerobes.[61–63]

The treatment is combined surgical and medical. We recommend ENT consultation. We could find no RCTs of antibiotic treatment. For severe infections, to cover the likely pathogens,[61–63] we recommend:

gentamicin <10 years: 7.5 mg/kg; ≥10 years: 6 mg/kg IV, daily PLUS EITHER
ticarcillin+clavulanate 50 + 1.7 mg/kg (max 3 + 0.1 g) IV, 6-hourly OR
piperacillin+tazobactam 100 + 12.5 mg/kg (max 4 + 0.5 g) IV, 8-hourly

Where there is extracranial extension, particularly when *Pseudomonas* is likely, we recommend using, on its own:

cefepime 50 mg/kg (max 2 g) IV, 8-hourly

Otitis externa

Otitis externa is a form of infected eczema which often follows persistent exposure of the ear canals to water. *Pseudomonas aeruginosa* and *S. aureus* are the most common organisms isolated, as well as other Gram-negative bacilli and occasionally fungi. We found 17 RCTs of topical treatment of otitis externa in children. Topical antibiotics and topical corticosteroids were equally effective, but were not compared with placebo or no treatment.

We recommend that a health professional should remove debris or exudate by dry aural toilet, using mechanical suction under direct vision or by dry mopping with a cotton wool swab. The ear canal should not be syringed with water. Dry cleaning should be followed by instillation of topical corticosteroid and antibiotic combination drops. Recommended treatment is:

dexamethasone 0.05%+framycetin 0.5%+gramicidin 0.005% ear drops, three drops instilled into the ear, thrice daily for 3–7 days OR

flumethasone 0.02%+clioquinol 1% ear drops, three drops instilled into the ear, twice daily for 3–7 days

It is recommended to keep the ear dry for 2 weeks after treatment. More severe cases may be treated by insertion of a wick soaked in the corticosteroid and antibiotic combination. Indications for systemic antibiotics include fever, spread of inflammation to the pinna, and local folliculitis.

If otitis externa recurs, it may help to keep the ear canals dry using earplugs and shower caps during showering and swimming, and/or using Vaseline or other water repellents, e.g., placing a few drops of isopropyl alcohol in the ear canals after swimming.

Common cold and purulent rhinitis

The common cold is caused by viruses. Characteristically, it causes clear nasal discharge, which becomes mucopurulent and persists for about 5–7 days. Although bacteria can often be isolated from the mucopurulent nasal discharge, this does not indicate whether they are colonizing the nose or causing the discharge. Just because a child has green mucus, it does not mean that antibiotics should be given.

Antibiotics and the common cold

Question | For children with colds, do antibiotics compared with no antibiotics or placebo reduce the duration of purulent rhinitis or prevent complications?

Literature review | We found seven RCTs, a Cochrane review,[64] and a more recent meta-analysis by the Cochrane authors.[65]

The Cochrane analysis of six trials in adults and children found that antibiotics were no better than placebo in terms of cure or persistent symptoms, and adult patients who received antibiotics had significantly more adverse effects.[64] An updated meta-analysis[65] by the same authors found seven trials, four with data on benefits and four with data on harms of antibiotics. At 5–8 days antibiotics were beneficial (RR 1.18, 95% CI 1.05–1.33), with 7–15 patients needing to be treated to benefit one. Antibiotics caused a significant increase in adverse events (RR 1.46, 95% CI 1.10–1.94), mostly gastrointestinal effects. Although antibiotics are probably effective for acute purulent rhinitis, they can cause harm, usually in the form of gastrointestinal effects.

Most patients will get better without antibiotics. We feel the significant adverse effects outweigh the modest benefits.

We do not recommend antibiotics for children with colds, even if they have purulent rhinitis.

Vitamin C and the common cold

Question | For normal children, does prophylactic vitamin C prevent the common cold or reduce its severity? For children with colds, does treatment with vitamin C compared with no vitamin C or placebo reduce the duration or severity of illness?

Literature review | We found 30 RCTs, a non-Cochrane meta-analysis, and a Cochrane review[66] on prophylaxis. We found 7 RCTs on treatment of common colds with vitamin C and the same Cochrane review[66] also looked at treatment effects of vitamin C.

The Cochrane review of 29 RCTs of vitamin C prophylaxis, using ≥ 200 mg/day of vitamin C, found no overall benefit of prophylactic vitamin C in reducing the incidence of colds.[66] Twelve of the prophylaxis studies included children. However, prophylaxis shortened the duration of colds by about a day in children taking prophylactic vitamin C (from 7 to 6 days) and their colds were less severe.[66] A sub-group of 6 trials that involved a total of 642 adult marathon runners, skiers, and soldiers on subarctic exercises reported a pooled RR of 0.50 (95% CI 0.38–0.66). The consistent and statistically significant small benefits on duration and severity for those using regular vitamin C prophylaxis indicates that vitamin C plays some role in respiratory defense mechanisms. In a study of Navajo schoolchildren, prophylactic vitamin C had no effect on incidence, severity, or duration of colds, but children with high plasma ascorbic acid concentrations had longer mean illness (6.8 days versus 4.0 days, $p < 0.05$) than those with low levels.[67] This suggests that high doses of vitamin C might have harmful effects. Mega-dose vitamin C supplementation is discouraged because it is potentially harmful. Low-dose vitamin C prophylaxis or emphasizing the importance of citrus fruit or fresh orange juice for children is justified by the data. Vitamin C supplementation could also be justified in children exposed to brief periods of severe physical exercise, such as elite athletes.

Starting treatment with vitamin C after symptoms of a cold developed did not reduce the incidence or duration of colds in adults or children and is not recommended.[66]

Antihistamines and nasal decongestants and the common cold

Question | For children with colds, do antihistamines and/or nasal decongestants compared with no treatment or placebo reduce the duration or severity of illness?

Literature review | We found 22 RCTs of antihistamines alone, 5 of decongestants, and 13 of combined treatment with antihistamines and decongestants. We found a Cochrane review of antihistamines[68] and a Cochrane review of decongestants.[69]

Antihistamines alone did not alleviate nasal congestion, rhinorrhea, or sneezing in children or adults, while first-generation antihistamines increased drowsiness.[68] Decongestants alone have not been studied in children and are not recommended for young children with colds.[69] A single dose is moderately effective for short-term relief of nasal congestion in adults, but repeated use has not been shown to be beneficial.[69] Antihistamine–decongestant combinations are ineffective in young children.[68] In adults and older children, they show a small benefit in general recovery, and in nasal symptoms, of doubtful clinical significance.[68]

We do not recommend antihistamines, decongestants, or antihistamine–decongestant combinations for children with colds.

Zinc and the common cold

Question | For children with colds, does zinc compared with no treatment or placebo reduce the duration or severity of illness?

Literature review | We found 15 RCTs, a Cochrane review,[70] and a non-Cochrane meta-analysis[71] of zinc lozenges.

A Cochrane review of 10 studies of zinc gluconate lozenges for treatment of colds found no overall benefit on duration or severity.[70] However, a meta-analysis[71] showed a trend toward benefit with a non-significant reduction in symptoms at 7 days (OR 0.52, 95% CI 0.25–1.2), so a very large study might show a significant benefit. Subsequent studies of zinc lozenges have not confirmed any benefit. The only study in children found no benefit in terms of duration or severity of colds, but the zinc group had significant adverse effects of bad taste, mouth, tongue, or throat discomfort, nausea, and diarrhea.[72]

We do not recommend zinc for children with colds.

Sinusitis

Imaging studies have shown that about 40% of children[73] and a greater proportion of adults[74] with colds have changes consistent with sinusitis after 7 days. Most of the changes will resolve spontaneously.[73] Persistence of nasal symptoms and cough beyond 10 days in children has been suggested as an indicator of a probable diagnosis of acute sinusitis.[75] In a study of 2013 children with respiratory complaints, 135 had persistent symptoms after 10 days and 92.5% of the 135 had radiologic changes of sinusitis.[75] Fever $>39°C$ and purulent nasal discharge increase the probability of severe sinusitis. Bad breath is often reported, but facial pain and headache are less common in children.[73,75]

Imaging for sinusitis is controversial. Plain radiographs (Waters' view) looking for sinus opacification, air-fluid level, or marked mucosal thickening have a high sensitivity in children with persistent respiratory symptoms (88% in one study[76]) but low specificity, because asymptomatic radiologic sinus changes are common. There is no need to use computerized tomography, with its increased radiation and the significant attendant risk of malignancy, in the vast majority of children with suspected acute or chronic sinusitis. The combination of typical acute or chronic symptoms together with typical changes on plain radiographs merits a trial of antibiotics (see below).

Question | For children with acute sinusitis, do antibiotics compared with no antibiotics or placebo reduce the duration or severity of symptoms?

Literature review | We found 49 RCTs and a Cochrane review[77] of antibiotic use in adults with acute maxillary sinusitis. We found only 3 RCTs of antibiotics in children with acute sinusitis. We found 6 RCTs and a Cochrane review[78] of antibiotics for children with persistent nasal discharge. The definition of sinusitis and the quality of the studies varied.

In a Cochrane review of 49 RCTs of antibiotics for acute maxillary sinusitis in adults and children,[77] penicillin improved clinical cure rates compared to controls (RR 1.72, 95% CI 1.00–2.96) and there was a trend for amoxicillin to be effective (RR 2.06, 95% CI 0.65–6.53) but wide confidence intervals. Radiographic outcomes were improved by antibiotic treatment. Comparisons between classes of antibiotics showed no significant differences between antibiotics. Compared to amoxicillin-clavulanate, dropouts due to adverse effects were significantly lower for cephalosporin antibiotics (RR 0.47, 95% CI 0.30–0.73). Relapse rates within 1 month of successful therapy were 7.7%. We found only 3 RCTs in children with acute sinusitis which compared antibiotics with placebo.[76,79,80] A small RCT of children with radiologically confirmed sinusitis found that children treated with either amoxicillin or amoxicillin-clavulanate were more likely to be cured (67 and 64%, respectively) than children treated with placebo (43%).[76] A larger study of children with clinical sinusitis treated with the same antibiotics found no benefit,[79] and a study of cefuroxime for radiologic sinusitis was likewise negative.[80]

A Cochrane review of children with nasal discharge persisting for at least 10 days[78] found six studies (562 children). They concluded that for children with persistent nasal discharge or older children with radiographically confirmed sinusitis, the available evidence suggests that antibiotics given for 10 days will reduce the probability of persistence in the short to medium term. They found that the benefits were modest and around 8 children must be treated in order to achieve one additional cure (NNT 8, 95% CI 5–29).

We conclude that there is evidence of modest benefit in treating children with radiologically confirmed acute sinusitis with antibiotics. The organisms causing sinusitis are the same as those causing AOM. Recommended treatment is:

amoxicillin 40–50 mg/kg (max 1 g) orally, 12-hourly for 7–14 days

If penicillin-insensitive pneumococci are rare, we recommend:

amoxicillin 15 mg/kg (max 500 mg) orally, 8-hourly for 7–14 days

OR (if compliance is likely to be a problem)

amoxicillin 30 mg/kg (max 1 g) orally, 12-hourly for 7–14 days

If the patient is allergic to penicillin, we recommend:

cefdinir 7 mg/kg (max 300 mg) orally, 12-hourly for 7–14 days OR
cefpodoxime 5 mg/kg (max 200 mg) orally, 12-hourly for 7–14 days OR
cefuroxime 15 mg/kg (max 500 mg) orally, 12-hourly for 7–14 days

Children who fail to respond to amoxicillin alone are likely to be infected with a beta-lactamase-producing organism, *H. influenzae* or *M. catarrhalis*. Amoxicillin-clavulanate contains clavulanic acid which inhibits beta-lactamase enzymes. Recommended treatment is:

amoxicillin+clavulanate 22.5 + 3.2 mg/kg (max 875 + 125 mg) orally, 12-hourly for 7–14 days

Acute tonsillitis or pharyngitis

Acute sore throat is most often caused by viral infections. It is difficult to distinguish clinically between viral and bacterial causes of sore throat. A bacterial cause of acute sore throat, almost always group A streptococcus (GAS) (*S. pyogenes*), is more common in children aged 3–13 years (30–40%) than in children aged less than 3 years (5–10%) or adults (5–15%).[81,82]

Question | For children with acute sore throat or tonsillitis, do antibiotics compared with no antibiotics or placebo shorten the duration of illness or reduce the frequency of complications?

Literature review | We found 27 RCTs of antibiotic treatment for sore throat or tonsillitis and a Cochrane review.[82]

A Cochrane systematic review of antibiotics for sore throat found 27 studies, but only 3 were exclusively in children.[82] Throat soreness and fever were reduced by antibiotics by about one half. The greatest difference was seen at about 3–4 days (when the symptoms of about 50% of untreated patients had settled). By 1 week about 90% of treated and untreated patients were symptom-free. Antibiotics are effective: just under six people with a sore throat need to be treated with penicillin rather than placebo to cure one extra sore throat

at day 3 (this is sometimes referred to as the "number needed to treat" or NNT = 6).[82] Antibiotics are far more effective in those who have culture-confirmed streptococcal sore throats, with symptoms significantly reduced after both 3 and 7 days.[82] Interestingly, however, antibiotics were associated with a significant reduction in symptoms at day 3 even if the swab was negative for GAS (RR 0.78, 95% CI 0.63–0.97), suggesting that other bacteria may be important causes of sore throat.

Antibiotics compared to placebo reduced the incidence of AOM (RR 0.30, 95% CI 0.15–0.58), of acute sinusitis (RR 0.48, 95% CI 0.08–2.76), and of quinsy or peritonsillar abscess (RR 0.15, 95% CI 0.05–0.47), which occurs in 1–2% of untreated episodes of tonsillitis.[82]

Several studies found that antibiotics reduced acute rheumatic fever by more than three quarters (RR 0.22, 95% CI 0.02–2.08).[82] Acute rheumatic fever is now rare in industrialized countries, where the annual incidence of rheumatic fever (<1 case per 100,000) is greatly exceeded by the risk of a severe reaction to penicillin (15–40 per 100,000 treatment courses).[82] Prevention of rheumatic fever remains important in developing countries, but is no longer the main indication for antibiotic treatment of streptococcal pharyngitis in industrialized countries, except in high-risk populations such as indigenous communities.

The Cochrane review found a trend for antibiotics to protect against acute glomerulonephritis, but there were insufficient cases to be certain.[82]

In order to reduce antibiotic use, it would be helpful to find ways of limiting antibiotic use to children with sore throat who are most likely to benefit, mainly those with streptococcal sore throat. Culture of a throat swab or use of a reliable rapid detection kit are the most reliable ways to diagnose the presence of GAS, although even this has problems because some children may be chronic carriers of GAS but have a coincidental viral sore throat. Culture results are not available for 24–48 hours. Treatment options are to decide whether to give antibiotics immediately on the basis of a rapid test, to wait for a culture result, to treat empirically, to give a delayed prescription,[22] or to give no antibiotics. The decision about which children to treat empirically might be helped by clinical criteria, such as a scoring system, or laboratory criteria, such as rapid antigen detection tests.

Box 12.1 McIsaac scoring system for assessing sore throat.[84]

Temperature > 38°C		1 point
No cough		1 point
Tender anterior cervical lymphadenopathy		1 point
Tonsillar swelling or exudate		1 point
Age 3–14 years		1 point

Add points to give total score

Total score 0 or 1 point	No culture or antibiotic	(Risk of Group A streptococcal infection 2–6%)
Total score 2 or 3 points	Culture all, treat only if positive	(Risk 10–28%)
Total score 4 or 5 points	Culture all, treat all with penicillin	(Risk at least 38–63%)

Clinical criteria for diagnosis of streptococcal tonsillopharyngitis

Clinical scoring systems improve the accuracy of identifying a patient as having a streptococcal sore throat. The best known are the Centor criteria[83]: an adult with sore throat who has fever, absence of cough, swollen tender anterior cervical lymph nodes, and tonsillar erythema and exudate has a >80% chance of having a streptococcal sore throat.[83] However, <10% of adults with sore throat meet these four criteria, so the criteria are not very useful in the day-to-day management of patients with sore throat.

The McIsaac clinical score, based on the Centor criteria but with an age weighting, is more appropriate for children, with a sensitivity of 96.9% for diagnosing group A streptococcal infection in children aged 3–14 years (see Box 12.1).[84] Using these criteria, 59% of patients would have been considered at low risk (total score 0 or 1 point) and not treated with antibiotics and no swab sent, while 10.5% had the highest score (4 or 5 points) and would be treated with antibiotics immediately. A swab would be sent on the remaining 30% of patients and antibiotics given only if positive. The authors of the study reported that the proportion of patients receiving initial antibiotic prescriptions would have been reduced by 48% by following these score-based recommendations compared with observed physician prescribing ($p < 0.001$) without any increase in throat culture use.[84]

Rapid diagnosis of group A streptococcal infection

Rapid antigen detection tests are frequently used in pediatric practice in North America. When the likelihood of streptococcal sore throat is low, they have not been shown to be cost-effective, but they are more cost-effective if the risk is higher, e.g., a child aged 3–15 years old with sore throat, tonsillar erythema, and no cough.[85]

Antibiotic for sore throat: yes or no?

Because of the need to reduce unnecessary antibiotic use, it is not recommended to treat children with sore throat with empiric antibiotics without taking a throat swab for rapid diagnosis or culture.

We recommend empiric antibiotic therapy after taking a swab for the following indications:
· tonsillitis with 4 or 5 days of fever >38°C, no cough, tender anterior cervical lymphadenopathy, tonsillar swelling, or exudate, age 3–14 years;
· patients aged 3 years and older with sore throat in communities with a high incidence of acute rheumatic fever (e.g., some Australian Aboriginal and native American communities);
· existing rheumatic heart disease at any age;
· scarlet fever;
· peritonsillar cellulitis or abscess (quinsy).

Empiric antibiotic therapy is not recommended for:
· children <3 years old, even with fever and exudate, because viral infection, e.g., adenovirus, is much more likely;
· children with suspected glandular fever.

Which antibiotic for sore throat, not laboratory-confirmed as due to GAS?

About 90% of adults and 70% of children with sore throat do not have streptococcal pharyngitis.[81,82] There are several reasons for preferring oral penicillin as empiric treatment for sore throat, which is suspected but not confirmed by laboratory testing to be group A streptococcal:

- If six children are treated with antibiotics instead of no antibiotic, one extra child will be free of sore throat 3 days later.[82]
- Most sore throats improve anyway: 90% of treated and untreated patients are free of symptoms by 1 week.[82]
- Penicillin is less likely to select for resistance than broader spectrum agents such as cephalosporins and macrolides.
- Penicillin is superior to placebo, cheap, and effective.
- Twelve-hourly phenoxymethylpenicillin is effective in streptococcal pharyngitis[86] and is recommended because of greater compliance than with more frequent dosing regimens.

Recommended treatment for unproven streptococcal sore throat:

phenoxymethylpenicillin 10 mg/kg (max 500 mg) orally, 12-hourly

It is recommended that the penicillin be stopped after 24–48 hours if the throat swab does not grow a pathogenic streptococcus.

In poorly compliant patients or those intolerant of oral therapy, recommended treatment is:

benzathine penicillin: child 3 to <6 kg: 225 mg; 6 to <10 kg: 337.5 mg; 10 to <15 kg: 450 mg; 15 to <20 kg: 675 mg; >20 kg: 900 mg (1.5 million U) IM, as single dose

For patients allergic to penicillin, it is safe to give cephalosporins.[87] Recommended treatment:

cefuroxime 15 mg/kg (max 500 mg) orally, 12-hourly for 10 days OR
azithromycin 20 mg/kg (max 600 mg) orally, daily for 3 days[88] OR
roxithromycin 4 mg/kg (max 150 mg) orally, 12-hourly for 10 days

Which antibiotic for laboratory-proven group A streptococcal infection?

Question | For children with proven group A streptococcal infection, is any class of antibiotics compared with other antibiotics more effective? For children with proven group A streptococcal infection, is 5 days of antibiotics as effective as 10 days in terms of cure?

Literature review | We found 35 RCTs and 1 meta-analysis[89] comparing cephalosporins and penicillin in children. We found 22 RCTS and 1 meta-analysis[90] comparing short course (4–5 days) with 10 days of antibiotics.

Meta-analyses in adults[91] and children[89] have shown that cephalosporins are more effective than penicillin for bacteriologic and clinical cure of group A streptococcal tonsillopharyngitis. In 1998, the USFDA, in providing guidance for the pharmaceutical industry, stated that any antibiotic evaluated for efficacy in group A streptococcal tonsillopharyngitis must have a bacterial eradication rate of ≥85% (www.fda.gov/cder/guidance/index.htm). A meta-analysis in children[89] and a meta-analysis of shortened durations of antibiotic therapies compared to 10 days penicillin for this infection[90] did not find a single study since 1990, in which the bacterial cure rate was ≥85% using 10 days of penicillin. The change in bacteriologic efficacy for the penicillins has occurred despite the fact that *S. pyogenes* remains highly susceptible to penicillin.[92] Among the most widely noted explanations for this reduction in penicillin efficacy is the presence of increased frequency of beta-lactamase-producing normal flora in the tonsillopharynx (so-called copathogenicity) driven by antibiotic overuse.[92] These copathogens (*H. influenzae*, *Morax. catarrhalis*, *S. aureus*, and mouth anaerobes) are thought to shield or protect *S. pyogenes* from eradication in vivo despite its continued in vitro activity. The copathogen explanation has only circumstantial supportive evidence.

We conclude that for laboratory-proven *S. pyogenes* tonsillopharyngitis, use of a cephalosporin has a strong evidence base. Because no differences have been shown among first-, second-, and third-generation cephalosporins in *S. pyogenes* eradication, we recommend use of first-generation agents.

Recommended treatment for proven streptococcal sore throat:

cephalexin 20 mg/kg (max 500 mg) orally, 12-hourly for 10 days

In poorly compliant patients, recommended treatment is to shorten duration:

cefpodoxime 5 mg/kg (max 200 mg) orally, 12-hourly for 5 days OR

cefdinir 7 mg/kg (max 300 mg) orally, 12-hourly for 5 days

Which antibiotic for laboratory-proven group A streptococcal infection in a population at high risk for rheumatic fever?

Some populations, particularly children in developing countries and indigenous children in industrialized countries such as native Americans, Australian Aborigines and Maori, and Pacific Islanders in New Zealand, are at very high risk of rheumatic fever. They are also at increased risk of other non-suppurative complications of group A streptococcal infections, such as glomerulonephritis. A Cochrane review has shown that antibiotic treatment of acute streptococcal sore throat reduces the risk of acute rheumatic fever by 78% (RR 0.22, 95% CI 0.02–2.08).[82] All these studies were almost done using penicillin to treat streptococcal sore throat. There have been no studies comparing cephalosporins with penicillin for prevention of acute rheumatic fever. For this reason, many authorities working with disadvantaged populations at high risk of rheumatic fever continue to recommend penicillin to treat sore throat.

In this case, recommended treatment for streptococcal sore throat is:

phenoxymethylpenicillin 10 mg/kg (max 500 mg) orally, 12-hourly for 10 days

In poorly compliant patients or those intolerant of oral therapy, recommended treatment is:

benzathine penicillin: child 3 to <6 kg: 225 mg; 6 to <10 kg: 337.5 mg; 10 to <15 kg: 450 mg; 15 to <20 kg: 675 mg, >20 kg: 900 mg IM, as single dose

Glandular fever (infectious mononucleosis)

Primary infection with Epstein-Barr virus and occasionally other viruses may be associated with severe pharyngitis. Antibiotics are not routinely indicated. Some reports have suggested an association between glandular fever and group A streptococcal infection, although the role of antibiotics in such cases is unclear. Amoxicillin and ampicillin are contraindicated in glandular fever because they frequently precipitate a severe rash. This is usually not an indication of penicillin hypersensitivity. Parenteral corticosteroids are often recommended if there is imminent airways obstruction, although without formal evidence. We found no studies on the effect of corticosteroids on airways obstruction. We found one RCT on the effect of dexamethasone on pain in exudative tonsillitis due to infectious mononucleosis.[93] A single dose of dexamethasone 0.3 mg/kg (max 15 mg) orally reduced pain at 12 hours, but not later. Narcotic analgesics are contraindicated in glandular fever because of the danger of respiratory obstruction.

Recurrent pharyngitis and/or tonsillitis

Question | For children with recurrent tonsillopharyngitis, do antibiotics compared with no antibiotics or placebo reduce the frequency of episodes? For children with recurrent tonsillopharyngitis, does tonsillectomy compared to non-surgical treatment reduce the frequency of episodes?

Literature review | We found six RCTs that compared different antibiotic regimens but had no placebo group and four RCTs that compared antibiotic prophylaxis with placebo.[94–97] We found three RCTs[98–100] and a Cochrane review[101] that compared tonsillectomy with no surgery.

The literature on recurrent pharyngitis and/or tonsillitis is sparse. We found only four RCTs with weak methodology comparing antibiotics with placebo for recurrent tonsillitis. Two studies suggested that benzathine penicillin reduced the incidence of group A streptococcal infections,[94,95] one showed that azithromycin was ineffective[96] and one showed that cefpodoxime reduced the frequency of sore throats.[97] On the basis of the limited evidence, we recommend prophylactic antibiotics are not used because of lack of proof of efficacy and because of concerns about inducing antibiotic resistance. We recommend that each individual episode be treated as discussed on pp. 177–8).

A Cochrane review of tonsillectomy for recurrent tonsillitis found only two trials and is out of date.[101] A study of "severely affected" children who had seven or more well-documented, clinically important, adequately treated episodes of throat infection in the preceding year, or five or more such episodes in each of the two preceding years, or three or more such episodes in each of the three preceding years, found that tonsillectomy reduced the number and severity of subsequent episodes of throat infection for at least 2 years.[98] On the other hand, in each follow-up year many subjects in the non-surgical groups had fewer than three episodes of infection, and most episodes among subjects in the non-surgical groups were mild. Surgery-related complications occurred in 14% of children and were reported as readily managed or self-limited. The authors conclude that their results warrant the election of tonsillectomy for children meeting the trial's stringent eligibility criteria, but also provide support for non-surgical management.[98] For mild to moderately affected children with fewer infections, most have very few infections in the next year without surgery and the at-best modest benefits of surgery do not appear to justify the risks.[99,100] We recommend considering tonsillectomy only for the most severely affected children with recurrent tonsillitis.

Croup (acute laryngotracheobronchitis)

Croup or viral laryngotracheobronchitis presents with a coryzal prodrome, hoarseness (or husky voice in those old enough to speak), inspiratory or biphasic stridor, and a barking "brassy" or seal-like cough.[102] Children with concurrent large airways involvement are wheezy. Croup is caused by viruses, most commonly parainfluenza viruses, but also other respiratory viruses including rhinoviruses, respiratory syncytial virus (RSV), and influenza. Croup is most common in 1–3-year-old children and is generally self-limiting, with a duration of 2–5 days.[102] Some children get recurrent episodes of spasmodic croup, which can have an allergic basis. Antibiotics are not indicated for croup.[102]

In mild cases, no treatment is necessary, but we strongly recommend early reevaluation. It should be remembered that croup often gets worse at night.

In moderate to severe cases (e.g., a history of very noisy breathing at night, difficulty with breathing, or the presence of stridor on examination) corticosteroids are often used and epinephrine (adrenaline) or humidification may be added. Is there evidence for these interventions?

Question | For children with acute laryngotracheobronchitis (croup), do inhaled or systemic corticosteroids compared with no steroids or placebo reduce the duration or severity of illness? Does inhaled epinephrine (adrenaline) compared with no epinephrine or placebo improve outcome? Do mist tents or humidification of air compared with no treatment improve outcome?

Literature review | We found 31 RCTs and a Cochrane review[103] of corticosteroid therapy for croup or laryngotracheobronchitis. We found 7 RCTs of epinephrine and 4 RCTs and a Cochrane review[104] of mist or humidification.

A Cochrane review of 31 RTCs found that glucocorticoid treatment was associated with an improvement in clinical score at 6 and 12 hours, but this improvement was no longer significant at 24 hours.[103] Patients treated with glucocorticoids were half as likely to return to hospital or be readmitted. On average, steroid-treated patients spent 12 hours less in accident and emergency or hospital.[103]

Nebulized epinephrine is superior to placebo for short-term relief of croup symptoms (three studies) and is comparable in efficacy to nebulized budesonide.[105]

Mist tents were not found in a Cochrane review[104] of three RCTs or a later study[106] to provide any significant benefit in croup.

Various corticosteroid regimens have been employed.

Examples include:

> **dexamethasone 0.3 mg/kg orally or IV** OR
> **prednisolone or prednisone 1 mg/kg orally** OR
> **budesonide 2 mg by nebulizer**

Repeat doses are usually not required, but can be considered if response to single-dose therapy is suboptimal at 24 hours. Failure to respond may rarely be due to bacterial tracheitis.

In more severe cases with significant airway obstruction or fatigue, treatment in hospital may be required with an initial dose of nebulized epinephrine.[104] Recommended treatment is:

> **epinephrine (adrenaline) 0.05 mL/kg/dose (max 0.5 mL) of 1:100 solution diluted up to 3 mL OR 0.5 mL/kg/dose (max 5 mL) 1:1000 solution, by nebulizer** PLUS EITHER
> **dexamethasone 0.6 mg/kg orally** (or IM or IV if vomiting) OR
> **prednisolone or prednisone 1 mg/kg orally**

Maintenance doses and frequency vary with the severity of the condition and the response to treatment.

Hydrocortisone should not be used due to lack of evidence and short duration of action.

Influenza

Influenza is caused by influenza A and B viruses.[107] The risk of catching influenza can be reduced by immunization, which needs to be given annually because of regular mutation of the virus ("antigenic drift"). Recommendations on which children should be routinely immunized vary from children at increased risk of severe disease, e.g., children with cyanotic congenital heart disease or chronic lung disease, to recommending that all children be immunized annually.[107]

During influenza epidemics, children with fever >38° and cough have a high probability of influenza, but other viral infections can present identically.[107] The decision to use antivirals should preferably be based on proof of influenza infection, e.g., positive immunofluorescence of nasopharyngeal secretions for influenza. Amantadine and rimantadine are effective and inexpensive but are only active against influenza A strains. They may be cost-effective during times when public health antibiotics have identified influenza A as the strain circulating during a season. Neuraminidase inhibitors, which are effective against both strains, reduce the duration of illness by just over a day in previously healthy children and reduce the time to return to normal activity.[108] Oseltamivir reduces complications of influenza, particularly otitis media.[108] Zanamavir is currently given by inhalation only, limiting its use to older children. Treatment with a neuraminidase inhibitor is of no benefit unless commenced within 48 hours of the patient developing symptoms. Resistance is an increasing problem and has emerged during therapy. For this reason, although prophylaxis with neuraminidase inhibitors is effective in adults, we do not recommend prophylaxis of children outside a pandemic situation. If treatment is given, we recommend:

> oseltamivir 2 mg/kg (max 75 mg) orally,
> 12-hourly for 5 days OR
> zanamivir (child >5 yr) 10 mg by inhalation,
> 12-hourly for 5 days

Antibacterials are not indicated in an otherwise healthy person. In those at special risk (e.g., children with chronic heart or lung disease) secondary bacterial infection may require treatment as for community-acquired pneumonia, using antibiotics active against staphylococcal as well as pneumococcal pneumonia.

Avian influenza is caused by a sub-type of influenza A virus. It is occasionally transmitted to humans via close contact with infected birds (especially chickens, but also ducks and geese). Occasional cases of human-to-human transmission have been reported (at the time of writing). There is the possibility of further virus mutation resulting in increased human-to-human transmission, with the potential for an influenza pandemic. If avian influenza is suspected, the local health department must be notified. Information is available from the World Health Organization (WHO) and the Centers for Disease Control (CDC) Web sites:

http://www.who.int/csr/disease/avian_influenza/
   updates/en/

http://www.cdc.gov/flu/avian/gen-info/avian-
   influenza.htm.

Pertussis

Pertussis (whooping cough) is caused by *Bordetella pertussis* and occasionally by *Bordetella parapertussis*.[109] Other organisms such as viruses and *Chlamydia* can cause a pertussis-like illness. Pertussis generally manifests as a persistent illness, usually afebrile, characterized by one or more of:

· paroxysms of coughing;
· inspiratory whoop without other apparent cause;
· post-tussive vomiting;
· persistent cough lasting more than 2 weeks.

A nasopharyngeal aspirate should be sent for culture and/or polymerase chain reaction (PCR) testing. Serology can be very helpful in older children and young adults. It is much less useful in infants, for whom direct detection of the organism in a nasopharyngeal aspirate is the diagnostic modality of choice.[109] Relevant public health authorities should be notified of cases of clinical or proven pertussis.

Treatment of pertussis

Question | For children with pertussis, do antibiotics compared with no antibiotics or placebo reduce infectivity or reduce symptoms?

Literature review | We found 10 RCTs and a Cochrane review[110] of antibiotic treatment.

A Cochrane review[110] found 10 antibiotic treatment trials of variable quality. Short-term antibiotics (azithromycin for 3 days, clarithromycin for 7 days, or erythromycin estolate for 7 days) were as effective as long-term antibiotic treatment (erythromycin estolate or erythromycin for 14 days) in eradicating *B. pertussis* from the nasopharynx, and there were fewer side effects with short-term treatment. Neither short- or long-term antibiotics altered the subsequent clinical course of the illness. Azithromycin is preferred to erythromycin in babies <1 month old because of a reported association between erythromycin and hypertrophic pyloric stenosis.[111] Recommended treatment is:

> **azithromycin child <6 months: 10 mg/kg orally, daily for 5 days**
> **child ≥6 months: 10 mg/kg (max 500 mg) orally on day 1, then 5 mg/kg (max 250 mg) orally, daily for a further 4 days** OR
> **clarithromycin child >1 month: 7.5 mg/kg (max 500 mg) orally, 12-hourly for 7 days** OR
> **erythromycin child >1 month: 10 mg/kg (max 250 mg) orally, 6-hourly for 7 days**

Prophylaxis against pertussis

Question | For children exposed to pertussis, do prophylactic antibiotics compared with no antibiotics or placebo prevent infection?

Literature review | We found two studies and a Cochrane review[110] of prophylactic antibiotics.

A Canadian study of household contacts found that erythromycin estolate prevented culture-positive pertussis in household contacts of patients with pertussis but did not prevent clinical pertussis.[112] The Cochrane review found only two studies and concluded that there is insufficient evidence to determine the benefit of prophylactic treatment of pertussis contacts.[110] Current recommendations for chemoprophylaxis of all household and child contacts with erythromycin or another macrolide are made despite the lack of evidence of efficacy. Prophylaxis is probably most justified for unimmunized or partially immunized babies <6 months old, because they have the highest risk of severe disease,[109] and so any benefits are likely to outweigh harms of treatment. If giving chemoprophylaxis, the regimens (including duration) for prophylaxis are the same as for treatment (see pp. 181–2).

It is important to check the immunization status of children in the household and to catch up missed doses of pertussis vaccine.

Prevention of pertussis

Prevention is primarily through immunization with either whole cell pertussis vaccines or acellular vaccines, which contain three or more purified components of *B. pertussis*. In unimmunized populations, pertussis infects mainly schoolchildren, who in turn may infect babies <6 months who are at greatest risk of death or complications.[109] A primary childhood course plus one or more booster doses protect against pertussis for a number of years. However, continued circulation of *B. pertussis*, with adults as an important source of childhood infections, has caused many countries to consider immunizing adolescents and adults, for whom acellular vaccines are highly immunogenic.[113]

Lower respiratory tract infections

Bronchiolitis

Bronchiolitis is the name of a pathologic condition (inflammation of the bronchioles) which is often used to describe a clinical entity.[114] In Europe and Australia, the term is used to describe children <18 months old and usually <1 year with a clinical illness characterized by cough, crackles (with or without wheeze), and hyperinflation, and with radiographic changes of hyperinflation and patchy consolidation.[114] In North America, the term is often used for a child <2 years old with an acute episode of wheeze (with or without crackles) during the RSV season (fall to mid-winter), which means there is considerable overlap with asthma.[114] This means that clinical studies need to be interpreted bearing in mind these differences in definition.

RSV causes over 70% of episodes of bronchiolitis, with the rest caused by other viruses, including rhinovirus, human metapneumovirus, parainfluenza, and influenza viruses.[114] RSV is the major respiratory pathogen of young children and the major cause of lower respiratory infections in infants. The peak incidence is between 1 and 6 months of age. It occurs worldwide, with annual epidemics in winter or in the rainy season in temperate climates. RSV is transmitted by close contact with contaminated fingers or fomites, but may also be spread by coarse aerosols produced by coughing or sneezing. The attack rate can be extremely high in day-care centers. Babies with chronic cardiorespiratory disease, babies born prematurely, the immunocompromised, and the elderly are at increased risk of severe RSV infection.[114]

Death from bronchiolitis is extremely rare and is usually due to hypoxia. The modern use of pulse oximetry to monitor oxygenation has resulted in better use of supplemental oxygen and improved survival.[114]

Treatment of bronchiolitis
Ribavirin for bronchiolitis

Question | In babies with bronchiolitis, does nebulized ribavirin compared with placebo or no treatment reduce clinical severity or duration of hospitalization?
Literature review | We found 12 RCTs and a Cochrane review.[115]

Initial excitement about the role of nebulized ribavirin in treating RSV infection has been tempered by the realization that the benefits are at best marginal[115] and offset by concerns about toxicity to staff, notably potential teratogenicity for pregnant women, and about cost. The vast majority of infants with RSV bronchiolitis recover without treatment. The cumulated results of three small trials on ventilated patients suggest that ribavirin may reduce the duration of mechanical ventilation by a mean of 1.8 days, but trials have not been able to show reductions in duration of hospitalization or in mortality.[115] Long-term follow-up studies have not shown any benefit in terms of pulmonary function or incidence of recurrent wheezing.[115]

> **We do not recommend nebulized ribavirin either for ventilated or for unventilated children with RSV bronchiolitis, but we recommend considering nebulized ribavirin to treat children with severe defects of immunity, e.g., oncology patients or children with T-cell immunodeficiency.**

Bronchodilators for bronchiolitis

Question | In babies with bronchiolitis, do bronchodilators compared with placebo or no treatment reduce clinical severity or duration of hospitalization?
Literature review | We found 22 RCTs and a Cochrane review.[116]

Analysis of the role of bronchodilators in bronchiolitis is complicated by the definitional problems described above. A Cochrane review of 22 clinical trials (1428 infants) with bronchiolitis found a statistically significant but clinically modest improvement in the overall average clinical score with bronchodilator use, but no significant improvement in oxygenation. Bronchodilator recipients showed no improvement in the rate of hospital admission after treatment as outpatients or duration of hospitalization for inpatients. The authors acknowledged that the inclusion of studies that enrolled infants with recurrent wheezing might have biased the results in favor of bronchodilators.[116]

> **We do not recommend bronchodilators for children with bronchiolitis.**

Epinephrine (adrenaline) for bronchiolitis

Question | In babies with bronchiolitis, does nebulized epinephrine (adrenaline) compared with bronchodilators or placebo or no treatment reduce clinical severity or duration of hospitalization?
Literature review | We found 14 RCTs and a Cochrane review.[117]

A Cochrane review[117] of 14 studies comparing epinephrine with placebo or bronchodilators found minimal evidence of benefit and some evidence of harm by causing increased pallor and tachycardia. Limited evidence suggested that outpatient use of nebulized epinephrine might be favorable compared with salbutamol and placebo, but the benefits were minor and there was no reduction in hospital admission.[117]

> **We do not recommend nebulized epinephrine for children with bronchiolitis.**

Corticosteroids for bronchiolitis

Question | In babies with bronchiolitis, do systemic corticosteroids compared with placebo or no treatment reduce clinical severity or duration of hospitalization?
Literature review | We found 13 RCTs and a Cochrane review of systemic corticosteroids.[118]

A Cochrane review of 13 trials (1198 children) showed no benefit of systemic (oral, IM, or IV) corticosteroids in acute bronchiolitis.[118]

We do not recommend systemic corticosteroids for children with bronchiolitis.

Chest physiotherapy for bronchiolitis

A Cochrane review of three studies found no evidence that chest physiotherapy improves outcome in children <2 years with bronchiolitis.[119]

Surfactant for mechanically ventilated children with bronchiolitis

A Cochrane review found three studies of surfactant for 79 babies being mechanically ventilated for bronchiolitis.[120] Surfactant decreased duration of mechanical ventilation by 2.6 days and duration of intensive care by 3.3 days, although the reviewers felt that the studies have overestimated the benefits.

Antibiotics for bronchiolitis

Question | In children with acute bronchiolitis, do antibiotics compared with no antibiotics or placebo improve outcome?

Literature review | We found two poor-quality RCTs and no meta-analyses.

The incidence of bacteremia is <1% in RSV bronchiolitis and even lower (<0.5%) in children without risk factors for severe RSV infection.[121] We could find only one RCT of ampicillin or placebo for babies with bronchiolitis.[122] The main outcome, duration of illness, was no different.[122] In another RCT of antibiotics for children with pneumonia or bronchiolitis from any cause, antibiotics had no effect on outcome in an RSV-positive sub-group.[123] Although there is weak evidence that antibiotics are unnecessary and no evidence of benefit, antibiotics are frequently prescribed for children with bronchiolitis and often continued even when the child is known to be RSV-positive.[121]

We do not recommend antibiotics routinely for children with bronchiolitis.

Children are more likely to be bacteremic if they have nosocomial RSV infection (6.5% of all RSV infections in one study[121]), cyanotic congenital heart disease (6.6%), or are admitted to intensive care (2.9%), and so empiric antibiotic therapy might be considered for these groups until cultures are back.[121] The organisms causing bacteremia are most often *S. pneumoniae*, *H. influenzae*, and *S. aureus*.[121]

If antibiotics are used, we recommend:

cefotaxime 25 mg/kg IV, 8-hourly OR
ceftriaxone 25 mg/kg IV, daily until culture results are available

Prevention of bronchiolitis

There are no effective RSV vaccines currently available, although there has been much recent research on live attenuated vaccines and sub-unit vaccines, which may be licensed in future.

RSV immunoglobulin

Hyperimmune polyclonal RSV immunoglobulin derived from blood donations has been shown to reduce the incidence of RSV hospitalization and admission to the intensive care unit, but not mechanical ventilation, when given prophylactically to babies and infants with bronchopulmonary dysplasia and to preterm babies without bronchopulmonary dysplasia.[124] RSV immunoglobulin is contraindicated in children with congenital heart disease because it caused severe cyanotic episodes and poor outcome after surgery. It is expensive, has to be given by monthly infusion, and is not readily available.

Palivizumab

A humanized mouse monoclonal antibody to RSV, palivizumab, is more effective and less costly than RSV immunoglobulin, but its cost is still very high. It is given by IM injection each month during periods of anticipated risk of RSV. It reduces the risk of hospitalization from about 10% to about 5% for both preterm babies, babies with bronchopulmonary dysplasia, and babies with congenital heart disease.[124,125] It has not been shown to decrease the risk of mechanical ventilation for RSV infection, to reduce long-term morbidity, or to save lives.

Question | For babies at increased risk of severe RSV infection, is palivizumab compared to no treatment cost-effective?

Literature review | We found nine cost-effectiveness analyses of palivizumab.

We found nine cost-effectiveness analyses of palivizumab. None of them found that palivizumab was cost-effective, even for selected babies at high risk of severe RSV infection, such as extremely low-birth weight babies or babies with congenital heart disease. Despite the lack of evidence of cost-effectiveness, the American Academy of Pediatrics recommends its use for selected high-risk babies.[126] We do not feel that the evidence supports the use of palivizumab unless cost is not a consideration.

We do not recommend the use of palivizumab.

Acute bronchitis

Question | For children with acute bronchitis, do antibiotics compared to no antibiotics or placebo speed recovery?

Literature review | We found eight RCTs of antibiotic use for acute bronchitis in children and a Cochrane review.[127]

Acute bronchitis is inflammation of the major bronchi and sometimes trachea, causing cough, and usually associated with an acute viral URTI.[127] A Cochrane review found that antibiotics reduce cough and feeling ill by about half a day,[127] statistically but probably not clinically significant. We recommend that children with acute bronchitis should not be given antibiotics routinely.

Chronic bronchitis

There is a group of children with recurrent moist cough who do not have bronchiectasis or asthma. The exact prevalence is unknown, but the prevalence of chronic cough reported in a large European study was 3% of school-aged children and 9% in the preschool-age group.[128] A Cochrane review[129] found only two moderate quality RCTs (140 children) comparing 7 days treatment with erythromycin[130] or amoxicillin-clavulanate[131] with placebo. Antibiotic treatment reduced the proportion of children not cured at follow-up (OR 0.13, 95% CI 0.06–0.32), which mean that only three children needed to be treated to cure one. Although the data are weak, antibiotics are likely to be beneficial in the treatment of children with chronic moist cough.

Pneumonia

In neonates, most early-onset pneumonia (in the first 2–3 days after birth) is caused by organisms acquired from the maternal perineal flora, with group B streptococcus (*S. agalactiae*) and Gram-negative bacilli the most common pathogens. After the neonatal period, most cases are viral in origin, but bacterial pneumonia can occur and may be life-threatening.[132]

Diagnosis of pneumonia

Pneumonia is a clinical and radiologic diagnosis. In infants, tachypnea, fever, and cough are the cardinal signs, but one or more may be absent in pneumonia. Additional signs of respiratory distress (chest recession, grunting, nasal flaring) may be present. There are few clinical signs or symptoms that distinguish viral from *Mycoplasma* from bacterial pneumonia. The most reliable distinguishing sign is wheeze, which is strongly correlated with viral pneumonia.[133] However, *Mycoplasma pneumoniae* and *Chlamydia pneumoniae* can also cause a pneumonitis which presents with wheeze, and although these organisms classically affect children >5 years old, they can also cause disease in children aged 2–5 years.[132,134]

Community-acquired pneumonia
Organisms causing community-acquired pneumonia

S. pneumoniae is the commonest cause of acute bacterial pneumonia in children.[132,135] The evidence for this statement does not come from positive laboratory data, because positive blood cultures are rare in pneumonia and the significance of elevated pneumococcal antibody titers is uncertain. The best evidence comes from the reduction in the incidence of pneumonia that followed the introduction of effective pneumococcal vaccines. The incidence of radiologic pneumonia fell by about 20% after the introduction of conjugate pneumococcal vaccines,[136] which is a reasonable evidence that 20% of radiologic pneumonia was due to pneumococci. This has been called the "vaccine probe" measure of the incidence of a disease. Less common causes of pneumonia include non-typeable *H. influenzae* (particularly in those with underlying lung disease), *H. influenzae* type b in unimmunized populations, *M. pneumoniae*,[134] *C. pneumoniae*,[134] and *S. aureus*.[132] *C. trachomatis* should be considered in afebrile infants up to 3 months of age with cough and pneumonitis, particularly if there is concomitant eye discharge and/or a history of maternal vaginal discharge (both present in about 50% of cases).[137]

Investigations for community-acquired pneumonia

Blood cultures are recommended but are positive in only about 10% of children with pneumonia. If pleural fluid is present, it should be aspirated, if possible, for diagnostic purposes. Rapid antigen testing for viruses using immunofluorescent techniques or ELISA can be very helpful, but finding a virus does not exclude mixed viral and bacterial infections. Acute viral serology is generally unhelpful, although finding a single high *M. pneumoniae* titer on an acute serum sample can direct therapy.[136] Bacterial antigen testing and bacterial serology are largely unhelpful in management decisions.

Antibiotic treatment of community-acquired pneumonia

Treatment will depend on local epidemiology and on availability of antibiotics. Antibiotic regimens should be as narrow as possible to treat the likely organisms. These include *S. pneumoniae* and *H. influenzae*, while it may be necessary to use antibiotics effective against *S. aureus* and *M. pneumoniae*.

S. aureus pneumonia is rare but severe. It is characterized by systemic toxicity and often radiographic changes of empyema and/or pneumatoceles. If *S. aureus* pneumonia is suspected, empiric therapy should include antistaphylococcal antibiotics (see p. 188). The possibility of community-acquired MRSA (cMRSA) should be considered whenever *S. aureus* is suspected, especially in risk groups for cMRSA, such as Maori-Polynesian or other indigenous groups.[138]

M. pneumoniae infection is more common once school age is reached.[134]

Oral antibiotics are preferred in mild pneumonia and are used to complete the treatment in more serious cases. Children with moderate to severe pneumonia usually require parenteral therapy, at least initially. Infants and children with preexisting cardiac or pulmonary disease require earlier and more intensive treatment than previously healthy children.

The following recommendations are based on consensus opinion because good evidence is not available.

Birth to 1 week

The pneumonia is usually caused by a maternally acquired pathogen. Recommended treatment is:

benzylpenicillin 60 mg (100,000 U)/kg IV, 12-hourly for 7 days PLUS
gentamicin 2.5–3 mg/kg (<30 weeks' gestation) OR 3.5 mg/kg (>30 weeks' gestation) IV, daily for 7 days

[NB: Herpes simplex virus (HSV) pneumonitis may present between days 3 and 7. The diagnosis can be made by sending a nasopharyngeal aspirate for rapid diagnosis using HSV immunofluorescence and viral culture. If positive for HSV, treat with:

acyclovir 20 mg/kg IV, 8-hourly for 14 days
(21 days if encephalitis also present)]

1 week to <4 months

Treatment for *C. trachomatis* and *Bord. pertussis* should be considered at this age. If patient is afebrile and only mildly or moderately ill, recommended treatment is:

azithromycin 10 mg/kg orally, daily for 5 days OR
(if child >1 month old)
clarithromycin 7.5 mg/kg orally, 12-hourly for 7 days OR
erythromycin 10 mg/kg orally or IV, 6-hourly for 7–14 days.

[In babies <1 month old, erythromycin is not recommended because of concerns that it may cause pyloric stenosis, and clarithromycin is not recommended because safety data are not available.]

If the patient is febrile or *C. trachomatis* has been excluded, use:

benzylpenicillin 30 mg (50,000 U)/kg IV, 6-hourly for 7 days

For severe disease (systemic toxicity and/or oxygen dependence), use:

cefotaxime 25 mg/kg IV, 8-hourly for 7 days OR
cefuroxime 50 mg/kg 2 g IV, 6-hourly for 7 days

If *S. aureus* is confirmed, see "Staphylococcal pneumonia," below.

4 months to <5 years

Most cases are viral, but because it is difficult to exclude bacterial infection, particularly pneumococcal infection, antibacterial therapy is recommended.

For mild disease, recommended treatment is:

amoxicillin 45–50 mg/kg (max 1 g) orally, 12-hourly for 7 days

If penicillin-insensitive pneumococci are rare, we recommend:

amoxicillin 15 mg/kg (max 500 mg) orally, 8-hourly for 5 days
OR (if compliance is likely to be a problem)
amoxicillin 30 mg/kg (max 1 g) orally, 12-hourly for 5 days

If the patient is allergic to penicillin, we recommend:

cefdinir 7 mg/kg (max 300 mg) orally, 12-hourly for 5 days OR
cefpodoxime 5 mg/kg (max 200 mg) orally, 12-hourly for 5 days OR
cefuroxime 15 mg/kg (max 500 mg) orally, 12-hourly for 5 days

For moderate disease (e.g., lobar or lobular consolidation, pleural effusion), children should be hospitalized and treatment should also cover atypical organisms (*M. pneumoniae, C. pneumoniae*). Recommended treatment is:

benzylpenicillin 30 mg (50,000 U)/kg IV, 6-hourly for 7 days PLUS EITHER
azithromycin 10 mg/kg orally, daily for 5 days OR
roxithromycin 4 mg/kg orally, 12-hourly for 7 days

For severe disease (large pleural effusion, systemic toxicity, and/or oxygen dependence), we recommend hospitalization and treatment using:

cefotaxime 25 mg/kg IV, 8-hourly for 7 days OR
THE COMBINATION OF
ceftriaxone 25 mg/kg IV, daily for 7 days PLUS
di/flucl/oxa/nafcillin 50 mg/kg IV, 6-hourly for 7 days

The addition of cover against atypical organisms should be considered. We recommend:

azithromycin 10 mg/kg/day IV, daily for 7 days

If staphylococcal pneumonia is suspected on clinical grounds (e.g., very severe disease, large pleural effusion, pneumatoceles) or ethnicity (increased incidence in Maori-Polynesian, Aboriginal, and other indigenous children), see "Staphylococcal pneumonia," below.

5–15 years

While *S. pneumoniae* is the commonest organism, *M. pneumoniae* is also prominent in this age group, but occurs in 3–4-yearly epidemics.

For mild disease, recommended treatment:

amoxicillin 45–50 mg/kg (max 1 g) orally, 12-hourly for 7 days

If penicillin-insensitive pneumococci are rare, we recommend:

amoxicillin 15 mg/kg (max 500 mg) orally, 8-hourly for 7 days
OR (if compliance is likely to be a problem)
amoxicillin 30 mg/kg (max 1 g) orally, 12-hourly for 7 days

If the patient is allergic to penicillin, we recommend:

cefdinir 7 mg/kg (max 300 mg) orally, 12-hourly for 7 days OR
cefpodoxime 5 mg/kg (max 200 mg) orally, 12-hourly for 7 days OR
cefuroxime 15 mg/kg (max 500 mg) orally, 12-hourly for 7 days

If also intending to treat for *M. pneumoniae or C. pneumoniae*, we recommend adding:

azithromycin 10 mg/kg (max 400 mg) orally, daily for 5 days OR
clarithromycin 7.5 mg/kg (max 250 mg) orally, 12-hourly for 7 days OR
roxithromycin 4 mg/kg (max 150 mg) orally, 12-hourly for 7 days

For more serious disease, we recommend hospitalization, and using:

benzylpenicillin 30 mg (50,000 U)/kg (max 1.2 g or 2 million U) IV, 6-hourly for 7 days PLUS
azithromycin 10 mg/kg (max 400 mg) orally, daily for 5 days OR
clarithromycin 12.5 mg/kg (max 500 mg) orally, 12-hourly for 7 days OR
roxithromycin 4 mg/kg (max 150 mg) orally, 12-hourly for 7 days

Staphylococcal pneumonia

Staphylococcal pneumonia may occur as a primary infection or secondary to right-sided endocarditis, influenza, measles, or aspiration. It is commonly severe in children and may be either community- or hospital-acquired.

Recently, there has been an increase in the incidence of severe community-acquired pneumonia caused by community strains of MRSA, in many parts of the world.[138] These strains are more prevalent in some populations (e.g., intravenous drug users and indigenous children) and are genetically distinct from hospital-acquired MRSA strains. Sometimes they are clinically more aggressive, causing severe soft tissue infections and necrotizing pneumonia, generally because they carry the gene for the virulence factor, Panton-Valentine leukocidin. They are usually susceptible to macrolides, such as clindamycin, and to trimethoprim+sulfamethoxazole. Appropriate susceptibility testing of all *S. aureus* isolates is crucial. Antibiotic therapy for these new cMRSA strains should be guided by microbiologic susceptibility data, and specialist advice may be necessary. In contrast, in many other clinical settings, the presence of *S. aureus* or MRSA in sputum culture may simply represent colonization.

For non-MRSA staphylococcal pneumonia, recommended treatment is:

di/flucl/oxa/nafcillin 50 mg/kg (max 2 g) IV, 6-hourly OR
cephalothin 50 mg/kg (max 2 g) IV, 6-hourly OR
cephazolin 25 mg/kg (max 1 g) IV, 8-hourly

When cMRSA is suspected, e.g., because child from ethnic group with high incidence[133] or because of accompanying soft tissue infection, recommended treatment is:

clindamycin 10 mg/kg (max 450 mg) IV, 8-hourly

For patients with immediate penicillin hypersensitivity and severely ill patients with suspected staphylococcal pneumonia, until antibiotic susceptibility data are available, recommended treatment is:

vancomycin <12 years: 30 mg/kg (max 1 g) IV, 12-hourly, 12 years or older: 25 mg/kg (max 1 g) IV, 12-hourly

For severely ill patients with suspected MRSA staphylococcal pneumonia, vancomycin should be given together with the beta-lactam regimen until susceptibility data are known. We recommend:

vancomycin <12 years: 30 mg/kg (max 1 g) IV, 12-hourly, 12 years or older: 25 mg/kg (max 1 g) IV, 12-hourly TOGETHER WITH
di/flucl/oxa/nafcillin 50 mg/kg (max 2 g) IV, 6-hourly OR WITH
cephalothin 50 mg/kg (max 2 g) IV, 6-hourly OR WITH
cephazolin 25 mg/kg (max 1 g) IV, 8-hourly

It is usually possible to complete antibiotic therapy with oral antibiotics, based on sensitivities if available. A suitable oral antibiotic for non-MRSA pneumonia would be:

cefuroxime 10 mg/kg (max 500 mg) orally, 12-hourly

For cMRSA, if sensitive, we recommend:

clindamycin 10 mg/kg (max 450 mg) orally, 8-hourly AND
rifampicin 10 mg/kg (max 400 mg) orally, daily

Trimethoprim-sulfamethoxazole is an alternative agent to treat susceptible cMRSA.

The optimum duration of therapy is unknown and may vary from child to child, but 7–14 days is usually effective.

Although some recent studies have suggested that linezolid may be more effective than vancomycin in patients with MRSA pneumonia, these studies suffer from significant flaws in methodology. Vancomycin, therefore, remains the treatment of choice for MRSA pneumonia, except for pneumonia caused by vancomycin-intermediate strains of *S. aureus* (VISA or hetero-VISA) when linezolid should be used.

Hospital-acquired pneumonia

Hospital-acquired or nosocomial pneumonia is defined as pneumonia that is not incubating at the time of admission to hospital and develops in a patient hospitalized for longer than 48 hours. Pneumonia in immunocompromised patients will be considered separately, below.

The pathogens causing hospital-acquired pneumonia differ from those causing community-acquired pneumonia. Hospitalized patients frequently develop oropharyngeal colonization with Gram-negative bacilli and may also be exposed to multiresistant hospital pathogens such as methicillin-resistant *S. aureus* (MRSA), and multi-drug-resistant (MDR) organisms including enterobacteria, *P. aeruginosa*, *Acinetobacter* species, and *Stenotrophomonas maltophilia*. RSV infection is usually acquired from hands of staff.[114] Other respiratory viruses and fungi that can be inhaled are potentially important causes. Prevention of nosocomial pneumonia is complex and has been addressed in a consensus guideline.[139]

We recommend that antibiotics are not justified in the following situations:

· When bacteria are cultured from sputum or endotracheal aspirates, but the child does not have pneumonia: this represents colonization only and does not justify a diagnosis of hospital-acquired pneumonia;
· When there is post-operative atelectasis: this should be managed with physiotherapy, and antibiotic therapy is not indicated, irrespective of sputum culture results;
· When a child with asthma has temporary atelectasis.

In the presence of pneumonia, sputum culture may give some indication of the bacterial agent(s) responsible and their antibiotic susceptibilities, although the accuracy of sputum culture in predicting the organisms causing pneumonia has not been proven. Use of bronchoalveolar lavage, endotracheal aspirates, and protected specimen brush can be valuable in identifying organisms and may provide evidence to stop or reduce therapy with broad-spectrum antibiotics.

Therapy can be stratified according to the risk of acquiring MDR organisms:

Low risk of MDR organisms: Patients hospitalized in a low-risk ward for any duration or short-term <5 days in a high-risk area (e.g., intensive care) should have therapy aimed at *S. pneumoniae* and non-MDR Gram-negative bacilli.

For low-risk patients with mild disease (well enough to take oral antibiotics), we recommend:

amoxicillin+clavulanate 22.5 + 3.2 mg/kg (max 875 + 125 mg) orally, 12-hourly for 7 days

If patient is unable to take oral therapy, we recommend:

benzylpenicillin 30 mg (50,000 U)/kg (max 1.2 g or 2 million U) IV, 6-hourly PLUS gentamicin <10 years: 7.5 mg/kg; ≥10 years: 6 mg/kg IV, daily

We recommend to switch to amoxicillin+clavulanate (as above) when patient is able to tolerate oral therapy.

In mildly ill patients allergic to penicillin, recommended treatment is:

cefuroxime 10 mg/kg (max 500 mg) orally, 12-hourly for 7 days OR moxifloxacin 10 mg/kg (max 400 mg) orally, daily for 7 days

For patients with moderate to severe pneumonia, recommended treatment is:

ceftriaxone 25 mg/kg (max 1 g) IV, daily OR cefotaxime 25 mg/kg (max 1 g) IV, 8-hourly OR ticarcillin+clavulanate 50 + 1.7 mg/kg (max 3 + 0.1 g) IV, 6-hourly OR THE COMBINATION OF benzylpenicillin 30 mg (50,000 U)/kg (max 1.2 g or 2 million U) IV, 6-hourly PLUS gentamicin <10 years: 7.5 mg/kg; ≥10 years: 6 mg/kg IV, daily

We recommend switching to oral therapy (as for patients with mild disease) when there has been significant improvement.

In patients with anaphylactic penicillin allergy, recommended treatment is:

moxifloxacin 10 mg/kg (max 400 mg) orally or IV, daily for 7 days

High risk of MDR organisms: Patients hospitalized for 5 days or longer in high-risk areas are more likely to have MDR infection. Because survival is improved by early appropriate therapy, a broader-spectrum initial regimen is recommended.

There is little published evidence to guide treatment options. The following regimens are likely to be equivalent, but local protocols should be developed based on the sensitivities of local colonizing and infecting organisms. When broad-spectrum antibiotics are used, their use should be reviewed regularly and they should be stopped as soon as possible. There is evidence that the response to appropriate antimicrobial therapy for ventilator-associated pneumonia occurs within the first 6 days and that prolonged therapy results in colonization and reinfection with resistant organisms. Treatment for 7 days is recommended, except for *P. aeruginosa*, *Acinetobacter* species, or *S. maltophilia* when up to 14 days' treatment may be needed.

For patients with hospital-acquired pneumonia in high-risk wards (e.g., intensive care unit, high-dependency units, known specific resistance problem) for 5 days or longer, recommended treatment is:

> **cefepime 50 mg/kg (max 2 g) IV, 8-hourly** OR
> **piperacillin+tazobactam 100 + 12.5 mg/kg (max 4 + 0.5 g) IV, 8-hourly** OR
> **ticarcillin+clavulanate 50 + 1.7 mg/kg (max 3 + 0.1 g) IV, 6-hourly**

Combination therapy using an aminoglycoside has shown a strong trend to reduced mortality for hospital-acquired pneumonia due to MDR organisms in critically ill adult patients. In children with severe pneumonia, consider adding to the above regimen:

> **gentamicin <10 years: 7.5 mg/kg; ≥10 years: 6 mg/kg IV, daily**

If Gram-positive cocci are seen on Gram stain and/or the hospital has a high prevalence of MRSA, add vancomycin to the above regimen, and discontinue it if cultures are negative after 48 hours:

> **vancomycin <12 years: 30 mg/kg (max 1 g) IV, 12-hourly, 12 years or older: 25 mg/kg (max 1 g) IV, 12-hourly**

Carbapenems should be reserved for children with organisms resistant to all other antibiotics. If indicated by susceptibility testing, recommended treatment is:

> **meropenem 25 mg/kg (max 1 g) IV, 8-hourly** OR
> **imipenem-cilastatin 25 mg/kg (max 1 g) IV, 6-hourly**

Pneumonia in the immunocompromised child

Children with underlying immunocompromise are at risk of infections with opportunist organisms. Children with defective humoral immunity (low antibodies) are most at risk of bacterial pneumonia with *S. pneumoniae* and untypeable *H. influenzae*. Children with defective cellular immunity (T cell) are at risk of *Pneumocystis carinii* (*P. jiroveci*) pneumonia (PCP) and infections with viruses such as CMV and fungi. Children with HIV infection or severe combined immunodeficiency may be susceptible to all the above organisms.

The type of immunodeficiency should be considered when deciding on treatment. Every attempt should be made to identify a causative organism. Induced sputum, bronchoscopy, fine needle aspiration, and/or open lung biopsy may be necessary to establish a specific diagnosis if examination of sputum or tracheal aspirates is unhelpful. The opinion of a clinical microbiologist or an infectious diseases physician should be sought.

Pneumocystis jiroveci (previously *Pneumocystis carinii*) pneumonia (PCP)

The classic presentation of PCP is with non-productive cough, fever, tachypnea, and dyspnea increasing in severity over a period of 2–3 weeks.[140] Oxygen saturation is often low, but cyanosis is a late sign. Children can present, however, with a more fulminant presentation.[140]

Mild to moderate PCP

Mild to moderate PCP is defined as PaO_2 >70 mm Hg in room air, alveolar-arterial gradient <35 mm Hg, and oxygen saturation >94% in room air. Recommended treatment is:

> **trimethoprim+sulfamethoxazole 5 + 25 mg/kg to 7 + 35 mg/kg orally, 8-hourly for 21 days**

If sulfamethoxazole is contraindicated, recommended treatment is:

> **dapsone 2 mg/kg (max 100 mg) orally, daily for 21 days** PLUS
> **trimethoprim 5 mg/kg (max 300 mg) orally, 8-hourly for 21 days**

Severe PCP

Severe disease is defined as PaO_2 <70 mm Hg in room air, alveolar-arterial gradient >35 mm Hg, and oxygen saturation <94% in room air. Recommended treatment is:

trimethoprim+sulfamethoxazole 5 + 25 mg/kg orally or IV, 6-hourly for a total of 21 days

If allergic to trimethoprim+sulfamethoxazole, desensitization is recommended. If unresponsive to trimethoprim+sulfamethoxazole, recommended treatment is:

pentamidine 4 mg/kg (max 300 mg) IV, daily for 21 days

Corticosteroids for PCP

A Cochrane review of six studies of adults with PCP complicating HIV infection showed that giving corticosteroids in addition to antibiotics reduces the need for mechanical ventilation and saves lives.[141] Improved survival with corticosteroid adjunctive therapy has been confirmed in two RCTs in children.[142,143] As adjunctive therapy for PCP, we recommend:

methylprednisolone 1 mg/kg (max 40 mg) IV, 6–12-hourly

Fungal pneumonia

Fungi are often cultured from sputum, which usually represents colonization. In the immunocompromised patient with pneumonia, however, sputum fungal cultures may represent true infection, although the presence of deep fungal infection should be confirmed by bronchoalveolar lavage or biopsy. For the treatment of fungal pneumonia, specialist advice is essential. Duration of treatment is dictated by clinical response and resolution of the immunosuppression. A Cochrane review found that lipid-soluble amphotericin preparations tended to be more effective than conventional amphotericin for invasive fungal infection, although this did not reach statistical significance, and there was a non-significant trend toward improved mortality with lipid-soluble preparations.[144] They also caused less nephrotoxicity, but are far more expensive.

Aspergillus and lung disease

Question | For children with pulmonary *Aspergillus* infection, are azoles more effective than amphotericin B?
Literature review | We found three RCTs,[145–147] a non-Cochrane meta-analysis, and a Cochrane review of

use of azoles in bronchopulmonary aspergillosis in asthma.[148] We found no RCTs comparing azoles with amphotericin B for pulmonary aspergillosis. We found one large RCT of voriconazole versus amphotericin B for invasive aspergillosis,[149] and a Cochrane review.[150] We found one RCT comparing conventional amphotericin B with amphotericin B colloidal dispersion for invasive aspergillosis.[151]

Allergic bronchopulmonary aspergillosis

In asthmatic children and children with cystic fibrosis, finding *Aspergillus* in the sputum in association with pulmonary infiltrates, raised serum IgE and/or IgG precipitins to *Aspergillus* species, is referred to as allergic bronchopulmonary aspergillosis. This condition is thought to be primarily an inflammatory condition and is managed with corticosteroids, with or without antifungals. A Cochrane review found only three RCTs of azoles in bronchopulmonary aspergillosis, two of them involving itraconazole and one ketoconazole.[145–147] Voriconazole has not been studied in this setting. Itraconazole was found to modify the immunologic activation associated with allergic bronchopulmonary aspergillosis (reduced eosinophilia and IgE) and improved clinical outcome, at least over a period of 16 weeks.[147,148] Improvement in lung function has not been shown.[148] In one trial, the number of exacerbations requiring oral corticosteroids was increased with itraconazole,[147] and there is potential concern about adrenal suppression when using inhaled steroids with itraconazole.[148]

Recommended treatment for bronchopulmonary aspergillosis, in addition to corticosteroids, is:

itraconazole 5 mg/kg (max 200 mg) orally, 12-hourly

Invasive pulmonary aspergillosis

Invasive pulmonary aspergillosis occurs most often in immunocompromised children with prolonged severe neutropenia, is usually rapidly progressive, and requires systemic antifungal treatment. An RCT compared voriconazole with conventional amphotericin B for confirmed and presumed invasive *Aspergillus* infections in 391 patients 12 years or older with mainly hematologic malignancies or stem cell transplants.[149] The study authors reported that voriconazole had significant benefit at 12 weeks, in terms of response to therapy and mortality.[149] A Cochrane review commented, however, that conventional amphotericin B was used without adequate attention to reducing its adverse effects by premedication and hydration.[150] This resulted in a marked difference in the duration of treatment on trial drugs (77 days with voriconazole versus 10 days with amphotericin B), and they felt precluded meaningful comparisons of the benefits and harms of the two drugs.[150]

Liposomal preparations of amphotericin have not been shown to be more effective than conventional amphotericin B for invasive aspergillosis. An RCT found that amphotericin B colloidal dispersion was as effective as conventional amphotericin B and less toxic.[151] Recommended treatment for pulmonary aspergillosis is:

voriconazole 6 mg/kg IV, 12-hourly for two doses, then 4 mg/kg IV, 12-hourly for at least 7 days, then 4 mg/kg up to 200 mg orally, 12-hourly OR liposomal amphotericin 3–5 mg/kg IV, daily OR amphotericin B desoxycholate 1 mg/kg IV, daily

Caspofungin, a recently introduced drug with activity against both *Candida* and *Aspergillus*, is very expensive. There are no RCTs of caspofungin in invasive aspergillosis. A retrospective study suggested that salvage treatment with caspofungin plus voriconazole may be superior to voriconazole alone for patients with invasive aspergillosis not responding to an amphotericin B-based regimen.[152] We do not recommend using caspofungin except for salvage therapy and after expert advice from a microbiologist or infectious diseases physician.

Candida pneumonia

Question | For children with pulmonary candidiasis, is therapy with an azole as effective as amphotericin B or as caspofungin?

Literature review | We found 10 RCTs comparing azoles or caspofungin with amphotericin B treatment of candidiasis in non-neutropenic patients, and 1 non-Cochrane meta-analysis in adults.[153]

Isolation of *Candida* species from the respiratory tract is seldom of significance, as this organism frequently colonizes the respiratory tract, particularly of neonates and older children ventilated in intensive care units.

A definitive diagnosis of candidal pneumonia rests on histologic evidence of fungal invasion of lung tissue, as well as radiologic changes.

For proven candidiasis, a non-Cochrane meta-analysis showed fluconazole is as effective as conventional amphotericin B and less toxic.[153] The combination of fluconazole and amphotericin has not been shown to be superior to fluconazole alone.[154] Conventional amphotericin B has not been shown to be inferior in efficacy to caspofungin[155] or liposomal amphotericin, which are much more expensive, although liposomal amphotericin may be preferred to conventional amphotericin if the child has significant renal toxicity. Voriconazole is as effective as giving amphotericin B followed by fluconazole,[156] but has not been shown to be superior to fluconazole, and is far more expensive. Prior fluconazole therapy is a risk factor for fluconazole-resistant candidiasis,[157] so amphotericin B is preferred for children who have previously received fluconazole.

For fluconazole-naïve children, we recommend:

fluconazole 6 mg/kg IV, daily

For children with fluconazole-resistant *Candida* and children who have already received fluconazole, if they are at low risk for renal impairment, we recommend:

amphotericin 1 mg/kg IV, daily

For such children, if they have preexisting renal impairment or at high risk of developing it, we recommend:

liposomal amphotericin 3 mg/kg IV, daily OR *voriconazole 6 mg/kg IV, 12-hourly for two doses, then 4 mg/kg 12-hourly

[*It is recommended that voriconazole levels be monitored.]

Cryptococcus pneumonia

Cryptococcus neoformans may cause primary community-acquired pneumonia with single or multiple pulmonary nodules in the normal host and in patients with defects in cellular immunity. The serum cryptococcal antigen is usually positive and the organism can sometimes be cultured from respiratory tract specimens. Recommended treatment is:

amphotericin B desoxycholate 1 mg/kg IV, daily for 2–4 weeks WITH OR WITHOUT

flucytosine 25 mg/kg IV or orally, 6-hourly for 2 weeks

Alternatively, or for continuation after amphotericin, use:

fluconazole 12 mg/kg (max 800 mg) orally or IV as a single dose, then 24 hours later, 6 mg/kg (max 400 mg) orally, daily for at least 4 weeks of therapy

Aspiration pneumonia

Aspiration pneumonia often involves anaerobes such as *Bacteroides fragilis* or mouth flora such as *S. milleri*. There are few antibiotic trials. Clindamycin and penicillin are equivalent in efficacy in children.[158] *S. aureus* infection is rare in aspiration and is adequately treated by clindamycin, which is also recommended if there is penicillin allergy. If aspiration has resulted in a lung abscess, treat as for lung abscess, below. For empiric treatment of aspiration pneumonia, recommended treatment is:

clindamycin 10 mg/kg (max 450 mg) IV or orally, 8-hourly OR the combination of benzylpenicillin 30 mg (50,000 U)/kg (max 1.2 g or 2 million U) IV, 6-hourly PLUS metronidazole 12.5 mg/kg (max 500 mg) IV, 12-hourly OR 10 mg/kg (max 400 mg) orally, 12-hourly

We recommend adding a third-generation cephalosporin if Gram-negative bacilli are found in the sputum or Gram-negative pneumonia is suspected. In adults, ampicillin+sulbactam is as effective as clindamycin+cephalosporin.[159]

When the child has improved, we recommend switching to oral therapy:

clindamycin 10 mg/kg (max 450 mg) orally, 8-hourly OR amoxicillin+clavulanate 22.5 + 3.2 mg/kg (max 875 + 125 mg) orally, 12-hourly

For uncomplicated aspiration pneumonia, a total of 7 days of therapy is usually adequate.

Lung abscess

Lung abscess in children is most commonly a complication of dental sepsis but can occur secondary to aspiration or as a complication of severe, necrotizing pneumonia.[160] Patients with altered conscious states (e.g., from anesthesia or postictal) and/or with swallowing difficulties are at increased risk. Septic emboli are occasionally a cause in patients with right-sided endocarditis. Rarely, lung abscesses can occur as a complication of septic thrombophlebitis of the internal jugular vein (Lemierre syndrome). It is not unusual to find no obvious cause of a lung abscess. The usual organisms are mouth flora, such as *S. milleri* and anaerobes.

If the cause is necrotizing pneumonia, pathogens such as *S. aureus* (see p. 188) and *Klebsiella pneumoniae* should be considered.

Whenever possible, an attempt should be made to identify the causal organism, using bronchoscopy, or surgical or interventional radiology techniques such as guided fine needle aspiration to obtain diagnostic specimens.

Clindamycin was superior in a small trial in adults.[161] For empiric antibiotic therapy, we recommend:

clindamycin 10 mg/kg (max 450 mg) IV or orally, 8-hourly OR the combination of benzylpenicillin 30 mg (50,000 U)/kg (max 1.2 g or 2 million U) IV, 6-hourly PLUS metronidazole 12.5 mg/kg (max 500 mg) IV, 12-hourly OR 10 mg/kg (max 400 mg) orally, 12-hourly

We recommend adding a third-generation cephalosporin if Gram-negative bacilli are found in the sputum or Gram-negative pneumonia is suspected. In adults, ampicillin+sulbactam is as effective as clindamycin+cephalosporin.[159]

Antibiotic therapy is generally required for at least 10–14 days, but we recommend continuing until any sputum is no longer purulent and the abscess cavity is free of fluid (in some cases this may require up to 4 weeks of treatment).

Pleural empyema

Parapneumonic effusions can be pyogenic (empyemas), can be due to other organisms such as *M. pneumoniae* or *M. tuberculosis*, or may have noninfectious causes. Pleural empyema affects nearly 1 of every 150 children hospitalized with pneumonia.[162] Pleural empyema is usually secondary to acute bacterial pneumonia, although may also result from hematogenous spread. The causative organisms are the same as for pneumonia, but the frequency is different. In a large retrospective US series,[163] the commonest organisms were *S. aureus* (35%), *S. pneumoniae* (30%), and *S. pyogenes* (20%). Untypeable *H. influenzae* is also represented in many series, while *H. influenzae* type b is an important cause in unimmunized populations.[164,165] *M. pneumoniae* can cause small to moderate pleural effusions.[166]

Diagnosis of pleural empyema

Question | In a child with pleural effusion, are pleural fluid parameters reliable for diagnosing empyema?
Literature review | We found seven studies comparing pleural fluid pH, lactase dehydrogenase (LDH) and glucose, and a meta-analysis.[167]

Thoracocentesis is almost always indicated in suspected pleural empyema to make the diagnosis and because the Gram stain and culture results guide specific therapy while the consistency of the pleural fluid may help in decisions about surgery.

Analysis of the pleural fluid pH, LDH, and glucose levels in parapneumonic effusions is potentially useful in diagnosing empyema and guiding decisions on the need for drainage. A meta-analysis of seven studies reporting values for pleural fluid pH, LDH, or glucose used area under the ROC curve (AUC) as a measure of sensitivity and specificity.[167] Pleural fluid pH had the highest diagnostic accuracy for all patients with parapneumonic effusions (AUC = 0.92) compared with pleural fluid glucose (AUC = 0.84) or LDH (AUC = 0.82). After excluding patients with purulent effusions, pH (AUC = 0.89) retained the highest diagnostic accuracy. Pleural fluid pH decision thresholds varied between 7.21 and 7.29 depending on cost-prevalence considerations.[167]

Antibiotic treatment of pleural empyema
In the only RCT of antibiotic treatment for pleural empyema, cefuroxime was equivalent to dicloxacillin+chloramphenicol.[168]

For empiric antibiotic treatment, we recommend:

cefuroxime 50 mg/kg (max 2 g) IV, 8-hourly OR cefotaxime 50 mg/kg (max 2 g) IV, 8-hourly

When cMRSA is suspected, e.g., because child from ethnic group with high incidence,[139] we recommend adding to the above treatment:

clindamycin 10 mg/kg (max 450 mg) IV, 8-hourly

For patients with anaphylactic penicillin allergy and severely ill patients, until antibiotic susceptibility data are available, recommended treatment is:

vancomycin <12 years: 30 mg/kg (max 1 g) IV, 12-hourly, 12 years or older: 25 mg/kg (max 1 g) IV, 12-hourly PLUS cefotaxime 50 mg/kg (max 2 g) IV, 8-hourly

Operative therapy for pleural empyema

Question | For children with pleural empyema, does primary surgical treatment compared with primary non-operative therapy (antibiotics and thoracentesis/chest tube drainage) speed recovery?
Literature review | We found 67 studies of operative or non-operative management of pediatric empyema, 8 studies comparing the two, a non-Cochrane meta-analysis[169] but only 1 RCT and a Cochrane review.[170]

The evidence regarding immediate surgical versus non-surgical intervention for empyema is weak. A non-Cochrane meta-analysis[169] found 67 observational studies, but children were not randomized to operative or non-operative management in any study. Data were aggregated from reports of children initially treated non-operatively (3418 cases from 54 studies) and of children treated with a primary operative approach (363 cases from 25 studies). The primary operative group had a lower aggregate inhospital mortality rate (0% versus 3.3%), reintervention rate (2.5% versus 23.5%), length of stay (10.8 days versus 20.0 days), duration of tube thoracostomy (4.4 days versus 10.6 days), and duration of antibiotic therapy (12.8 days versus 21.3 days), compared with patients who underwent non-operative therapy. Although these results look impressive, it should be remembered that non-randomized studies are prone to selection bias.

A Cochrane review[170] found only one RCT. In this study, 20 adults with empyema that was loculated or had pH < 7.2 were randomized to immediate surgery using video-assisted thoracoscopic surgery or to chest tube drainage combined with streptokinase.[171] The surgical group had a significantly higher primary treatment success, shorter chest tube duration (5.8 days versus 9.8 days), and shorter hospital stay (8.7 days versus 12.8 days).

The limited data seem to favor immediate surgery for large empyemas.

Fibrinolytic therapy for pleural empyema

A meta-analysis of three small RCTs (total 104 patients) comparing fibrinolytic therapy with streptokinase or urokinase against saline favored fibrinolytic therapy, but results were not always consistent.[172] A subsequent large RCT of 454 patients found that intrapleural streptokinase had no benefit over placebo and was associated with an increase in serious adverse events.[173]

Prevention of pleural empyema

Two non-Cochrane meta-analyses suggest that prophylactic antibiotics are indicated to reduce the risk of empyema in patients with chest drains inserted for trauma.[174,175] The antibiotics used should cover *S. aureus*.[171]

Bronchiectasis

Bronchiectasis is irreversible dilatation of the subsegmental airways, causing chronic, recurrent cough, and sputum production.[176,177] Bronchiectasis may follow severe childhood pneumonia, and its incidence has fallen in industrialized countries, as measles, pertussis, and tuberculosis have become rare.[176,177] Nevertheless, bronchiectasis may rarely result from severe pneumonia due to adenovirus or other viruses. Bronchiectasis remains more common in developing countries and in some indigenous groups in industrialized countries. There are diseases in which bronchiectasis may occur as a result of failure to clear the airways due to increased viscosity of secretions as in cystic fibrosis (see below), reduced ciliary activity (ciliary dysmotility syndromes), or defective immunity.[176,177] These need to be excluded.

In non-CF bronchiectasis, the commonest organisms isolated from sputum are untypeable *H. influenzae*, *S. pneumoniae*, and *P. aeruginosa*.[176,177] Physiotherapy and intermittent courses of oral or inhaled antibiotics for exacerbations are often recommended.

Antibiotics for bronchiectasis

Question | In children with bronchiectasis not due to cystic fibrosis, do prolonged antibiotics compared with no antibiotics or placebo improve outcome?

Literature review | We found six RCTs on prolonged antibiotic treatment of non-cystic fibrosis (non-CF) bronchiectasis and a Cochrane review.[178]

A Cochrane review of six studies of antibiotics used for 4 weeks to 1 year showed that prolonged antibiotics had significant clinical benefit in terms of response to treatment, but they did not decrease the number of exacerbations.[178] The review was limited by the diversity of the trials. An individual decision for each patient will be needed regarding the benefits versus risks of long-term oral antibiotics. If used, the choice of antibiotic therapy should reflect the sensitivities of organisms isolated from sputum cultures. Studies of inhaled antibiotics have mostly been of tobramycin for non-CF patients colonized with *Pseudomonas*.[179,180] They suggest an effect in reducing the density of sputum colonization, but with little demonstrable effect on patient's well-being or lung function.

Physical therapy for bronchiectasis

Although physiotherapy is always recommended, the evidence for its efficacy in non-CF bronchiectasis is scanty. We found eight RCTs on physical therapy, but most studies were in adults. There is, however, good evidence of short-term benefit in cystic fibrosis,[181] and it seems reasonable to extrapolate this to non-CF bronchiectasis. If physiotherapy is used, a Flutter device is preferred to percussion or active breathing techniques.[182] Exercise training improves lung function in bronchiectasis and should be encouraged.[183]

Cystic fibrosis

Antibiotics for cystic fibrosis
Infants

Question | In infants with cystic fibrosis, do prophylactic antistaphylococcal antibiotics compared with no antibiotics or placebo improve outcome?

Literature review | We found four RCTs on antistaphylococcal antibiotic use in infants and a Cochrane review.[184]

It was traditionally taught that infants acquired *S. aureus* before they acquired *Pseudomonas* and that early antistaphylococcal therapy was beneficial. A Cochrane review of four studies involving 401 patients showed that prophylactic antistaphylococcal therapy can delay colonization with *S. aureus*, but the clinical benefits were uncertain.[184] In addition, there was a trend toward a lower cumulative isolation rate of *P. aeruginosa* in the prophylaxis group at 2 and 3 years but toward a higher rate from 4 to 6 years.[184] On the basis of this evidence, some clinics recommend prophylactic antistaphylococcal antibiotics from diagnosis until 2 years of age, and others recommend antibiotic treatment only if the child develops a moist cough, whether or not chest examination is normal. It is often not possible to get a microbiologic diagnosis because of difficulties in obtaining an adequate sputum sample from infants. If no sample is available, to treat both *S. aureus* and *H. influenzae*, we recommend

amoxicillin+clavulanate 22.5 + 3.2 mg/kg orally, 12-hourly

To treat *S. aureus* alone, use:

di/flucl/oxa/nafcillin 12.5 mg/kg orally, 6-hourly

If the moist cough persists despite the above treatment, consider admission for intravenous antibiotics.

Initial *Pseudomonas* colonization

Question | In children with cystic fibrosis who become newly colonized with *Pseudomonas*, does early antibiotic treatment compared with no antibiotic or placebo reduce long-term colonization?

Literature review | We found three studies of early antibiotic treatment of patients newly colonized with *Pseud. aeruginosa* and a Cochrane review.[185]

There is limited evidence that early antibiotic treatment of patients newly colonized with *P. aeruginosa* can reduce the proportion that become chronically colonized. A Cochrane review found 15 studies but only three RCTs (69 participants) of people with cystic fibrosis recently colonized with *P. aeruginosa* and comparing combinations of inhaled, oral, or intravenous antibiotics with placebo or usual treatment (or both) or other combinations of inhaled, oral, or intravenous antibiotics. There was evidence from two RCTs reported to be of questionable methodologic

quality that treatment of early *P. aeruginosa* infection with inhaled tobramycin results in microbiologic eradication of the organism from respiratory secretions more often than placebo and that this effect may persist for up to 12 months.[185] One small RCT of oral ciprofloxacin and nebulized colistin versus usual treatment[186] suggested that treatment of early infection results in microbiologic eradication of *P. aeruginosa* more often than usual treatment after 2 years (RR 0.24, 95% CI 0.06–0.96). There is insufficient evidence to determine whether antibiotic strategies for the eradication of early *P. aeruginosa* decrease mortality or morbidity, improve quality of life, or are associated with adverse effects compared to placebo or standard treatment.

Because avoiding chronic *Pseudomonas* colonization is important and the risks of short-term antibiotics are very low, we recommend that antibiotics active against *Pseudomonas* be given when patients become newly colonized with *P. aeruginosa* and repeated with each early recurrence in an attempt to prevent chronic colonization. The choice of antibiotic should ideally be based on susceptibility testing, but if not yet available, recommended empiric therapy:

ciprofloxacin 10 mg/kg (max 500 mg) orally, 12-hourly for 3 weeks PLUS EITHER tobramycin: child <5 years: 40 mg by inhalation, 12-hourly; child 5–10 years: 80 mg, 12-hourly; >10 years and adult: 160 mg, 12-hourly OR gentamicin: child <5 years: 40 mg by inhalation, 12-hourly; child 5–10 years: 80 mg, 12-hourly; >10 years and adult: 160 mg, 12-hourly

[NB: Single doses, not per kilogram. Dilute 40 and 80 mg doses of tobramycin or gentamicin to 4 mL with 0.9% saline.]

The antibiotics should be changed if the *Pseudomonas* is found to be resistant. If colonization and respiratory symptoms persist despite the above treatment, consider admission for intravenous antipseudomonal antibiotics.

Elective admission ("tune-ups") for cystic fibrosis

Some cystic fibrosis clinics bring children into hospital on a regular basis even when well for physiotherapy and antibiotics. These elective admissions are sometimes called "tune ups."

Question | In children with cystic fibrosis, do regular elective admissions compared with treating children only when symptomatic improve outcome?

Literature review | We found three studies and a Cochrane review.[187]

A Cochrane review included only two studies (79 participants) in the review.[187] Differences in study design and objectives meant that data could not be pooled for meta-analysis. Neither study demonstrated significant differences in outcome measures between intervention and comparison groups. We conclude that the evidence for regular elective admissions is weak.

Nebulized antibiotics for cystic fibrosis

Question | In children with cystic fibrosis, does intermittent or long-term treatment with nebulized antibiotics compared to no treatment or placebo improve outcome?

Literature review | We found 14 RCTs, 2 non-Cochrane meta-analyses,[188,189] and a Cochrane review.[190]

A Cochrane review found 14 eligible trials (1100 participants) and 13 (985 participants) compared a nebulized antipseudomonal antibiotic with placebo or usual treatment.[190] Tobramycin was studied in 8 trials. Follow-up ranged from 1 to 32 months. Lung function measured as forced expired volume in 1 second (FEV_1) was better in the treated group than in control group in nine studies. Resistance to antibiotics increased more in the antibiotic-treated group than in placebo group. Tinnitus and voice alteration were more frequent with tobramycin than placebo. The authors conclude that nebulized antipseudomonal antibiotics improve lung function, but more evidence is needed to determine if this benefit is maintained as well as to determine the significance of development of antibiotic-resistant organisms.[190]

In the USA, the usual adolescent or adult dose of tobramycin is 300 mg, but lower doses are often used elsewhere. If it is decided to use nebulized antibiotics, we recommend:

tobramycin <5 years: 40 mg, 5–10 years: 80 mg, >10 years: 160 mg, nebulized, 12-hourly

[NB: Single doses, not per kilogram. Dilute 40 and 80 mg doses to 4 mL with 0.9% saline.]

OR

gentamicin <5 years: 40 mg, 5–10 years: 80 mg, >10 years: 160 mg, nebulized, 12-hourly

[NB: Single doses, not per kilogram. Dilute 40 and 80 mg doses to 4 mL with 0.9% saline.]

Exacerbations in children with cystic fibrosis colonized with *Pseudomonas*

Treatment of exacerbations of colonized children with antipseudomonal antibiotics should be based on sensitivities. Duration should depend on clinical response, but 10–14 days of treatment is often used. The antibiotics may be given orally (ciprofloxacin), nebulized, or intravenously, or a combination of these. It should be noted that cefotaxime and ceftriaxone have no useful activity against *Pseudomonas* species. Ceftazidime and cefepime, on the other hand, have excellent antipseudomonal activity as long as organisms remain sensitive.

A Cochrane analysis showed no difference between single and combination intravenous antibiotics, but there was considerable heterogeneity of the 27 trials, and the authors felt the results were inconclusive.[191] There is no evidence that combinations of inhaled and intravenous antibiotics are more effective, but they are often used. The optimum mode of delivery will depend on the child's clinical situation. The choice of antibiotics should always depend on the sensitivities of the organisms cultured from sputum.

Burkholderia cepacia

In the 1980s, it was recognized that *B. cepacia* (previously called *P. cepacia*) was an opportunistic lung pathogen in cystic fibrosis and was associated with increased rates of morbidity and mortality.[192–195] The clinical course of patients colonized with *B. cepacia* is variable, and it is not clear whether *B. cepacia* colonization causes deterioration or that patients do not become colonized until they are already deteriorating from other causes. We could find no RCTs of treatment of patients colonized with *B. cepacia*. *B. cepacia* is inherently resistant to many antibiotics, and treatment must be based on sensitivities.

Macrolides

Macrolides can modify host immune response and may have benefits in diseases where the host immune response contributes to pathology. A Cochrane review found two studies, one in adults and one in children, suggesting that 6 months of oral azithromycin produced small but significant improvements in lung function.[196] The authors of the Cochrane review argued against widespread use of azithromycin until further studies are available. Because azithromycin is expensive and long-term use will drive macrolide and possibly multidrug resistance, we think this is wise advice.

Physical therapy for cystic fibrosis

There is good evidence that physiotherapy provides short-term benefit in cystic fibrosis.[181] A Flutter device is preferred to percussion or active breathing techniques.[182] A Cochrane review of seven studies provided limited evidence that aerobic or anaerobic physical training improves exercise capacity, strength, and lung function.[197]

Hypertonic saline for cystic fibrosis

A Cochrane review of 14 trials showed that nebulized hypertonic saline improves short-term mucociliary clearance and appears to increase lung function.[198] Two subsequent RCTs of long-term nebulized hypertonic saline for 2 years showed improved mucus clearance, improved lung function, and fewer respiratory exacerbations.[199,200] We found two published studies comparing hypertonic saline with recombinant deoxyribonuclease (rhDNase) in cystic fibrosis, and one abstract. In one study in children, hypertonic saline was not as effective as rhDNase, although there was variation in individual response. The mean FEV_1 increased by 16% with daily rhDNase, 14% with alternate-day rhDNase, and 3% with hypertonic saline.[201] A crossover study comparing hypertonic saline with rhDNase found that both treatments improved lung function to the same extent.[202] Hypertonic saline is considerably cheaper than rhDNase and appears to give comparable benefit, but is not always well tolerated in young children. We recommend a trial of therapy of hypertonic saline before using rhDNase.

rhDNase for cystic fibrosis

A Cochrane review of rhDNase in cystic fibrosis identified 14 eligible trials (2397 participants) and 3 additional studies that examined the health-care cost from one of the clinical trials.[203] Eleven studies compared rhDNase to placebo, 1 compared daily rhDNase with hypertonic saline and alternate-day rhDNase[201] and 2 compared daily rhDNase with hypertonic saline. Study duration varied from 6 days to 2 years. Lung function measured by spirometry improved in the treated groups, with significant differences at 1 month, 3 months, 6 months, and 2 years. There was no excess of adverse effects except voice alteration and rash. Insufficient data were available to analyze differences in antibiotic treatment, inpatient stay, and quality of life. On the other hand, hypertonic saline has not been clearly shown to be inferior to rhDNase; there is individual variation and saline is much cheaper.

We recommend a trial of therapy of hypertonic saline before using rhDNase.

Severe acute respiratory syndrome

Severe acute respiratory syndrome (SARS) is caused by the SARS-associated coronavirus and is primarily transmitted by respiratory droplet transmission.[204] Some infected adults shed masses of virus, while most do not. The therapeutic use of nebulizers generated aerosols, which disseminated the organism and spread the disease. SARS is relatively mild in children, which suggests an important immunologic component to the pathogenesis of disease. At the time of writing, the last reported cases occurred in China in 2004. If SARS reemerges, precautions will need to be resumed. Strict infection control, respiratory and personal contact precautions are necessary to prevent person-to-person transmission. If SARS is suspected, the local health department must be notified. For information on SARS, readers are referred to the WHO Web site: http://www.who.int/csr/sars/en/ or the CDC Web site: http://www.cdc.gov/niosh/topics/SARS/.

Tuberculosis (TB)

TB often presents very differently in children from adults. In children, TB is usually the primary infection and is of very low infectivity to others, unless the child has military TB or adult-type open TB. The main differences are shown in Table 12.1.

Adults with pulmonary TB classically present with "open TB" with cavitating lesions. They are "smear positive" with acid-fast bacilli visible on sputum microscopy. In contrast, if children present with pulmonary TB (as opposed to being diagnosed on screening), it is usually with complications of hilar

Table 12.1 Differences between adult and pediatric pulmonary TB.

Category	Adult	Child
Type of infection	Reactivation	Primary
Organism load	Large	Small
Infectivity	High	Very low
Risk of miliary disease	Low	High

Adapted from Reference 205.

lymphadenopathy. The hilar nodes can compress the major bronchus causing wheeze or even hypostatic pneumonia, can rupture into the bronchus causing tuberculous pneumonia, or can rupture into the pleural cavity causing empyema.

An important distinction is drawn between TB infection and TB disease. Early after inhaling the organism, the patient is infected, but has not yet developed any clinical manifestations. A patient who remains well with no clinical disease is said to have TB infection; i.e., infection is latent. A patient who develops signs or symptoms has TB disease.

Diagnosis of TB

Because it is rare to see or culture *M. tuberculosis* in children (apart from adolescents with adult-type "open TB" cavitatory pulmonary disease), the diagnosis in children generally relies on demonstrating the host immune response to the organism. The classic method is using tuberculin skin testing (TST), although interferon-gamma assays are generating much interest.

TST and TB

TST is the traditional technique for distinguishing TB-infected from TB-uninfected persons from those who have TB infection or TB disease. False negatives can occur in very young babies, in children who are malnourished or immunocompromised extremely unwell with TB, e.g., with miliary disease. False positives can occur due to infection with cross-reacting non-tuberculous mycobacteria (see p. 202). Interpretation of TST requires consideration of prevalence and the purpose for testing.

A systematic review found that for the general US population, TST was sensitive and specific for diagnosing TB infection (latent infection) and 100% sensitive for diagnosing TB disease.[206] The authors concluded that the operating characteristics of the tuberculin test are superior to those of nearly all commonly used screening and diagnostic tests.[206]

Although the Red Book[207] says to ignore previous BCG immunization in interpreting TSTs, a meta-analysis showed that the tuberculin skin response is more likely to be positive if the child has had BCG vaccine and the size of the response is likely to be increased up to 15 mm but not usually greater for 5 years or more after BCG.[208] The Red Book Committee recommends giving chemoprophylaxis to asymptomatic children with a TST response of 10–14 mm, even if they had BCG.[207] However, other authorities would not give chemoprophylaxis to a child who had received BCG unless the TST was 15 mm or greater (see Table 12.2), an approach that will reduce the number of children (particularly refugee children) given prophylaxis and seems logical on the basis of the evidence.[208]

Table 12.2 Working definitions of positive TST.

Induration	Tuberculin Positive
5 mm or greater	Child contact of person with infectious TB disease
	Child thought to have TB disease
	Immunosuppressed child, e.g., HIV, or on steroids or cytotoxics
10 mm or greater	Child < 4 years old
	Child any age with chronic disease, e.g., diabetes, malnutrition, renal failure
	Child born (or parents born) in region with high prevalence of TB
	Child who has traveled to region with high prevalence of TB
	Child frequently exposed to adults at high risk of TB
15 mm or greater	Child > 4 years old with no risk factors
	Child who has received BCG vaccine in last 5 years

Interferon-gamma assays and TB

Until recently, TSTs were the only way to diagnose latent TB. In vitro tests have now been developed, based on the detection of interferon-gamma produced by T cells in response to TB infection. A systematic review of 75 studies suggested that the better interferon-gamma-based tests may have some advantages over TST, in terms of higher specificity, better correlation with exposure to *M. tuberculosis*, and less cross-reactivity due to BCG or non-tuberculous mycobacteria.[209] On the other hand, they are expensive, and there is less evidence for children, for persons who are immunocompromised, who have extrapulmonary TB or non-tuberculous mycobacterial infection and in TB endemic countries.[209] Because the interferon-gamma-based tests are not affected by prior BCG immunization they can be used in situations where the results of TSTs are likely to be confounded by prior BCG vaccination, e.g., contact tracing, immigrant screening, and surveillance programs.[210]

Nucleic acid detection and TB

Because infection in children is pauci-bacterial, there is a need for highly sensitive tests to detect *M. tuberculosis*. The use of PCR techniques to amplify nucleic acid held great promise in TB, although the promise has not entirely been fulfilled. Although PCR can be useful, it is still not sensitive enough for a negative PCR to exclude infection. For example, according to a meta-analysis of 14 studies,[211] the sensitivity of PCR of the CSF in diagnosing tuberculous meningitis is only 56%. The sensitivity and specificity of PCR is also not consistently good enough to recommend its routine use for smear-negative pulmonary TB.[212] However, by sequencing the product, PCR techniques can distinguish between *M. tuberculosis* and atypical mycobacterial infection.[213] In addition, by looking at gene mutations, PCR can be used to predict the sensitivity of an isolate of *M. tuberculosis* to antituberculous drugs.[214]

Treatment of TB
Treatment of latent TB infection

Question | In otherwise healthy children with latent TB infection, does chemoprophylaxis using one or more antituberculous drugs compared with no chemoprophylaxis or placebo reduce the risk of TB disease?

Literature review | We found 11 RCTs of chemoprophylaxis and a Cochrane review.[215]

Patients with latent TB infection (no signs or symptoms) may progress to develop active TB disease. Risk factors include young age, particularly children <4 years old, recent infection within the previous 2 years, and immunosuppression. A Cochrane review of 11 trials of non-HIV infected children[215] showed that isoniazid chemoprophylaxis reduced the proportion of children and young adults with latent TB who progressed to active TB by 60% (95% CI 48–69%). There was no difference between 6 and 12 months of isoniazid, so although some authorities recommend 6 months of isoniazid[216] and others recommend 9 months,[207] there seems little evidence to support continuing for 9 months. Six months of rifampin (rifampicin) can be used as an alternative, e.g., for isoniazid-resistant TB, but there are fewer data on its efficacy.

After active TB has been excluded, children with a positive tuberculin skin test or TB-specific interferon-gamma release assay who should be considered for chemoprophylaxis are:
· young children (the risk of progression increases with decreasing age[215]);
· children with HIV infection (long-term preventive therapy is protective, although the effect may decline with time[217]);
· close contacts of a patient with smear-positive pulmonary TB;
· recent tuberculin converters;
· prior to the commencement of immunosuppressive therapy (including with corticosteroids or tumor necrosis factor inhibitors such as infliximab and etanercept);
· children with underlying medical conditions such as diabetes and chronic renal failure.
    Recommended treatment is:

isoniazid 10 mg/kg (max 300 mg) orally, daily for 6 months

Supplemental pyridoxine is recommended for adults (25 mg) and for breast-fed babies (5 mg, if no syrup available can crush a 25-mg tablet, make up to 5 mL with water, and give 1 mL).
    The Red Book[207] states that directly observed twice-weekly isoniazid for 9 months is an alternative if daily

therapy is not possible. This regimen lacks supportive data, but may be the only practical approach if compliance is a problem. Use:

> **isoniazid 15 mg/kg (max 900 mg) orally, twice-weekly for 9 months**

Treatment of TB disease

M. tuberculosis is a slow-growing intracellular organism, and treatment for less than 6 months is associated with a lower success rate.[218]

Standard short-course therapy for 6 months is suitable to treat pulmonary TB and also cervical lymphadenitis due to TB,[218] provided that:

· any organisms cultured are susceptible to isoniazid, rifampicin, and pyrazinamide;
· the patient is able to tolerate all drugs in the regimen;
· isoniazid and rifampicin are taken for the full 6 months and pyrazinamide for at least the first 2 months;
· cavitation is absent on the initial chest film and sputum cultures are negative after 2 months of treatment.

Standard short-course therapy is unsuitable if resistance to isoniazid or rifampicin is documented or is suspected on epidemiologic grounds, or if pyrazinamide cannot be used in the first 2 months. If standard short-course therapy is unsuitable, treatment for 9–12 months will be required.

Question | For children with TB disease, does intermittent therapy compared with daily therapy cure infection?

Literature review | We found 27 observational studies, 8 RCTs, and a Cochrane meta-analysis.[219]

A Cochrane meta-analysis[219] considered only one trial comparing daily therapy with intermittent dosing[220] to be eligible and thus concluded that there is insufficient evidence. Two RCTs in children, one in South Africa[221] and one in India,[222] found no difference in relapse rates between children treated with daily or intermittent dosing, but no difference in compliance.[221]

The weight of evidence from RCTs and from many observational studies suggests that intermittent dosing is associated with a low relapse rate comparable to daily dosing. Because of resource implications and to improve compliance, intermittent dosing regimens are often used. Daily therapy is sometimes preferred in children in industrialized countries but intermittent

(thrice-weekly) regimens may be used for reasons of compliance and resources to treat older children. Intermittent regimens are recommended only if directly observed therapy (DOT) is available. Dosage should be reviewed if weight changes significantly during therapy.

Daily regimen

For the daily regimen, recommended treatment is:

> **isoniazid 10 mg/kg (max 300 mg) orally, daily for 6 months** PLUS
> **rifamp(ic)in 10 mg/kg (max 600 mg) orally, daily for 6 months** PLUS
> **pyrazinamide 25 mg/kg (max 2 g) orally, daily for 2 months**

Because of concerns about its effect on vision, ethambutol is not recommended for children <6 years old. If used instead of or as well as pyrazinamide, the dose of ethambutol is 15 mg/kg daily for 2 months, but stop earlier if the organism is shown to be sensitive to isoniazid and rifampicin.

Thrice-weekly regimen (with DOT)

For the thrice-weekly regimen, recommended treatment is:

> **isoniazid 15 mg/kg (max 600 mg) orally, thrice weekly for 6 months** PLUS
> **rifamp(ic)in 15 mg/kg (max 600 mg) orally, thrice weekly for 6 months** PLUS
> **pyrazinamide 50 mg/kg (max 3 g) orally, thrice weekly for 2 months**

Because of concerns about its effect on vision, ethambutol is not recommended for children <6 years old. If used instead of or as well as pyrazinamide, the dose of ethambutol is 30 mg/kg thrice weekly for 2 months, but stop earlier if the organism is shown to be sensitive to isoniazid and rifampicin.

Extrapulmonary TB

Although there are few formal studies of duration of therapy, it is recommended that children with most forms of extrapulmonary TB, e.g., lymph node,[223] bone, pleural, can be treated with standard short-course therapy for 6 months.[207] Patients with miliary (disseminated) and CNS TB (tuberculous meningitis, tuberculoma, TB spine) should be treated for

12 months (2 months with three or four drugs, followed by 10 months of rifampicin and isoniazid). Prolongation of therapy should be considered for any child with TB that has not resolved after 6 months.[207]

Corticosteroids

Corticosteroids reduce mortality and severe residual disability in tuberculous meningitis in children.[224] They are also often used for children with tuberculous pleurisy,[225] endobronchial obstruction, pericardial effusion, and severe miliary TB, but there is no good evidence for or against these indications.

The usual dose is prednisone 1–2 mg/day up to 60 mg daily for 6–8 weeks (expert opinion), although some authors have recommended higher doses for theoretical reasons but without evidence that the benefits exceed the likely harms.

Directly observed therapy

The WHO and others have stressed the importance of DOT to improve compliance and reduce the risk of inducing resistance. A Cochrane meta-analysis was unable to show any significant benefit of DOT above self-treatment at home.[226] However, the six studies reviewed excluded patients at high risk of non-compliance. For the same reasons as the WHO, we still strongly advise using DOT whenever resources permit.

TB in pregnancy and breast-feeding

A pregnant woman with suspected TB should be treated with antituberculous medication urgently, because of the high risk of TB to the fetus. Isoniazid, rifampicin, and ethambutol all cross the placenta, but have not been reported to be teratogenic. Although US guidelines state that pyrazinamide is not recommended for routine use in pregnant women because of insufficient safety data, pyrazinamide is widely used in this situation in other countries.

Breast-feeding is considered to be safe for women who are being treated with isoniazid, rifampicin, and ethambutol because the low concentrations of these drugs in breast milk have not been shown to be toxic for the nursing infant. However, to prevent deficiency, it is recommended to give pyridoxine 5 mg on the days that the mother receives her isoniazid dose to babies who are being breast-fed by mothers who are taking isoniazid (with or without pyridoxine).

Prevention of TB

In a meta-analysis of RCTs, BCG vaccine given to newborns or infants was 74% effective against TB disease, 65% protective against death, and 64% against TB meningitis.[227] Better studies reported greater efficacy. Although the efficacy of BCG vaccine wanes with time,[228] we have no better vaccine at present. BCG is a live, attenuated vaccine (*M. bovis*) and is contraindicated for highly immunocompromised children.

Non-tuberculous mycobacterial infection

Non-tuberculous mycobacteria are environmental organisms, which can cause respiratory, cutaneous, or disseminated disease. Isolation of these organisms from respiratory secretions does not distinguish between colonization and infection. Defense to these organisms depends on T-cell function and in particular on interferon-gamma activity.

Question | For children with non-tuberculous mycobacterial infections, does treatment with three antimycobacterial drugs compared with two drugs cure infection?

Literature review | We found 48 studies and 2 RCTs in HIV-infected adults,[232,233] and 1 RCT in HIV-negative adults.[234]

The evidence on optimal treatment of non-tuberculous mycobacterial infections is weak. We could find only two RCTs comparing three drugs, with two drugs in HIV-infected adults[232,233] and one in HIV-negative adults.[234] These favored three-drug regimens, although the evidence was stronger in HIV-infected than HIV-negative patients.

Mycobacterium avium complex (MAC)

MAC can cause:
· cervical lymphadenitis, which is usually treated surgically;
· pulmonary MAC;
· disseminated MAC, which occurs in immunocompromised patients with impaired T-cell immunity, e.g., severe combined immunodeficiency, HIV, or in association with familial defects in the interferon-gamma receptor.[229–231]

For most drugs, with the exception of clarithromycin and azithromycin, there is poor correlation between in vitro susceptibility testing and clinical response to treatment of MAC.

The following recommendations are based largely on expert consensus opinion.[235–237]

For **pulmonary MAC**, a combination of three drugs is recommended.[235–237] Daily therapy is more effective than thrice-weekly regimens in severe cases.[236] Treatment duration (with all three drugs) depends on clinical, microbiological, and radiological responses, but should continue until the patient has been culture-negative for at least 12 months.

For the daily regimen, we recommend:

ethambutol 15 mg/kg (child ≥6 years) orally, daily PLUS EITHER
clarithromycin 12.5 mg/kg (max 500 mg) orally, 12-hourly OR
azithromycin 15 mg/kg (max 500 mg) orally, daily PLUS EITHER
rifamp(ic)in 10 mg/kg (max 600 mg) orally, daily OR
rifabutin 5 mg/kg (max 300 mg) orally, daily

For the thrice-weekly regimen, recommended treatment is:

ethambutol 25 mg/kg (child ≥6 years) orally, thrice weekly PLUS
rifamp(ic)in 10 mg/kg (max 600 mg) orally, thrice weekly PLUS EITHER
clarithromycin 12.5 mg/kg (max 500 mg) orally, 12-hourly, thrice weekly OR
azithromycin 10 mg/kg (max 600 mg) orally, thrice weekly

The addition of amikacin 25 mg/kg IM or streptomycin 25 mg/kg IM, thrice weekly for the first 2 months of treatment may be considered in some cases (e.g., macrolide resistance).

For **disseminated MAC**, use the daily regimen of clarithromycin (or azithromycin) plus ethambutol plus rifabutin recommended for pulmonary MAC. The rifabutin dose should be modified if the patient has HIV and is on concurrent protease inhibitor or non-nucleoside reverse transcriptase inhibitor therapy.

Mycobacterium kansasii

M. kansasii causes a chronic pulmonary infection that resembles TB. Organisms are resistant to pyrazinamide. For treatment, we recommend:

isoniazid 10 mg/kg (max 300 mg) orally, daily PLUS
rifamp(ic)in 10 mg/kg (max 600 mg) orally, daily PLUS
ethambutol child ≥6 years: 15 mg/kg orally, daily

Recommended treatment duration is 18 months, with at least 12 months of negative sputum cultures.

References

1 American Academy of Pediatrics Sub-committee on Management of Acute Otitis Media. Diagnosis and management of acute otitis media. *Pediatrics* 2004;113:451–65.

2 Gates GA, Avery C, Cooper JC, Hearne EM, Holt GR. Predictive value of tympanometry in middle ear effusion. *Ann Otol Rhinol Laryngol* 1986;95:46–50.

3 Le CT, Daly KA, Margolis RH, Lindgren BR, Giebink GS. A clinical profile of otitis media. *Arch Otolaryngol Head Neck Surg* 1992;118:1225–8.

4 Finitzo T, Friel-Patti S, Chinn K, Brown O. Tympanometry and otoscopy prior to myringotomy: issues in diagnosis of otitis media. *Int J Pediatr Otorhinolaryngol* 1992;24:101–10.

5 Watters GWR, Jones JE, Freeland AP. The predictive value of tympanometry in the diagnosis of middle ear effusions. *Clin Otolaryngol* 1997;22:343–5.

6 Jardine AH, Maw AR, Coulton S. Dry tap at myringotomy: a three-year study of 1688 children undergoing myringotomy. *Clin Otolaryngol* 1999;24:266–9.

7 Saeed K, Coglianese CL, McCormick DP, Chonmaitree T. Otoscopic and tympanometric findings in acute otitis media yielding dry tap at tympanocentesis. *Pediatr Infect Dis J* 2004;23:1030–4.

8 Paradise JL, Smith CG, Bluestone CD. Tympanometric detection of middle ear effusion in infants and young children. *Pediatrics* 1976;58:198–210.

9 Orchik DJ, Dunn JW, McNutt L. Tympanometry as a predictor of middle ear effusion. *Arch Otolaryngol* 1978;104:4–6.

10 Palmu AA, Syrjanen R. Diagnostic value of tympanometry using subject-specific normative values. *Int J Pediatr Otorhinolaryngol* 2005;69:965–71.

11 McCormick D, Lim-Melia E, Saeed K, Baldwin CD, Chonmaitree T. Otitis media: can clinical findings predict bacterial or viral etiology? *Pediatr Infect Dis J* 2000;19:256–8.

12 Bluestone CD, Stephenson JS, Martin LM. Ten-year review of otitis media pathogens. *Pediatr Infect Dis J* 1992;11:S7–11.

13 Del Beccaro MA, Mendelman PM, Inglis AF et al. Bacteriology of acute otitis media: a new perspective. *J Pediatr* 1992;120:81–4.

14 Jacobs MR, Dagan R, Applebaum PC, Burch DJ. Prevalence of antimicrobial-resistant pathogens in middle ear fluid: multinational study of 917 children with acute otitis media. *Antimicrob Agents Chemother* 1998;42:589–95.

15 Chonmaitree T, Howie VM, Truant AL. Presence of respiratory viruses in middle ear fluids and nasal wash specimens from children with acute otitis media. *Pediatrics* 1986;77:698–702.

16 Ruohola A, Meurman O, Nikkari S et al. Microbiology of acute otitis media in children with tympanostomy tubes: prevalences of bacteria and viruses. *Clin Infect Dis* 2006;43:1417–22.

17 Casey JR, Pichichero ME. Changes in frequency and pathogens causing acute otitis media in 1995–2003. *Pediatr Infect Dis J* 2004;9:824–8.

18 Syrjanen RK, Herva EE, Makela PH et al. The value of nasopharyngeal culture in predicting the etiology of acute otitis media in children less than two years of age. *Pediatr Infect Dis J* 2006;25:1032–6.

19 Takata GS, Chan LS, Shekelle P, Morton SC, Mason W, Marcy SM. Evidence assessment of management of acute otitis media: I. The role of antibiotics in treatment of uncomplicated acute otitis media. *Pediatrics* 2001;108:239–47.

20 Glasziou PP, Del Mar CB, Sanders SL, Hayem M. Antibiotics for acute otitis media in children. *The Cochrane Database of Systematic Reviews* 2004;(1):Art No CD000219.

21 Little P, Gould C, Williamson I, Moore M, Warner G, Dunleavey J. Pragmatic randomised controlled trial of two prescribing strategies for childhood acute otitis media. *BMJ* 2001;322:336–42.

22 Spurling GKP, Del Mar CB, Dooley L, Foxlee R. Delayed antibiotics for symptoms and complications of respiratory infections. *The Cochrane Database of Systematic Reviews* 2004;(4):Art No CD004417.

23 Kozyrskyj AL, Hildes-Ripstein GE, Longstaffe SE et al. Treatment of acute otitis media with a shortened course of antibiotics: a meta-analysis. *JAMA* 1998;279:1736–42.

24 Kozyrskyj AL, Hildes-Ripstein GE, Longstaffe SEA et al. Short course antibiotics for acute otitis media. *The Cochrane Database of Systematic Reviews* 2000;(2):Art No CD001095.

25 Flynn CA, Griffin GH, Schultz JK. Decongestants and antihistamines for acute otitis media in children. *The Cochrane Database of Systematic Reviews* 2004;(3):Art No CD001727.

26 Damoiseaux RA, Rovers MM, Van Balen FA, Hoes AW, de Melker RA. Long-term prognosis of acute otitis media in infancy: determinants of recurrent acute otitis media and persistent middle ear effusion. *Fam Pract* 2006;23:40–5.

27 Gebhart DE. Tympanostomy tubes in the otitis media prone child. *Laryngoscope* 1981;91:849–66.

28 Gonzalez C, Arnold JE, Woody EA et al. Prevention of recurrent acute otitis media: chemoprophylaxis versus tympanostomy tubes. *Laryngoscope* 1986;96:1330–4.

29 Le CT, Freeman DW, Fireman BH. Evaluation of ventilating tubes and myringotomy in the treatment of recurrent or persistent otitis media. *Pediatr Infect Dis J* 1991;10: 2–11.

30 Casselbrant ML, Kaleida PH, Rockette HE et al. Efficacy of antimicrobial prophylaxis and of tympanostomy tube insertion for prevention of recurrent acute otitis media: results of a randomized clinical trial. *Pediatr Infect Dis J* 1992;11:278–86.

31 Paradise JL, Bluestone CD, Rogers KD et al. Efficacy of adenoidectomy for recurrent otitis media in children previously treated with tympanostomy-tube placement: results of parallel randomized and non-randomized trials. *JAMA* 1990;263:2066–73.

32 Paradise JL, Bluestone CD, Colborn DK et al. Adenoidectomy and adenotonsillectomy for recurrent acute otitis media: parallel randomized clinical trials in children not previously treated with tympanostomy tubes. *JAMA* 1999;282:945–53.

33 Koivunen P, Uhari M, Luotonen J et al. Adenoidectomy versus chemoprophylaxis and placebo for recurrent acute otitis media in children aged under 2 years: randomised controlled trial. *BMJ* 2004;328:487.

34 Hammaren-Malmi S, Saxen H, Tarkkanen J, Mattila PS. Adenoidectomy does not significantly reduce the incidence of otitis media in conjunction with the insertion of tympanostomy tubes in children who are younger than 4 years: a randomized trial. *Pediatrics* 2005;116:185–9.

35 Williams RL, Chalmers TC, Stange KC, Chalmers FT, Bowlin SJ. Use of antibiotics in preventing recurrent acute otitis media and in treating otitis media with effusion: a meta-analytic attempt to resolve the brouhaha. *JAMA* 1993;270: 1344–51.

36 Teele DW, Klein JO, Word BM et al. Antimicrobial prophylaxis for infants at risk for recurrent acute otitis media. *Vaccine* 2000;19(suppl 1):S140–3.

37 Roberts JE, Rosenfeld RM, Zeisel SA. Otitis media and speech and language: a meta-analysis of prospective studies. *Pediatrics* 2004;113:e238–48.

38 Takata GS, Chan LS, Morphew T, Mangione-Smith R, Morton SC, Shekelle P. Evidence assessment of the accuracy of methods of diagnosing middle ear effusion in children with otitis media with effusion. *Pediatrics* 2003;112:1379–87.

39 American Academy of Family Physicians; American Academy of Otolaryngology-Head and Neck Surgery; American Academy of Pediatrics Sub-committee on Otitis Media with Effusion. Otitis media with effusion. *Pediatrics* 2004;113:1412–29.

40 Rosenfeld RM, Post JC. Meta-analysis of antibiotics for the treatment of otitis media with effusion. *Otolaryngol Head Neck Surg* 1992;106:378–86.

41 Rosenfeld RM, Mandel EM, Bluestone CD. Systemic steroids for otitis media with effusion in children. *Arch Otolaryngol Head Neck Surg* 1991;117:984–9.

42 Butler CC, van der Voort JH. Oral or topical nasal steroids for hearing loss associated with otitis media with effusion in children. *The Cochrane Database of Systematic Reviews* 2002;(4):Art No CD001935.

43 Lous J, Burton MJ, Felding JU, Ovesen T, Rovers MM, Williamson I. Grommets (ventilation tubes) for hearing loss associated with otitis media with effusion in children. *The Cochrane Database of Systematic Reviews* 2005;(1):Art No CD001801.

44 Rovers MM, Black N, Browning GG, Maw R, Zielhuis GA, Haggard MP. Grommets in otitis media with effusion:

an individual patient data meta-analysis. *Arch Dis Child* 2005;90:480–5.

45 Griffin GH, Flynn C, Bailey RE, Schultz JK. Antihistamines and/or decongestants for otitis media with effusion (OME) in children. *The Cochrane Database of Systematic Reviews* 2006;(4):Art No CD003423.

46 Acuin J, Smith A, Mackenzie I. Interventions for chronic suppurative otitis media. *The Cochrane Database of Systematic Reviews* 1998;(4):Art No CD000473.

47 WHO/CIBA Foundation Workshop. Prevention of hearing impairment from chronic otitis media. WHO/PDH/98.4, 1996.

48 Smith AW, Hatcher J, Mackenzie IJ et al. Randomised controlled trial of treatment of chronic suppurative otitis media in Kenyan schoolchildren. *Lancet* 1996;348:1128–33.

49 Macfadyen CA, Alcuin JM, Gamble C. Topical antibiotics without steroids for chronically discharging ears with underlying eardrum perforations. *The Cochrane Database of Systematic Reviews* 2005;(4):Art No CD004618.

50 Macfadyen CA, Acuin JM, Gamble C. Systemic antibiotics versus topical treatments for chronically discharging ears with underlying eardrum perforations. *The Cochrane Database of Systematic Reviews* 2006;(1)Art No CD005608.

51 Couzos S, Lea T, Mueller R, Murray R, Culbong M. Effectiveness of ototopical antibiotics for chronic suppurative otitis media in Aboriginal children: a community-based, multicentre, double-blind trial. *Med J Aust* 2003;179:185–90.

52 Jang CH, Park SY. Emergence of ciprofloxacin-resistant pseudomonas in chronic suppurative otitis media. *Clin Otolaryngol Allied Sci* 2004;29:321–3.

53 Roland PS, Hannley M, Friedman R et al. The development of antibiotic resistant organisms with the use of ototopical medications. *Otolaryngol Head Neck Surg* 2004;130(3, suppl):S89–94.

54 Agrawal S, Husein M, MacRae D. Complications of otitis media: an evolving state. *J Otolaryngol* 2005;34(suppl 1): S33–9.

55 Spratley J, Silveira H, Alvarez I, Pais-Clemente M. Acute mastoiditis in children: review of the current status. *Int J Pediatr Otorhinolaryngol* 2000;56:33–40.

56 Ginsburg CM, Rudoy R, Nelson JD. Acute mastoiditis in infants and children. *Clin Pediatr (Phila)* 1980;19:549–53.

57 Ogle JW, Lauer BA. Acute mastoiditis: diagnosis and complications. *Am J Dis Child* 1986;140:1178–82.

58 Nadal D, Herrmann P, Baumann A, Fanconi A. Acute mastoiditis: clinical, microbiological, and therapeutic aspects. *Eur J Pediatr* 1990;149:560–4.

59 Hoppe JE, Koster S, Bootz F, Niethammer D. Acute mastoiditis—relevant once again. *Infection* 1994;22:178–82.

60 Maroldi R, Farina D, Palvarini L et al. Computed tomography and magnetic resonance imaging of pathologic conditions of the middle ear. *Eur J Radiol* 2001;40:78–93.

61 Brook I. The role of anaerobic bacteria in acute and chronic mastoiditis. *Anaerobe* 2005;11:252–7.

62 Finegold SM. Anaerobic infections in otolaryngology. *Ann Otol Rhinol Laryngol Suppl* 1981;90:13–6.

63 Brook I. Aerobic and anaerobic bacteriology of chronic mastoiditis in children. *Am J Dis Child* 1981;135:478–9.

64 Arroll B, Kenealy T. Antibiotics for the common cold and acute purulent rhinitis. *The Cochrane Database of Systematic Reviews* 2005;(3):Art No CD000247.

65 Arroll B, Kenealy T. Are antibiotics effective for acute purulent rhinitis? Systematic review and meta-analysis of placebo controlled randomised trials. *BMJ* 2006;333:279–81.

66 Douglas RM, Hemila H, D'Souza R, Chalker EB, Treacy B. Vitamin C for preventing and treating the common cold. *The Cochrane Database of Systematic Reviews* 2004;(4):Art No CD000980.

67 Coulehan JL, Eberhard S, Kapner L, Taylor F, Rogers K, Garry P. Vitamin C and acute illness in Navajo school children. *N Engl J Med* 1976;295:973–7.

68 Sutter AI, Lemiengre M, Campbell H, Mackinnon HF. Antihistamines for the common cold. *The Cochrane Database of Systematic Reviews* 2003;(3):Art No CD001267.

69 Taverner D, Latte J, Draper M. Nasal decongestants for the common cold. *The Cochrane Database of Systematic Reviews* 2004;(3):Art No CD001953.

70 Marshall I. Zinc for the common cold. *The Cochrane Database of Systematic Reviews* 2006;(3):Art No CD001364.

71 Jackson JL, Lesho E, Peterson C. Zinc and the common cold: a meta-analysis revisited. *J Nutr* 2000;130(5S, suppl):1512S–5S.

72 Macknin ML, Piedmonte M, Calendine C, Janosky J, Wald E. Zinc gluconate lozenges for treating the common cold in children: a randomized controlled trial. *JAMA* 1998;279:1962–7.

73 Puhakka T, Makela MJ, Alanen A et al. Sinusitis in the common cold. *J Allergy Clin Immunol* 1998;102:403–8.

74 Gwaltney JM, Jr, Phillips CD, Miller RD, Riker DK. Computed tomographic study of the common cold. *N Engl J Med* 1994;330:25–30.

75 Ueda D, Yoto Y. The ten-day mark as a practical diagnostic approach for acute paranasal sinusitis in children. *Pediatr Infect Dis J* 1996;15:576–9.

76 Wald ER, Chiponis D, Ledesma-Medina J. Comparative effectiveness of amoxicillin and amoxicillin-clavulanate potassium in acute paranasal sinus infections in children: a double-blind placebo-controlled trial. *Pediatrics* 1986;77:795–800.

77 Williams JW, Jr, Aguilar C, Cornell J et al. Antibiotics for acute maxillary sinusitis. *The Cochrane Database of Systematic Reviews* 2003;(2):Art No CD000243.

78 Morris P, Leach A. Antibiotics for persistent nasal discharge (rhinosinusitis) in children. *The Cochrane Database of Systematic Reviews* 2002;(4):Art No CD001094.

79 Garbutt JM, Goldstein M, Gellman E, Shannon W, Littenberg B. A randomized, placebo-controlled trial of antimicrobial treatment for children with clinically diagnosed acute sinusitis. *Pediatrics* 2001;107:619–25.

80 Kristo A, Uhari M, Luotonen J, Ilkko E, Koivunen P, Alho OP. Cefuroxime axetil versus placebo for children with acute respiratory infection and imaging evidence of sinusitis: a randomized controlled trial. *Acta Paediatr* 2005;94:1208–13.

81 Pichichero ME. Evaluating the need, timing and best choice of antibiotic therapy for acute otitis media and tonsillopharyngitis infections in children. *Pediatr Infect Dis J* 2000;19(12, suppl):S131–40.

82 Del Mar CB, Glasziou PP, Spinks AB. Antibiotics for sore throat. *The Cochrane Database of Systematic Reviews* 2006;(4):Art No CD000023.

83 Centor RM, Whitherspoon JM, Dalton HP, Brody CE, Link K. The diagnosis of strep throat in adults in the emergency room. *Med Decis Making* 1981;1:239–46.

84 McIsaac WJ, White D, Tannenbaum D, Low DE. A clinical score to reduce unnecessary antibiotic use in patients with sore throat. *Can Med Assoc J* 1998;158:75–83.

85 Edmonson MB, Farwell KR. Relationship between the clinical likelihood of group A streptococcal pharyngitis and the sensitivity of a rapid antigen-detection test in a pediatric practice. *Pediatrics* 2005;115:280–5.

86 Gerber MA, Spadaccini LJ, Wright LL, Deutsch L, Kaplan EL. Twice-daily penicillin in the treatment of streptococcal pharyngitis. *Am J Dis Child* 1985;139:1145–8.

87 Pichichero ME. A review of evidence supporting the American Academy of Pediatrics recommendation for prescribing cephalosporin antibiotics for penicillin-allergic patients. *Pediatrics* 2005;115:1048–57.

88 Cohen R. Defining the optimum treatment regimen for azithromycin in acute tonsillopharyngitis. *Pediatr Infect Dis J* 2004;23(2, suppl):S129–34.

89 Casey JR, Pichichero ME. Meta-analysis of cephalosporin versus penicillin treatment of group A streptococcal tonsillopharyngitis in children. *Pediatrics* 2004;113:866–82.

90 Casey JR, Pichichero ME. Meta-analysis of short course antibiotic treatment for group A streptococcal tonsillopharyngitis. *Pediatr Infect Dis J* 2005;24:909–17.

91 Casey JR, Pichichero ME. Meta-analysis of cephalosporins versus penicillin for treatment of group A streptococcal tonsillopharyngitis in adults. *Clin Infect Dis* 2004;38:1526–34.

92 Pichichero ME. Pathogen shifts and changing cure rates for otitis media and tonsillopharyngitis. *Clin Pediatr (Phila)* 2006;45:493–502.

93 Roy M, Bailey B, Amre DK, Girodias JB, Bussieres JF, Gaudreault P. Dexamethasone for the treatment of sore throat in children with suspected infectious mononucleosis: a randomized, double-blind, placebo-controlled, clinical trial. *Arch Pediatr Adolesc Med* 2004;158:250–4.

94 Sirimanna KS, Madden GJ, Miles SM. The use of long-acting penicillin in the prophylaxis of recurrent tonsillitis. *J Otolaryngol* 1990;19:343–4.

95 Aksit S, Caglayan S, Dokucu G. Seasonal benzathine penicillin G prophylaxis for recurrent streptococcal pharyngitis in children. *Acta Paediatr Jpn* 1998;40:256–8.

96 Lildholdt T, Doessing H, Lyster M, Outzen KE. The natural history of recurrent acute tonsillitis and a clinical trial of azithromycin for antibiotic prophylaxis. *Clin Otolaryngol* 2003;28:371–3.

97 Mora R, Salami A, Mora F et al. Efficacy of cefpodoxime in the prophylaxis of recurrent pharyngotonsillitis. *Int J Pediatr Otorhinolaryngol* 2003;67(suppl 1):S225–8.

98 Paradise JL, Bluestone CD, Bachman RZ et al. Efficacy of tonsillectomy for recurrent throat infection in severely affected children: results of parallel randomized and non-randomized clinical trials. *N Engl J Med* 1984;310:674–83.

99 Paradise JL, Bluestone CD, Colborn DK, Bernard BS, Rockette HE, KursLasky M. Tonsillectomy and adenotonsillectomy for recurrent throat infection in moderately affected children. *Pediatrics* 2002;110:7–15.

100 van Staaij BK, van den Akker EH, Rovers MM, Hordijk GJ, Hoes AW, Schilder AG. Effectiveness of adenotonsillectomy in children with mild symptoms of throat infections or adenotonsillar hypertrophy: open, randomised controlled trial. *BMJ* 2004;7467:651.

101 Burton MJ, Towler B, Glasziou P. Tonsillectomy versus non-surgical treatment for chronic/recurrent acute tonsillitis. *The Cochrane Database of Systematic Reviews* 1999;(3):Art No CD001802.

102 Johnson D. Croup. *Clin Evid* 2005;14:310–27.

103 Russell K, Wiebe N, Saenz A et al. Glucocorticoids for croup. *The Cochrane Database of Systematic Reviews* 2004;(1):Art No CD001955.

104 Moore M, Little P. Humidified air inhalation for treating croup. *The Cochrane Database of Systematic Reviews* 2006;(3):Art No CD002870.

105 Fitzgerald D, Mellis C, Johnson M, Allen H, Cooper P, Van Asperen P. Nebulized budesonide is as effective as nebulized adrenaline in moderately severe croup. *Pediatrics* 1996;97:722–5.

106 Scolnik D, Coates AL, Stephens D, Da Silva Z, Lavine E, Schuh S. Controlled delivery of high vs low humidity vs mist therapy for croup in emergency departments: a randomized controlled trial. *JAMA* 2006;295:1274–80.

107 Nicholson KG, Wood JM, Zambon M. Influenza. *Lancet* 2003;362:1733–45.

108 Matheson NJ, Symmonds-Abrahams M, Sheikh A, Shepperd S, Harnden A. Neuraminidase inhibitors for preventing and treating influenza in children. *The Cochrane Database of Systematic Reviews* 2003;(3):Art No CD002744.

109 Crowcroft NS, Pebody RG. Recent developments in pertussis. *Lancet* 2006;367:1926–36.

110 Altunaiji S, Kukuruzovic R, Curtis N, Massie J. Antibiotics for whooping cough (pertussis). *The Cochrane Database of Systematic Reviews* 2005;(1):Art No CD004404.

111 Mahon BE, Rosenman MB, Kleiman MB. Maternal and infant use of erythromycin and other macrolide antibiotics as risk factors for infantile hypertrophic pyloric stenosis. *J Pediatr* 2001;139:380–4.

112 Halperin SA, Bortolussi R, Langley JM, Eastwood BJ, De Serres G. A randomized, placebo-controlled trial of erythromycin estolate chemoprophylaxis for household contacts of children with culture-positive *Bordetella pertussis* infection. *Pediatrics* 1999;104:e42.

113 Ward JI, Cherry JD, Chang SJ et al. Efficacy of an acellular pertussis vaccine among adolescents and adults. *N Engl J Med* 2005;53:1555–63.

114 Smyth RL, Openshaw PJ. Bronchiolitis. *Lancet* 2006;368:312–22.

115 Ventre K, Randolph A. Ribavirin for respiratory syncytial virus infection of the lower respiratory tract in infants and young children. *The Cochrane Database of Systematic Reviews* 2004;(4):Art No CD000181.

116 Gadomski AM, Bhasale AL. Bronchodilators for bronchiolitis. *The Cochrane Database of Systematic Reviews* 2006;(3):Art No CD001266.

117 Hartling L, Wiebe N, Russell K, Patel H, Klassen TP. Epinephrine for bronchiolitis. *The Cochrane Database of Systematic Reviews* 2004;(1):CD003123.

118 Patel H, Platt R, Lozano JM, Wang EEL. Glucocorticoids for acute viral bronchiolitis in infants and young children. *The Cochrane Database of Systematic Reviews* 2004;(3):Art No CD004878.

119 Perrotta C, Ortiz Z, Roque M. Chest physiotherapy for acute bronchiolitis in paediatric patients between 0 and 24 months old. *The Cochrane Database of Systematic Reviews* 2005;(2):Art No CD004873.

120 Ventre K, Haroon M, Davison C. Surfactant therapy for bronchiolitis in critically ill infants. *The Cochrane Database of Systematic Reviews* 2006;(3):Art No CD005150.

121 Bloomfield P, Dalton D, Karleka A, Kesson A, Duncan G, Isaacs D. Bacteraemia and antibiotic use in respiratory syncytial virus infections. *Arch Dis Child* 2004;89:363–7.

122 Field CM, Connolly JH, Murtagh G, Slattery CM, Turkington EE. Antibiotic treatment of epidemic bronchiolitis—a double-blind trial. *BMJ* 1966;5479:83–5.

123 Friis B, Andersen P, Brenoe E et al. Antibiotic treatment of pneumonia and bronchiolitis: a prospective randomised study. *Arch Dis Child* 1984;59:1038–45.

124 Wang EEL, Tang NK. Immunoglobulin for preventing respiratory syncytial virus infection. *The Cochrane Database of Systematic Reviews* 1999;(3):Art No CD001725.

125 The IMpactRSV Study Group. Palivizumab, a humanized respiratory syncytial virus monoclonal antibody, reduces hospitalization from respiratory syncytial virus infection in high-risk infants. *Pediatrics* 1998;102:531–7.

126 Meissner HC, Long SS, for the American Academy of Pediatrics Committee on Infectious Diseases and Committee on Fetus and Newborn. Revised indications for the use of palivizumab and respiratory syncytial virus immune globulin intravenous for the prevention of respiratory syncytial virus infections. *Pediatrics* 2003;112:1447–52.

127 Fahey T, Smucny J, Becker L, Glazier R. Antibiotics for acute bronchitis. *The Cochrane Database of Systematic Reviews* 2004;(4):Art No CD000245.

128 Spee-van der Wekke J, Meulmeester JF, Radder JJ, Verloove-Vanhorick SP. School absence and treatment in school children with respiratory symptoms in The Netherlands: data from the Child Health Monitoring System. *J Epidemiol Community Health* 1998;52:359–63.

129 Marchant JM, Morris P, Gaffney JT, Chang AB. Antibiotics for prolonged moist cough in children. *The Cochrane Database of Systematic Reviews* 2005;(4):Art No CD004822.

130 Darelid J, Lofgren S, Malmvall B-E. Erythromycin treatment is beneficial for longstanding *Moraxella catarrhalis*

associated cough in children. *Scand J Infect Dis* 1993;25:323–9.

131 Gottfarb P, Brauner A. Children with persistent cough—outcome with treatment and role of *Moraxella catarrhalis? Scand J Infect Dis* 1994;26:545–51.

132 Heath PT. Epidemiology and bacteriology of bacterial pneumonias. *Paediatr Respir Rev* 2000;1:4–7.

133 Isaacs D. Problems in determining the etiology of childhood pneumonia. *Pediatr Infect Dis J* 1989;8:l43–8.

134 Esposito S, Blasi F, Arosio C et al. Importance of acute *Mycoplasma pneumoniae* and *Chlamydia pneumoniae* infections in children with wheezing. *Eur Respir J* 2000;16:1142–6.

135 Esposito S, Bosis S, Cavagna R et al. Characteristics of *Streptococcus pneumoniae* and atypical bacterial infections in children 2–5 years of age with community-acquired pneumonia. *Clin Infect Dis* 2002;35:1345–52.

136 Black SB, Shinefield HR, Hansen J et al. Post-licensure evaluation of the effectiveness of seven valent pneumococcal conjugate vaccine. *Pediatr Infect Dis J* 2001;20:1105–7.

137 Darville T. *Chlamydia trachomatis* infections in neonates and young children. *Semin Pediatr Infect Dis* 2005;16:235–44.

138 Jeyaratnam D, Reid C, Kearns A, Klein J. Community associated MRSA: an alert to paediatricians. *Arch Dis Child* 2006;91:511–2.

139 Tablan OC, Anderson LJ, Besser R, Bridges C, Hajjeh R, for the CDC Healthcare Infection Control Practices Advisory Committee. Guidelines for preventing health-care-associated pneumonia, 2003. *MMWR Recomm Rep* 2004;53(RR-03):1–36.

140 Graham SM. Non-tuberculosis opportunistic infections and other lung diseases in HIV-infected infants and children. *Int J Tuberc Lung Dis* 2005;9:592–602.

141 Briel M, Bucher HC, Boscacci R, Furrer H. Adjunctive corticosteroids for *Pneumocystis jiroveci* pneumonia in patients with HIV-infection. *The Cochrane Database of Systematic Reviews* 2006;(3):Art No CD006150.

142 Sleasman JW, Hemenway C, Klein AS, Barrett DJ. Corticosteroids improve survival of children with AIDS and *Pneumocystis carinii* pneumonia. *Am J Dis Child* 1993;147:30–4.

143 Barone SR, Auito LT, Krilov LR. Increased survival of young infants with *Pneumocystis carinii* pneumonia and acute respiratory failure with early steroid administration. *Clin Infect Dis* 1994;19:212–3.

144 Johansen HK, Gotzsche PC. Amphotericin B lipid soluble formulations versus amphotericin B in cancer patients with neutropenia. *The Cochrane Database of Systematic Reviews* 2000;(3):Art No CD000969.

145 Shale DJ, Faux JA, Lane DJ. Trial of ketoconazole in non-invasive pulmonary aspergillosis. *Thorax* 1987;42:26–31.

146 Stevens DA, Lee JY, Schwartz HJ, Jerome D, Catanzaro A. A randomised trial of itraconazole in allergic bronchopulmonary aspergillosis. *N Engl J Med* 2000;342:756–62.

147 Wark PAB, Hensley MJ, Saltos N et al. Itraconazole reduces eosinophilic airway inflammation in allergic

bronchopulmonary aspergillosis. *Am J Respir Crit Care Med* 2001;163:A811.

148 Wark PAB, Gibson PG, Wilson AJ. Azoles for allergic bronchopulmonary aspergillosis associated with asthma. *The Cochrane Database of Systematic Reviews* 2004;(3):Art No CD001108.

149 Herbrecht R, Denning DW, Patterson TF et al. Voriconazole versus amphotericin B for primary therapy of invasive aspergillosis. *N Engl J Med* 2002;347:408–15.

150 Jørgensen KJ, Gøtzsche PC, Johansen HK. Voriconazole versus amphotericin B in cancer patients with neutropenia. *The Cochrane Database of Systematic Reviews* 2006;(1):Art No CD004707.

151 Bowden R, Chandrasekar P, White MH et al. A double-blind, randomized, controlled trial of amphotericin B colloidal dispersion versus amphotericin B for treatment of invasive aspergillosis in immunocompromised patients. *Clin Infect Dis* 2002;35:359–66.

152 Marr KA, Boeckh M, Carter RA, Kim HW, Corey L. Combination antifungal therapy for invasive aspergillosis. *Clin Infect Dis* 2004;39:797–802.

153 Kontoyiannis DP, Bodey GP, Mantzoros CS. Fluconazole vs. amphotericin B for the management of candidaemia in adults: a meta-analysis. *Mycoses* 2001;44:125–35.

154 Rex JH, Pappas PG, Karchmer AW et al. A randomized and blinded multicenter trial of high-dose fluconazole plus placebo versus fluconazole plus amphotericin B as therapy for candidemia and its consequences in non-neutropenic subjects. *Clin Infect Dis* 2003;36:1221–8.

155 Mora-Duarte J, Betts R, Rotstein C et al. Comparison of caspofungin and amphotericin B for invasive candidiasis. *N Engl J Med* 2002;347:2070–2.

156 Kullberg BJ, Sobel JD, Ruhnke M et al. Voriconazole versus a regimen of amphotericin B followed by fluconazole for candidaemia in non-neutropenic patients: a randomised non-inferiority trial. *Lancet* 2005;366:1435–42.

157 Nguyen MH, Peacock JE, Jr, Morris AJ et al. The changing face of candidemia: emergence of non-*Candida albicans* species and antifungal resistance. *Am J Med* 1996;100:617–23.

158 Jacobson SJ, Griffiths K, Diamond S et al. A randomized controlled trial of penicillin vs clindamycin for the treatment of aspiration pneumonia in children. *Arch Pediatr Adolesc Med* 1997;151:701–4.

159 Allewelt M, Schuler P, Bolcskei PL et al. Ampicillin+sulbactam vs clindamycin±cephalosporin for the treatment of aspiration pneumonia and primary lung abscess. *Clin Microbiol Infect* 2004;10:163–70.

160 Brook I. Anaerobic pulmonary infections in children. *Pediatr Emerg Care* 2004;20:636–40.

161 Levison ME, Mangura CT, Lorber B et al. Clindamycin compared with penicillin for the treatment of anaerobic lung abscess. *Ann Intern Med* 1983;98:466–71.

162 Lewis KT, Bukstein DA. Parapneumonic empyema in children: diagnosis and management. *Am Fam Physician* 1992;46:1443–55.

163 Chonmaitree T, Powell KR. Parapneumonic pleural effusion and empyema in children: review of a 19-year experience, 1962–1980. *Clin Pediatr (Phila)* 1983;22:414–9.

164 Alkrinawi S, Chernick V. Pleural fluid in hospitalized pediatric patients. *Clin Pediatr (Phila)* 1996;35:5–9.

165 Nelson JD. Pleural empyema. *Pediatr Infect Dis* 1985;4(3, suppl):S31–3.

166 Narita M, Tanaka H. Two distinct patterns of pleural effusions caused by *Mycoplasma pneumoniae* infection. *Pediatr Infect Dis J* 2004;23:1069.

167 Heffner JE, Brown LK, Barbieri C, DeLeo JM. Pleural fluid chemical analysis in parapneumonic effusions: a meta-analysis. *Am J Respir Crit Care Med* 1995;151:1700–8.

168 Palacios GC, Gonzalez SN, Perez FL, Cuevas SF, Solorzano SF. Cefuroxime vs a dicloxacillin/chloramphenicol combination for the treatment of parapneumonic pleural effusion and empyema in children. *Pulm Pharmacol Ther* 2002;15:17–23.

169 Avansino JR, Goldman B, Sawin RS, Flum DR. Primary operative versus non-operative therapy for pediatric empyema: a meta-analysis. *Pediatrics* 2005;115:1652–9.

170 Coote N, Kay E. Surgical versus non-surgical management of pleural empyema. *The Cochrane Database of Systematic Reviews* 2005;(4):Art No CD001956.

171 Wait MA, Sharma S, Hohn J, Dal-Nogare A. A randomized trial of empyema therapy. *Chest* 1997;111:1548–51.

172 Cameron R, Davies HR. Intra-pleural fibrinolytic therapy versus conservative management in the treatment of parapneumonic effusions and empyema. *The Cochrane Database of Systematic Reviews* 2004;(2):Art No CD002312.

173 Maskell NA, Davies CW, Nunn AJ et al. U.K. Controlled trial of intrapleural streptokinase for pleural infection. *N Engl J Med* 2005;352:865–74.

174 Evans JT, Green JD, Carlin PE, Barrett LO. Meta-analysis of antibiotics in tube thoracostomy. *Am Surg* 1995;61:215–9.

175 Fallon WF, Jr, Wears RL. Prophylactic antibiotics for the prevention of infectious complications including empyema following tube thoracostomy for trauma: results of meta-analysis. *J Trauma* 1992;33:110–6.

176 Dagli E. Noncystic fibrosis bronchiectasis. *Paediatr Respir Rev* 2000;1:64–70.

177 Selvadurai H. Investigation and management of suppurative cough in pre-school children. *Paediatr Respir Rev* 2006;7:15–20.

178 Evans DJ, Bara AI, Greenstone M. Prolonged antibiotics for purulent bronchiectasis. *The Cochrane Database of Systematic Reviews* 2003;(4):Art No CD001392.

179 Barker AF, Couch L, Fiel SB et al. Tobramycin solution for inhalation reduces sputum *Pseudomonas aeruginosa* density in bronchiectasis. *Am J Respir Crit Care Med* 2000;162:481–5.

180 Drobnic ME, Sune P, Montoro JB, Ferrer A, Orriols R. Inhaled tobramycin in non-cystic fibrosis patients with bronchiectasis and chronic bronchial infection with *Pseudomonas aeruginosa*. *Ann Pharmacother* 2005;39:39–44.

181 van der Schans C, Prasad A, Main E. Chest physiotherapy compared to no chest physiotherapy for cystic fibrosis. *The Cochrane Database of Systematic Reviews* 2000;(2):Art No CD001401.

182 Thompson CS, Harrison S, Ashley J, Day K, Smith DL. Randomised crossover study of the Flutter device and the active cycle of breathing technique in non-cystic fibrosis bronchiectasis. *Thorax* 2002;57:446–8.

183 Newall C, Stockley RA, Hill SL. Exercise training and inspiratory muscle training in patients with bronchiectasis. *Thorax* 2005;60:943–8.

184 Smyth A, Walters S. Prophylactic anti-staphylococcal antibiotics for cystic fibrosis. *The Cochrane Database of Systematic Reviews* 2003;(3):Art No CD001912.

185 Wood DM, Smyth AR. Antibiotic strategies for eradicating *Pseudomonas aeruginosa* in people with cystic fibrosis. *The Cochrane Database of Systematic Reviews* 2006;(1):Art No CD004197.

186 Valerius NH, Koch C, Hoiby N. Prevention of chronic *Pseudomonas aeruginosa* colonisation in cystic fibrosis by early treatment. *Lancet* 1991;338:725–6.

187 Breen L, Aswani N. Elective versus symptomatic intravenous antibiotic therapy for cystic fibrosis. *The Cochrane Database of Systematic Reviews* 2001;(4):Art No CD002767.

188 Mukhopadhyay S, Singh M, Cater JI, Ogston S, Franklin M, Olver RE. Nebulised antipseudomonal antibiotic therapy in cystic fibrosis: a meta-analysis of benefits and risks. *Thorax* 1996;51:364–8.

189 Mukhopadhyay S, Singh M, Ogston S, Ryan G, Smyth R. Systematic review of nebulized antibiotics in cystic fibrosis: evolution of protocol. *J R Soc Med* 1998;91(suppl 34): 25–9.

190 Ryan G, Mukhopadhyay S, Singh M. Nebulised antipseudomonal antibiotics for cystic fibrosis. *The Cochrane Database of Systematic Reviews* 2003;(3):Art No CD001021.

191 Elphick HE, Tan A. Single versus combination intravenous antibiotic therapy for people with cystic fibrosis. *The Cochrane Database of Systematic Reviews* 2005;(2):Art No CD002007.

192 Isles A, Maclusky I, Corey M et al. *Pseudomonas cepacia* infection in cystic fibrosis: an emerging problem. *J Pediatr* 1984;104:206–10.

193 Frangolias DD, Mahenthiralingam E, Rae S et al. *Burkholderia cepacia* in cystic fibrosis: variable disease course. *Am J Respir Crit Care Med* 1999;160:1572–7.

194 Muhdi K, Edenborough FP, Gumery L et al. Outcome for patients colonised with *Burkholderia cepacia* in a Birmingham adult cystic fibrosis clinic and the end of an epidemic. *Thorax* 1996;51:374–7.

195 Tablan OC, Martone WJ, Doershuk CF et al. Colonization of the respiratory tract with *Pseudomonas cepacia* in cystic fibrosis: risk factors and outcomes. *Chest* 1987;91:527–32.

196 Southern KW, Barker PM, Solis A. Macrolide antibiotics for cystic fibrosis. *The Cochrane Database of Systematic Reviews* 2003;(3):Art No CD002203.

197 Bradley J, Moran F. Physical training for cystic fibrosis. *The Cochrane Database of Systematic Reviews* 2002;(2):Art No CD002768.

198 Wark PAB, McDonald V, Jones AP. Nebulised hypertonic saline for cystic fibrosis. *The Cochrane Database of Systematic Reviews* 2005;(3):Art No CD001506.

199 Elkins MR, Robinson M, Rose BR et al. A controlled trial of long-term inhaled hypertonic saline in patients with cystic fibrosis. *N Engl J Med* 2006;354:229–40.

200 Donaldson SH, Bennett WD, Zeman KL et al. Mucus clearance and lung function in cystic fibrosis with hypertonic saline. *N Engl J Med* 2006;354:241–50.

201 Jones AP, Wallis CE, Kearney CE. Recombinant human deoxyribonuclease for cystic fibrosis. *The Cochrane Database of Systematic Reviews* 2003;(3):Art No CD001127.

202 Suri R, Metcalfe C, Lees B et al. Comparison of hypertonic saline and alternate-day or daily recombinant human deoxyribonuclease in children with cystic fibrosis: a randomised trial. *Lancet* 2001;358:1316–21.

203 Ballmann M, von der Hardt H. Hypertonic saline and recombinant human DNase: a randomised cross-over pilot study in patients with cystic fibrosis. *J Cystic Fibrosis* 2002;1: 35–7.

204 Zhong N, Zeng G. What we have learnt from SARS epidemics in China. *BMJ* 2006;333:389–91.

205 Mellis C. Pulmonary tuberculosis. In: Isaacs D, Moxon ER (eds.), *A Practical Approach to Pediatric Infections.* New York: Churchill Livingstone, 1996:157–66.

206 Rose DN, Schechter CB, Adler JJ. Interpretation of the tuberculin skin test. *J Gen Intern Med* 1995;10:635–42.

207 American Academy of Pediatrics. Tuberculosis. In: Pickering LK (ed.), *Red Book: 2003 Report of the Committee on Infectious Diseases*, 26th edn. Elk Grove Village, IL: American Academy of Pediatrics , 2003:642–60.

208 Wang L, Turner MO, Elwood RK, Schulzer M, FitzGerald JM. A meta-analysis of the effect of Bacille Calmette Guerin vaccination on tuberculin skin test measurements. *Thorax* 2002;57:804–9.

209 Pai M, Riley LW, Colford JM, Jr. Interferon-gamma assays in the immunodiagnosis of tuberculosis: a systematic review. *Lancet Infect Dis* 2004;4:761–76.

210 Mazurek GH, Jereb J, Lobue P et al. Guidelines for using the quantiferon-TB Gold test for detecting *Mycobacterium tuberculosis* infection, United States. *MMWR* 2005;54:49–55.

211 Pai M, Flores LL, Pai N, Hubbard A, Riley LW, Colford JM, Jr. Diagnostic accuracy of nucleic acid amplification tests for tuberculous meningitis: a systematic review and meta-analysis. *Lancet Infect Dis* 2003;3:633–43.

212 Sarmiento OL, Weigle KA, Alexander J, Weber DJ, Miller WC. Assessment by meta-analysis of PCR for diagnosis of smear-negative pulmonary tuberculosis. *J Clin Microbiol* 2003;41:3233–40.

213 Yam WC, Yuen KY, Kam SY et al. Diagnostic application of genotypic identification of mycobacteria. *J Med Microbiol* 2006;55:529–36.

214 Cavusoglu C, Turhan A, Akinci P, Soyler I. Evaluation of the Genotype MTBDR assay for rapid detection of rifampin and isoniazid resistance in *Mycobacterium tuberculosis* isolates. *J Clin Microbiol* 2006;44:2338–42.

215 Smieja MJ, Marchetti CA, Cook DJ, Smaill FM. Isoniazid for preventing tuberculosis in non-HIV infected persons. *The Cochrane Database of Systematic Reviews* 1999;(1):Art No CD001363.

216 British Thoracic Society. Chemotherapy and management of tuberculosis in the United Kingdom: recommendations 1998. *Thorax* 1998;53:536–48.

217 Woldehanna S, Volmink J. Treatment of latent tuberculosis infection in HIV infected persons. *The Cochrane Database of Systematic Reviews* 2004;(1):Art No CD000171.

218 Gelband H. Regimens of less than six months for treating tuberculosis. *The Cochrane Database of Systematic Reviews* 1999;(4):Art No CD001362.

219 Mwandumba HC, Squire SB. Fully intermittent dosing with drugs for treating tuberculosis in adults. *The Cochrane Database of Systematic Reviews* 2001;(4):Art No CD000970.

220 Hong Kong Chest Service/British Medical Research Council. Controlled trial of four thrice weekly regimens and a daily regimen all given for 6 months for pulmonary tuberculosis. *Lancet* 1981;1:171–4.

221 Te Water Naude JM, Donald PR, Hussey GD et al. Twice weekly vs. daily chemotherapy for childhood tuberculosis. *Pediatr Infect Dis J* 2000;19:405–10.

222 Kumar L, Dhand R, Singhi PD, Rao KL, Katariya S. A randomized trial of fully intermittent vs. daily followed by intermittent short course chemotherapy for childhood tuberculosis. *Pediatr Infect Dis J* 1990;9:802–6.

223 van Loenhout-Rooyackers JH, Laheij RJ, Richter C, Verbeek AL. Shortening the duration of treatment for cervical tuberculous lymphadenitis. *Eur Respir J* 2000;15:192–5.

224 Prasad K, Volmink J, Menon GR. Steroids for treating tuberculous meningitis. *The Cochrane Database of Systematic Reviews* 2000;(3):Art No CD002244.

225 Matchaba PT, Volmink J. Steroids for treating tuberculous pleurisy. *The Cochrane Database of Systematic Reviews* 2000;(1):Art No CD001876.

226 Volmink J, Garner P. Directly observed therapy for treating tuberculosis. *The Cochrane Database of Systematic Reviews* 2003;(1):Art No CD003343.

227 Colditz GA, Berkey CS, Mosteller F et al. The efficacy of bacillus Calmette-Guerin vaccination of newborns and infants in the prevention of tuberculosis: meta-analyses of the published literature. *Pediatrics* 1995;96:29–35.

228 Sterne JA, Rodrigues LC, Guedes IN. Does the efficacy of BCG decline with time since vaccination? *Int J Tuberc Lung Dis* 1998;2:200–7.

229 Newport MJ, Huxley CM, Huston C et al. A mutation in the interferon-gamma-receptor gene and susceptibility to mycobacterial infection. *N Engl J Med* 1996;335:1941–9.

230 Dupuis S, Doffinger R, Picard C et al. Human interferon gamma-mediated immunity is a genetically controlled continuous trait that determines the outcome of mycobacterial invasion. *Immunol Rev* 2000;178:129–37.

231 Dorman SE, Picard C, Lammas D et al. Clinical features of dominant and recessive interferon gamma receptor 1 deficiencies. *Lancet* 2004;364:2113–21.

232 Shafran SD, Singer J, Zarowny DP et al, for the Canadian HIV Trials Network Protocol 010 Study Group. A comparison of two regimens for the treatment of *Mycobacterium avium* complex bacteremia in AIDS: rifabutin, ethambutol, and clarithromycin versus rifampin, ethambutol, clofazimine, and ciprofloxacin. *N Engl J Med* 1996;335:377–83.

233 Benson CA, Williams PL, Currier JS et al. A prospective, randomized trial examining the efficacy and safety of clarithromycin in combination with ethambutol, rifabutin, or both for the treatment of disseminated *Mycobacterium avium* complex disease in persons with acquired immunodeficiency syndrome. *Clin Infect Dis* 2003;37:1234–43.

234 Research Committee of the British Thoracic Society. First randomised trial of treatments for pulmonary disease caused by *M. avium* intracellulare, *M. malmoense*, and *M. xenopi* in HIV negative patients: rifampicin, ethambutol and isoniazid versus rifampicin and ethambutol. *Thorax* 2001;56: 167–72.

235 Griffith DE, Brown BA, Girard WM, Griffith BE, Couch LA, Wallace RJ, Jr. Azithromycin-containing regimens for treatment of *Mycobacterium avium* complex lung disease. *Clin Infect Dis* 2001;32:1547–53.

236 Lam PK, Griffith DE, Aksamit TR et al. Factors related to response to intermittent treatment of *Mycobacterium avium* complex lung disease. *Am J Respir Crit Care Med* 2006;173:1283–9.

237 Therapeutic Guidelines Ltd. Mycobacterial infections. In: *Therapeutic Guidelines: Antibiotic*, 13th edn. Melbourne: Therapeutic Guidelines Ltd, 2006:158–69.

CHAPTER 13

Sexually transmitted and genital infections

13.1 Balanitis and balanoposthitis

Balanitis (inflammation of the glans penis), with or without posthitis (inflammation of the prepuce), is reported in 6% of uncircumcised and 3% of circumcised males.[1] Most cases are mild and recover without specific treatment. *Streptococcus pyogenes* is the most commonly reported organism cultured from skin swabs taken when the foreskin is retracted.[2] Infection causes pain, redness, and swelling, and may be associated with perianal cellulitis or other manifestations of group A streptococcal infection such as sore throat, rash, and fever. Toxic shock syndrome was reported in association with one case of staphylococcal balanitis.[3] In adults, bacterial causes are less common than *Candida albicans*.

If *S. pyogenes* is cultured, use:

phenoxymethylpenicillin 10 mg/kg (max 500 mg) orally, 6-hourly

Candidal balanitis occurs typically in sexually active, uncircumcised males, causing itchy, red, maculopapular lesions of the glans, with circumferential scale and satellite lesions. A combination of a topical antifungal and hydrocortisone is usually effective.

13.2 Vulvovaginitis

Vulvitis is local irritation of the vulva, and vaginitis is erythema and inflammation of the vaginal mucosa, usually with a vaginal discharge.[4] Vulvovaginitis is common in prepubertal girls[4] and presents with redness, local irritation, dysuria, and often vaginal discharge. It is often stated that poor hygiene is a cause of

The antibiotics and doses recommended in this chapter are based on those in *Therapeutic Guidelines: Antibiotic*, 13th edn, Therapeutic Guidelines Ltd, Melbourne, 2006.

Box 13.1 Causes of vulvovaginitis.

- Non-specific
- Worms
- Foreign body
- Group A streptococcus
- Group B streptococcus
- Gonorrhoea
- Chlamydia
- Candidiasis
- Trichomonas
- Bacterial vaginosis

vulvovaginitis, and in one study, poor hygiene and pinworms were the major reported cause.[5] The lack of a control group casts doubt on this claim, and controlled studies have not found any increase in poor hygiene in patients compared with controls.[6,7] Similarly, although bubble baths are often blamed,[8] they were used more commonly by controls than patients in one controlled study.[6] These examples illustrate the importance of including a control group before talking of associations as being risk factors for a disease or causes of the disease.

Potentially pathogenic organisms can be grown often from the vagina of girls with vulvovaginitis, and are blamed often.[8,9] Culturing organisms does not mean they are causing the problem, however, since normal girls can carry most of the same organisms.[6,7] When a controlled study was performed, potential pathogens were no more common in girls with vulvovaginitis than in controls.[6] One uncontrolled study found *S. pyogenes* in cultures from 21% of girls with vulvovaginitis.[9]

A number of associations with and possible causes of vulvovaginitis are given in Box 13.1.

Non-specific vulvovaginitis

We recommend that non-specific vulvovaginitis, with no cause found, should not be treated with specific agents, but only symptomatically. In a study of 50 girls with vulvovaginitis who presented to specialist pediatric services, only 10 had a probable infectious cause found.[6]

Vulvovaginitis due to foreign body

Foreign body characteristically results in foul-smelling discharge and requires an examination under anesthetic.[4,5]

Vulvovaginitis due to Enterobius (pinworms or threadworms)

Worm infestation with Enterobius (pinworms or threadworms) can cause a vulvovaginitis characterized by itch, including nighttime itch, redness, and scanty or no vaginal discharge.[9] The diagnosis can be confirmed by placing sticky tape, to which the eggs adhere, on the anal mucosa. If confirmed or strongly suspected, we recommend:

mebendazole 100 mg (child ≤10 kg: 50 mg) orally, as a single dose OR
pyrantel 10 mg/kg (max 750 mg) orally, as a single dose

Group A streptococcus vulvovaginitis

Group A streptococcus can cause vulvovaginitis alone, or with perianal cellulitis, and/or with other manifestations of streptococcal infection, such as rash, fever, or sore throat.[9,10] There is even one report of glomerulonephritis in association with group A streptococcal vulvovaginitis.[11] The peak age of group A streptococcal vulvovaginitis is around 5 years.[9,10] Erythema is usually prominent.[9,10]

If *S. pyogenes* is cultured, use:

phenoxymethylpenicillin 10 mg/kg (max 500 mg) orally, 6-hourly

Group B streptococcus (GBS) vulvovaginitis

Colonization with GBS is common, usually asymptomatic, and does not correlate with sexual activity.[12] A retrospective study of adolescent girls and young women who grew a pure growth of GBS found that 12 of 13 had purulent vaginal discharge and concluded that they had GBS vulvovaginitis.[13] However, their swabs were taken because of symptoms, and the presence of GBS, which colonizes up to 30% of normal women, may have been coincidental and not causal. Most au-

thorities would, however, treat an adolescent with purulent vaginal discharge who grew GBS with penicillin.

We recommend:

phenoxymethylpenicillin 10 mg/kg (max 500 mg) orally, 6-hourly

Neisseria gonorrhoeae vaginal infection

Vaginal infection with *N. gonorrhoeae* is almost always symptomatic and results in a purulent green vaginal discharge, at least when it is a result of sexual abuse.[14,15] Beyond the neonatal period, gonorrhea is always sexually acquired. In prepubertal girls it is acquired through child sexual abuse, and isolation of the organism is an absolute indication to make enquiries about child sexual abuse.[16] The possibility of sexual abuse should be considered in any case for gonorrhea in a child of any age, from the neonatal period until adolescence.

The diagnosis of gonococcal infection can be suspected from gram stain and must be confirmed by culture of the organism.[16] Although non-culture techniques such as polymerase chain reaction (PCR) are sensitive and specific,[17] they are no better than culture, which is rapid and definitive. PCR for *N. gonorrhoeae* should be used on only urogenital specimens, and never on eye or throat specimens, when non-pathogenic Neisseriae can cause false-positive results. Where it is critical not to get false positives, as in likely medicolegal cases, culture is the only acceptable test.[18] It is recommended to examine and take swabs from the oropharynx and anus as additional potential areas of infection.

Penicillin-resistance of *N. gonorrhoeae* is common, and eradication of unsuspected pharyngeal or anorectal infection is important.

Question | For the treatment of children with uncomplicated gonorrhea, is one antibiotic compared with others more effective?

Literature review | We found 23 RCTs of ceftriaxone, 9 RCTs and a review[19] of ciprofloxacin, 7 RCTs of cefixime, 4 RCTs of ofloxacin, 3 RCTs of cefotaxime, and 3 RCTs of azithromycin.

A single dose of IM ceftriaxone has been studied most widely, and in 23 RCTs was 98–100% effective in treating uncomplicated gonorrhea and eradicating the organism, even when *N. gonorrhoeae* is penicillin-resistant. Ceftriaxone is the gold standard therapy to which other antibiotics are compared.

A single dose of IM cefotaxime was no different from IM ceftriaxone in three studies. Oral ciprofloxacin was found in a review to be effective,[19] but a study from the Philippines reported 32% treatment failures when treating female sex workers with oral ciprofloxacin compared with 4% with oral cefixime, because of the emergence of ciprofloxacin resistance.[20] Resistance to quinolones will also affect treatment with ofloxacin or gatifloxacin, but in the absence of quinolone resistance, ciprofloxacin, ofloxacin, and gatifloxacin have all been shown to be as effective as ceftriaxone. Oral cefixime[20–23] and oral azithromycin[24–26] are both >95% effective in curing uncomplicated gonorrhea, including penicillin-resistant strains and in resource-poor settings.

We recommend:

ceftriaxone ≤45 kg: 125 mg, >45 kg: 250 mg IM, as a single dose OR
cefotaxime 25 mg/kg (max 1 g) IM, as a single dose OR
cefixime 20 mg/kg (max 800 mg) orally, as a single dose OR
azithromycin 20 mg/kg (max 1 g) orally, as a single dose

Because of increasing resistance, oral ciprofloxacin and other quinolones are no longer recommended, unless a sensitive strain has been identified.

The above treatment is ineffective against *Chlamydia*, with the exception of azithromycin (see below).[27] We recommend excluding *Chlamydia* infection and, if it is not possible to exclude it, giving empiric treatment for *Chlamydia* infection (see below).

Chlamydia trachomatis vulvovaginitis

C. trachomatis infection is sexually acquired. Infection is often asymptomatic,[27] but the detection of *C. trachomatis* in a child with vulvovaginitis is an indication for treatment and, if the child is prepubertal, for child sexual abuse enquiries and possible action.[16]

C. trachomatis may be detected by non-culture techniques such as PCR or LCR (ligase chain reaction), which are highly sensitive, can be used on urine as well as genital secretions,[17,18,28] and may thus be valuable in non-invasive screening for *Chlamydia*.[28] LCR and PCR are more often positive than culture for *Chlamydia*, which means they are either more sensitive or detecting false positives (or both).[17,18,28] However, none

of the non-culture tests is approved or recommended by the manufacturers for rectogenital specimens from children.[18] In addition to medical implications, the identification of *Chlamydia*, especially in a young child, also has legal implications. Because of the legal implications, the test needs to have the highest specificity, which is more important than sensitivity in this situation. Data on the specificity of these tests in prepubertal children are insufficient to permit their use at this time. Tests that are appropriate for screening a sexually active adult in a STD (sexually transmitted disease) clinic may not be appropriate for evaluating a child victim of suspected sexual abuse. Although missing possible sexual abuse is a major concern, the ramifications of a false-positive test for an STD, which can lead to erroneous accusations of sexual abuse, must also be considered.[18]

If *Chlamydia* is identified by PCR or LCR on vaginal secretions of a girl with vulvovaginitis, we recommend treatment, but also recommend performing culture to confirm *Chlamydia* infection if the child is prepubertal or sexual abuse is suspected. Azithromycin is >95% effective, even in a resource-poor setting,[25] and doxycycline is >90%.[25] We recommend:

azithromycin 20 mg/kg (max 1 g) orally, as a single dose OR
doxycycline (>8 years): 2.5 mg/kg (max 100 mg) orally, 12-hourly for 7 days

Sexual partners should be traced and treated, if possible.

Vulvovaginal candidiasis

Vulvovaginal candidiasis is rare in prepubertal girls with vulvovaginitis,[6–9] but becomes increasingly common thereafter. Up to 75% of women of child-bearing age develop acute vulvovaginal candidiasis, which becomes chronic in 5–10%.[29–32]

Effective topical preparations include nystatin and azoles (clotrimazole, econazole, miconazole), which are comparable in efficacy.[33] Topical clotrimazole is 95% effective in treating acute candidal vulvovaginitis.[34] Oral itraconazole is as effective as topical clotrimazole, but fluconazole is somewhat less effective.[34] In an RCT which looked at recurrence rates after 6 months, the most successful treatment with a cure rate of 81% was miconazole vaginal cream with oral nystatin.[35] Occasionally, topical therapy may itself cause irritation. Nystatin, although marginally less effective, is generally better tolerated than the imidazoles.[33] We recommend:

topical clotrimazole vaginal cream or pessary OR
topical nystatin vaginal cream or pessary

The use of preparations that also contain topical steroids can relieve irritation.

If the patient is intolerant of topical therapy or would prefer to use oral therapy, or infection recurs and the patient is not pregnant, 1-day treatment with either fluconazole[34] or itraconazole[36] is effective. We recommend:

fluconazole 4 mg/kg (max 150 mg) orally, as a single dose OR
itraconazole 5 mg/kg (max 200 mg) orally 12-hourly for 1 day (best taken with an acid drink such as Coca Cola to improve absorption)

If the initial treatment fails, we recommend reviewing the diagnosis and seeking specialist advice.

Symptomatic sexual partners (usually balanitis in the uncircumcised male) should be treated with a topical antifungal plus a topical corticosteroid (see Section 13.1, p. 211).

Trichomonas vulvovaginitis

Trichomoniasis is an STD of post-menarchal girls and women.[37] Symptomatic women complain of vaginal discharge, pruritus, and irritation. Signs of infection include pale yellow to gray-green vaginal discharge (42%), fishy or musty odor (50%), and edema or erythema (22–37%).[37] The discharge is classically described as frothy, but it is actually frothy in only about 10% of patients.[37] Colpitis macularis (strawberry cervix) is a specific clinical sign for this infection, but is detected with reliability only by colposcopy and rarely during routine examination. Other complaints may include dysuria and lower abdominal pain. Most adolescents and women with trichomoniasis also have bacterial vaginosis.[37,38] Nearly half of all women with *Trichomonas vaginalis* are asymptomatic.[37]

Male partners are usually asymptomatic, but can develop urethritis, and rarely epidydimitis or prostatitis.[37] Empiric treatment of partners is indicated. Investigation for other sexually transmitted infections should be considered. Metronidazole and tinidazole are both effective in >95% of cases.[37] We recommend:

metronidazole 50 mg/kg (max 2 g) orally, as a single dose OR
tinidazole 50 mg/kg (max 2 g) orally, as a single dose

In one study, 20 patients with clinically refractory trichomoniasis (failure to respond to therapy with oral metronidazole using at least 500 mg twice a day for 7 days) were treated with high doses of oral and vaginal tinidazole (2–3 g orally plus 1–1.5 g intravaginally for 14 days). The cure rate was 92% and no patients discontinued therapy due to side effects.[39]

Bacterial vaginosis

Bacterial vaginosis is a condition of sexually active adolescents and women, characterized by changes in vaginal flora. The clinical diagnosis requires three of the following: a white, non-inflammatory, vaginal discharge; vaginal pH >4.5; a fishy odor before or after adding 10% hydrogen peroxide (the "whiff test"); presence of "clue cells" on microscopy of vaginal secretions (squamous epithelial cells covered with bacteria resulting in ragged edges).[40–42] Bacterial vaginosis in pregnancy is associated with preterm birth,[41] but meta-analyses of trials of treating bacterial vaginosis with antibiotics have consistently failed to show a reduction in preterm births.[42]

Metronidazole vaginal gel is as effective as oral metronidazole and is associated with fewer gastrointestinal complaints.[43] We recommend:

metronidazole 0.75% gel intravaginally, once daily for 5 days

13.3 Epididymo-orchitis

Acute epididymo-orchitis can cause swelling, redness, and pain in the testis and/or epididymis. It is rare in young children[44,45] and needs to be distinguished clinically from testicular torsion.[46] Boys with epididymo-orchitis are more likely to have a tender epididymis and some scrotal swelling and redness without pain, whereas boys with torsion are more likely to have a tender testicle and an absent cremasteric reflex.[46] High-resolution ultrasound with an experienced investigator is able to exclude torsion reliably,[45] so that routine surgical exploration is seldom necessary.

Testicular swelling can also occur with edema due to nephrotic syndrome, due to malignancy, and as a manifestation of Henoch–Schonlein purpura.

Epididymo-orchitis can occur in infancy and in boys aged 10–15 years.[44,45] It is rare to find a cause, although there may be underlying urinary tract problems and urine cultures occasionally grow a pathogen, such as *Escherichia coli*. Urinalysis and urine culture should be performed on all children with acute epididymo-orchitis.[45]

In adolescents and young men, acute epididymo-orchitis is usually either a complication of genitourinary infection with enteric Gram-negative bacteria or a complication of a sexually transmitted urethral infection, such as *C. trachomatis*[47,48] or *N. gonorrhoeae*.[47] Rarely, it occurs by hematogenous spread as a complication of a systemic infection. Genitourinary tuberculosis may present as epididymo-orchitis, with scrotal pain, swelling, and often sinuses.[49]

For mild to moderate infection from a probable urinary tract source, we recommend:

> **cephalexin 12.5 mg/kg (max 500 mg) orally, 12-hourly for 14 days** OR
> **trimethoprim 4 mg/kg (max 150 mg) orally, 12-hourly for 14 days**

If resistance to the above drugs is suspected or proven, we recommend:

> **norfloxacin 10 mg/kg (max 400 mg) orally, 12-hourly for 14 days**

If infection is thought to be sexually acquired, *C. trachomatis* (D–K serovars) or *N. gonorrhoeae* are usually involved, although in men who are the insertive partner during anal intercourse, epididymitis can be caused by sexually transmitted enteric organisms (e.g., *E. coli*). We recommend taking appropriate specimens (urethral exudate or swab or first-void urine) before starting empiric therapy with:

> **ceftriaxone ≤45 kg: 125 mg, >45 kg: 250 mg IM, as a single dose** PLUS EITHER
> **doxycycline 2.5 mg/kg (max 100 mg) orally, 12-hourly for 14 days** OR
> **roxithromycin 4 mg/kg (max 150 mg) orally, 12-hourly for 14 days**

If adherence to 2 weeks of doxycycline or roxithromycin is unlikely, there are theoretical grounds for using azithromycin 25 mg/kg (max 1 g) orally on days 1 and 8, although no clinical trial has assessed this.

13.4 *Neisseria gonorrhoeae* infections

Infection with *N. gonorrhoeae*[50] can occur at the following ages:
· *Neonatal*: Usually ophthalmic, but can cause vaginitis, scalp abscess, or disseminated bacteremic disease involving joints and meninges
· *Prepubertal* (usually due to child sexual abuse): Vaginitis, less commonly pelvic inflammatory disease (PID), hepatitis, rarely anorectal, and tonsillopharyngeal
· *Sexually active adolescents*: Girls may be asymptomatic or develop urethritis, endocervicitis, and salpingitis, and boys usually develop symptomatic urethritis. Rectal and pharyngeal infections are often asymptomatic.

For diagnosis and rationale for treatment, see p. 212. For uncomplicated infection, we recommend:

> **ceftriaxone ≤45 kg: 125 mg, >45 kg: 250 mg IM, as a single dose** OR
> **cefotaxime 25 mg/kg (max 1 g) IM, as a single dose** OR
> **cefixime 20 mg/kg (max 800 mg) orally, as a single dose** OR
> **azithromycin 20 mg/kg (max 1 g) orally, as a single dose**

13.5 Syphilis

Congenital syphilis can cause still birth, preterm birth, hydrops fetalis, and intrauterine growth retardation. Other manifestations at birth or developing in early infancy include bullous rash, anemia, hepatosplenomegaly, edema, snuffles, and osteitis presenting as pseudoparalysis of a limb or limbs. Late manifestations of untreated congenital syphilis include Hutchinson triad of Hutchinson teeth (notched central incisor), sensorineural deafness, and interstitial keratitis, and also saddle nose, rhagades (fissured skin around the mouth), anterior shin bowing, and Clutton joints (symmetric painless swelling of the knees).[51,52]

Acquired primary syphilis results in chancres, which are painless indurated ulcers of the mucous membranes or skin at the site of infection, usually the genitalia.[53]

Secondary syphilis, which develops 1–2 months later, causes a generalized maculopapular rash usually involving palms and soles, papular lesions called condyloma lata in moist areas around the vulva or anus, and regional or generalized lymphadenopathy. The patient may have systemic manifestations such as fever, malaise, arthralgia, sore throat, and splenomegaly.[53]

Disease then becomes latent, with serologic evidence of infection but no clinical manifestations, although the symptoms of secondary syphilis may recur. Late syphilis can be tertiary, with gumma formation and aortitis from cardiovascular syphilis, or can cause neurosyphilis, which is particularly likely in association with human immunodeficiency virus (HIV) infection.[53]

The diagnosis of syphilis is usually made serologically,[53,54] although dark ground microscopy and PCR on clinical specimens are also valuable.[55]

Specific serologic tests for *Treponema pallidum* are the fluorescent treponemal antibody absorption and the *T. pallidum* particle agglutination tests. These antibody tests remain reactive for life, even after successful treatment, so should not be used to indicate response to treatment.[53,54] False positives can occur with other treponemal disease including yaws and rat-bite fever and with Lyme disease.[53,54]

Non-specific (non-treponemal) tests are the Venereal Disease Research Laboratory (VDRL), the rapid plasma reagin test (RPR), and the automated reagin test (ART). They are cheap and rapid and give quantitative results, which are useful to monitor response to treatment. They are usually used for screening for syphilis, and specific tests are done if the non-specific test is positive. False negatives can occur in early primary disease, latent disease, and late congenital syphilis, while false positives can occur in a number of other conditions including EBV infection, SLE, and lymphoma.[53,54]

If in doubt about serology results, which can be very confusing, we recommend asking advice from a microbiologist. The need for long-term follow-up with repeat serology and the frequent presence of complicating factors makes it desirable to seek specialist advice, particularly for patients who are pregnant, have HIV infection, or are allergic to penicillin.

Treatment of syphilis

Penicillin remains the drug of choice for syphilis, and there are few alternatives. A single dose of oral azithromycin was as effective as benzathine penicillin in early syphilis in three trials.[56–58] A small study found that ceftriaxone and penicillin G were equally effective for primary and secondary syphilis,[59] while a pilot study found ceftriaxone to be as effective as penicillin G for HIV-infected patients with neurosyphilis, but differences in the two groups limited comparisons between them.[60] Penicillin desensitization should be performed whenever practicable for patients who are allergic to penicillin. If drugs other than penicillin are used, careful follow-up is recommended.

Pregnancy and congenital syphilis

Pregnant patients should be treated with penicillin in the dosage schedule recommended for non-pregnant patients at a similar stage of the disease.[51,52,61] We recommend desensitizing patients who are allergic to penicillin or seeking specialist advice. Tetracyclines should never be used in pregnancy or in the newborn, and erythromycin does not reliably treat an infected fetus.

If a mother with positive serology or active syphilis receives adequate penicillin treatment before 28 weeks' gestation (and her partner is adequately treated simultaneously) and she is not reinfected, the risk of congenital syphilis is low, but the baby should still be examined and investigated at birth, and the placenta examined by direct immunofluorescence and silver stains.[51,52]

Cord blood is inadequate for screening.[51,52] All infants of seropositive mothers should be examined carefully, and a quantitative non-treponemal syphilis antibody test (VDRL or RPR) should be done on baby's and mother's blood.[51,52]

Because of the risk from untreated congenital syphilis,[51,52,61] the baby should be treated empirically unless all the following apply:

· Mother was adequately treated (with an appropriate penicillin regimen, not with a non-penicillin such as erythromycin).

· Mother was treated >1 month before delivery (treatment failures can occur).

· Mother's antibody titers fell after treatment and remain low at delivery (reinfection can occur).

· The baby's physical examination is normal.

· The baby's VDRL or RPR is low and no higher than the mother's.

· Follow-up is assured.

If the mother's titer has risen fourfold, or the baby's titer is fourfold higher than the mother's, or the baby's examination is abnormal, it is recommended to perform liver function tests, long bone radiographs, and a CSF (cerebrospinal fluid) microscopy and VDRL on the baby.[51,52,61]

All newborns of mothers with syphilis should be investigated and treated in consultation with a specialist. For the treatment of congenital syphilis, we recommend:

> **benzylpenicillin (aqueous crystalline penicillin G) 30 mg/kg or 50,000 U/kg IV, 12-hourly for 7 days, then 8-hourly for 3 days OR**
> **procaine penicillin 30 mg/kg or 50,000 U/kg IM, daily for 10 days**

There have been two small studies that suggest that a single dose of benzathine penicillin (50,000 U/kg IM) may be adequate to treat asymptomatic babies at risk of syphilis.[62,63] A South African study of asymptomatic babies whose mothers had VDRL titers of 32 or more found that 4 of 8 untreated babies developed congenital syphilis, but none of 11 given benzathine penicillin.[62] A North American study found that a single dose of benzathine penicillin and 10 days of procaine penicillin were equally effective, although neither was 100% effective.[63] IV benzylpenicillin for 10 days is kinder than 10 days of IM procaine penicillin, is known to be effective, including treating and preventing neurosyphilis (procaine penicillin may not give adequate CSF levels[61]), and is the recommended treatment of choice for congenital syphilis.[51,52,61]

Early syphilis

Early syphilis is defined as primary (chancre), secondary (rash or condylomata lata), or latent (asymptomatic syphilis confirmed to be <2 years duration, based on serology results). We recommend:

> **benzathine penicillin 30 mg/kg or 50,000 U/kg (max 1.5 g or 2.4 million U) IM, as a single dose OR**
> **procaine penicillin 30 mg/kg or 50,000 U/kg (max 1.5 g or 2.4 million U) IM, daily for 10 days**

For nonpregnant patients who are allergic to penicillin and in whom desensi-tization is not possible, azithromycin has been shown to be effective in RCTs in industrialized[56] and developing countries.[57,58] Ceftriaxone appears to be as effective, but data are more limited.[59,60] There are no RCTs of tetracyclines in syphilis. We recommend:

> **azithromycin 50 mg/kg (max 2 g) orally, as a single dose**

Careful clinical and serologic follow-up is essential.

Pregnant patients who are allergic to penicillin should be desensitized and treated with penicillin.

We recommend advising the patient to avoid sexual activity until lesions are healed. Sexual contacts within the last 3 months should have the same treatment even if their serology is negative.

HIV-infected patients with early syphilis are at increased risk for neurological complications.[64–66] They should be evaluated clinically and serologically at 6-monthly intervals for at least 2 years after therapy. If, at any time, clinical symptoms develop or nontreponemal titers rise fourfold, a repeat CSF examination should be performed and treatment administered accordingly.[66] Some specialists recommend additional treatments in HIV-positive patients (e.g., benzathine penicillin administered at 1-week intervals for 3 weeks, as recommended for late syphilis).[66]

Late latent syphilis

Late latent syphilis is defined as latent syphilis of >2 years or indeterminate duration, in the absence of tertiary syphilis. Specialist advice should be sought regarding the need for and interpretation of lumbar puncture. This is particularly important for situations with treatment failure or HIV infection. For treatment, use:

> **benzathine penicillin 30 mg/kg or 50,000 U/kg (max 1.5 g or 2.4 million U) IM, once weekly for three doses**

We recommend a CSF examination before treatment for HIV-infected patients with late latent syphilis or syphilis of unknown duration, because of the increased risk of neurosyphilis with HIV infection.[66] If the CSF examination is normal, treat with benzathine penicillin as above, but if abnormal we recommend to treat and manage as for neurosyphilis[66] (see p. 218).

Tertiary syphilis and neurosyphilis

Tertiary syphilis includes cardiovascular syphilis and gummata. Neurosyphilis is diagnosed on CSF findings. Specialist advice should be sought. Use:

> **benzylpenicillin 60 mg/kg or 100,000 U/kg (max 2.4 g or 4 million U) IV, 4-hourly for 14 days** OR **procaine penicillin 60 mg/kg or 100,000 U/kg (max 2.4 g or 4 million U) IM, daily for 14 days**

When treating cardiovascular or neurosyphilis, prednisolone 0.5 mg/kg (max 20 mg) orally, 12-hourly for three doses may be administered with penicillin to reduce the likelihood of a Jarisch–Herxheimer reaction.[53]

13.6 Genital herpes simplex virus (HSV) infection

Genital herpes is sexually acquired and characterized by vesicular or ulcerative lesions of the genitalia and sometimes the perineum, although infection may be asymptomatic.[67] It can be caused by HSV-1 or -2. The diagnosis is made by viral culture from swabs of the genitalia or by rapid diagnostic tests, such as immunofluorescence or PCR.[68,69] Patients should have a full screen for sexually transmissible infections (including HIV serology) on their first presentation.

Oral acyclovir reduces systemic symptoms and shortens viral shedding in first episode genital herpes, but does not reduce the incidence of subsequent recurrences.[70] We could find no studies comparing valacyclovir or famciclovir with acyclovir for acute genital HSV infection. However, the evidence from studies of recurrent genital herpes suggests that the three drugs are therapeutically equivalent. Ease of administration, availability, and cost should be considered when choosing therapy.

Initial acute episode of genital herpes

For a first clinical episode, after taking a swab for culture, immunofluorescence, or PCR, we recommend:

> **acyclovir 10 mg/kg (max 400 mg) orally, 6-hourly for 7 days (preferred in pregnancy)** OR (only if >12 years)
> **famciclovir 250 mg orally, 8-hourly for 7 days** OR (only if >12 years)
> **valacyclovir 1 g orally, 12-hourly for 7 days**

Recurrent genital herpes

Infrequent but severe recurrences can be treated with episodic therapy, commenced at the onset of prodromal symptoms or within a day. Acyclovir is as effective as famciclovir[71] and valacyclovir.[72] Studies on duration of therapy have shown effective treatment with 2 days of acyclovir,[73] 3 days of valacyclovir,[74] and a single day of patient-initiated famciclovir.[75] We recommend:

> **acyclovir 20 mg/kg (max 800 mg) orally, 8-hourly for 2 days (preferred in pregnancy)** OR (only if >12 years)
> **famciclovir 1 g orally, 12-hourly for 1 day** OR (only if >12 years)
> **valacyclovir 500 mg orally, 12-hourly for 3 days**

Suppressive treatment may be indicated for frequent, severe recurrences. Suppression reduces recurrences by 70–80%.[76] Transmission of HSV can still occur. We recommend:

> **acyclovir 5 mg/kg (max 200 mg) orally, 12-hourly** OR (only if >12 years)
> **famciclovir 250 mg orally, 12-hourly (500 mg orally, 12-hourly in immunocompromised patients)** OR (only if >12 years)
> **valacyclovir 500 mg orally, daily (1 g orally, daily in immunocompromised patients)**

If frequent breakthrough infections occur during prophylaxis, higher doses may be successful. Treatment may be interrupted every 6 months to determine the natural history of the disease in any given patient, and can be restarted in the event of frequent recurrences.

13.7 Human papillomavirus (HPV) infection

HPV infection in the genital tract is largely asymptomatic and transient.[77] It can be detected only by cellular changes seen by cytology of the Papanicolaou (Pap) smear or at colposcopy, or by HPV DNA testing.[77] There are 30–40 HPV genotypes that infect the genital area. These are divided into high-risk (or oncogenic) and low-risk genotypes.[77]

HPVs cause cervical cancer. Persistent infection with one of the oncogenic genotypes is a prerequisite for the development of high-grade cervical intraepithelial neoplasia (CIN2 or CIN3), which is the precursor to cervical cancer.[77] Genotypes 16 and 18 are the most important genotypes, responsible for 70% of cervical cancers, and have been incorporated into HPV vaccines.[78,79] Low-grade cervical dysplasia (CIN1) is benign.[77]

Infection of males with oncogenic HPV can rarely result in cancer of the penis.[77]

Low-risk HPV genotypes 6 and 11 cause more than 90% of genital warts (condylomata acuminata) in both sexes, but do not cause cervical cancer.[77] However, the presence of genital warts indicates sexual activity and a risk of exposure to oncogenic HPV. It is important for all female patients with genital warts to have regular Pap smears.[77] The presence of anogenital warts may be an indicator of child sexual abuse, and affected children should be examined and tested for other sexually transmitted infections.[77]

Vaccines have been developed using virus-like particles. One vaccine[79] contains HPV 16 and 18, while another vaccine[78] contains HPV 6, 11, 16, and 18. Both vaccines have been shown in RCTs to be highly effective.[78,79] These vaccines will be introduced routinely for schoolgirls and possibly schoolboys and uninfected sexually active young women in industrialized countries.[77]

13.8 Pelvic inflammatory disease

The term "pelvic inflammatory disease" denotes a spectrum of inflammatory disorders of the female genital tract, including endometritis, chorioamnionitis, intraamniotic syndrome, salpingitis, oophoritis, tuboovarian abscess, and pelvic peritonitis.[80,81] Infections can vary from mild to life-threatening. Empiric treatment for PID is recommended in sexually active young women with uterine or adnexal tenderness or cervical motion tenderness if no other cause can be identified.[81]

Pelvic infection in females is usually sexually acquired or results from complications associated with pregnancy. Infection is usually polymicrobial. A meta-analysis of 34 studies of variable quality published between 1966 and 1992 showed that a number of treatment regimens were effective.[82] A subsequent RCT showed that 14 days of azithromycin was at least as effective as regimens using metronidazole+doxycycline+cefoxitin+probenecid or doxycycline+amoxycillin/clavulanate for up to 21 days.[83] A number of different regimens are recommended by the CDC (Centers for Disease Control and Prevention) for both ambulatory and parenteral treatment, while acknowledging that the evidence for them is scanty.[84]

For severe infections, we recommend:

azithromycin 12.5 mg/kg (max 500 mg) IV, daily for 1–2 days, then azithromycin 10 mg/kg (max 400 mg) orally, daily for 14 days OR
cefotetan 40 mg/kg (max 2 g) IV, 12-hourly OR THE COMBINATION OF
amoxi/ampicillin 50 mg/kg (max 2 g) IV, 6 hourly PLUS
gentamicin 6 mg/kg IV, daily PLUS metronidazole 12.5 mg/kg (max 500 mg) IV, 12-hourly

For mild to moderate infection, we recommend:

azithromycin 10 mg/kg (max 400 mg) orally, daily for 14 days OR
amoxicillin+clavulanate 22.5 + 3.2 mg/kg (max 875 + 125 mg) orally, 12-hourly for 14 days PLUS doxycycline 2.5 mg/kg (max 100 mg) orally, 12-hourly for 14 days

13.9 Post-sexual assault prophylaxis

Following sexual assault, the victim should be assessed and examined by an expert. Evidence-based guidelines have been published.[85] The examiner may decide to conduct tests for STDs, although this is not inevitable. Approximately 5% of sexually abused children acquire an STD as a result of the abuse.[85,86]

Universal screening of post-pubertal patients for STDs is recommended,[87] but more selective criteria may be appropriate for testing prepubertal patients.[85] For example, the yield of positive gonococcal cultures is low in asymptomatic prepubertal children, especially when the history indicates only fondling.[88] Vaginal samples are adequate for STD testing in prepubertal children, whereas cervical samples are recommended in post-pubertal children.[85,86]

It is recommended to test before initiating any prophylactic treatment, for legal as well as treatment reasons.[85,86] The most specific and sensitive tests should be used when evaluating children for STDs. Cultures are considered the "gold standard" for diagnosing *C. trachomatis* (cell culture) and *N. gonorrhoeae* (bacterial culture). New tests such as nucleic acid amplification tests (e.g., PCR) may be more sensitive in detecting vaginal *C. trachomatis*, but data are limited regarding the use of these test in prepubertal children.[18,85,86] When child sexual abuse is suspected and STD testing is indicated, vaginal/urethral samples and/or rectal swabs for isolation of *C. trachomatis* and *N. gonorrhoeae* are recommended. In addition, vaginal swabs for isolation of *T. vaginalis* may be obtained. Testing for other STDs, including HIV, hepatitis B, hepatitis C, and syphilis, is based on the presence of symptoms and signs, patient/family wishes, detection of another STD, and physician discretion. Venereal warts, caused by HPV infection, are clinically diagnosed without testing. Any genital or anal lesions suspicious for herpes should be confirmed with a culture, distinguishing between HSV-1 and -2. Guidelines for treatment are published by the CDC.[84]

Post-sexual assault antibiotic prophylaxis

Antibiotic prophylaxis is not generally recommended, unless the person committing the assault is known to be suffering from or at high risk of a sexually transmitted infection. If it is decided to give prophylaxis, we recommend:

> **ceftriaxone ≤45 kg: 125 mg, >45 kg: 250 mg IM, as a single dose PLUS**
> **azithromycin 20 mg/kg (max 1 g) orally, as a single dose PLUS EITHER**
> **metronidazole 50 mg/kg (max 2 g) orally, as a single dose OR**
> **tinidazole 50 mg/kg (max 2 g) orally, as a single dose**

Post-sexual assault HIV prophylaxis

An estimate of the pooled risk of acquiring HIV after a single act with an HIV-infected person, based on observational studies,[89–91] is given in Table 13.1. Knowledge of the risk helps when deciding or counseling about prophylaxis. Although efficacy of post-exposure prophylaxis against HIV infection is unknown for sexual abuse, prophylaxis is effective in needlestick injuries (see Section 8.9, p. 112) and is recommended for unprotected receptive or insertive anal or vaginal intercourse if the person committing the assault is known or suspected to be infected with HIV.[92] Initiation of prophylaxis should be the responsibility of, or be un-

Table 13.1 Estimated risk of acquisition of HIV according to exposure to a single sexual act.

Route of Exposure	Risk per 1000 Exposures
Receptive anal intercourse	5
Receptive penile vaginal intercourse	1
Insertive anal intercourse	0.65
Insertive penile vaginal intercourse	0.5
Receptive oral intercourse	0.1
Insertive oral intercourse	0.05

Adapted from References 89–91.

dertaken after taking advice from, an experienced HIV physician.[92]

If it is decided to give HIV prophylaxis, we recommend:

> **lamivudine 4 mg/kg (max 150 mg) AND**
> **zidovudine 8 mg/kg (max 300 mg) orally,**
> **12-hourly for 4 weeks or until source shown to be HIV negative PLUS EITHER**
> **lopinavir 300 mg/m^2 (max 400 mg) AND**
> **ritonavir 75 mg/m^2 (max 100 mg), orally,**
> **12-hourly (Kaletra) for 4 weeks or until source shown to be HIV negative OR**
> **nelfinavir <13 years 55 mg/kg (max 2 g) orally,**
> **12-hourly; >12 years 1250 mg orally, 12-hourly for 4 weeks or until source shown to be HIV negative**

Post-sexual assault hepatitis B virus (HBV) prophylaxis

If the child is not fully immunized against HBV, or their vaccine status is unknown, we recommend hepatitis B immunoglobulin and a course of hepatitis B vaccine.[87]

References

1 Herzog LW, Alvarez SR. The frequency of foreskin problems in uncircumcised children. *Am J Dis Child* 1986;140:254–6.

2 Orden B, Martin R, Franco A, Ibanez G, Mendez E. Balanitis caused by group A beta-hemolytic streptococci. *Pediatr Infect Dis J* 1996;15:920–1.

3 Daher A, Fortenberry JD. Staphylococcus-induced toxic shock following balanitis. *Clin Pediatr (Phila)* 1995;34:172–4.

4 Jones R. Childhood vulvovaginitis and vaginal discharge in practice. *Fam Pract* 1996;13:369–72.

5 Pierce A, Hart C. Vulvovaginitis: causes and management. *Arch Dis Child* 1992;67:509–12.

6 Jaquiery A, Stylionopoulus A, Hogg G, Grover S. Vulvovaginitis: clinical features, aetiology and microbiology of genital tract. *Arch Dis Child* 1999;81:64–7.

7 Cuadros J, Mazon A, Martinez R et al. The aetiology of paediatric inflammatory vulvovaginitis. *Eur J Pediatr* 2004;163:105–7.

8 Merkley K. Vulvovaginitis and vaginal discharge in the pediatric patient. *J Emerg Nurs* 2005;31:400–2.

9 Stricker T, Navratil F, Sennhauser FH. Vulvovaginitis in prepubertal girls. *Arch Dis Child* 2003;88:324–6.

10 Mogielnicki NP, Schwartzman JD, Elliott JA. Perineal group A streptococcal disease in a pediatric practice. *Pediatrics* 2000;106:276–81.

11 Nair S, Schoeneman MJ. Acute glomerulonephritis with group A streptococcal vulvovaginitis. *Clin Pediatr (Phila)* 2000;39:721–2.

12 Honig E, Mouton JW, van der Meijden WI. The epidemiology of vaginal colonisation with group B streptococci in a sexually transmitted disease clinic. *Eur J Obstet Gynecol Reprod Biol* 2002;105:177–80.

13 Schuchat A. Epidemiology of group B streptococcal disease in the united states: shifting paradigms. *Clin Microbiol Rev* 1998;11:497–513.

14 Siegel RM, Schubert CJ, Myers PA, Shapiro RA. The prevalence of sexually transmitted diseases in children and adolescents evaluated for sexual abuse in Cincinnati: rationale for limited STD testing in prepubertal girls. *Pediatrics* 1995;96:1090–4.

15 Ingram DL, Everett VD, Flick LA, Russell TA, White-Sims ST. Vaginal gonococcal cultures in sexual abuse evaluations: evaluation of selective criteria for preteenaged girls. *Pediatrics* 1997;99:E8.

16 Kellogg N. American academy of pediatrics committee on child abuse and neglect: the evaluation of sexual abuse in children. *Pediatrics* 2005;116:506–12.

17 Kellogg ND, Baillargeon J, Lukefahr JL, Lawless K, Menard SW. Comparison of nucleic acid amplification tests and culture techniques in the detection of *Neisseria gonorrhoeae* and *Chlamydia trachomatis* in victims of suspected child sexual abuse. *J Pediatr Adolesc Gynecol* 2004;17:331–9.

18 Hammerschlag MR. Appropriate use of non-culture tests for the detection of sexually transmitted diseases in children and adolescents. *Semin Pediatr Infect Dis* 2003;14:54–9.

19 Echols RM, Heyd A, O'Keeffe BJ, Schacht P. Single-dose ciprofloxacin for the treatment of uncomplicated gonorrhea: a worldwide summary. *Sex Transm Dis* 1994;21:345–52.

20 Aplasca De Los Reyes MR, Pato-Mesola V, Klausner JD et al. A randomized trial of ciprofloxacin versus cefixime for treatment of gonorrhea after rapid emergence of gonococcal ciprofloxacin resistance in the Philippines. *Clin Infect Dis* 2001;32:1313–8.

21 Handsfield HH, McCormack WM, Hook EW, III, et al., for the Gonorrhea Treatment Study Group. A comparison of single-dose cefixime with ceftriaxone as treatment for uncomplicated gonorrhea. *N Engl J Med* 1991;325:1337–41.

22 Portilla I, Lutz B, Montalvo M, Mogabgab WJ. Oral cefixime versus intramuscular ceftriaxone in patients with uncomplicated gonococcal infections. *Sex Transm Dis* 1992;19:94–8.

23 Plourde PJ, Tyndall M, Agoki E et al. Single-dose cefixime versus single-dose ceftriaxone in the treatment of antimicrobial-resistant *Neisseria gonorrhoeae* infection. *J Infect Dis* 1992;166:919–22.

24 Handsfield HH, Dalu ZA, Martin DH, Douglas JM, Jr, McCarty JM, Schlossberg D, for the Azithromycin Gonorrhea Study Group. Multicenter trial of single-dose azithromycin vs. ceftriaxone in the treatment of uncomplicated gonorrhea. *Sex Transm Dis* 1994;21:107–11.

25 Rustomjee R, Kharsany AB, Connolly CA, Karim SS. A randomized controlled trial of azithromycin versus doxycycline/ciprofloxacin for the syndromic management of sexually transmitted infections in a resource-poor setting. *J Antimicrob Chemother* 2002;49:875–8.

26 Steingrimsson O, Olafsson JH, Thorarinsson H, Ryan RW, Johnson RB, Tilton RC. Single dose azithromycin treatment of gonorrhea and infections caused by *C. trachomatis* and *U. urealyticum* in men. *Sex Transm Dis* 1994;21:43–6.

27 Biro FM, Reising SF, Doughman JA, Kollar LM, Rosenthal SL. A comparison of diagnostic methods in adolescent girls with and without symptoms of *Chlamydia* urogenital infection. *Pediatrics* 1994;93:476–80.

28 Macmillan S, McKenzie H, Templeton A. Parallel observation of four methods for screening women under 25 years of age for genital infection with *Chlamydia trachomatis*. *Eur J Obstet Gynecol Reprod Biol* 2003;107:68–73.

29 Deligeoroglou E, Salakos N, Makrakis E, Chassiakos D, Hassan EA, Christopoulos P. Infections of the lower female genital tract during childhood and adolescence. *Clin Exp Obstet Gynecol* 2004;31:175–8.

30 Kent HL. Epidemiology of vaginitis. *Am J Obstet Gynecol* 1991;165:1168–75.

31 Sobel JD. Pathogenesis and treatment of recurrent vulvovaginal candidiasis. *Clin Infect Dis* 1992;14:S148–53.

32 Fidel PL, Jr. Immunity in vaginal candidiasis. *Curr Opin Infect Dis* 2005;18:107–11.

33 Emele FE, Fadahunsi AA, Anyiwo CE, Ogunleye O. A comparative clinical evaluation of econazole nitrate, miconazole, and nystatin in the treatment of vaginal candidiasis. *West Afr J Med* 2000;19:12–15.

34 Woolley PD, Higgins SP. Comparison of clotrimazole, fluconazole and itraconazole in vaginal candidiasis. *Br J Clin Pract* 1995;49:65–6.

35 Dennerstein GJ, Langley R. Vulvovaginal candidiasis: treatment and recurrence. *Aust N Z J Obstet Gynaecol* 1982;22:231–3.

36 Urunsak M, Ilkit M, Evruke C, Urunsak I. Clinical and mycological efficacy of single-day oral treatment with itraconazole (400 mg) in acute vulvovaginal candidosis. *Mycoses* 2004;47:422–7.

37 Schwebke JR, Burgess D. Trichomoniasis. *Clin Microbiol Rev* 2004;17:794–803.

38 James JA, Thomason JL, Gelbart SM, Osypowski P, Kaiser P, Hanson L. Is trichomoniasis often associated with bacterial

vaginosis in pregnant adolescents? *Am J Obstet Gynecol* 1992;166:859–63.

39 Sobel J, Nyirjesy P, Brown W. Tinidazole therapy for metronidazole-resistant vaginal trichomoniasis. *Clin Infect Dis* 2001;33:1341–6.

40 Joesoef MR, Schmid G. Bacterial vaginosis. *Clin Evid* 2005;13:1968–78.

41 Yudin MH. Bacterial vaginosis in pregnancy: diagnosis, screening, and management. *Clin Perinatol* 2005;32:617–27.

42 Varma R, Gupta JK. Antibiotic treatment of bacterial vaginosis in pregnancy: multiple meta-analyses and dilemmas in interpretation. *Eur J Obstet Gynecol Reprod Biol* 2006;124:10–4.

43 Hanson JM, McGregor JA, Hillier SL et al. Metronidazole for bacterial vaginosis: a comparison of vaginal gel vs. oral therapy. *J Reprod Med* 2000;45:889–96.

44 Gierup J, von Hedenberg C, Osterman A. Acute non-specific epididymitis in boys: a survey based on 48 consecutive cases. *Scand J Urol Nephrol* 1975;9:5–7.

45 Haecker FM, Hauri-Hohl A, von Schweinitz D. Acute epididymitis in children: a 4-year retrospective study. *Eur J Pediatr Surg* 2005;15:180–6.

46 Kadish HA, Bolte RG. A retrospective review of pediatric patients with epididymitis, testicular torsion, and torsion of testicular appendages. *Pediatrics* 1998;102:73–6.

47 Bowie WR. Approach to men with urethritis and urologic complications of sexually transmitted diseases. *Med Clin North Am* 1990;74:1543–57.

48 Wagenlehner FM, Weidner W, Naber KG. Chlamydial infections in urology. *World J Urol* 2006;24:4–12.

49 Ferrie BG, Rundle JS. Tuberculous epididymo-orchitis: a review of 20 cases. *Br J Urol* 1983;55:437–9.

50 Woods CR. Gonococcal infections in neonates and young children. *Semin Pediatr Infect Dis* 2005;16:258–70.

51 Isaacs D, Moxon ER. *Handbook of Neonatal Infections: A Practical Guide.* London: WB Saunders, 1999.

52 Doroshenko A, Sherrard J, Pollard AJ. Syphilis in pregnancy and the neonatal period. *Int J STD AIDS* 2006;17:221–7.

53 Hyman EL. Syphilis. *Pediatr Rev* 2006;27:37–9.

54 Farnes SW, Setness PA. Serologic tests for syphilis. *Postgrad Med* 1990;87:37–41.

55 Palmer HM, Higgins SP, Herring AJ, Kingston MA. Use of PCR in the diagnosis of early syphilis in the United Kingdom. *Sex Transm Infect* 2003;79:479–83.

56 Hook EW, III, Martin DH, Stephens J, Smith BS, Smith K. A randomized, comparative pilot study of azithromycin versus benzathine penicillin G for treatment of early syphilis. *Sex Transm Dis* 2002;29:486–90.

57 Riedner G, Rusizoka M, Todd J et al. Single-dose azithromycin versus penicillin G benzathine for the treatment of early syphilis. *N Engl J Med* 2005;353:1236–44.

58 Kiddugavu MG, Kiwanuka N, Wawer MJ et al. Effectiveness of syphilis treatment using azithromycin and/or benzathine penicillin in Rakai, Uganda. *Sex Transm Dis* 2005;32:1–6.

59 Schofer H, Vogt HJ, Milbradt R. Ceftriaxone for the treatment of primary and secondary syphilis. *Chemotherapy* 1989;35:140–5.

60 Marra CM, Boutin P, McArthur JC et al. A pilot study evaluating ceftriaxone and penicillin G as treatment agents for neurosyphilis in human immunodeficiency virus-infected individuals. *Clin Infect Dis* 2000;30:540–4.

61 American Academy of Pediatrics. Syphilis. In: Pickering LK (ed.), *Red Book: 2003 Report of the Committee on Infectious Diseases*, 26th edn. Elk Grove Village, IL: American Academy of Pediatrics, 2003:595–607.

62 Radcliffe M, Meyer M, Roditi D, Malan A. Single-dose benzathine penicillin in infants at risk of congenital syphilis—results of a randomised study. *S Afr Med J* 1997;87:62–5.

63 Paryani SG, Vaughn AJ, Crosby M, Lawrence S. Treatment of asymptomatic congenital syphilis: benzathine versus procaine penicillin G therapy. *J Pediatr* 1994;125:471–5.

64 Smith NH, Musher DM, Huang DB et al. Response of HIV-infected patients with asymptomatic syphilis to intensive intramuscular therapy with ceftriaxone or procaine penicillin. *Int J STD AIDS* 2004;15:328–32.

65 Zhou P, Gu Z, Xu J, Wang X, Liao K. A study evaluating ceftriaxone as a treatment agent for primary and secondary syphilis in pregnancy. *Sex Transm Dis* 2005;32:495–8.

66 Karumudi UR, Augenbraun M. Syphilis and HIV: a dangerous duo. *Expert Rev Anti Infect Ther* 2005;3:825–31.

67 Jungmann E. Genital herpes. *Clin Evid* 2005;14:1937–49.

68 Coyle PV, Desai A, Wyatt D, McCaughey C, O'Neill HJ. A comparison of virus isolation, indirect immunofluorescence and nested multiplex polymerase chain reaction for the diagnosis of primary and recurrent herpes simplex type 1 and type 2 infections. *J Virol Methods* 1999;83:75–82.

69 Baker DA. Diagnosis and treatment of viral STDs in women. *Int J Fertil Womens Med* 1997;42:107–14.

70 Mertz GJ, Critchlow CW, Benedetti J et al. Double-blind placebo-controlled trial of oral acyclovir in first-episode genital herpes simplex virus infection. *JAMA* 1984;252:1147–51.

71 Tyring SK, Douglas JM, Jr, Corey L, Spruance SL, Esmann J, for the Valaciclovir International Study Group. A randomized, placebo-controlled comparison of oral valacyclovir and acyclovir in immunocompetent patients with recurrent genital herpes infections. *Arch Dermatol* 1998;134:185–91.

72 Chosidow O, Drouault Y, Leconte-Veyriac F et al. Famciclovir vs. aciclovir in immunocompetent patients with recurrent genital herpes infections: a parallel-groups, randomized, double-blind clinical trial. *Br J Dermatol* 2001;144:818–24.

73 Wald A, Carrell D, Remington M et al. Two-day regimen of acyclovir for treatment of recurrent genital herpes simplex virus type 2 infection. *Clin Infect Dis* 2002;34:944–8.

74 Leone PA, Trottier S, Miller JM. Valacyclovir for episodic treatment of genital herpes: a shorter 3-day treatment course compared with 5-day treatment. *Clin Infect Dis* 2002;34:958–62.

75 Aoki FY, Tyring S, Diaz-Mitoma F, Gross G, Gao J, Hamed K. Single-day, patient-initiated famciclovir therapy for recurrent genital herpes: a randomized, double-blind, placebo-controlled trial. *Clin Infect Dis* 2006;42:8–13.

76 Gupta R, Wald A. Genital herpes: antiviral therapy for symptom relief and prevention of transmission. *Expert Opin Pharmacother* 2006;7:665–75.

77 Dunne EF, Markowitz LE. Genital human papillomavirus infection. *Clin Infect Dis* 2006;43:624–9.

78 Villa LL, Costa RL, Petta CA et al. Prophylactic quadrivalent human papillomavirus (types 6, 11, 16, and 18) L1 virus-like particle vaccine in young women: a randomised double-blind placebo-controlled multicentre phase II efficacy trial. *Lancet Oncol* 2005;6:271–8.

79 Harper DM, Franco EL, Wheeler CM et al. Sustained efficacy up to 4.5 years of a bivalent L1 virus-like particle vaccine against human papillomavirus types 16 and 18: follow-up from a randomised control trial. *Lancet* 2006;367:1247–55.

80 Ross J. Pelvic inflammatory disease. *Clin Evid* 2006;15:2176–82.

81 American Academy of Pediatrics. Pelvic inflammatory disease. In: Pickering LK (ed.), *Red Book: 2003 Report of the Committee on Infectious Diseases*, 26th edn. Elk Grove Village, IL: American Academy of Pediatrics, 2003:468–72.

82 Walker CK, Kahn JG, Washington AE, Peterson HB, Sweet RL. Pelvic inflammatory disease: metaanalysis of antimicrobial regimen efficacy. *J Infect Dis* 1993;168:969–78.

83 Bevan CD, Ridgway GL, Rothermel CD. Efficacy and safety of azithromycin as monotherapy or combined with metronidazole compared with two standard multidrug regimens for the treatment of acute pelvic inflammatory disease. *J Int Med Res* 2003;31:45–54.

84 Centers for Disease Control and Prevention; Workowski KA, Berman SM. Sexually transmitted diseases treatment guidelines, 2006. *MMWR Recomm Rep* 2006;55(RR-11):1–94. Available at http://www.ncbi.nlm.nih.gov/entrez/query.fcgi? db=pubmed &cmd=Retrieve&dopt=AbstractPlus&list_uids =16888612& query_hl=32&itool=pubmed_docsum.

85 Kellogg N, for the American Academy of Pediatrics Committee on Child Abuse and Neglect. The evaluation of sexual abuse in children. *Pediatrics* 2005;116:506–12. Aviable at http://pediatrics.aappublications.org/cgi/content/full/116/2/506.

86 Hammerschlag MR. Sexually transmitted diseases in sexually abused children: medical and legal implications. *Sex Transm Infect* 1998;74:167–74.

87 American Academy of Pediatrics. Sexually transmitted diseases. In: Pickering LK (ed.), *Red Book: 2003 Report of the Committee on Infectious Diseases*, 26th edn. Elk Grove Village, IL: American Academy of Pediatrics, 2003:157–67.

88 Siegel RM, Schubert CJ, Myers PA, Shapiro RA. The prevalence of sexually transmitted diseases in children and adolescents evaluated for sexual abuse in Cincinnati: rationale for limited STD testing in prepubertal girls. *Pediatrics* 1995;96:1090–4.

89 European Study Group on Heterosexual Transmission of HIV. Comparison of female to male and male to female transmission of HIV in 563 stable couples. *BMJ* 1992;304:809–13.

90 Varghese B, Maher JE, Peterman TA, Branson BM, Steketee RW. Reducing the risk of sexual HIV transmission: quantifying the per-act risk for HIV on the basis of choice of partner, sex act, and condom use. *Sex Transm Dis* 2002;29:38–43.

91 Leynaert B, Downs AM, De Vincenzi I , for the European Study Group on Heterosexual Transmission of HIV. Heterosexual transmission of HIV: variability of infectivity throughout the course of infection. *Am J Epidemiol* 1998;148:88–96.

92 Smith DK, Grohskopf LA, Black RJ et al. Antiretroviral post-exposure prophylaxis after sexual, injection-drug use, or other non-occupational exposure to HIV in the United States. *MMWR* 2005;54(RR02):1–20. Available at http://www.ncbi.nlm.nih.gov/entrez/query.fcgi?orig_db=PubMed&db=PubMed&cmd=Search&term=MMWR%5BJour%5D+AND+54%5Bvolume%5D+AND+1%5Bpage%5D+AND+2005%5Bpdat%5D+AND+Smith+DK%5Bauth-or%5D.

CHAPTER 14
Skin and soft tissue infections

Evidence-based practice guidelines on the management of skin and soft tissue infections have been developed by the Infectious Disease Society of America.[1]

14.1 Bites: dog, cat, and human bites

Bites often become infected. The rate of infection is highest for cat and human bites. In a Cochrane review of prophylactic antibiotics, the rates of infection without antibiotics were 67% for cat bites and 47% for human bites.[2] The rate for dog bites was 5.5% in the Cochrane review,[2] but 16% in a meta-analysis of prophylactic antibiotics for dog bites.[3]

A study of human and animal bites in children found that most wounds were polymicrobial and were infected with both aerobic and anaerobic organisms.[4] The most frequent isolates in both types of bite wounds were *Staphylococcus aureus*, anaerobic cocci, and bacteroides spp. *Pasteurella multocida* and *Pseudomonas fluorescens* were present only in animal bites, while group A streptococci were present only in human bites. Beta-lactamase-producing organisms were common. This study demonstrates the polymicrobial aerobic–anaerobic nature of human and animal bite wounds.

In a study of infected cat and dog bites, *Pasteurella* species were the most frequent isolates from both dog bites (50%) and cat bites (75%): *P. canis* was the most common isolate from dog bites, and *P. multocida* from cat bites.[5] Other common aerobes included streptococci, staphylococci, Moraxella, and Neisseria. Common anaerobes included fusobacterium, bacteroides, porphyromonas, and prevotella.

Thorough wound cleaning and debridement of devitalized tissue is advised, with operative wound exploration if necessary.[6] This advice follows basic microbiologic principles, although we could not find any controlled trials.

Prophylactic antibiotics for dog, cat, and human bites

Question | For children with dog, cat, or human bites, do prophylactic antibiotics compared with no prophylactic antibiotics or placebo reduce the risk of infection?

Literature review | We found eight RCTs and one Cochrane review[2] of prophylactic antibiotics for mammalian bites. We found a non-Cochrane meta-analysis of trials of prophylactic antibiotics for dog bites.[3] We found one RCT of prophylactic antibiotics for cat bites[7] and one RCT for human bites to the hand.[8]

The Cochrane review of prophylactic antibiotics for bites from mammals (animals and humans) found eight RCTs, which met the search criteria, six of them included dog bites.[2] For dog bites, there was no statistically significant reduction of infection rate after the use of prophylactic antibiotics (10/225 or 4%) compared to the control group (13/238 or 5.5%; OR 0.74, 95% CI 0.30–1.85). However, a separate meta-analysis of dog bites, including two additional studies, which did not meet Cochrane criteria, reached a different conclusion.[3] The estimated cumulative incidence of infection in controls in the eight studies was 16%. The relative risk for infection in patients given antibiotics compared with controls was 0.56 (95% CI 0.38–0.82), and about 14 patients must be treated to prevent one infection.[3] The evidence for prophylactic antibiotics for dog bites is fairly weak.

The Cochrane review identified one small RCT of oxacillin for cat bites.[7] The infection rate in the control group was 67% (4/6) compared with none of five in the prophylactic antibiotic group ($p = 0.045$). Material

---

The antibiotics and doses recommended in this chapter are based on those in *Therapeutic Guidelines: Antibiotic*, 13th edn, Therapeutic Guidelines Ltd, Melbourne, 2006.

obtained from three of the four infected patients grew *P. multocida*.[7]

The Cochrane review identified only one human study, of bites to the hand, in which patients received oral or parenteral antibiotics or no antibiotics.[8] The infection rate in the antibiotic group (0/33) was significantly lower than the infection rate in the control group (7/15 or 47%; OR 0.02, 95% CI 0–0.33).

Time since the bite is also important. An RCT compared amoxicillin-clavulanate with placebo in full-thickness animal bite wounds in a series of 185 consecutive patients.[9] In wounds less than 9 hours old, no significant benefit was found with antibiotic. The infection rate was reduced significantly in wounds presenting 9–24 hours after injury, although the numbers were small.

Antibiotics may not be necessary for mild dog bites not involving tendons or joints that can be adequately debrided and irrigated within 8 hours.

We recommend prophylactic antibiotics in the following circumstances:

· cat bites;
· human bites;
· bites from dogs and other mammals with delayed presentation (≥8 hours);
· bite wounds that cannot be debrided adequately;
· bites on hands, feet, or face;
· bites involving underlying structures, such as bones, joints, or tendons;
· bites in immunocompromised patients.

If the wound is obviously infected, a wound swab should be taken, and consideration should be given to delaying primary wound closure.[6]

For oral antibiotics, we recommend:

amoxicillin+clavulanate 22.5 + 3.2 mg/kg (max 875 + 125 mg) orally, 12-hourly for 5 days

If there is likely to be delay in starting oral antibiotics and there is a need to start treatment urgently, we recommend:

procaine penicillin 50 mg (80,000 U)/kg (max 1.5 g or 2.4 million U) IM, as a single dose, followed by oral amoxicillin+clavulanate, as above

or alternatively:

clindamycin 10 mg/kg orally or IV, 8-hourly

For severe and penetrating injuries, it is advised to commence with parenteral treatment,[1,6,10] to change to oral antibiotics (amoxicillin-clavulanate unless cultures dictate differently) when improving, and continue antibiotics (IV+oral) for a total of 14 days.[10] We recommend:

metronidazole 10 mg/kg (max 400 mg) orally, 12-hourly PLUS EITHER
ceftriaxone 25 mg/kg (max 1 g) IV, daily OR
cefotaxime 25 mg/kg (max 1 g) IV, 8-hourly

Alternatively, as a single preparation, use:

piperacillin+tazobactam 100 + 12.5 mg/kg (max 4 + 0.5 g) IV, 8-hourly OR
ticarcillin+clavulanate 50 + 1.7 mg/kg (max 3 + 0.1 g) IV, 6-hourly OR
ampicillin+sulbactam 50 mg/kg (max 2 g) IV, 6-hourly[6] (not licensed for children)

For patients with anaphylactic penicillin allergy, we recommend:

metronidazole 10 mg/kg (max 400 mg) IV or orally, 12-hourly PLUS
ciprofloxacin 10 mg/kg (max 500 mg) IV or orally, 12-hourly

The recommendations regarding prophylactic antibiotics for bites from other mammals such as rats and raccoons are less clear-cut, because they have not been studied so systematically. However, because the risk of spirochetal infection following rat bite is about 10%, some authorities recommend penicillin prophylaxis.[11] The need for immunization should always be considered (see below).

Human immunodeficiency virus (HIV) prophylaxis should be considered for children exposed to HIV by a bite (see p. 112).

Immunization of the child with a mammalian bite

The major considerations for prevention by immunization are rabies, tetanus, and hepatitis B.

Bats and raccoons are known to carry rabies (or Lyssavirus in Australia), and if a child is bitten by an animal that might be rabid, we recommend strong consideration of post-exposure prophylaxis against rabies.[1,6,11–13]

For children who have received their primary immunizations including tetanus, a dose of tetanus toxoid (or dT or DTP) is advised only if the child has not had a fourth dose. For children who have had fewer than three doses of tetanus, a dose of tetanus toxoid is recommended. Tetanus toxoid is recommended for unimmunized children and if immunization status is unknown. Tetanus immunoglobulin should be considered for unimmunized or partially immunized children, depending on the severity of the bite.[1,6,11–13]

The risk of hepatitis B should be assessed. We recommend giving vaccine and immunoglobulin to unimmunized children exposed to hepatitis B virus (see p. 93).

14.2 Bites: reptile bites

Reptile bites from sharks,[14] alligators,[15] and large reptiles[16] are associated with water-loving, Gram-negative bacilli, including Vibrios, Aeromonas, Klebsiella, *Escherichia coli*, and anaerobes. All reptile bites, including snake bites, should prompt the clinician to consider the child's tetanus status. Antibiotic prophylaxis is advised for most reptile bites, because of the high rate of wound infection.[6,15]

For oral prophylaxis, we recommend:

ciprofloxacin 10 mg/kg (max 500 mg) orally, 12-hourly

For severe bites requiring hospitalization, we recommend:

ciprofloxacin 10 mg/kg (max 400 mg) IV, 12-hourly OR
cefotaxime 50 mg/kg (max 2 g) IV, 8-hourly

14.3 Anthrax

Bacillus anthracis is an aerobic Gram-positive, spore-forming bacillus. It produces exotoxins, which cause hemorrhage, edema, and necrosis. Natural infection occurs as a zoonosis, from contact with infected animals or contaminated animal products, such as hides, wool, or meat. Anthrax can also be spread by bioterrorism. Anthrax can be cutaneous, inhalational, or gastrointestinal.[17–19]

In cutaneous anthrax, a pruritic papule or vesicle at the entry site develops 1–12 days after contact, and enlarges and ulcerates in 1–2 days, forming a painless ulcer with a black scab (eschar). There is a variable degree of surrounding edema, hyperemia, and regional lymphadenopathy. The eschar generally separates and sloughs after 12–14 days. Swelling surrounding the lesion can be minor or severe (i.e., malignant edema). Mild-to-moderate fever, headaches, and malaise often accompany the illness. Cultures of untreated lesions, depending on the stage of evolution, have positive results >80% of the time.[17–19]

There are no RCTs of therapy of cutaneous anthrax. Most published data indicate that penicillin is effective therapy and will "sterilize" most lesions after a few hours to 3 days, but does not accelerate healing.[17–19] Its value seems to be primarily reducing mortality from as high as 20% to 0%. In vitro and animal studies suggest that ciprofloxacin and doxycycline should be effective.[17–19]

For naturally occurring anthrax, penicillin is effective in >90% of children.[20] We recommend:

phenoxymethylpenicillin (penicillin V) 10 mg/kg (max 500 mg) orally, 6-hourly for 7–10 days

For bioterrorism-associated cutaneous disease, it is recommended to use ciprofloxacin 10–15 mg/kg (max 500 mg) orally, 12-hourly, or doxycycline 2.5 mg/kg (max 100 mg) orally, 12-hourly until susceptibility data are known.[17–19] The rationale is that genetically altered *B. anthracis* might be resistant to penicillin. So far, there is no evidence of penicillin-resistant bioterrorist strains, and there are animal studies but no clinical evidence in humans to support the use of ciprofloxacin and doxycycline.[17–19]

Initiation of intravenous therapy depends on the severity of the illness, particularly the degree of edema.

14.4 Boils, furuncles, and carbuncles

Acute boils, furuncles, and carbuncles

Furuncles (or "boils") are infections of the hair follicle with suppuration that extends through the dermis into the subcutaneous tissue, forming a small abscess. Furuncles differ from folliculitis, in which inflammation is more superficial and pus is present in the epidermis. Furuncles or boils can occur anywhere on hairy skin. When infection extends to involve several adjacent follicles, producing a coalescent inflammatory mass with pus draining from multiple follicular orifices, the lesion is called a carbuncle. Carbuncles tend to develop on the back of the neck and are especially likely to occur in diabetic persons. Boils and carbuncles are usually caused by *S. aureus*, although *Streptococcus pyogenes* can also be a cause. The isolation of a pure growth of an unusual organism, such as *E. coli* or *Pseudomonas*, from a child's boil should prompt consideration of chronic granulomatous disease (CGD).[21]

Outbreaks of furunculosis caused by *S. aureus* (methicillin-sensitive or MRSA) can occur in families and other settings such as sports teams. Inadequate personal hygiene and close contact with others with furuncles are important risk factors. In some cases, fomites may harbor the organism and facilitate transmission. Recommendations to control outbreaks include bathing with antibacterial soaps, such as chlorhexidine; thorough laundering of clothing, towels, and bed wear; separate use of towels and washcloths; and attempted eradication of staphylococcal carriage among colonized persons (see p. 228).[1]

Small lesions may be treated with drainage alone. For large lesions, in addition to surgical incision and drainage, we recommend:

> **di/flucl/oxa/nacillin 12.5 mg/kg (max 500 mg) orally, 6-hourly for 5 days** OR
> **cephalexin 25 mg/kg (max 1 g) orally, 8-hourly for 5 days**

For patients with anaphylactic penicillin allergy and for patients where community-associated methicillin-resistant *S. aureus* (cMRSA) is suspected because of ethnic background or local epidemiology, we recommend:

> **clindamycin 10 mg/kg (max 450 mg) orally, 8-hourly for 5 days**

The boil or furuncle should be lanced, if possible, and ongoing treatment should be based on culture and susceptibility.

Recurrent furunculosis (recurrent boils)

Some children have recurrent attacks of furunculosis. Most of these children have no demonstrable immune deficiency, and they and their family are well prior to onset.[22–24] Other family members often have boils before or after the child, which may be because some strains are more virulent but may also suggest a familial tendency to boils. Recurrent furunculosis is strongly associated with eczema, because the skin excoriation is a focus for infection.[22–24] Rare but important associations are diseases with defective neutrophil function, such as CGD[21] and hyper-IgE syndrome (Job syndrome). An association has been described with low serum iron,[25] but there are no studies showing that correcting iron deficiency improves furunculosis. For most children, the only identifiable predisposing factor is the presence of *S. aureus* in the anterior nares or, occasionally, elsewhere, such as the perineum.[22] The prevalence of nasal staphylococcal colonization in the general population is 20–40%, but why some carriers develop recurrent skin infections and others do not is unclear.[1]

We recommend taking swabs from any boils and from the nose to identify the organism and sensitivities, a nitroblue tetrazolium test or equivalent to exclude CGD, and a serum IgE if clinically indicated. More sophisticated neutrophil function tests are not widely available and not usually indicated.

Question | For children with recurrent furunculosis, do topical or oral antibiotics compared with no antibiotics reduce the frequency of recurrences?

Literature review | We found one RCT of nasal mupirocin[26] and two RCTs of oral antibiotics[27,28] for furunculosis due to methicillin-sensitive *S. aureus*. We found six RCTs and a Cochrane review[29] for MRSA.

Recurrent furunculosis with methicillin-sensitive *Staphylococcus aureus*

We found one RCT of 34 immunocompetent subjects with recurrent skin infections, who were carriers of methicillin-sensitive *S. aureus*.[26] After an initial 5-day course of twice daily nasal mupirocin ointment for all patients, 17 patients continued to apply a 5-day course of nasal mupirocin every month for 1 year, and the other 17 patients applied a placebo ointment. The overall numbers of skin infections were 26 in the mupirocin group and 62 in the placebo group ($p < 0.002$). Colonization was eradicated in 8 of the 17 mupirocin-treated patients but only 2 of the placebo group. One of the 10 patients free of colonization during the 12-month treatment period had skin infections, but all 24 patients with positive cultures had boils ($p < 0.01$). Staphylococci resistant to mupirocin were observed in 1 patient. No adverse effects of mupirocin were reported.[26]

The efficacy of nine different antibiotics used in different non-randomized regimens for eradicating nasal colonization with methicillin-sensitive *S. aureus* was investigated in a retrospective study. Clindamycin and ofloxacin were the most effective.[30] In an RCT, 22 otherwise healthy adults with recurrent furunculosis were randomized to low-dose (150 mg/day) oral clindamycin or placebo.[27] Seven of 11 placebo-treated patients (64%) but only 2 of 11 in the clindamycin group (18%) had a recurrent abscess within 3 months.[27] Six of the 9 patients who responded to clindamycin treatment did not have a recurrent infection for at least 9 months after discontinuing antibiotic therapy. All patients tolerated the regimen without side effects.[27] Rifampin has good tissue penetration, and even a short course might be useful to eradicate colonization. In an RCT, the addition of rifampin (rifampicin) to ofloxacin (or to vancomycin for MRSA) significantly improved cure from staphylococcal infections.[28] The study did not look at colonization.[28] Two observational studies suggested that a short course of rifampin, either alone[31] or in combination with other antistaphylococcal antibiotics,[32] could eradicate colonization and prevent recurrent boils in 50% or more of patients.

For patients with recurrent staphylococcal skin infections due to methicillin-sensitive *S. aureus*, we recommend treating any acute furuncles (see Section 14.4, p. 226). We then recommend using nasal mupirocin:

mupirocin 2% nasal ointment intranasally, 2 times daily for 5 days, and repeated monthly for 1 year

We recommend treating symptomatic household contacts in the same way as the index child. Some would recommend giving topical mupirocin to all household carriers, even if they were asymptomatic, to try to eradicate the organism.

Some authorities also recommend hygiene measures, such as washing daily with an antiseptic wash or soap containing triclosan 1% or chlorhexidine 2%, paying particular attention to hair-bearing areas, for at least 5 days, and washing clothes, towels, and sheets in hot water on two separate occasions.[10] There is no evidence to back these recommendations.

Because of ease of administration and although there is only weak evidence from observational studies,[31,32] a short course of oral antibiotics is often more acceptable than nasal mupirocin, or can be tried if mupirocin fails. We recommend:

rifampicin 10 mg/kg (max 600 mg) orally, daily for 7 days PLUS ONE OF
clindamycin 10 mg/kg (max 450 mg) orally, 8-hourly for 7 days OR
di/flucl/oxa/nafcillin 12.5 mg/kg (max 500 mg) orally, 6-hourly for 7 days OR
cephalexin 25 mg/kg (max 1 g) orally, 8-hourly for 7 days

If lesions continue to recur despite good compliance, we recommend:

clindamycin 4 mg/kg (max 150 mg) orally, daily for 3 months

Recurrent furunculosis with MRSA

MRSA is more difficult to eradicate than methicillin-sensitive *S. aureus*. A Cochrane meta-analysis of six trials (384 participants) found no evidence that topical or systemic antibiotics, including mupirocin, were effective in eradicating MRSA nasal colonization.[29]

For MRSA, we do not recommend mupirocin. We recommend that ensuring the isolate is susceptible to the drug or drugs used in any oral antibiotic regimen. MRSA will be resistant to di/flucl/oxa/ nafcillin, but may be sensitive to other antibiotics including clindamycin, fusidic acid, or trimethoprim/sulfamethoxazole.

14.5 Cellulitis

Cellulitis is a diffuse, spreading skin infection, and the term excludes infections associated with underlying suppurative foci, such as cutaneous abscesses, necrotizing fasciitis (NF), septic arthritis, and osteomyelitis.[1] The spreading, tender erythema may be associated with one or more of fever, lymphangitis, lymphadenopathy, and systemic toxicity. As the rash progresses, blistering may occur.[1] The causative organism in spontaneous, rapidly spreading cellulitis is almost always *S. pyogenes*. Wound-associated purulent cellulitis is more likely to be associated with *S. aureus*. *Haemophilus influenzae* type b (Hib) was an important cause of facial cellulitis (particularly, periorbital or buccal) in childen <4 years old, but has disappeared in countries that routinely immunize against Hib,[33] although may still be important in countries that do not.

Erysipelas is a severe form of cellulitis distinguished clinically by the following two features: the lesions are raised above the level of the surrounding skin, and there is a clear line of demarcation between involved and uninvolved tissue.[34] Erysipelas is almost always caused by beta-hemolytic streptococci, usually group A (*S. pyogenes*), although similar lesions can be caused by serogroup C or G streptococci. Rarely, group B streptococci or *S. aureus* may be the cause.

Swartz gives an extensive differential diagnosis for cellulitis.[35] The conditions in childhood that cause the most problem clinically are missing an underlying osteomyelitis or NF. It may require a bone scan or other imaging to exclude osteomyelitis (see Chapter 11). Ultrasound and/or magnetic resonance imaging (MRI) scan can help decide whether there is NF (see Section 14.9, p. 231).

Antibiotic treatment of cellulitis and erysipelas

We could find only five RCTs of antibiotic treatment of cellulitis, and no antibiotic was clearly superior to any other. Blood cultures are positive in only 4% of adult patients,[35] and serology is rarely back quickly enough to guide therapy.

For oral therapy, to treat *S. pyogenes* or *S. aureus*, we recommend:

di/flucl/oxa/nafcillin 12.5 mg/kg (max 500 mg) orally, 6-hourly for 7–10 days OR
cephalexin 25 mg/kg (max 1 g) orally, 8-hourly for 7–10 days OR, if cMRSA likely,
clindamycin 10 mg/kg (max 450 mg) orally, 8-hourly for 7 days

If *S. pyogenes* is confirmed, or suspected due to clinical presentation or local disease patterns, e.g. in some indigenous communities, we recommend:

phenoxymethylpenicillin 10 mg/kg (max 500 mg) orally, 6-hourly for 10 days OR
cephalexin 25 mg/kg (max 1 g) orally, 8-hourly for 7–10 days OR
procaine penicillin 50 mg (80,000 U)/kg (max 1.5 g or 2.4 million U) IM, daily for at least 3 days

For patients with anaphylactic penicillin allergy, we recommend:

clindamycin 10 mg/kg (max 450 mg) orally, 8-hourly for 7 days

It should be noted that the erythema may be slow to resolve and may even progress for the first 24–48 hours, even as the child becomes afebrile and improves. It is reassuring if the erythema is somewhat less intense at this time and starts to clear centrally.[1,35]

For severe cellulitis with significant systemic features, or if the patient is not responding to oral therapy after 48 hours, we recommend commencing IV therapy and continuing IV until the patient is afebrile and the erythematous rash has improved. This may take anything from 2 days to 2 weeks. The patient can then change to oral therapy (as above for cellulitis and erysipelas).

To treat infection with either streptococci or staphylococci, we recommend:

di/flucl/oxa/nafcillin 50 mg/kg (max 2 g) IV, 6-hourly OR
cephazolin 50 mg/kg (max 2 g) IV, 8-hourly OR
cephalothin 2 g 50 mg/kg (max 2 g) IV, 6-hourly

For patients with anaphylactic penicillin allergy and for patients where cMRSA is suspected because of ethnic background or local epidemiology (see p. 188), we recommend:

clindamycin 10 mg/kg (max 400 mg) IV, 8-hourly OR
vancomycin <12 years: 30 mg/kg (max 1 g) IV, 12-hourly; 12 years and older: 25 mg/kg (max 1 g) IV, 12-hourly

If there is significant systemic toxicity, consider the possibility of underlying myonecrosis or NF(see Section 14.9, p. 231).

14.6 Cutaneous larva migrans

The larvae of the dog and cat hookworms, *Ancylostoma braziliense* and *Agropyron caninum*, can cause a skin eruption in humans, called cutaneous larva migrans. This is different from visceral larva migrans and abdominal larva migrans, both of which are caused by Toxocara, the roundworms of dogs and cats. Human hookworms, *A. duodenale* and *Necator americanus*, can cause local pruritus and a different, papulo-vesicular rash lasting 1–2 weeks at the site of entry, usually the feet.

After penetrating the epidermis, the dog or cat hookworm larva is unable to enter the bloodstream or lymphatics, and instead burrows just below the corium, traveling up to an inch a day. Papules mark the site of entry and advancing end of the larva, and the tunneling larva causes slightly elevated, red, serpiginous wavy lines that are intensely itchy. Vesicles may form along the course of the tunnels, and scaling develops as the lesions age. The most common sites in children are the buttocks and the dorsum of the feet, but any area can be affected. The eruption generally disappears after 1–2 months, but may persist for 6 months or longer. Diagnosis is clinical. Biopsy may show an inflammatory, eosinophilic infiltrate but not the parasite, while serologic assays are available only in research laboratories.

There are no controlled trials of therapy, but observational studies favor topical treatment. Larvae can be eliminated in >95% of cases with topical 15% thiabendazole, which can easily be made from the oral preparation, if not commercially available, by crushing 500-mg tablets in a water-soluble base.[36,37] We recommend:

thiabendazole 15% cream, topically, 8–12-hourly for 5–10 days

Oral treatment may be needed for children who do not respond or who relapse. Both ivermectin and albendazole are very effective,[38] but children are less likely to relapse after treatment with ivermectin.[38] We recommend:

ivermectin (children >5 years) 200 μg/kg orally, as a single dose OR
albendazole 400 mg (children <10 kg: 200 mg) orally, daily for 3 days

Cryotherapy is painful and has an unacceptably high failure rate.[36,39]

14.7   Folliculitis

Folliculitis is inflammation of the hair follicles due to an infection or irritation in which the inflammation is more superficial than in a furuncle or boil and pus is present in the epidermis.[1]

Folliculitis is most often due to *S. aureus* infection, but this should be confirmed by culture, as the condition can also be caused by *Pseudomonas aeruginosa* (usually from hot tubs or spas),[40–42] yeasts like Malassezia,[43] and viruses like herpes simplex virus or varicella-zoster virus.[44] A non-infective variant known as eosinophilic folliculitis can occur in HIV infection.[45]

Staphylococcal infection can be treated as for staphylococcal impetigo (see Section 14.8, below). If skin swabs grow *P. aeruginosa*, the most important treatment measure is to identify the source and cease contact until the water supply has been treated[41,42].

14.8   Impetigo

In affluent communities, impetigo is most commonly caused by *S. aureus* and less commonly by *S. pyogenes* (group A streptococcus), although sometimes both organisms occur together. *S. pyogenes* is usually the primary pathogen in disadvantaged circumstances, such as remote Australian indigenous communities, and causes non-bullous or crusted impetigo, characterized by yellow, crusting lesions. It may be associated with scabies, and complications include glomerulonephritis (see Chapter 17) and rheumatic fever (see Chapter 3). Bullous impetigo, which causes round, itchy blisters, is caused by *S. aureus*.

Impetigo is mainly a disease of young children, but may be seen at any age. The condition is contagious and can spread from person to person in child care facilities, in schools, and in crowded, underprivileged communities.[46]

We found a Cochrane review[46] and also a non-Cochrane systematic review[47] of treatment of impetigo. Both found that topical antibiotics were at least as good as oral antibiotics at curing impetigo, and that topical mupirocin was better than oral erythromycin.[46,47] Also, there was no significant difference between different topical agents, including mupirocin and fusidic acid.[46,47] The Cochrane review found that oral penicillin was not as effective as most other antibiotics, but included studies of patients with impetigo due to *S. aureus* as well as *S. pyogenes*.[46]

If cultures are not back, it seems reasonable in settings other than remote communities to use a regimen that will treat both *S. aureus* and *S. pyogenes*. For mild or localized infections, we recommend:

mupirocin 2% topically, 8-hourly

For widespread or recurrent infections, cephalexin and dicloxacillin are equally effective.[48] We recommend:

> **cephalexin 12.5 mg/kg (max 250 mg) orally, 6-hourly OR**
> **di/flucl/oxa/nafcillin 12.5 mg/kg (max 250 mg) orally, 6-hourly**

For patients with anaphylactic penicillin allergy and for patients where cMRSA is suspected because of ethnic background (see p. 188) or is proven, we recommend:

> **clindamycin 10 mg/kg (max 450 mg) orally, 8-hourly for 5 days**

In situations where *S. pyogenes* is highly likely, and there is a relatively high risk of major complications like glomerulonephritis and rheumatic fever, such as in indigenous communities, we recommend:

> **phenoxymethylpenicillin 10 mg/kg (max 500 mg) orally, 6-hourly OR**
> **benzathine penicillin 900 mg = 1.2 million units (children 3 to <6 kg: 225 mg; 6 to <10 kg: 337.5 mg; 10 to <15 kg: 450 mg; 15 to <20 kg: 675 mg) IM, as a single dose**

With recurrent or resistant impetigo, chronic carriage of *S. aureus* is possible. We recommend taking swabs from the nose and/or perineum, depending on the location of the impetigo. If swabs are positive, consider treating the whole family and close contacts (see pp. 227–8).

14.9 Necrotizing skin and soft tissue infections

Diagnosis: distinguishing necrotizing skin and soft tissue infections from cellulitis

Necrotizing skin and soft tissue infections tend to be deeper than other skin infections like cellulitis and may involve the fascial and/or muscle compartments. They cause major destruction of tissue and can be fatal.[1] Critically ill patients with skin and soft tissue infections may have underlying necrosis of the soft tissues (NF) or muscle (myonecrosis). Extensive necrosis is referred to as gangrene.

Infection can develop from an initial break in the skin related to trauma or surgery, and can involve just one organism (usually *S. pyogenes*, or more rarely *Clostridium perfringens* causing gas gangrene or *S. aureus*, including MRSA) or can be polymicrobial (usually mixed aerobic and anaerobic bacteria). Penetrating and crush injuries are particularly likely to cause these infections, but life-threatening *S. pyogenes* NF can occur spontaneously or following varicella (chicken pox).

A number of syndromes of necrotizing soft tissue infections have been described on the basis of etiology, microbiology, and anatomic location, but there is a common initial approach in terms of the diagnosis, antimicrobial treatment, and decision to use operative management.[1,49,50] The initial concern is usually to distinguish between cellulitis and a necrotizing infection. The clinical features that suggest the presence of a necrotizing infection are described in reviews[1,49,50] and shown in Box 14.1.

What is the evidence that these clinical criteria truly distinguish necrotizing infection from cellulitis (with histologic proof as the "gold standard")? A North American surgical team developed a model from a comparison between proven NF patients and matched

---

Box 14.1 Clinical features described as suggestive of a necrotizing skin and soft tissue infection.[1,49,50]

· Pain: severe and constant
· *Bullae
· *Purple skin discoloration (sometimes described as ecchymosis or bruising)
· Skin necrosis
· Gas in the soft tissues (palpable crepitus or *gas on radiograph)
· *Edema extending beyond the margin of erythema
· *Cutaneous anesthesia
· Systemic toxicity; e.g., high fever, hypotension, shock, and delirium
· Rapid spread

*Denotes clinical features shown to be more common in necrotizing infection than in cellulitis.[51]

non-NF controls.[52] They then used the model to compare retrospectively 31 NF patients with 328 non-NF patients.[51] NF patients had a significantly lower mean admission systolic BP (124 mm Hg versus 136 mm Hg, $p = 0.007$) and higher mean admission respiratory rate (20 versus 18 breaths per minute, $p = 0.009$), but no significant difference in temperature or heart rate. Two NF patients (7%) and 2 non-NF patients (1%) presented with hypotension (SBP <90 mm Hg, $p = NS$). No threshold for any vital sign significantly distinguished NF from non-NF patients.

Physical examination of both NF and non-NF patients revealed a combination of tenderness, erythema, warmth, swelling, and fluctuance. NF patients differed from non-NF patients with respect to the presence of tense edema (23% versus 3%, $p = 0.0002$), bullae (16% versus 3%, $p = 0.006$), purplish skin discoloration (10% versus 1%, $p = 0.02$), and sensory or motor deficit (13% versus 3%, $p = 0.03$). Skin necrosis was present in 6% of NF patients and 2% of non-NF patients ($p = NS$). Seven of 22 NF patients (32%) had gas on plain radiograph, versus 6 of 224 non-NF patients (3%) ($p < 0.0001$). No patient had crepitus, so radiographic evidence of gas was present in about a third of patients, but no clinical evidence of gas. This study did not look at pain severity.[51]

Laboratory criteria may help distinguish NF from non-NF patients. A retrospective study compared laboratory results in 145 NF patients with 309 patients with severe cellulitis or abscesses. A score based on total white cell count, hemoglobin, sodium, glucose, serum creatinine, and C-reactive protein had good positive and negative predictive value in this population, although may not be so useful in clinical practice, as the results are likely to be abnormal in severe cellulitis.[53] The serum creatine phosphokinase (creatine kinase, CK) is rarely raised in cellulitis in contrast to NF: in one series, 5% of patients with erysipelas had a serum CK >600 IU/L.[54] In another series,[55] serum CK was >200 IU/L in 75% of patients with group A streptococcal NF and >600 IU/L in 61%. However, in the same study,[55] serum CK was >200 IU/L in 26% of patients with NF due to other organisms, and none of these had a CK >600 IU/L. Patients with group A streptococcal NF had a higher mortality. An elevated CK is, therefore, useful for supporting a diagnosis of NS, particularly group A streptococcal NF, but a normal CK does not exclude the diagnosis.

Can imaging reliably differentiate between cellulitis and NF? Computed tomography (CT) scan, ultrasound, and MRI for the imaging of necrotizing soft tissue infection have been intensely studied and reviewed.[56] Authors have reported features that they consider to be indicative of NF, but these are difficult to verify objectively. MRI is probably the most sensitive modality, but its sensitivity often exceeds its specificity, resulting in overestimation of the extent of deep fascial involvement.[56] However, absence of deep fascial involvement on MRI effectively excludes NF. While imaging can be an invaluable adjunct to diagnosis, it may not be readily available and is certainly not cheap. In patients with a suspicion of NF, operative debridement should not be delayed while waiting for an MRI scan.

Treatment of necrotizing skin and soft tissue infections

Surgery for necrotizing skin and soft tissue infections

The principle of treatment is a combination of surgical removal of necrotic tissue and early antibiotics.[57] We could find 156 review articles on surgery for NF, but not surprisingly no RCTs.

Antibiotics for necrotizing skin and soft tissue infections

The recommended antibiotic treatment of choice for group A streptococcal and for clostridial necrotizing infections is clindamycin plus penicillin.[1] This recommendation is based on susceptibility but not on clinical trials.

For *S. pyogenes* NF, or for proven clostridial infection, we recommend:

**benzylpenicillin 60 mg (100,000 U)/kg (max 2.4 g or 4 million U) IV, 4-hourly PLUS
clindamycin 15 mg/kg (max 600 mg) IV, 8-hourly**

For empiric therapy, meropenem is used until Gram-negative organisms have been excluded. We recommend:

**clindamycin 15 mg/kg (max 600 mg) IV, 8-hourly PLUS
meropenem 25 mg/kg (max 1 g) IV, 8-hourly**

Although penicillin is often added, this is not likely to improve the efficacy of the above regimen, so we do not recommend it.

Intravenous immunoglobulin for necrotizing skin and soft tissue infections

Intravenous immunoglobulin (IVIG) contains antibodies against streptococcal superantigens,[58] and although IVIG has been used in patients with severe streptococcal infections,[59–62] there have been no RCTs of the use in streptococcal toxic shock or NF. Reports have been case reports,[59] uncontrolled case series,[61,62] or have used historic controls.[60] Recommendations to use or to consider using IVIG are based on the severity of the illness, the difficulty in doing RCTs (so there is a lack of evidence of efficacy rather than evidence of lack of efficacy), and the likelihood that benefit will outweigh harm. If used, the recommended dose[63] is:

> **normal immunoglobulin 1–2 g/kg IV, repeated on days 2 and 3 if indicated**

Hyperbaric oxygen for necrotizing skin and soft tissue infections

A review[64] found seven studies reporting the results of hyperbaric oxygen in the treatment of necrotizing skin and soft tissue infections; all the studies were uncontrolled, retrospective, and observational studies. The review concluded that the results were inconsistent, with some studies claiming that hyperbaric oxygen can improve patient survival and decrease the number of debridements required to achieve wound control, whereas others failed to show any beneficial effect.[64]

14.10 Pediculosis capitis (head lice)

Pediculosis capitis or infestation with head lice is extremely common in child care and schools throughout the world.[65,66] One of the major problems with control has been the emergence of resistance to pediculicides, such as permethrin and malathion.

Question | For children with head lice, are topical pediculicides compared with wet combing compared with no treatment or placebo effective at eradicating head lice?

Literature review | We found 19 RCTs and a Cochrane review[67] of interventions for head lice.

We found 19 RCTs, a 2001 Cochrane review,[67] and treatment guidelines,[68] but one of the major problems was whether the findings are applicable when there is resistance to pediculicides. The Cochrane review found only four eligible studies[67] and found that pediculicides were effective compared with no treatment, but did not favor any one pediculicide.

The emergence of pediculicide resistance has driven studies of physical methods of lice removal, paricularly using fine tooth combs. We found four RCTs comparing wet combing with conditioner. Two studies strongly found that wet combing using fine tooth combs and conditioner ("Bug Busting") was far more effective than using a pediculicide.[69,70] In contrast, one RCT found that wet combing was less effective than a pediculicide[71] and another found that adding wet combing to a pediculicide did not improve eradication.[72]

> **Because it is safe, cheap, and often effective, and avoids the risk of resistance and toxicity from using pediculicides, we recommend wet combing plus conditioner as the initial treatment of choice for head lice.**

14.11 Perianal cellulitis

Perianal cellulitis has been recognized to be caused commonly by group A beta-hemolytic streptococci for many years,[73] although other reported causes include S. aureus,[74] pinworms,[75] and polymicrobial synergistic gangrene in immunocompromised children.[76] Streptococcal perianal cellulitis occurs mainly in children ages 6 months to 10 years.[73,77,78] It causes sharply circumscribed perianal erythema, with or without itching, anal fissures, pain on defecation, constipation, rectal bleeding, and mucopurulent anal discharge.[78]

The disorder can be associated with guttate psoriasis[79] and with vulvovaginitis in prepubertal girls (see Section 13.2, p. 211), and with balanoposthitis in boys[79] (see Section 13.1, p. 211). Infection sometimes spreads in families or in day care.[75]

Treatment of perianal streptococcal cellulitis has never been prospectively evaluated. Effective treatment of sporadic cases with oral penicillin,[80] erythromycin,[81] or mupirocin cream alone[82] has been reported, but recurrence rates may be as high as 40–50%.[73]

We recommend:

phenoxymethylpenicillin (penicillin V) 10 mg/kg (max 500 mg) orally, 6-hourly

14.12 Pyomyositis

Pyomyositis is the presence of pus within individual muscle groups.[83−86] Local muscle trauma is thought to predispose to pyomyositis, but a clear history of trauma is often not obtained. Because it is most commonly reported in the tropics, this condition is often called tropical pyomyositis,[83] but cases are also reported in temperate climates, often in children without underlying risk factors.[84−86]

The most common organism by far in both tropical and temperate settings is *S. aureus*,[83−86] which can be methicillin-sensitive or methicillin-resistant (often cMRSA).[83] Occasionally, *S. pneumoniae* or a Gram-negative enteric bacillus is responsible.[83−86] Blood culture results are positive in 5–30% of cases.[83−86]

Children usually present with pain in a single muscle or muscle group, muscle spasm, and fever, although occasionally the presentation is more indolent, with fever but little pain.[81−83] The disease most often occurs in an extremity, but any muscle group can be involved, including the psoas or trunk muscles. An iliopsoas abscess classically presents with hip pain and difficulty walking, which mimics septic arthritis, although children with iliopsoas abscess tend to hold the hip rigid, while children with septic arthritis hold it flexed in the neutral position.[87]

Pyomyositis may coexist with septic arthritis and/or osteomyelitis (see Chapter 11). The diagnosis of pyomyositis can be made with ultrasound, CT, or MRI scan, which will delineate the extent of the lesion and whether or not there is also septic arthritis.

Ultrasound- or CT-guided percutaneous drainage can be both therapeutic and diagnostic.[83−86]

For empiric therapy, in the absence of any other indications, we recommend:

di/flucl/oxa/nafcillin 50 mg/kg (max 2 g) IV, 6-hourly OR
cephalothin 50 mg/kg (max 2 g) IV, 6-hourly OR
cephazolin 50 mg/kg (max 2 g) IV, 8-hourly

When cMRSA infection is suspected, because of local prevalence and/or ethnicity, or when sensitive cMRSA is proven, we recommend:

clindamycin 10 mg/kg (max 450 mg) IV, 8-hourly
THEN (if susceptible)
clindamycin 10 mg/kg (max 450 mg) orally, 8-hourly

For patients with anaphylactic penicillin allergy, or with probable or proven hospital-acquired MRSA, we recommend:

vancomycin <12 years: 30 mg/kg (max 1 g); 12 years and older: 25 mg/kg (max 1 g) IV, 12-hourly

If *S. aureus* is not susceptible to macrolides, and patient is allergic to penicillin, base oral therapy following vancomycin on proven susceptibility. Suitable oral options may be trimethoprim+sulfamethoxazole or doxycycline.

14.13 Scabies

Scabies is a common parasitic infection caused by the mite *Sarcoptes scabiei* variety *hominis*. The worldwide prevalence may be as high as 300 million cases yearly.[88,89] Scabies is spread by close physical contact between infected persons. Human scabies is not acquired from animals. Scabies occurs in both sexes, at all ages, in all ethnic groups, and at all socioeconomic levels. In an epidemiologic study in the UK, scabies was more prevalent in urban areas, among women and children, and in winter.[66]

Scabies causes itchy, linear, or serpiginous lesions with burrows. In infants, the eruption may be more vesicular, and can occur on the head, neck, palms, and soles, as well as elsewhere on the body and limbs. In older children and adults, lesions are more often confined to the interdigital spaces, wrists, elbows, axilla, areolae, waist, umbilicus, thighs, buttocks, and genitalia.[88,90] However, scabies can occur above the neck in elderly and in malnourished persons. Lesions can become secondarily infected, leading to pyoderma or impetigo.

A crusted form of scabies called Norwegian scabies can occur in immunocompromised persons, including those with congenital immune deficiency or HIV infection.[91,92] In crusted (Norwegian) scabies, the mite population on the patient is very high due to a poor host response.

The diagnosis of scabies is primarily clinical.[88,91] In a report from a sub-Saharan region with a high prevalence of scabies (13%), the presence of diffuse itching and visible lesions associated with either at least two typical locations of scabies or a household member with itching had 100% sensitivity and 97% specificity for the diagnosis.[90] Diagnostic tests involve skin scraping with a blade or biopsy, but have a relatively low sensitivity.[88] Empiric treatment is reasonable for patients with classical clinical findings. However, empiric treatment is not recommended for persons with generalized itching, even after exposure (e.g., staff), unless they have a typical eruption.[88]

Topical treatment for scabies

Permethrin and lindane are the two most studied topical treatments for scabies. A Cochrane review[89] found four randomized trials comparing these agents. A single overnight application of permethrin was found to be more effective than lindane and less toxic.[89] However, there was considerable heterogeneity among studies in the meta-analysis, and a different author examined the same data and concluded that if clinical cure was the outcome, there was no significant treatment advantage for permethrin.[93]

Reversible neurotoxicity has been described following an overdose of topical lindane,[94] and the potential of lindane for neurotoxicity, especially if giving repeated applications, has caused sufficient concern that the product is no longer available in the UK or Australia. Although it costs more than lindane, 5% permethrin is recommended by the Centers for Disease Control and Prevention as first-line topical therapy for scabies.[95] Mass treatment with permethrin has also been effective in controlling scabies in communities in which it is endemic.[95,96]

Other topical treatments include benzyl benzoate (not available in the USA) and crotamiton. Limited data from an RCT suggest that crotamiton is less effective after 4 weeks than permethrin (61% versus 89% cure).[97] In Vanuatu, in the South Pacific, where scabies is a major public health problem, 10% benzyl benzoate was as effective as a single oral dose of ivermectin (51% versus 56%) but more likely to cause burning or stinging (33% versus 7%).[98] In France, where permethrin is not available, benzyl benzoate is considered first-line local treatment, mainly on the basis of professional experience. The Cochrane review concluded that data were insufficient to compare the effectiveness of either benzyl benzoate or crotamiton with lindane or permethrin.[89]

There are insufficient data to recommend sulfur, topical ivermectin, or tea tree oil, which have been suggested as treatments. Pyrethrin aerosol spray, which has been used to treat scabies, can cause severe and even fatal asthma.[88]

For the topical treatment of scabies, permethrin 5% cream is at least as effective as other agents, safer, and cheap. Benzyl benzoate is effective in scabies if used correctly, but it is more irritating than is permethrin. We recommend:

> **permethrin 5% cream (adult and child >6 month) topically; leave on the skin for 8–14 hours (usually overnight) and reapply to hands if they are washed** OR
> **benzyl benzoate 25% emulsion (child <2 years: dilute with 3 parts of water; child 2–12 years: dilute with equal parts of water) topically; leave on the skin for 24 hours and reapply to hands if they are washed**

A second dose 1 week later improves cure rate.[88]

If secondary bacterial infection is present, also treat for impetigo (see Section 14.9).

Treatment of scabies in babies

The recommended treatment[63,99] of scabies in babies is:

> **permethrin 5% cream topically to the entire skin surface; include scalp, avoid eyes and mouth, cover hands in mittens to avoid the child ingesting the medication, leave on for 8 hours**

Although there are limited safety data on permethrin in babies <6 months old, this must be balanced against the high morbidity of untreated scabies. If the clinician judges the risks of treatment with permethrin to outweigh the benefit, alternatives are:

> **sulfur 10% in white soft paraffin topically, daily for 2–3 days (child <2 months: sulfur 5% in white soft paraffin)** OR
> **crotamiton 10% cream topically, daily for 2–3 days**

Oral treatment for scabies

Topical treatments may cause local reactions, especially when the skin is excoriated or eczematous, and there is a potential risk from percutaneous absorption. Oral ivermectin is an alternative.[100] Several controlled trials have assessed the efficacy of a single dose of ivermectin (200 μg/kg) for the treatment of scabies. Ivermectin is superior to placebo (74% versus 15% cure).[101] In small studies, no significant differences in clinical cure rates were found between ivermectin and 10% benzyl benzoate,[98] or between ivermectin and lindane.[102] In one RCT,[103] a single dose of oral ivermectin was less effective (70% cure) than a single overnight application of 5% permethrin (98% cure), but a second dose of ivermectin 2 weeks later increased the cure rate to 95%. The lower efficacy of single-dose ivermectin could reflect the lack of ovicidal action of the drug.

Ivermectin is potentially neurotoxic and costly. No serious adverse effects were noted in a program of mass treatment with ivermectin for children with scabies in the Solomon Islands.[104] However, encephalopathy has been reported in heavily infected patients with onchocerciasis, who are treated with ivermectin.[105] One study reported an excess risk of death among elderly patients who received ivermectin for scabies,[106] but this observation has not been confirmed in other studies, including studies of nursing home residents.[107]

Treatment of crusted (Norwegian) scabies

There are no RCTs of the treatment of crusted (Norwegian) scabies, and the optimum treatment is uncertain.[108] A retrospective study using historic controls found that the mortality from Norwegian scabies in Northern Australia fell from 4.3 to 1.1%, coincident with but not necessarily because of the introduction of multiple dosing with oral ivermectin.[88] The following recommendations are empiric.[63] Ivermectin therapy is effective and should be given in association with more frequent scabicide dosing, but is not recommended in children <5 years of age. To reduce scaling, topical keratolytics (e.g., salicylic acid 5–10% in sorbolene cream, or lactic acid 5% plus urea 10% in sorbolene cream) can be applied daily after washing on days when scabicides are not applied.[63]

For less severe crusted scabies, we recommend:

ivermectin 200 μg/kg (child >5 years) orally, as single doses 1 week apart

For moderate crusted scabies, use:

ivermectin 200 μg/kg (child >5 years) orally, on days 1, 2, and 8 (i.e., three single doses)

For severe crusted scabies, use:

ivermectin 200 μg/kg (child >5 years) orally, on days 1, 2, 8, 9, and 15 (i.e., five single doses), with two further doses on days 22 and 29 for extremely severe cases

Scabies in HIV-infected individuals may be resistant to repeated attempts at topical therapy.[109] There are no RCTs, and advice is empiric.[63,109] We recommend:

ivermectin 200 μg/kg orally, weekly until scrapings are negative and there is no further clinical evidence of infestation

14.14   Water-related infections

Wound infections, cellulitis, or sepsis associated with water, e.g. in fishermen, swimmers, or aquarium owners, may be associated with water-loving Gram-negative bacilli, including Vibrios, Aeromonas, Klebsiella, *E. coli*, and anaerobes (see also Section 14.2, p. 226).[110] There is little difference between the organisms following exposure to fresh water from a river, brackish water, or salt water, although *Mycobacterium marinum* is particularly associated with fish tanks.[111]

For empiric treatment, we recommend:

ciprofloxacin 10 mg/kg (max 500 mg) orally, 12-hourly

or for systemic therapy:

cefotaxime 50 mg/kg (max 2 g) IV, 8-hourly OR ciprofloxacin 10 mg/kg (max 400 mg) IV, 12-hourly

Coral cuts

Coral cuts are often infected with *S. pyogenes*, but infection may also occur with marine pathogens. For mild infection, we recommend treating as for impetigo (see Section 14.8, p. 230), and if unresponsive or severe, treating as for severe cellulitis (see p. 229), until culture results are back.

Mycobacterium marinum infections

M. marinum causes a localized papular or nodular skin lesion associated with exposure to fresh water, often from a fish tank or aquarium ("fish-tank granuloma" or "swimming-pool granuloma"). Diagnosis is often made by biopsy, and antibiotic therapy may not be required if a single lesion is successfully excised. There have been no controlled trials that compare the multiple treatment regimens for *M. marinum*, but a review of the literature suggested that treatment with two of clarithromycin, ethambutol, and rifampicin was most likely to be successful.[111] It is suggested to treat for 1–2 months after the resolution of all lesions (typically 3–6 mo in total).[111] We recommend:

> **clarithromycin 12.5 mg/kg (max 500 mg) orally, 12-hourly** PLUS EITHER
> **ethambutol 15 mg/kg (child ≥6 years) orally, daily** OR
> **rifamp(ic)in 10 mg/kg (max 600 mg) orally, daily**

14.15   Wound infections

Surgical site infections

Post-operative surgical site infections may settle with drainage and cleaning. Cultures should be obtained. Topical antibiotics are not recommended because they can select for the emergence of resistant organisms and can cause skin reactions.

For mild-to-moderate infection with surrounding cellulitis, we recommend:

> **di/flucl/oxa/nafcillin 12.5 mg/kg (max 500 mg) orally, 6-hourly** OR
> **cephalexin 12.5 mg/(max 500 mg) orally, 6-hourly**

Alternatively, if Gram-negative organisms are suspected or known to be involved, we recommend:

> **amoxycillin+clavulanate 22.5 + 3.2 mg/kg (max 875 + 125 mg) orally, 12-hourly**

For more severe infections, particularly where systemic symptoms are present, we recommend:

> **di/flucl/oxa/nafcillin 50 mg/kg (max 2 g) IV, 6-hourly** OR
> **cephalothin 50 mg/kg (max 2 g) IV, 6-hourly** OR
> **cephazolin 50 mg/kg (max 2 g) IV, 8-hourly**

If Gram-negative organisms are suspected or known to be involved, we recommend adding:

> **gentamicin 4–6 mg/kg (child <10 years: 7.5 mg/kg; ≥10 years: 6 mg/kg) IV, daily**

Alternatively, it is possible to use a single preparation, which has advantages of ease of administration, but disadvantages of increased cost and probably increased risk of selecting for resistant organisms:

> **piperacillin+tazobactam 100 + 12.5 mg/kg (max 4 + 0.5 g) IV, 8-hourly** OR
> **ticarcillin+clavulanate 50 + 1.7 mg/kg (max 3 + 0.1 g) IV, 6-hourly**

If MRSA is proven (or suspected), or for patients with anaphylactic penicillin allergy, we recommend:

> **vancomycin <12 years: 30 mg/kg (max 1 g); 12 years and older: 25 mg/kg (max 1 g) IV, 12-hourly**

For subsequent oral therapy, see Section 14.12 pyomyositis.

Wound infections related to vascular access

Vascular-access devices are the most common iatrogenic factor predisposing patients to skin and soft tissue infections. Many patients with intravenous catheters have additional factors that increase their risk of infection, such as neutropenia or defects of cellular or humoral immunity. Intravenous vascular-access devices are almost universal for patients who are undergoing cancer therapy; for stem cell, marrow, and solid organ transplant recipients; and for intensive care patients. Many of these catheters remain in place for prolonged periods, and the risk of cutaneous infections varies with the device, the duration of catheter placement, and the severity of immune suppression.

Cutaneous infections associated with catheter placement include entry-site infections (inflammation from the entry site to the first subcutaneous cuff), tunnel infections (inflammation involving the skin and soft tissues surrounding the catheter tunnel from the catheter cuff to the venous entrance), or vascular port-pocket infections.[112] Blood cultures are positive in 30–40% of tunnel and port-pocket infections, but rarely positive when catheter infection is limited to the entry site.[112]

Gram-positive organisms cause two-thirds of all vascular device infections, particularly coagulase-negative staphylococci and *S. aureus*, but other causes include Gram-negative bacilli, fungi, and atypical mycobacteria.[112] The prevalence of infection due to Gram-positive pathogens justifies recommending the use of empiric intravenous vancomycin for treatment of clinically serious catheter-associated infections.[112] Most entry-site infections can be treated effectively with appropriate antimicrobial therapy without catheter removal.[112] It is recommended to remove the catheter in tunnel or port-pocket infections.[112] Catheter-site infections caused by fungi or non-tuberculosis mycobacteria will not resolve without catheter removal and debridement of devitalized soft tissues.[113] One case series reported cure of all tunnel infections caused by non-tuberculous mycobacteria, using combination antimicrobial therapy for 3–6 weeks plus catheter removal and debridement of the infected soft tissue.[113]

Treatment should be based on cultures. For empiric therapy, pending culture results, we recommend:

vancomycin <12 years: 30 mg/kg (max 1 g); 12 years and older: 25 mg/kg (max 1 g) IV, 12-hourly

Post-traumatic wound infections

Antibiotics are often used in the early treatment of contaminated wounds following traumatic injuries, such as muscular, skeletal, and soft tissue trauma, crush injuries, penetrating injuries, and stab wounds. Careful cleaning and debridement of wounds is important to prevent infection, and immobilization and elevation reduce edema. The most common pathogens are *S. aureus*, *S. pyogenes*, *C. perfringens*, and aerobic Gram-negative bacilli.[1] For penetrating foot injuries through footwear, *P. aeruginosa* is commonly implicated (see p. 157).

In all cases, a patient's tetanus immunisation status should be assessed. For wounds caused by bites, see Section 14.1, p. 224.

Clean wounds

Antibiotics are not usually necessary for clean wounds. If it is decided to give empiric antibiotics to treat the above organisms, because management is delayed (≥8 hours) or debridement is difficult, we recommend:

di/flucl/oxa/nafcillin 12.5 mg/kg (max 500 mg) orally, 6-hourly OR
cephalexin 12.5 mg/(max 500 mg) orally, 6-hourly OR
amoxicillin+clavulanate 22.5 + 3.2 mg/kg (max 875 + 125 mg) orally, 12-hourly

For patients with anaphylactic penicillin allergy, or if *Pseudomonas* infection is a risk, we recommend:

ciprofloxacin 10 mg/kg (max 500 mg) orally, 12-hourly PLUS
clindamycin 10 mg/kg (max 450 mg) orally, 8-hourly for 5 days

Contaminated wounds

For contaminated wounds, it is important to prevent gas gangrene due to clostridial infection. Metronidazole and clindamycin provide adequate prophylaxis. We recommend:

di/flucloxacillin 50 mg/kg (max 2 g) IV, 6-hourly PLUS
gentamicin 4–6 mg/kg (child <10 years: 7.5 mg/kg; ≥10 years: 6 mg/kg) IV, daily PLUS
metronidazole 12.5 mg/kg (max 500 mg) IV, 12-hourly

Alternatively, use:

metronidazole 12.5 mg/kg (max 500 mg) IV, 12-hourly PLUS EITHER
cephalothin 50 mg/kg (max 2 g) IV, 6-hourly OR
cephazolin 50 mg/kg (max 2 g) IV, 8-hourly

Another possibility is:

clindamycin 15 mg/kg (max 600 mg) IV or orally, 8-hourly PLUS
gentamicin 4–6 mg/kg (child <10 yr: 7.5 mg/kg; ≥10 years: 6 mg/kg) IV, daily

For subsequent oral therapy, use an oral regimen as for clean wounds (see above).

References

1 Stevens DL, Bisno AL, Chambers HF et al. Infectious Diseases Society of America. Practice guidelines for the diagnosis and management of skin and soft-tissue infections. *Clin Infect Dis* 2005;41:1373–406.

2 Medeiros I, Saconato H. Antibiotic prophylaxis for mammalian bites. *The Cochrane Database of Systematic Reviews* 2001;(2):Art No CD001738.

3 Cummings P. Antibiotics to prevent infection in patients with dog bite wounds: a meta-analysis of randomized trials. *Ann Emerg Med* 1994;23:535–40.

4 Brook I. Microbiology of human and animal bite wounds in children. *Pediatr Infect Dis J* 1987;6:29–32.

5 Talan DA, Citron DM, Abrahamian FM, Moran GJ, Gold-stein EJ. Bacteriologic analysis of infected dog and cat bites. Emergency medicine animal bite infection study group. *N Engl J Med* 1999;340:85–92.

6 American Academy of Pediatrics. Bite wounds. In: Pickering LK (ed.), *Red Book: 2003 Report of the Committee on Infectious Diseases*, 26th edn. Elk Grove Village, IL: American Academy of Pediatrics, 2003:183–6.

7 Elenbaas RM, McNabney WK, Robinson WA. Evaluation of prophylactic oxacillin in cat bite wounds. *Ann Emerg Med* 1984;13:155–7.

8 Zubowicz VN, Gravier M. Management of early human bites of the hand: a prospective randomized study. *Plast Reconstr Surg* 1991;88:111–4.

9 Brakenbury PH, Muwanga C. A comparative double blind study of amoxycillin/clavulanate vs placebo in the prevention of infection after animal bites. *Arch Emerg Med* 1989;6:251–6.

10 Therapeutic Guidelines Ltd. *Therapeutic Guidelines: Antibiotic*, 13th edn. Melbourne: Therapeutic Guidelines Ltd, 2006.

11 American Academy of Pediatrics. Rat-bite fever. In: Pickering LK (ed.), *Red Book: 2003 Report of the Committee on Infectious Diseases*, 26th edn. Elk Grove Village, IL: American Academy of Pediatrics 2003:521–3.

12 *Australian Immunisation Handbook*, 8th edn. Canberra: Commonwealth Publishing, 2003. Available at http://www.immunise.health.gov.au/internet/immunise/publishing.nsf/Content/handbook03.

13 Department of Health. *Immunisation Against Infectious Disease: "The Green Book"*. London: UK Department of Health, 1996, revised 2006. Available at http://www.dh.gov.uk/PolicyAndGuidance/HealthAndSocialCareTopics/GreenBook/fs/en.

14 Royle JA, Isaacs D, Eagles G et al. Infections after shark attacks in Australia. *Pediatr Infect Dis J* 1997;16:531–2.

15 Howard RJ, Burgess GH. Surgical hazards posed by marine and freshwater animals in Florida. *Am J Surg* 1993;166:563–7.

16 Montgomery JM, Gillespie D, Sastrawan P, Fredeking TM, Stewart GL. Aerobic salivary bacteria in wild and captive Komodo dragons. *J Wildl Dis* 2002;38:545–51.

17 Inglesby TV, Henderson DA, Bartlett JG et al. Anthrax as a biological weapon: medical and public health management. Working Group on Civilian Biodefense. *JAMA* 1999;281:1735–45.

18 Dixon TC, Meselson M, Guillemin J, Hanna PC. Anthrax. *N Engl J Med* 1999;341:815–26.

19 Centers for Disease Control and Prevention (CDC). Update: investigation of bioterrorism-related anthrax and interim guidelines for exposure management and antimicrobial therapy, October 2001. *MMWR* 2001;50:909–19.

20 Oncul O, Ozsoy MF, Gul HC, Kocak N, Cavuslu S, Pahsa A. Cutaneous anthrax in Turkey: a review of 32 cases. *Scand J Infect Dis* 2002;34:413–6.

21 Liese J, Kloos S, Jendrossek V et al. Long-term follow-up and outcome of 39 patients with chronic granulomatous disease. *J Pediatr* 2000;137:687–93.

22 Hedstrom SA. Recurrent staphylococcal furunculosis. Bacteriological findings and epidemiology in 100 cases. *Scand J Infect Dis* 1981;13:115–9.

23 Wong HB. The child with recurrent boils. *J Singapore Paediatr Soc* 1988;30:25–30.

24 Hedstrom SA. Treatment and prevention of recurrent staphylococcal furunculosis: clinical and bacteriological follow-up. *Scand J Infect Dis* 1985;17:55–8.

25 Weijmer MC, Neering H, Welten C. Preliminary report: furunculosis and hypoferraemia. *Lancet* 1990;336:464–6.

26 Raz R, Miron D, Colodner R, Staler Z, Samara Z, Keness Y. A 1-year trial of nasal mupirocin in the prevention of recurrent staphylococcal nasal colonization and skin infection. *Arch Intern Med* 1996;156:1109–12.

27 Klempner MS, Styrt B. Prevention of recurrent staphylococcal skin infections with low-dose oral clindamycin therapy. *JAMA* 1988;260:2682–5.

28 Van der Auwera P, Meunier-Carpentier F, Klastersky J. Clinical study of combination therapy with oxacillin and rifampin for staphylococcal infections. *Rev Infect Dis* 1983;5(suppl 3):S515–22.

29 Loeb M, Main C, Walker-Dilks C, Eady A. Antimicrobial drugs for treating methicillin-resistant *Staphylococcus aureus* colonization (review). *The Cochrane Database of Systematic Reviews* 2003;(4):Art No CD003340.

30 Lipsky BA, Pecoraro RE, Ahroni JH, Peugeot RL. Immediate and long-term efficacy of systemic antibiotics for eradicating nasal colonization with *Staphylococcus aureus*. *Eur J Clin Microbiol Infect Dis* 1992;11:43–7.

31 Mashhood AA, Shaikh ZI, Qureshi SM, Malik SM. Efficacy of rifampicin in eradication of carrier state of *Staphylococcus aureus* in anterior nares with recurrent furunculosis. *J Coll Physicians Surg Pak* 2006;16:396–9.

32 Hoss DM, Feder HM, Jr. Addition of rifampin to conventional therapy for recurrent furunculosis. *Arch Dermatol* 1995;131:647–8.

33 Fisher RG, Benjamin DK, Jr. Facial cellulitis in childhood: a changing spectrum. *South Med J* 2002;95:672–4.

34 Bisno AL, Stevens DL. Streptococcal infections in skin and soft tissues. *N Engl J Med* 1996;334:240–5.

35 Swartz MN. Clinical practice. Cellulitis. *N Engl J Med* 2004;350:904–12.

36 Davies HD, Sakuls P, Keystone JS. Creeping eruption. A review of clinical presentation and management of 60 cases presenting to a tropical disease unit. *Arch Dermatol* 1993;129:588–91.

37 Katz R, Hood WR. Topical tiabendazole for creeping eruption. *Arch Dermatol* 1966;94:643–5.

38 Caumes E, Carriere J, Datry A, Gaxotte P, Danis M, Gentilini M. A randomized trial of ivermectin versus albendazole for the treatment of cutaneous larva migrans. *Am J Trop Med Hyg* 1993;49:641–4.

39 Jelineck T, Maiwald H, Northdurft HD, Loscher T. Cutaneous larva migrans in travelers: synopsis of histories, symptoms and treatment of 98 patients. *Clin Infect Dis* 1994;19:1062–6.

40 Centers for Disease Control and Prevention. *Pseudomonas dermatitis/folliculitis* associated with pools and hot tubs—Colorado and Maine, 1999–2000. *JAMA* 2001;285:157–8.

41 Gustafson TL, Band JD, Hutcheson RH, Schaffner W. *Pseudomonas folliculitis*: an outbreak and review. *Rev Infect Dis* 1983;5:1–8.

42 Ratnam S, Hogan K, March SB, Butler RW. Whirlpool-associated folliculitis caused by *Pseudomonas aeruginosa*: report of an outbreak and review. *J Clin Microbiol* 1986;23:655–9.

43 Gupta AK, Batra R, Bluhm R, Boekhout T, Dawson TL, Jr. Skin diseases associated with Malassezia species. *J Am Acad Dermatol* 2004;51:785–98.

44 Boer A, Herder N, Winter K, Falk T. Herpes folliculitis: clinical, histopathological, and molecular pathologic observations. *Br J Dermatol* 2006;154:743–6.

45 Rajendran PM, Dolev JC, Heaphy MR, Jr, Maurer T. Eosinophilic folliculitis: before and after the introduction of antiretroviral therapy. *Arch Dermatol* 2005;141:1227–31.

46 Koning S, Verhagen AP, van Suijlekom-Smit LW, Morris A, Butler CC, van der Wouden JC. Interventions for impetigo. *The Cochrane Database of Systematic Reviews* 2004;(2):Art No CD003261.

47 George A, Rubin G. A systematic review and meta-analysis of treatments for impetigo. *Br J Gen Pract* 2003;53:480–7.

48 Dillon HC, Jr. Treatment of staphylococcal skin infections: a comparison of cephalexin and dicloxacillin. *J Am Acad Dermatol* 1983;8:177–81.

49 Ahrenholz DH. Necrotizing soft-tissue infections. *Surg Clin North Am* 1988;68:199–214.

50 Lewis RT. Necrotizing soft-tissue infections. *Infect Dis Clin North Am* 1992;6:693–703.

51 Wall DB, Klein SR, Black S, de Virgilio C. A simple model to help distinguish necrotizing fasciitis from non-necrotizing soft tissue infection. *J Am Coll Surg* 2000;191:227–31.

52 Wall DB, de Virgilio C, Black S, Klein SR. Objective criteria may assist in distinguishing necrotizing fasciitis from non-necrotizing soft tissue infection. *Am J Surg* 2000;179:17–21.

53 Wong CH, Khin LW, Heng KS, Tan KC, Low CO. The LRINEC (Laboratory Risk Indicator for Necrotizing Fasciitis) score: a tool for distinguishing necrotizing fasciitis from other soft tissue infections. *Crit Care Med* 2004;32:1535–41.

54 Simonart T, Simonart JM, Derdelinckx I et al. Value of standard laboratory tests for the early recognition of group A beta-hemolytic streptococcal necrotizing fasciitis. *Clin Infect Dis* 2001;32:E9–12.

55 Simonart T, Nakafusa J, Narisawa Y. The importance of serum creatine phosphokinase level in the early diagnosis and microbiological evaluation of necrotizing fasciitis. *J Eur Acad Dermatol Venereol* 2004;18:687–90.

56 Wong CH, Wang YS. The diagnosis of necrotizing fascitis. *Curr Opin Infect Dis* 2005;18:101–6.

57 Schroeder JL, Steinke EE. Necrotizing fasciitis—the importance of early diagnosis and debridement. *AORN J* 2005;82:1031–40.

58 Darenberg J, Soderquist B, Normark BH, Norrby-Teglund A. Differences in potency of intravenous polyspecific immunoglobulin G against streptococcal and staphylococcal superantigens: implications for therapy of toxic shock syndrome. *Clin Infect Dis* 2004;38:836–42.

59 Lamothe F, D'Amico P, Ghosn P et al. Clinical usefulness of intravenous human immunoglobulins in invasive group A streptococcal infections: case report and review. *Clin Infect Dis* 1995;21:1469–70.

60 Kaul R, McGeer A, Norrby-Teglund A et al. Intravenous immunoglobulin therapy for streptococcal toxic shock syndrome—a comparative observational study. The Canadian Streptococcal Study Group. *Clin Infect Dis* 1999;28:800–7.

61 Haywood CT, McGeer A, Low DE. Clinical experience with 20 cases of group A streptococcus necrotizing fasciitis and myonecrosis: 1995 to 1997. *Plast Reconstr Surg* 1999;103:1567–73.

62 Norrby-Teglund A, Muller MP, McGeer A et al. Successful management of severe group A streptococcal soft tissue infections using an aggressive medical regimen including intravenous polyspecific immunoglobulin together with a conservative surgical approach. *Scand J Infect Dis* 2005;37:166–72.

63 Therapeutic Guidelines Ltd. *Therapeutic Guidelines: Antibiotic*, 13th edn. Melbourne: Therapeutic Guidelines Ltd, 2006.

64 Jallali N, Withey S, Butler PE. Hyperbaric oxygen as adjuvant therapy in the management of necrotizing fasciitis. *Am J Surg* 2005;189:462–6.

65 Gratz N. *Human Lice—Their Prevalence, Control and Resistance to Insecticides*. WHO/CTD/WHOPES/97.8. Geneva: World Health Organization, 1997.

66 Downs AMR, Harvey I, Kennedy CTC. The epidemiology of head lice and scabies in the UK. *Epidemiol Infect* 1999;122:471–7.

67 Dodd CS. Interventions for treating headlice. *The Cochrane Database of Systematic Reviews* 2001;(2):Art No CD001165.

68 Frankowski BL, Weiner LB. Committee on School Health the Committee on Infectious Diseases. American Academy of Pediatrics. Head lice. *Pediatrics* 2002;110:638–43.

69 Plastow L, Luthra M, Powell R, Wright J, Russell D, Marshall MN. Head lice infestation: bug busting vs. traditional treatment. *J Clin Nurs* 2001;10:775–83.

70 Hill N, Moor G, Cameron MM et al. Single blind, randomised, comparative study of the Bug Buster kit and over the counter pediculicide treatments against head lice in the United Kingdom. *BMJ* 2005;331:384–7.

71 Roberts RJ, Casey D, Morgan DA, Petrovic M. Comparison of wet combing with malathion for treatment of head lice in the UK: a pragmatic randomised controlled trial. *Lancet* 2000;356:540–4.

72 Meinking TL, Clineschmidt CM, Chen C et al. An observer-blinded study of 1% permethrin creme rinse with and

without adjunctive combing in patients with head lice. *J Pediatr* 2002;141:665–70.

73 Amren DP, Anderson AS, Wannamaker LW. Perianal cellulitis associated with group A streptococci. *Am J Dis Child* 1966;112:546–52.

74 Montemarano AD, James WD. *Staphylococcus aureus* as a cause of perianal dermatitis. *Pediatr Dermatol* 1993;10:259–62.

75 Mattia AR. Perianal mass and recurrent cellulitis due to *Enterobius vermicularis. Am J Trop Med Hyg* 1992;47:811–5.

76 Williamson M, Thomas A, Webster DJ, Young HL. Management of synergistic bacterial gangrene in severely immunocompromised patients. Report of four cases. *Dis Colon Rectum* 1993;36:862–5.

77 Kokx NP, Comstock JA, Facklam RR. Streptococcal perianal disease in children. *Pediatrics* 1987;80:659–63.

78 Barzilai A, Choen HA. Isolation of group A streptococci from children with perianal cellulitis and from their siblings. *Pediatr Infect Dis J* 1998;17:358–60.

79 Patrizi A, Costa AM, Fiorillo, Neri I. Perianal streptococcal dermatitis associated with guttate psoriasis and/or balanoposthitis: a study of five cases. *Pediatr Dermatol* 1994;11:168–71.

80 Krol AL. Perianal streptococcal cellulitis. *Pediatr Dermatol* 1990;7:97–100.

81 Rehder PA, Eliezer ET, Lane AT. Perianal cellulitis: cutaneous group A streptococcal disease. *Arch Dermatol* 1988;124:702–4.

82 Medina S, Gomez MI, De Misa RF, Ledo A. Perianal streptococcal cellulitis: treatment with topical mupirocin. *Dermatology* 1992;185:219.

83 Sissolak D, Weir WR. Tropical pyomyositis. *J Infect* 1994;29:121–7.

84 Gubbay AJ, Isaacs D. Pyomyositis in children. *Pediatr Infect Dis J* 2000;19:1009–12; quiz 1013.

85 Frank G, Mahoney HM, Eppes SC. Musculoskeletal infections in children. *Pediatr Clin North Am* 2005;52:1083–106.

86 Bocchini CE, Hulten KG, Mason EO, Jr, Gonzalez BE, Hammerman WA, Kaplan SL. Panton-Valentine leukocidin genes are associated with enhanced inflammatory response and local disease in acute hematogenous *Staphylococcus aureus* osteomyelitis in children. *Pediatrics* 2006;117:433–40.

87 Parbhoo A, Govender S. Acute pyogenic psoas abscess in children. *J Pediatr Orthop* 1992;12:663–6.

88 Chosidow O. Clinical practices. Scabies. *N Engl J Med* 2006;354:1718–27.

89 Walker GJA, Johnstone PW. Interventions for treating scabies. *The Cochrane Database of Systematic Reviews* 2000;(3):Art No CD000320.

90 Mahe A, Faye O, N'Diaye HT et al. Definition of an algorithm for the management of common skin diseases at primary health care level in sub-Saharan Africa. *Trans R Soc Trop Med Hyg* 2005;99:39–47.

91 Roberts LJ, Huffam SE, Walton SF, Currie BJ. Crusted scabies: clinical and immunological findings in seventy-eight patients and a review of the literature. *J Infect* 2005;50:375–81.

92 Guldbakke KK, Khachemoune A. Crusted scabies: a clinical review. *J Drugs Dermatol* 2006;5:221–7.

93 Bigby M. A systematic review of the treatment of scabies. *Arch Dermatol* 2000;136:387–9.

94 Bhalla M, Thami GP. Reversible neurotoxicity after an overdose of topical lindane in an infant. *Pediatr Dermatol* 2004;21:597–9.

95 Centers for Disease Control and Prevention. *Scabies Fact Sheet.* Atlanta: Centers for Disease Control and Prevention, 2005. Available at http://www.cdc.gov/ncidod/dpd/parasites/scab ies/factsht_scabies.htm.

96 Carapetis JR, Connors C, Yarmirr D, Krause V, Currie BJ. Success of a scabies control program in an Australian aboriginal community. *Pediatr Infect Dis J* 1997;16:494–9.

97 Taplin D, Meinking TL, Chen JA, Sanchez R. Comparison of crotamiton 10% cream (Eurax) and permethrin 5% cream (Elimite) for the treatment of scabies in children. *Pediatr Dermatol* 1990;7:67–73.

98 Brooks PA, Grace RF. Ivermectin is better than benzyl benzoate for childhood scabies in developing countries. *J Paediatr Child Health* 2002;38:401–4.

99 American Academy of Pediatrics. Scabies. In: Pickering LK (ed.), *Red Book: 2003 Report of the Committee on Infectious Diseases*, 26th edn. Elk Grove Village, IL: American Academy of Pediatrics, 2003:547–9.

100 Meinking TL, Taplin D, Hermida JL, Pardo R, Kerdel FA. The treatment of scabies with ivermectin. *N Engl J Med* 1995;333:26–30.

101 Macotela-Ruiz E, Pena-Gonzalez G. Tratamiento de la escabiasis con ivermectina por via oral. *Gac Med Mex* 1993;129:201–5.

102 Chouela EN, Abeldano AM, Pellerano G et al. Equivalent therapeutic efficacy and safety of ivermectin and lindane in the treatment of human scabies. *Arch Dermatol* 1999;135:651–5.

103 Usha V, Gopalakrishnan Nair TV. A comparative study of oral ivermectin and topical permethrin cream in the treatment of scabies. *J Am Acad Dermatol* 2000;42: 236–40.

104 Lawrence G, Leafasia J, Sheridan J et al. Control of scabies, skin sores and haematuria in children in the Solomon Islands: another role for ivermectin. *Bull World Health Organ* 2005;83:34–42.

105 Gardon J, Gardon-Wendel N, Demanga-Ngangue, Kamgno J, Chippaux JP, Boussinesq M. Serious reactions after mass treatment of onchocerciasis with ivermectin in an area endemic for Loa loa infection. *Lancet* 1997;350: 18–22.

106 Barkwell R, Shields S. Deaths associated with ivermectin treatment of scabies. *Lancet* 1997;349:1144–5.

107 del Giudice P, Marty P, Gari-Toussaint M, Le Fichoux Y. Ivermectin in elderly patients. *Arch Dermatol* 1999;135: 351–2.

108 Burkhart CG, Burkhart CN. Optimal treatment for scabies remains undetermined. *J Am Acad Dermatol* 2001;45: 637–8.

109 Taplin D, Meinking TL. Treatment of HIV-related scabies with emphasis on the efficacy of ivermectin. *Semin Cutan Med Surg* 1997;16:235–40.

110 Oliver JD. Wound infections caused by *Vibrio vulnificus* and other marine bacteria. *Epidemiol Infect* 2005;133:383–91.

111 Lewis FM, Marsh BJ, von Reyn CF. Fish tank exposure and cutaneous infections due to *Mycobacterium marinum*: tuberculin skin testing, treatment, and prevention. *Clin Infect Dis* 2003;37:390–7.

112 Mermel LA, Farr BM, Sherertz RJ et al. Guidelines for the management of intravascular catheter-related infections. *Clin Infect Dis* 2001;32:1249–72.

113 Gaviria JM, Garcia PJ, Garrido SM, Corey L, Boeckh M. Non-tuberculous mycobacterial infections in hematopoietic stem cell transplant recipients: characteristics of respiratory and catheter-related infections. *Biol Blood Marrow Transplant* 2000;6:361–9.

CHAPTER 15

Systemic sepsis

Severe sepsis has been defined in adults and older children as the systemic response to an infection, as manifested by organ dysfunction, hypoperfusion, or hypotension, and two or more of fever, tachycardia, tachypnea, and elevated white cell count.[1] Consensus definitions of sepsis, severe sepsis, septic shock, and the systemic inflammatory response syndrome in neonates and children have been published.[2] Antibiotics to cover the most likely pathogens, sometimes loosely called "broad spectrum" antibiotics, are only one aspect of the management of septic shock. Other interventions to preserve tissue perfusion and oxygenation are given in Section 15.3, p. 245 and in Boxes 15.1 and 15.2.

15.1 Antibiotic therapy for severe sepsis

Question | For children with severe sepsis, is one antibiotic regimen more effective compared to other regimens in terms of mortality or morbidity?

Literature review | We reviewed 801 RCTs of sepsis or sepsis syndrome in children, but none compared antibiotic choices for immunocompetent children with severe sepsis, other than those comparing once daily with multiple dose aminoglycosides. We found one review.[3]

The choice of empiric antibiotics will be guided to an extent by the spectrum of organisms causing infection locally, and also by clinical criteria, such as the presence of rash or accompanying soft tissue infection. Nevertheless, it is surprising and disappointing how little published data are available on the antibiotic treatment of severe sepsis. We found a so-called "evidence-based" review, but because the review was severely limited by the small number of trials and absence of relevant RCTs, most of the recommendations were based on consensus.[3] We found one RCT that found no difference between IV penicillin and IV cefuroxime in the empiric treatment of 154 children aged 3 months to 15 years, mostly with moderately severe

infections such as pneumonia, other lower respiratory infections, and other common acute infections warranting hospitalization and parenteral antimicrobials.[4] Our recommendations are, therefore, based on the organisms infecting children in epidemiologic studies of severe sepsis, but may need to be varied depending on local circumstances.

Organism unknown, meningitis not excluded

For empiric therapy of severe sepsis with no obvious source of infection in children 0–3 months of age, when meningitis has not been excluded, we recommend:

> **amoxi/ampicillin 50 mg/kg IV, 6-hourly** PLUS
> **cefotaxime 50 mg/kg IV, 6-hourly** PLUS
> **vancomycin 15 mg/kg IV, 6-hourly**

This regimen provides effective treatment for the likely infant pathogens acquired through the respiratory route, such as *Haemophilus influenzae* type b, pneumococcus, and meningococcus, but also bowel/urinary-tract-derived pathogens such as *Escherichia coli* and other Gram-negative bacilli. Enterococci and Listeria, neonatally acquired organisms that can cause postneonatal sepsis, are inherently resistant to cefotaxime, hence the use of ampicillin. Vancomycin is used because meningitis caused by strains of pneumococcus insensitive to penicillin does not respond adequately to ampicillin. Vancomycin also provides cover for MRSA infection, either community- or hospital-acquired, and should be used if there are risk factors, such as ethnicity, soft tissue infection, or prior colonization.

Children aged >3 months are more likely to be infected with *Staphylococcus aureus*, and an antistaphylococcal antibiotic is indicated. Recommended antibiotics are:

> **di/flucl/oxa/nafcillin 50 mg/kg (max 2 g) IV, 6-hourly** PLUS
> **vancomycin 15 mg/kg (max 500 mg) IV, 6-hourly**

Organism unknown, meningitis excluded

For empiric therapy of severe sepsis with no obvious source of infection in children 0–3 months of age when meningitis has been excluded, recommended antibiotics to cover respiratory and gastrointestinal or urinary tract pathogens are:

amoxi/ampicillin 50 mg/kg IV, 6-hourly PLUS
gentamicin 7.5 mg/kg IV, daily

For children aged 4 months and older, to cover Gram-negative and *S. aureus* infection, recommended antibiotics are:

di/flucl/oxa/nafcillin 50 mg/kg (max 2 g) IV, 6-hourly PLUS EITHER
cefotaxime 50 mg/kg (max 2 g) IV, 6-hourly OR
ceftriaxone 50 mg/kg (max 2 g) IV, daily

Skin or soft tissue source of infection

For severe sepsis resulting from a skin infection (including cellulitis), *S. aureus* and/or *Streptococcus pyogenes* are the most likely pathogens. Recommended treatment is:

di/flucl/oxa/nafcillin 50 mg/kg (max 2 g) IV, 6-hourly

For patients with non-anaphylactic penicillin allergy, we recommend:

cephalothin 50 mg/kg up (max 2 g) IV, 6-hourly OR
cephazolin 50 mg/kg (max 2 g) IV, 8-hourly

For patients with anaphylactic penicillin allergy, we recommend:

clindamycin 10 mg/kg (max 450 mg) IV or orally, 8-hourly OR
vancomycin <12 years: 30 mg/kg (max 1 g) IV, 12-hourly, 12 years or older: 25 mg/kg (max 1 g) IV, 12-hourly

If there is fresh- or saltwater contamination, to cover Vibrios etc. (see Section 14.14, p. 236), we recommend adding:

cefotaxime 50 mg/ kg (max 2g) IV, 8-hourly OR
ciprofloxacin 10 mg/kg (max 400 mg) IV, 12-hourly

15.2 Fluid therapy in severe sepsis

It has been known for some time that vigorous fluid resuscitation improves survival in pediatric septic shock. An observational study compared the outcome of children with septic shock given <20, 20–40, or >40 mL/kg in the first hour after emergency department presentation.[5] Rapid fluid resuscitation >40 mL/kg in the first hour was associated with improved survival, decreased occurrence of persistent hypovolemia, and no increase in the risk of cardiogenic pulmonary edema or adult respiratory distress syndrome.[5]

Question | In children with septic shock, does the use of colloids for fluid resuscitation in comparison to crystalloids reduce mortality or morbidity?

Literature review | We found 53 RCTs, Cochrane review,[6] and a non-Cochrane review[7] comparing colloids with crystalloids in critically ill patients. We found 1 RCT comparing colloid to crystalloid in pediatric septic shock.[7]

Colloids have been used in intensive care for some years, and there is laboratory and animal data to support their use in sepsis. Early systematic reviews comparing colloid and crystalloid in critically ill patients caused alarm, because albumin appeared to be harmful compared with saline. However, the trials in these reviews were small, and more recent systematic reviews, notably the latest Cochrane review,[6] have found that colloids are no worse and no better than crystalloids. Nineteen trials of albumin or plasma protein fraction (7576 patients) reported no effect on mortality (RR 1.02, 95% 95% CI 0.93–1.11). There was no difference between hydroxyethyl starch and crystalloids, between modified gelatin and crystalloid, between dextran and a crystalloid, or between dextran in hypertonic crystalloid and isotonic crystalloid. This Cochrane review has been criticized by intensivists, for the quality of the studies included in the meta-analysis, which nevertheless fulfill the strict Cochrane criteria for inclusion.

Albumin might affect endothelial permeability and redox balance to a different extent to artificial colloids. It is unclear from the above studies, however, whether albumin differs from other colloids, particularly synthetic ones, in outcome.

In a non-Cochrane review of fluid resuscitation for severe sepsis, the authors concluded that albumin decreased pulmonary edema and respiratory dysfunction compared with crystalloid, while hydroxyethyl starch induced abnormalities of hemostasis.[7]

In the only pediatric RCT, from India, 31 children with septic shock were resuscitated with saline and 29 with gelatin polymer.[8] There was no difference in mortality (29% with saline and 31% with gelatin), and no difference in plasma volume or hemodynamic stability.

The SAFE study[9] was published subsequent to both the Cochrane review[6] and the non-Cochrane review.[7] In the SAFE study, 6997 adult intensive care patients needing fluid resuscitation for any cause were randomized to receive albumin or saline on admission.[9] The mortality of the albumin and saline groups was virtually identical (RR 0.99). A sub-group analysis, however, found that that there was a trend for patients with sepsis to be less likely to die within 28 days if they received albumin rather than saline (RR 0.87, 95% CI 0.74–1.02, $p = 0.09$). Interestingly, patients with trauma were more likely to die if they received albumin rather than saline.

The colloid versus crystalloid controversy continues, but to date the evidence does not favor either. Considering that colloids are considerably more expensive than are crystalloids, there seems little reason not to use saline. In a setting where resources are scarce, saline is preferable. The critical factor is that timely and vigorous resuscitation with either colloid or crystalloid improves prognosis in septic shock, and that failure to resuscitate adequately with fluids can lead to refractory shock.

We recommend resuscitating children with severe sepsis intravenously using at least 40 mL/kg in the first hour of either crystalloid or colloid.

15.3 Vasopressors and inotropes in septic shock

Question | In children with septic shock refractory to intravenous fluid resuscitation, do vasopressors or inotropes compared with standard therapy reduce mortality or morbidity?

Literature review | We found seven observational studies, one RCT,[10] and two non-Cochrane reviews.[11,12]

In hypovolemic, cardiogenic, and obstructive forms of shock, the primary defect is a fall in cardiac output lead-ing to tissue hypoperfusion. In septic shock, however, there is a complex interaction between pathological vasodilatation (warm shock), hypovolemia, toxic myocardial depression, and altered distribution of blood flow.[11] Vasopressors such as norepinephrine (noradrenaline) and dopamine vary in their inotropic effect.

We found one RCT which showed that the vasopressor/inotrope milrinone improved cardiac function in children with non-hyperdynamic septic shock, who also received catecholamines.[10] We found two evidence-based reviews of vasopressor and inotropic support in septic shock.[11,12] Neither review could find any other RCTs, and their recommendations were mainly reached by consensus. The recommendations, modified from one of the reviews,[11] and the strength of the evidence are given in Box 15.1.

Vasopressors/inotropes are used often if intravenous fluids do not correct shock. A Cochrane review found

---

Box 15.1 Recommendations on vasopressor or inotropic support for children with septic shock.

1 Monitor arterial blood pressure continuously using an arterial catheter (weak evidence).

2 Give adequate fluid resuscitation (weak evidence).

3 If adequate fluid challenge does not restore arterial pressure and tissue perfusion, give vasopressor or inotrope support (weak evidence, see Box 15.2).

4 Either norepinephrine (noradrenaline) or dopamine is the vasopressor/inotrope of choice to correct hypotension. There is no evidence that using both norepinephrine and dopamine is superior than dopamine alone (weak evidence).

5 Low-dose dopamine should not be used routinely for renal protection (one good RCT[13]).

6 Epinephrine (adrenaline) and phenylephrine should not be first-line vasopressor/inotropes in septic shock (weak evidence).

7 Vasopressin may be considered in patients with refractory shock despite adequate fluids and high-dose vasopressor/inotropes (weak evidence).

8 Dobutamine is the agent of choice for patients with low cardiac output despite adequate fluid resuscitation (weak evidence).

9 Inotropes should not be used to increase cardiac output above physiologic levels (good evidence from two RCTs[14,15]).

Modified from Reference 11.

only eight studies comparing vasopressor to placebo, vasopressor to intravenous fluids, or one vasopressor regime with another, using mortality as the outcome.[16] There was insufficient evidence that vasopressin was better than placebo or that a particular vasopressor was superior to other agents in the treatment of shock.

On the other hand, there is one observational study, suggesting that children with septic shock refractory to fluids will respond to inotrope and/or vasopressor therapy.[17] In a study of 50 children with refractory septic shock, the overall 28-day survival was 80%. The children were categorized according to hemodynamic state: those with a low cardiac index responded to an inotrope with or without a vasopressor, those with a high cardiac index and low systemic vascular resistance responded to vasopressor alone, and those with both vascular and cardiac dysfunction responded to combined inotrope and vasopressor therapy.[17]

15.4 Glycemic control in severe sepsis

Hypoglycemia is associated with poor neurologic outcome, and it is obviously important to correct hypoglycemia associated with sepsis. Some septic patients, however, have hyperglycemia, and it is less clear that this should be corrected. There is some evidence that the maintenance of good glycemic control in adults with septic shock improves prognosis, but no good evidence in children.[12]

15.5 Corticosteroids in septic shock

Question | In children with septic shock from any cause, do corticosteroids compared with no steroids or placebo reduce mortality or morbidity?
Literature review | We found no RCTs of corticosteroids in children with septic shock. We found 15 RCTs and a Cochrane review of corticosteroids in adults with septic shock.[18]

A Cochrane review of the use of corticosteroids in adults with septic shock from any cause[18] found 15 RCTs (2023 patients). Corticosteroids did not change 28-day, all-cause mortality (RR 0.92, 95% CI 0.75–1.14) or hospital mortality (RR 0.89, 95% CI 0.71–1.11). Corticosteroids did, however, reduce intensive care unit mortality (RR 0.83, 95% CI 0.70–0.97), and increased the proportion of shock reversal by day 7 (RR 1.22, 95% CI 1.06–1.40) and by day 28 (RR 1.26, 95% CI 1.04–1.52), without increasing the rate of gastroduodenal bleeding, superinfection, or hyperglycemia.

There are no comparable data on corticosteroid use in children. A study of adrenal function in children with septic shock found absolute adrenal insufficiency with catecholamine-resistant shock in 18% and relative adrenal insufficiency in 26% of children.[19] Efficacy studies are needed. Some pediatric intensivists already use intravenous hydrocortisone at a dose of 25 mg/m^2 6-hourly (100 mg/m^2/day in four divided doses) to treat children with septic shock, but the evidence is weak.

15.6 Intravenous immunoglobulins in severe sepsis

Question | In children with septic shock from any cause, do intravenous immunoglobulins (IVIG) compared with no IVIG reduce mortality or morbidity?
Literature review | We found 27 RCTs of IVIG in septic shock, of which 2 were in children. We found a Cochrane review of IVIG in adults with septic shock.[20]

A Cochrane review of the use of IVIG in septic shock[20] found 27 eligible studies of polyclonal immunoglobulin preparations and specific antibodies, such as monoclonal antibodies (see Section 15.7, p. 247). The overall mortality was reduced in 492 patients who received polyclonal IVIG (RR 0.64, 95% CI 0.51–0.80). A sub-analysis showed that sepsis-related mortality, i.e., deaths caused by sepsis, was significantly reduced in 161 patients who received polyclonal IVIG (RR 0.35, 95% CI 0.18–0.69). For the two high-quality trials on 91 patients of polyclonal IVIG, there was a 70% reduction in mortality, but the confidence intervals were wide (RR 0.30, 95% CI 0.09–0.99). The authors commented that although polyclonal IVIG significantly reduced mortality, all the trials were small and the totality of the evidence is insufficient to support a robust conclusion of benefit.

We recommend considering using IVIG in children with severe and refractory septic shock.

15.7 Monoclonal antibodies in severe sepsis (antiendotoxins and anticytokines)

In the Cochrane review of the use of immunoglobulins,[20] mortality was not reduced among 2826 patients who received monoclonal antibodies, such as antiendotoxins in five good-quality studies (RR 0.97, 95% CI 0.88–1.07), or 4318 patients who received anticytokines (RR 0.93, 95% CI 0.86–1.01). A few studies measured secondary outcomes (deaths from sepsis or length of hospitalization), but no differences in the intervention and control groups were identified in patients receiving antiendotoxin or anticytokine monoclonal antibodies.

15.8 Activated protein C in severe sepsis

In septic shock, there is consumption of coagulation factors including protein C. Although recombinant activated protein C (drotrecogin alfa) reduces mortality from septic shock in adults,[21] it has proven to be of no value in children. A large RCT of activated protein C in children with severe sepsis was halted early by the Data Monitoring Committee because of lack of efficacy (Eli Lilly, 2005).

15.9 Naloxone in severe sepsis

A Cochrane review found six RCTs of naloxone in septic shock.[22] The mean arterial pressure was significantly higher in the naloxone groups than in the placebo groups (weighted mean difference: +9.33 mm Hg; 95% CI 7.07–11.59). Higher blood pressure, however, does not necessarily equate with improved tissue perfusion. The mortality was lower in the naloxone group, but not statistically significantly (OR 0.59, 95% CI 0.21–1.67). The clinical role of naloxone remains unclear.

15.10 Nitric oxide antagonists in severe sepsis

There are theoretical grounds for believing that it might be effective to inhibit nitric oxide synthase. However, the use of a nitric oxide synthase inhibitor in adults and children with septic shock was associated with increased mortality.[23]

15.11 Colony stimulating factors (G-CSF and GM-CSF) in severe sepsis

Recombinant granulocyte colony stimulating factor (G-CSF, filgrastim) was safe but ineffective in reducing mortality in patients with pneumonia and sepsis.[24] We could find no studies of the use of granulocyte macrophage colony stimulating factor (GM-CSF) to treat pediatric septic shock.

15.12 Extracorporeal membrane oxygenation (ECMO) in severe sepsis

Not surprisingly, there are no RCTs of the use of ECMO in septic shock. In one small series, four of nine children with refractory septic shock survived, and the authors concluded that near-fatal septic shock was not a contraindication to ECMO.[25]

15.13 Early goal-directed therapy in severe sepsis

Goal-directed therapy involves adjustments of cardiac preload, after-load, and contractility to balance oxygen delivery with oxygen demand. It has been used successfully in an RCT of adults with septic shock. In this study, mortality was reduced from 46.5% with standard therapy to 30.5% with 6 hours of early goal-directed therapy.[26]

15.14 Sepsis bundles

A "sepsis bundle" is a group of interventions designed to improve the outcome of systemic sepsis. The principle is that patients are assessed to see which of a number of recommended investigations have been performed and which interventions instigated. If it can be demonstrated that compliance with the recommendations in the sepsis bundle is associated with improved outcome, this provides evidence for promotion of the package of interventions as likely to improve outcome. It is not a randomized intervention and is open to selection bias, but it is a reasonable approach given the complexity of intensive care.

The use of sepsis bundles to prevent ventilator-associated pneumonia in a number of adult intensive care units reduced the mean incidence by 44.5%.[27] Sepsis care bundles for systemic sepsis in adults are used to encourage early monitoring and treatment of patients. One sepsis bundle[28] recorded whether or not the following targets were achieved at 6 hours:

- serum lactate measured;
- antibiotics given within an hour of taking blood cultures;
- 0.5 L of fluid given in the first 30 minutes;
- vasopressors for mean arterial pressure <65 mm Hg despite fluid resuscitation;
- inotropes and/or blood transfusion to target Hb 7–9 g/dL.

At 24 hours, the targets were:

- serum glucose <8.3 mmol/L;
- plateau pressure average <30 cm H_2O if ventilated;
- drotrecogin alfa considered for severe sepsis (but note that this would not be used in children, see above);
- steroids for septic shock ;
- APACHE II score;
- predicted mortality.

The rate of compliance with the 6-hour sepsis bundle was 52%. The mortality was more than twice as high in the patients for whom the sepsis bundle was not used, compared with the patients in whom it was used (49% versus 23%, RR 2.12, 95% CI 1.20–3.76) despite similar age and severity of sepsis. Compliance with the 24-hour sepsis bundle was achieved in only 30% of eligible candidates (21/69). Hospital mortality was higher in the patients in whom the bundle was not used (50% versus 29%), although the difference did not reach statistical significance (RR 1.76, 95% CI 0.84–3.64, $p = 0.16$). These data suggest that compliance with sepsis bundles, particularly the early measures, reduces the mortality from sepsis.[28] Sepsis bundles appropriate to children need to be developed and evaluated.

15.15   Recommendations on the management of severe sepsis in children

The evidence for the recommendations given in Box 15.2 is based on the evidence given above. There have also been RCTs in adults, described in two overview papers,[30,31] and are difficult to evaluate individually because of the complex nature of intensive care of the patient with septic shock. Clearly, there are several interventions that are urgent: correction of hypoglycemia

Box 15.2 Recommendations for the initial management of severe sepsis with shock in children.

1 ABC: establish and maintain airway, breathing, and circulation.

2 Administer oxygen. Intubate and ventilate if necessary to maintain adequate gas exchange.

3 If the patient is hypotensive or there is evidence of organ hypoperfusion (e.g., lactate >4 mmol/L or oliguria), administer at least 20 mL/kg of crystalloid (or colloid equivalent) rapidly, and over 40 mL/kg in the first hour.

4 Correct hypoglycemia.

5 Take blood cultures and other appropriate cultures (e.g., urine, sputum, wounds, and possibly CSF).

6 Administer appropriate antibiotics (see below) **immediately** after obtaining blood cultures.

7 Correction of hypotension is a high priority. Use inotropes and/or vasopressors (dopamine, noradrenaline, or occasionally vasopressin) for hypotension not responding to initial fluid resuscitation. Titrate dose to maintain blood pressure and adequate organ perfusion.

8 Control the source of sepsis where possible. This may require surgical or percutaneous drainage, with appropriate samples collected.

9 Low-dose corticosteroid therapy (hydrocortisone 25 mg/m² IV, 6-hourly) may be an option in refractory shock, but its use remains controversial in children.

10 Continuing fluid replacement (0.9% sodium chloride or 4% albumin) may be required to maintain an adequate central venous pressure and adequate tissue perfusion in sepsis.

Adapted with permission from Reference 29.

(intervention 4 in Box 15.2) is almost as urgent as 1–3. Antibiotics need to be given as soon as possible, and any delay could be detrimental.

15.16   Management of specific infections

Meningococcal infection

Clinical diagnosis of meningococcal infection
The differential diagnosis of a child with fever and petechiae or purpura is discussed in Chapter 6 (see Section 6.8, p. 62). About 10% of children with fever

and rash have serious bacterial infection and about 7% have meningococcal infection.[32–37] In a UK case series of 233 children presenting with non-blanching rash, 26 (11%) had meningococcal disease.[38] Children with meningococcal infection were more likely than non-infected children to be assessed as "ill" (not otherwise defined), to be pyrexial ($>38.5°C$), have purpura, and a capillary refill time <2 seconds.[38]

The management of a well-looking child with petechiae and fever is less clear-cut. The basis for deciding which children need urgent treatment and admission to hospital is discussed in Section 6.7, p. 60.

Not all children with meningococcal infection present with rash. How does the primary care physician or the pediatrician identify children with meningococcal infection without rash? The signs and symptoms of meningococcal infection in infants <1 year and young children aged 1–4 years have been described in detail in a British paper that illustrates the natural history of meningococcal infection.[39]

Parents generally describe a sudden change in the child's mood or condition. A quarter of all children with meningococcal infection have had symptoms of a cold or upper respiratory tract infection in the 2 weeks prior to being diagnosed with meningococcal infection, but parents still report a sudden change in the child's behavior or overall condition at what is thought to be the onset of meningococcal infection.[39]

The earliest signs and symptoms of meningococcal infection are non-specific, and may equally well be seen in children with viral infections. Early signs in young children include fever, irritability, vomiting, diarrhea, and anorexia.

After a median of about 4 hours, young children with meningococcal infection may look pale, have cold hands and feet, and those who can talk may complain of limb pains.[39] During the next few hours, they may become drowsy and develop rapid or labored breathing.

If a rash develops, it is on average about 8 hours after the onset of the illness. This rash is characteristically purpuric, meaning it consists of purple dots or bruises due to bleeding into the skin, which do not blanch (go white) on pressure. Less commonly, a less specific, non-blanching rash mimicking a viral rash can occur, and may only develop into the classic purpuric rash over several hours.[36] Interestingly, parents are often advised to compress the rash using a glass tumbler, to see if the skin blanches, and if so, to seek urgent medical advice. A literature search failed to find any evidence that this reliably identifies children with petechiae or with meningococcal infection.[40]

Young children aged 1–4 years in the British study were admitted to hospital a median of 13 hours after the onset of the illness. By this time, most but not all were clearly unwell with fever, tachycardia, tachypnea, and often with rash, shock, and impaired consciousness. The terminal signs of unconsciousness, delirium, or convulsions were seen at about 24 hours.[39]

We use a term "toxicity" or "toxic child" to describe febrile children who are non-specifically unwell. The signs of toxicity are decreased alertness and arousal, altered breathing, blue lips, cold peripheries, weakness, high-pitched cry, and decreased fluid intake and/or urine output (see p. 57). Studies have shown that febrile children who are judged as being toxic are more likely to have serious bacterial infection.[41–46]

We recommend that all toxic children with fever and rash be sent to hospital urgently (and see p. 250 for recommendations on pre-hospital antibiotics).

We recommend that it is safest to send a non-toxic child with fever and rash to hospital for assessment, especially if the examiner is relatively inexperienced at assessing sick children.

Prehospital antibiotic treatment of meningococcal infection

The current generally recommended management of a patient in whom *Neisseria meningitidis* infection is suspected on clinical grounds[47] is to give an immediate intramuscular dose of an antibiotic, usually penicillin (see Table 15.1), and arrange urgent transfer to hospital for further treatment. It is also recommended, if possible, that blood cultures or aspirates from skin lesions are collected prior to administration of the antibiotics and sent with the patient to hospital. Although it is intuitive that early antibiotic therapy would reduce mortality, the evidence is limited.

Table 15.1 Dose of benzylpenicillin prior to hospitalization for suspected meningococcal sepsis.

Age of Child	Benzylpenicillin IV or IM
< 1 year	300 mg (500,000 U)
1–9 years	600 mg (1,000,000 U)
≥10 years	1200 mg (2,000,000 U)

Question | For children with meningococcal infection, do preadmission antibiotics compared with no antibiotics reduce mortality?

Literature review | We found 15 observational studies and one non-Cochrane systematic review[48] of the effect of preadmission antibiotics on mortality from meningococcal disease.

We found no RCTs of emergency antibiotic treatment of suspected meningococcal infection, and nor are any likely to be done. Most studies are observational, and these compare patients given preadmission antibiotics with those not given antibiotics. The great problem is confounding by severity: the sickest patients are those who are most likely to be given parenteral antibiotics. A systematic review[48] found that patients given oral antibiotics compared with those not given oral antibiotics (i.e., given no antibiotics or parenteral antibiotics) had a markedly reduced risk of dying from meningococcal infection, with a risk ratio of 0.17 (95% CI 0.07–0.44). Presumably, they were given oral antibiotics because they were not very ill, rather than oral antibiotics being protective. One primary care-based study suggested reduced morbidity and mortality from parenteral antibiotics,[49] while two others found that preadmission parenteral antibiotics were associated with an increase in mortality.[50,51]

It is plausible that parenteral antibiotics could cause harm, by rapid killing of meningococci causing massive release of endotoxin, leading to shock. In a study of patients with severe meningococcal infection, however, plasma endotoxin levels were high on admission, before antibiotics were given, and did not rise after antibiotics were given.[52]

At present, although the evidence on the benefit of early parenteral antibiotics for suspected meningococcal infection is not strong and may never improve, we think they are more likely to be beneficial than harmful.

We recommend giving parenteral antibiotics to any child seen outside hospital with suspected meningococcal infection (see Table 15.1), and we recommend staying with the child until he or she is admitted to hospital.

In patients with penicillin allergy, or in remote areas where further parenteral therapy may be substantially delayed (>6 hours), we recommend:

ceftriaxone 50 mg/kg (max 2 g) IV or IM

Emergency Department management of meningococcal infection

A case-control study comparing fatal and non-fatal cases of meningococcal infection in children found three factors independently associated with risk of dying. These were failure to be looked after by a pediatrician, failure of adequate supervision of junior staff, and failure of hospital staff to give adequate inotropes.[53]

Hospital antibiotic treatment of meningococcal infection

For the treatment of acute (or chronic) meningococcemia, we recommend:

benzylpenicillin 30 mg (50,000 U)/kg (max 1.2 g or 2 million U) IV, 4-hourly for 5 days

For patients with non-anaphylactic penicillin allergy, we recommend:

ceftriaxone 100 mg/kg (max 4 g) IV, daily for 5 days OR
cefotaxime 50 mg/kg (max 2 g) IV, 6-hourly for 5 days

For patients with anaphylactic penicillin or cephalosporin allergy, we recommend:

ciprofloxacin 10 mg/kg (max 400 mg) IV, 12-hourly for 5 days

Corticosteroids in meningococcal infection

Question | In children with septic shock due to meningococcal infection, do corticosteroids compared to no corticosteroids or placebo reduce morbidity or mortality?

Literature review | We found no RCTs of corticosteroids in children with septic shock due to meningococcal infection. We found one non-Cochrane systematic review of corticosteroids for meningococcal infection[54] and 15 RCTs and a Cochrane review of corticosteroids in adults with septic shock from any cause.[18]

We discussed the use of steroids in pediatric septic shock from any infection given in Section 15.5. A non-Cochrane systematic review found no papers that directly studied the use of corticosteroids in children with meningococcal shock.[54] The review concluded that high-dose corticosteroids (30 mg/kg of methyl-prednisolone or equivalent) were detrimental to adults with severe septic shock from any infection,[55] but that the use of low-dose corticosteroids (200–300 mg/day of hydrocortisone in adults, equivalent to 5–6 mg/kg/day or 25 mg/m^2 hydrocortisone IV 6-hourly in children) was promising.[56–58]

Three papers on adrenal function did not find that children with meningococcal infection developed adrenal failure, but did show what may be an inadequate adrenal response to infection.[59–61] The authors of the review concluded that the reasonable evidence of benefit from low-dose corticosteroids in adults with severe sepsis[56–58] plus the evidence of suboptimal adrenal response in children with meningococcal infection[59–61] supported the use of hydrocortisone replacement therapy in children with meningococcal shock dependent on catecholamines.[54]

We feel that the data are insufficient and would prefer to see RCT data before recommending the use of low-dose corticosteroids in children with meningococcal infection.

Adjunctive therapy with monoclonal antibodies and cytokines in meningococcal infection

There is no evidence to support the use of antibodies against endotoxin in children with meningococcal infection, nor of the use of recombinant human activated protein C, also known as drotrecogin alfa.[62,63]

Chemoprophylaxis for meningococcal infection

The secondary attack rate in household contacts is increased to 4.2 per 1000 for meningococcal disease[64] (see p. 138). Antibiotic chemoprophylaxis of close contacts of meningococcal cases is recommended, and is also given to the patient (the "index" case) if penicillin is used, because parenteral penicillin does not eradicate carriage. A non-Cochrane systematic review of the effectiveness of prophylactic antibiotics[65] found no high-quality prospective studies, but four retrospective observational studies and one small trial comparing children who did or did not receive chemoprophylaxis. The outcome was secondary cases of meningococcal infection occurring 1–30 days after the index case. Chemoprophylaxis reduced the risk of meningococcal infection for household contacts by an impressive 89%: the risk ratio was 0.11 (95% CI 0.02–0.58), and 218 contacts had to take prophylactic antibiotics to

prevent one case of meningococcal infection. In contrast, the data in day care settings were insufficient to judge whether or not chemoprophylaxis is indicated.

A Cochrane review of chemoprophylaxis[66] found no RCTs and no secondary cases, so could not comment on the effectiveness of chemoprophylaxis. It found that ciprofloxacin, minocycline, and rifamp(ic)in were effective at eradicating nasal carriage of meningococcus at 1 week, but only rifampin (RR 0.20, 95% CI 0.14–0.29) and ciprofloxacin (RR 0.03, 95% CI 0.00–0.42) still proved effective at 1–2 weeks. Rifampin continued to be effective compared to placebo for up to 4 weeks after treatment, but resistant isolates were seen following prophylactic treatment. No trials evaluated ceftriaxone against placebo, but ceftriaxone was more effective than rifampin after 1–2 weeks of follow-up (RR 5.93, 95% CI 1.22–28.68).

Because there were no cases of meningococcal disease during follow-up in any of the trials, effectiveness regarding prevention of future disease cannot be directly assessed.

We recommend *N.meningitidis* (meningococcus) prophylaxis for household contacts using:

> **rifamp(ic)in: neonate <1 month 5 mg/kg; child 10 mg/kg (max 600 mg); adult 600 mg, orally, 12-hourly for 2 days (preferred option for children) OR**
> **ciprofloxacin (adult and child ≥12 years) 500 mg orally, child 12.5 mg/kg (max 500 mg) as a single dose OR**
> **ceftriaxone 250 mg (child 125 mg) IM as a single dose (preferred option during pregnancy)**

Rifamp(ic)in is associated with multiple drug interactions, stains contact lenses orange, and is not recommended for persons with severe liver disease. Because they cause cartilage damage in laboratory animals, there are theoretical concerns about quinolones causing skeletal problems in children, although data do not suggest this is a real clinical problem.[67]

Immunization against meningococcal infection

Both conjugate and polysaccharide vaccines are available against meningococci. No conjugate or polysaccharide vaccine is effective against *N.meningitidis* group B. Polysaccharide vaccines have been developed, which incorporate the other serogroups A, C, W-135, and Y. These polysaccharide vaccines are relatively poorly immunogenic in infancy, and do not produce lasting immunity because the antibody response is generated without T-cell involvement. A conjugate vaccine against serogroup C has been very successful in reducing group C meningococcal disease in the UK[68] and Australia.[69] In the USA, where serogroups B, C, and Y are each responsible for 30% of cases, a conjugate vaccine against A, C, W-135, and Y has been licensed and is recommended for children from 11 to 12 years and for adolescents.[70]

Staphylococcal toxic shock syndrome

Staphylococcal toxic shock syndrome is a toxin-mediated disease characterized by fever, hypotension, a diffuse sunburnlike erythema, cerebral dysfunction with impaired consciousness, and sometimes convulsions, thrombocytopenia, and multisystem involvement often including evidence of hepatic and renal impairment.[70] The source of the toxin-producing strain of *S. aureus* may be apparent, such as an infected wound or burn, osteomyelitis, or bacterial tracheitis; may be occult, such as a tampon; or there may be asymptomatic carriage of the organism, with no apparent focus of infection. Aggressive resuscitation and treatment of the source are important aspects of therapy.

There is in vitro evidence that clindamycin reduces toxin production,[71] particularly for streptococcal toxins (see below, streptococcal toxic shock syndrome), but no good evidence that using clindamycin alone or adding it to other antibiotics improves outcome. Clindamycin is recommended if there is a high incidence of community-acquired MRSA and vancomycin should be used if hospital-acquired MRSA is likely, because of prior hospitalization or colonization.

Recommended treatment:

**clindamycin 15 mg/kg (max 600 mg) IV, 8-hourly OR
di/flucl/oxa/nafcillin 50 mg/kg (max 2 g IV), 6-hourly OR
cephalothin 50 mg/kg (max 2 g) IV, 6-hourly OR
cephazolin 50 mg/kg (max 2 g) IV, 8-hourly OR
vancomycin <12 years: 30 mg/kg (max 1 g) IV, 12-hourly, 12 years or older: 25 mg/kg (max 1 g) IV, 12-hourly**

A Cochrane review[20] found that polyclonal IVIG reduces mortality in patients with sepsis and septic shock.

There is no direct evidence to support the use of IVIG in staphylococcal toxic shock syndrome, but its use could be considered in patients responding poorly to antibiotics and with persistent hypotension. Recommended dose:

normal immunoglobulin 1–2 g/kg IV

Streptococcal sepsis including streptococcal toxic shock syndrome

Streptococcal toxic shock syndrome has been defined as the isolation of a group A streptococcus (*S. pyogenes*), hypotension, and two of renal impairment, coagulopathy, liver involvement, adult respiratory distress syndrome, generalized rash, or soft tissue necrosis.[70] It may be less common in children than adults, but when it occurs, it can be fulminant.[72–75]

There is in vitro evidence that clindamycin reduces toxin production by group A streptococci,[71] but no good evidence from clinical trials that it improves outcome. It should not be used alone because a few strains are resistant.[75] Recommended antibiotics:

**benzylpenicillin 45 mg/kg (max 1.8 g) IV, 4-hourly PLUS
clindamycin 15 mg/kg (max 600 mg) IV, 8-hourly**

For patients hypersensitive to penicillin (excluding anaphylactic hypersensitivity), substitute for benzylpenicillin:

**cephalothin 50 mg/kg (max 2 g) IV, 6-hourly OR
cephazolin 50 mg/kg (max 2 g) IV, 8-hourly**

In streptococcal toxic shock syndrome, there is one RCT[73] of 21 patients with streptococcal toxic shock syndrome that found IVIG 1 g/kg on day 1 and 0.5 g/kg on days 2 and 3 was associated with a significant reduction in organ failure and a non-significant reduction in mortality. Although the evidence is not strong, the condition is rare, making large studies difficult. We recommend using IVIG:

normal immunoglobulin 1–2 g/kg IV, repeated on days 2 and 3 if hypotension persists

References

1 Calandra T, Cohen J. The international sepsis forum consensus conference on definitions of infection in the intensive care unit. *Crit Care Med* 2005;33:1538–48.

2 Goldstein B, Giroir B, Randolph A; International Consensus Conference on Pediatric Sepsis. International pediatric sepsis consensus conference: definitions for sepsis and organ dysfunction in pediatrics. *Pediatr Crit Care Med* 2005;6: 2–8.

3 Bochud PY, Bonten M, Marchetti O, Calandra T. Antimicrobial therapy for patients with severe sepsis and septic shock: an evidence-based review. *Crit Care Med* 2004;32(suppl 11):S495–512.

4 Vuori-Holopainen E, Peltola H, Kallio MJ; SE-TU Study Group. Narrow- versus broad-spectrum parenteral antimicrobials against common infections of childhood: a prospective and randomized comparison between penicillin and cefuroxime. *Eur J Pediatr* 2000;159:878–84.

5 Carcillo JA, Davis AL, Zaritsky A. Role of early fluid resuscitation in pediatric septic shock. *JAMA* 1991;266:1242–5.

6 Roberts I, Alderson P, Bunn F, Chinnock P, Ker K, Schierhout G. Colloids versus crystalloids for fluid resuscitation in critically ill patients. *The Cochrane Database of Systematic Reviews* 2004;(4):Art No CD000567.

7 Vincent JL, Gerlach H. Fluid resuscitation in severe sepsis and septic shock: an evidence-based review. *Crit Care Med* 2004;32(suppl 11):S451–4.

8 Upadhyay M, Singhi S, Murlidharan J, Kaur N, Majumdar S. Randomized evaluation of fluid resuscitation with crystalloid (saline) and colloid (polymer from degraded gelatin in saline) in pediatric septic shock. *Indian Pediatr* 2005;42:223–31.

9 The SAFE Study Investigators. A comparison of albumin and saline for fluid resuscitation in the intensive care unit. *N Engl J Med* 2004;350:2247–56.

10 Barton P, Garcia J, Kouatli A et al. Hemodynamic effects of IV milrinone lactate in pediatric patients with septic shock: a prospective double-blinded, randomize, placebo-controlled interventional study. *Chest* 1996;109:1302–12.

11 Beale RJ, Hollenberg SM, Vincent J-L, Parrillo JE. Vasopressor and inotropic support in septic shock: an evidence-based review. *Crit Care Med* 2004;32(suppl):S455–65.

12 Carcillo JA, Fields AI. Clinical practice parameters for hemodynamic support of pediatric and neonatal patients in septic shock. *Crit Care Med* 2002;30:1365–78.

13 Bellomo R, Chapman M, Finfer S et al. Low-dose dopamine in patients with early renal dysfunction: a placebo-controlled randomized trial. *Lancet* 2000;356:2139–43.

14 Hayes MA, Timmins AC, Yau EH et al. Elevation of systemic oxygen delivery in the treatment of critically ill patients. *N Engl J Med* 1994;330:1717–22.

15 Gattioni L, Brazzi L, Pelosi P et al. A trial of goal-oriented hemodynamic therapy in critically ill patients. *N Engl J Med* 1995;333:1025–32.

16 Müllner M, Urbanek B, Havel C, Losert H, Waechter F, Gamper G. Vasopressors for shock. *The Cochrane Database of Systematic Reviews* 2004;(3):Art No CD003709.

17 Ceneviva G, Paschall JA, Maffei F, Carcillo JA. Hemodynamic support in fluid-refractory pediatric septic shock. *Pediatrics* 1998;102:e19.

18 Annane D, Bellissant E, Bollaert PE, Briegel J, Keh D, Kupfer Y. Corticosteroids for treating severe sepsis and septic shock.

The Cochrane Database of Systemic Reviews 2004;(1):Art No CD002243.

19 Pizarro CF, Troster MEJ, Damiani D, Carcillo JA. Absolute and relative adrenal insufficiency in children with septic shock. *Crit Care Med* 2005;33:855–9.

20 Alejandria MM, Lansang MA, Dans LF, Mantaring JBV. Intravenous immunoglobulin for treating sepsis and septic shock. *The Cochrane Database of Systematic Reviews* 2002;(1):Art No CD001090.

21 Rice TW, Bernard GR. Drotrecogin alfa (activated) for the treatment of severe sepsis and septic shock. *Am J Med Sc* 2004;328:205–14.

22 Boeuf B, Poirier V, Gauvin F et al. Naloxone for shock. *The Cochrane Database of Systematic Reviews* 2003;(3):Art No CD004443.

23 Lopez A, Lorente JA, Steingrub J et al. Multi-center, randomized, placebo-controlled, double-blind study of the nitric oxide synthase inhibitor 546C88: effect on survival in patients with septic shock. *Crit Care Med* 2004;32:2–30.

24 Root RK, Lodato RF, Patrick W et al. Multicenter, double-blind, placebo-controlled study of the use of filgrastim in patients hospitalized with pneumonia and severe sepsis. *Crit Care Med* 2003;31:367–73.

25 Beca J, Butt W. Extracorporeal membrane oxygenation for refractory septic shock in children. *Pediatrics* 1994;93:726–9.

26 Rivers E, Nguyen B, Havstad S et al. Early goal-directed therapy in the treatment of severe sepsis and septic shock. *N Engl J Med* 2001;345:1368–77.

27 Resar R, Pronovost P, Haraden C, Simmonds T, Rainey T, Nolan T. Using a bundle approach to improve ventilator care processes and reduce ventilator-associated pneumonia. *Jt Comm J Qual Patient Saf* 2005;31:243–8.

28 Gao F, Melody T, Daniels DF, Giles S, Fox S. The impact of compliance with 6-hour and 24-hour sepsis bundles on hospital mortality in patients with severe sepsis: a prospective observational study. *Crit Care* 2005;9:R764–70.

29 Therapeutic Guidelines Ltd. *Therapeutic Guidelines: Antibiotic*, version 13. Melbourne: Therapeutic Guidelines Ltd., 2006:257.

30 Poulton B. Advances in the management of sepsis: the randomised controlled trials behind the Surviving Sepsis Campaign recommendations. *Int J Antimicrob Agents* 2006;27:97–101.

31 Dellinger RP, Carlet JM, Masur H et al. Surviving Sepsis Campaign guidelines for management of severe sepsis and septic shock. *Crit Care Med* 2004;32:858–73.

32 Van Nguyen Q, Nguyen EA, Weiner LB. Incidence of invasive bacterial disease in children with fever and petechiae. *Pediatrics* 1984;74:77–80.

33 Baker RC, Seguin JH, Leslie N, Gilchrist MJ, Myers MG. Fever and petechiae in children. *Pediatrics* 1989;84:1051–5.

34 Mandl KD, Stack AM, Fleisher GR. Incidence of bacteremia in infants and children with fever and petechiae. *J Pediatr* 1997;131:398–404.

35 Brogan PA, Raffles A. The management of fever and petechiae: making sense of rash decisions. *Arch Dis Child* 2000;83: 506–7.

36 Nielsen HE, Andersen EA, Andersen J et al. Diagnostic assessment of haemorrhagic rash and fever. *Arch Dis Child* 2001;85:160–5.

37 Carpenter CT, Kaiser AB. Purpura fulminans in pneumococcal sepsis: case report and review. *Scand J Infect Dis* 1997;29:479–83.

38 Wells LC, Smith JC, Weston VC, Collier J, Rutter N. The child with a non-blanching rash: how likely is meningococcal disease? *Arch Dis Child* 2001;85:218–22.

39 Thompson MJ, Ninis N, Perera R et al. Clinical recognition of meningococcal disease in children and adolescents. *Lancet* 2006;367:397–403.

40 Parikh A, Maconochie I. What is the use of the glass test? *Arch Dis Child* 2003;88:1135.

41 McCarthy PL, Sharpe MR, Spiesel SZ et al. Observation scales to identify serious illness in young children. *Pediatrics* 1982;70: 802–9.

42 Hewson PH, Humphries SM, Roberton DM, McNamara JM, Robinson MJ. Markers of serious illness in infants under 6 months old presenting to a children's hospital. *Arch Dis Child* 1990;65:750–6.

43 Bonadio WA, Hegenbarth M, Zachariason M. Correlating reported fever in young infants with subsequent temperature patterns and rate of serious bacterial infections. *Pediatr Infect Dis J* 1990;9:158–60.

44 Baker MD, Avner JR, Bell LM. Failure of infant observation scales in detecting serious illness in febrile, 4- to 8-week-old infants. *Pediatrics* 1990;85:1040–3.

45 Teach SJ, Fleisher GR. Efficacy of an observation scale in detecting bacteremia in febrile children three to thirty-six months of age, treated as outpatients. Occult Bacteremia Study Group. *J Pediatr* 1995;126:877–81.

46 Neto G. Fever in the young infant. In: Moyer VA (ed.), *Evidence-Based Pediatrics and Child Health.* London: BMJ Books, 2000:178–88.

47 Bilukha OO, Rosenstein N; Centers for Disease Control and Prevention. Prevention and control of meningococcal disease: recommendations of the Advisory Committee on Immunization Practices (ACIP). *MMWR* 2005;54(RR-7):1–21.

48 Hahne SJM, Charlett A, Purcell B et al. Effectiveness of antibiotics given before admission in reducing mortality from meningococcal disease: systematic review. *bmj.com* 2006; 332:1299.

49 Cartwright K, Reilly S, White D, Stuart J. Early treatment with parenteral penicillin in meningococcal disease. *BMJ* 1992;305:143–7.

50 Norgard B, Sorensen HT, Jensen ES, Faber T, Schonheyder HC, Nielsen GL. Pre-hospital parenteral antibiotic treatment of meningococcal disease and case fatality: a Danish population-based cohort study. *J Infect* 2002;45:144–51.

51 Harnden A, Ninis N, Thompson M et al. Parenteral penicillin for children with meningococcal disease before hospital admission: case-control study. *BMJ* 2006;332:1295–8.

52 Brandtzaeg P, Kierulf P, Gaustad P et al. Plasma endotoxin as a predictor of multiple organ failure and death in systemic meningococcal disease. *J Infect Dis* 1989;159:195–204.

53 Ninis N, Phillips C, Bailey L et al. The role of healthcare delivery in the outcome of meningococcal disease in children: case-control study of fatal and non-fatal cases. *bmj.com* 2005;330:1475.

54 Branco RG, Russell RR. Should steroids be used in children with meningococcal shock? *Arch Dis Child* 2005;90: 1195–6.

55 Bone RC, Fisher CJ, Jr, Clemmer TP et al. A controlled clinical trial of high-dose methylprednisolone in the treatment of severe sepsis and septic shock. *N Engl J Med* 1987;317: 653–8.

56 Annane D, Sebille V, Charpentier C et al. Effect of treatment with low doses of hydrocortisone and fludrocortisone on mortality in patients with septic shock. *JAMA* 2002;288:862–71.

57 Yildiz O, Doganay M, Aygen B et al. Physiological-dose steroid therapy in sepsis. *Crit Care* 2002;6:251–9.

58 Bollaert PE, Charpentier C, Levy B et al. Reversal of late septic shock with supraphysiologic doses of hydrocortisone. *Crit Care Med* 1998;26:645–50.

59 Bone M, Diver M, Selby A et al. Assessment of adrenal function in the initial phase of meningococcal disease. *Pediatrics* 2002;110:563–9.

60 De Kleijn ED, Joosten KF, Van Rijn B et al. Low serum cortisol in combination with high adrenocorticotrophic hormone concentrations are associated with poor outcome in children with severe meningococcal disease. *Pediatr Infect Dis J* 2002;21:330–6.

61 Riordan FA, Thomson AP, Ratcliffe JM et al. Admission cortisol and adrenocorticotrophic hormone levels in children with meningococcal disease: evidence of adrenal insufficiency? *Crit Care Med* 1999;27:2257–61.

62 Fischer M, Hilinski J, Stephens DS. Adjuvant therapy for meningococcal sepsis. *Pediatr Infect Dis J* 2005;24:177–8.

63 de Kleijn ED, de Groot R, Hack CE et al. Activation of protein C following infusion of protein C concentrate in children with severe meningococcal sepsis and purpura fulminans: a randomized, double-blinded, placebo-controlled dose-finding study. *Crit Care Med* 2003;31:1839–47.

64 Meningococcal Disease Surveillance Group. Analysis of endemic meningococcal disease by serogroup and evaluation of chemoprophylaxis. *J Infect Dis* 1976;134:201–4.

65 Purcell B, Samuelsson S, Hahne SJM et al. Effectiveness of antibiotics in preventing meningococcal disease after a case: systematic review. *bmj.com* 2004;328:1339.

66 Fraser A, Gafter-Gvili A, Paul M, Leibovici L. Antibiotics for preventing meningococcal infections. *The Cochrane Database of Systematic Reviews* 2005(1):Art No CD004785.

67 Trotter CL, Andrews NJ, Kaczmarski EB, Miller E, Ramsay ME. Effectiveness of meningococcal serogroup C conjugate vaccine 4 years after introduction. *Lancet* 2004;364: 365–7.

68 http://www.health.gov.au/internet/wcms/publishing.nsf/content/cda-cdi2902d.htm. Accessed June 14, 2006.

69 Committee on Infectious Diseases. Prevention and control of meningococcal disease: recommendations for use

of meningococcal vaccines in pediatric patients. *Pediatrics* 2005;116:496–505.

70 Chuang YY, Huang YC, Lin TY. Toxic shock syndrome in children: epidemiology, pathogenesis, and management. *Paediatr Drugs* 2005;7:11–25.

71 Mascini EM, Jansze M, Schouls LM, Verhoef J, Van Dijk H. Penicillin and clindamycin differentially inhibit the production of pyrogenic exotoxins A and B by group A streptococci. *Int J Antimicrob Agents* 2001;18:395–8.

72 Pichichero ME. Group A beta-hemolytic streptococcal infections. *Pediatr Rev* 1998;19:291–302.

73 Darenberg J, Ihendyane N, Sjolin J et al. Intravenous immunoglobulin G therapy in streptococcal toxic shock syndrome: a European randomized, double-blind, placebo-controlled trial. *Clin Infect Dis* 2003;37:333–40.

74 American Academy of Pediatrics. Committee on Infectious Diseases. Severe invasive group A streptococcal infections: a subject review. *Pediatrics* 1998;101:136–40.

75 Davies HD, Matlow A, Scriver SR et al. Apparent lower rates of streptococcal toxic shock syndrome and lower mortality in children with invasive group A streptococcal infections compared with adults. *Pediatr Infect Dis J* 1994;13:49–56.

CHAPTER 16
Tropical infections and travel

16.1 Travel

We have not included a chapter specifically covering travel medicine, but have instead dealt with traveler's diarrhea in Chapter 7, and will cover individual infections in this and other chapters.

For travel advice, the following Web sites are useful:
http://www.cdc.gov/travel
http://www.who.int/topics/travel/en
http://www.travax.nhs.uk

16.2 Brucellosis

Brucellosis is a zoonotic disease, which occurs worldwide in tropical and temperate countries.[1] Humans catch it by exposure to domesticated or wild animals through unpasteurized milk or milk products, or contact with carcasses or secretions.

The most common clinical manifestations are fever, arthralgia or arthritis, malaise, weight loss, hepatosplenomegaly, and lymphadenopathy.[2–4] The onset is often insidious with ongoing fevers and sweats, although children may present more acutely. Back pain due to lumbar spondylitis is common in adults. Serious complications include endocarditis, meningitis, and osteomyelitis.

The diagnosis is usually made by growing brucella from blood or from bone marrow, CSF, or other tissues. Serology using serum agglutination test (SAT) or enzyme-linked immunosorbent assay (ELISA) is more sensitive for acute brucellosis (42–98%) than for chronic infection (23–64%).[4,5] Polymerase chain reaction (PCR) on blood and other tissues, if available, is generally >90% sensitive and >90% specific.[6,7]

We found six RCTs comparing different antibiotic regimens to treat brucellosis in children. In a large multicenter RCT in Kuwait involving 1100 children, monotherapy with oral oxytetracycline, doxycycline, or rifampin showed comparable results with low relapse rates (9% or less) regardless of duration.[8] Trimethoprim-sulfamethoxazole (TMP-SMX) alone had a 30% relapse rate. In combined oral therapy, rifampin plus oxytetracycline, rifampin plus TMP-SMX, and oxytetracycline plus TMP-SMX showed comparable results with low relapse rates ranging from 4 to 8% in patients receiving therapy for 3 or 5 weeks, while no relapses occurred in patients treated for 8 weeks.[8] Four of the other studies used doxycycline plus streptomycin as the comparator: two found that doxycycline plus rifampicin was inferior,[9,10] while one found that the regimens were equivalent, except perhaps for spondylitis.[11] Ceftriaxone was inferior to doxycycline plus streptomycin.[12] Finally, an RCT mainly in adults found more treatment failures with doxycycline plus rifampin than with TMP-SMX plus rifampin.[13] Regimens using invasive therapy, such as streptomycin and gentamicin (which has been studied in adults),[14] have not shown advantages over oral regimens. There have been no studies of quinolones to treat brucellosis in children, and studies in adults are inconclusive.[15]

To treat brucellosis in children, we recommend:

doxycycline (child >8 years) 2.5 mg/kg (max 100 mg) orally, 12-hourly for 8 weeks OR the combination of
trimethoprim+sulfamethoxazole 6 + 30 mg/kg (max 240 + 1200 mg) orally, 12-hourly for 8 weeks PLUS
rifampicin 15 mg/kg (max 600 mg) orally, daily for 8 weeks

For children with endocarditis, meningitis, or osteomyelitis, it is recommended to give parenteral streptomycin or gentamicin for the first 7–14 days, together with doxycycline (or with TMP-SMX if <8 years old) plus rifamp(ic)in.[16] The oral antibiotics should be continued, often for several months.[16]

16.3 Hydatid disease

Hydatid disease in children results from infection with the sheep or cattle tapeworm, *Echinococcus granulosus*. Hydatid disease is common in some parts of the world where the disease is endemic, and extremely rare in others. Dogs and other mammals act as intermediate hosts by swallowing protoscolices of the parasite. They pass embryonated eggs in their feces, which the sheep or cattle swallow. Humans can be infected, and cysts develop in various organs, but humans do not pass on the infection. The commonest places for cysts to grow and cause problems are the liver[17] and the lung.[18] They can also develop elsewhere, such as the central nervous system (CNS),[19] the heart, kidneys, spleen, or thyroid. Commonly, cysts are extremely slow growing and come to notice because they occupy space, e.g., convulsions from cranial hydatid or jaundice from hepatic cyst pressing on bile duct, or because the cyst ruptures.

The diagnosis of hydatid disease may be made histologically (scolices seen in fluid from liver cyst, in sputum, or in CNS cyst), but positive echinococcus serology can support a diagnosis of hydatid disease, while negative serology effectively excludes it.[18]

The imidazoles, albendazole and mebendazole, are effective against echinococcus, but may not penetrate large cysts adequately.

Hepatic hydatid cysts

The classic treatment for hepatic cysts is surgical, although there have been recent studies of percutaneous drainage. An RCT found that only 2 of 11 hepatic cysts treated with albendazole reduced in size compared with all 22 treated with percutaneous drainage, with or without albendazole.[20] A systematic review concluded that chemotherapy alone was not as effective as surgery, but there were insufficient studies to distinguish between definitive surgery and percutaneous drainage with or without an imidazoles.[21] This was also the conclusion of a Cochrane review of the "PAIR" technique.[17] PAIR is performed under ultrasound or sometimes computed tomography guidance, and involves percutaneous drainage of the cysts with a fine needle or catheter, aspiration of the contents, instillation of scolicidal substances (e.g., hypertonic saline or absolute alcohol), and reaspiration. An RCT showed that percutaneous drainage plus albendazole was at least as effective as surgery, shortened hospital stay and was associated with fewer complications.[22]

The limited current evidence favors percutaneous aspiration and albendazole. Although it is sometimes recommended to use praziquantel before surgery or if there is cyst spillage, we could find no evidence to support this recommendation. We recommend:

albendazole 7.5 mg/kg (max 400 mg) orally, 12-hourly for 1–6 months

Patients on prolonged albendazole therapy require regular monitoring of liver function tests and white cell count.

Pulmonary hydatid disease

Pulmonary cysts may be picked up as an incidental finding on chest radiograph, or the cyst may rupture into a bronchus, in which case the child may cough up fluid with the appearance of "grape skins," and may develop wheeze, urticaria, or even anaphylaxis.[23,24] Alternatively, the cyst can rupture into the pleural cavity and cause a pleural effusion.[24,25] Hydatid lung cysts are more common in boys than girls (1.6–3:1),[18,24] are often large, unilateral, and right sided, may cause pneumothorax (15% of children in one study[18]) and are associated with hepatic cysts in 10–33% of children[18,24] but 79% of adults.[24]

Treatment of asymptomatic infection is usually not required. We could find no studies comparing medical with surgical management of hydatid lung cysts. In one study, 82 children with lung cysts were treated with albendazole or mebendazole, without surgery.[26] Lung cysts were cured in 34%, improved in 34%, and treatment failed in 32%. Albendazole was more likely than mebendazole to result in improvement. The children who failed had larger cysts (mean 7.3 cm) than those who improved or resolved (5.3 cm).

If it is decided to treat medically, with or without surgery, we recommend:

albendazole 7.5 mg/kg (max 400 mg) orally, 12-hourly

16.4 Malaria

There are four species of the malarial parasite Plasmodium that infect humans, of which *Plasmodium falciparum* is the most pathogenic and most resistant to antimalarials. About 2 billion people are exposed to *P. falciparum* malaria annually, resulting in over 500 million clinical attacks and about a million deaths, predominantly in children less than 5 years living in sub-Saharan Africa.[27] Malaria is also a problem for children returning or immigrating to industrialized countries from tropical regions. Despite the availability of good preventive measures, >10,000 cases of malaria were reported from 1985 to 2001 in US travelers.[28] An estimated 20% of all cases of malaria imported to the USA and Europe occur in children.[28,29]

Diagnosis of malaria begins with clinical suspicion. In nonimmune children, malaria typically presents with high fever that might be accompanied by sweats, chills, rigors, and headache.[30] Symptoms and signs may be more subtle in partially immune children. Young children are more likely to have signs and symptoms attributable to severe anemia, such as pallor or heart failure. Children may develop cough and tachypnea, mimicking respiratory infection. Other systemic symptoms include nausea, vomiting, diarrhea, abdominal pain, back pain, and arthralgia, while signs include hepatomegaly, splenomegaly, and jaundice.[30] Cerebral malaria can progress rapidly from altered sensorium and confusion to convulsions, coma, hypertonia with opisthotonus, decerebrate post-uring, and death.[31] Partially immune children who migrate from endemic areas are often asymptomatic or have isolated splenomegaly.[32]

Malaria should be considered in any patient who has visited a malarious area and presents with fever. A blood sample collected into an EDTA tube should be sent to an appropriate laboratory for examination, including thick and thin films. Thick blood smears help to determine when infection is present, but a single negative blood film or negative antigen test does not exclude the diagnosis of malaria, particularly if antimalarials or antibiotics have been taken recently, because some antibiotics have modest antimalarial activity.[28] Thin blood smears aid in identifying the species of parasite. Antigen and nucleic acid detection tests are available in some specialized laboratories. Rapid antigen tests perform variably, but probably have the same sensitivity as a blood smear.[28] PCR is highly sensitive, but not widely available.[28] In addition, we recommend screening refugees who have recently arrived from an endemic area with a blood film for malarial parasites.[32]

Treatment of acute malaria should include careful supportive care, and intensive care measures should be available for treating children with complicated *P. falciparum* malaria.

Treatment of malaria

Treatment of uncomplicated *Plasmodium falciparum* malaria

The antimalarials of choice will depend on local epidemiology (which Plasmodium species are prevalent) and on local resistance patterns. There is a new class of artemisinin (qinghaosu) derivatives, used as artemether, artesunate, and dihydroartemisinin-piperaquine, which have been studied intensely.

The CDC currently advises oral chloroquine for *P. falciparum* infections acquired in the few areas without chloroquine-resistant strains, which include Central America, west of the Panama Canal, Haiti, the Dominican Republic, and most of the Middle East.[33] For pediatric *P. falciparum* infections acquired in areas with chloroquine-resistant strains, they offer three treatment options: quinine sulfate (together with doxycycline, tetracycline, or clindamycin), atovaquone-proguanil, and mefloquine.[33] For children <8 years old, doxycycline and tetracycline are generally not indicated, so quinine is recommended, alone or with clindamycin and atovaquone-proguanil. The third option, mefloquine, is associated with a higher rate of severe neuropsychiatric reactions when used at treatment doses, and is recommended by CDC only when the quinine sulfate combination or atovaquone-proguanil options cannot be used.[33] CDC advises that, in rare instances, doxycycline or tetracycline can be used in combination with quinine in children <8 years old if other treatment options are not available or are not tolerated, and the benefit of adding doxycycline or tetracycline is judged to outweigh the risk.[33] To date, the CDC do not recommend artemesinin derivatives.

Question | For children with uncomplicated falciparum malaria, do the artemesinin derivatives compared with standard antimalarial regimens reduce mortality or morbidity?

Literature review | We found 41 RCTs and a Cochrane review[34] of artemisinin derivatives in adults and children with uncomplicated falciparum malaria. We found 11 RCTs of artemisinin derivatives in children with uncomplicated falciparum malaria. We found 16 RCTs and a non-Cochrane meta-analysis[35] of the addition of artemesinin derivatives to standard antimalarial therapy. We found a non-Cochrane systematic review of trials of any antimalarial therapy.[36]

A Cochrane review of artemesinin derivatives for treating uncomplicated falciparum malaria in adults and children[34] found 41 trials (over 5000 patients), but variation in study design and quality made synthesis of the data problematic. Compared with standard antimalarial treatments, artemisinin drugs showed fast parasite clearance and high cure rates at follow-up, provided the duration of treatment with artemisinin drugs was adequate.

We found 11 RCTs in children of combinations of antimalarials, which included one of the artemisinin (qinghaosu) derivatives. The trials were carried out in areas of high resistance to conventional antimalarials in Southeast Asia, Africa, and Bangladesh.[37–47] Dihydroartemisinin-piperaquine was >99% effective in two studies,[46,47] had fewer adverse effects than mefloquine+artesunate,[47] and is cheaper.[46,47] Mefloquine+artesunate was 100% effective in Bangladesh[43] and Lao.[47] Amodiaquine+artesunate and artemether+lumefantrine were >94–100% effective at clearing parasitemia and preventing relapse,[37–43,45] except in Nigeria[44] where they were 82.5–87% effective. Regimens using chloroquine with sulfadoxine and pyrimethamine[42,43] or using amodiaquine alone[37,41] were only about 60% effective.

A non-Cochrane meta-analysis of the addition of 1 or 3 days of artesunate to standard treatment of *P. falciparum* malaria[35] found 16 randomized trials (5948 patients), of which only two exclusively studied children. Adding 3 days of artesunate to standard treatment reduced parasitologic failure by 70–80% at days 14 and 28. One day of artesunate was not as effective.[35]

A non-Cochrane systematic review of trials of antimalarials in adults and children[36] found a steady increase in the past 20 years in failure rates reported for chloroquine due to the emergence of chloroquine resistance. Treatment failure rates with sulphadoxine-pyrimethamine were very high in the 1970s and early 1980s, reflecting trials only from Southeast Asia where resistance was emerging, and there has since been a steady increase in treatment failure rates reported from Africa.[36] In contrast, the recrudescence rates

for quinine reported over the past 30 years have remained roughly constant.[36] Mefloquine failure rates have increased over the past decade, reflecting the emergence of resistance in Southeast Asia, despite an increase in dosage used (from 15 to 25 mg/kg).[36] Treatment failure rates with artemisinin and its derivatives in combinations (mainly with mefloquine) have remained constantly low, since trials began in the early 1990s.[36]

If a child is admitted with malaria, we recommend seeking advice from an expert and consulting the CDC[33] or WHO[48] Web sites. Artemesinin derivatives appear to be safe and effective, although mefloquine+artesunate is not recommended because of the psychiatric adverse reactions with mefloquine.

For uncomplicated *P. falciparum* malaria acquired in an area of chloroquine resistance, we recommend:

artemether+lumefantrine (20 + 120 mg tablets) child 5–14 kg: 1 tablet; 15–24 kg: 2 tablets; 25–34 kg: 3 tablets; >34 kg: 4 tablets, orally with fatty food, six doses at 0, 8, 24, 36, 48, and 60 hours OR dihydroartemisinin-piperaquine 2.1 + 16.8 mg/kg orally, once daily for 3 days (tablets are 40 + 320 mg; for children, these can be crushed and given with syrup) OR THE COMBINATION OF quinine sulfate 10 mg/kg (max 600 mg) orally, 8-hourly for 7 days PLUS EITHER clindamycin 10 mg/kg (max 450 mg) orally, 8-hourly for 7 days OR doxycycline child >8 years: 2.5 mg/kg (max 100 mg) orally, 12-hourly for 7 days

In developing countries, cost and availability are important considerations. A comparative trial in the Central African Republic, where artemesinin compounds are not yet available, found that amodiaquine with sulfadoxine-pyrimethamine was 100% effective in uncomplicated malaria and chloroquine with sulfadoxine-pyrimethamine 92.8% effective.[49]

For uncomplicated *P. falciparum* malaria acquired in an area where there is no chloroquine resistance, we recommend:

chloroquine 10 mg base/kg (max 620 mg base = 4 tablets) orally, initially, then 5 mg base/kg (max 310 mg base = 2 tablets) for three doses, one 6 hours later and one each on days 2 and 3

Treatment of severe malaria (*P. falciparum*)

Severe malaria is diagnosed[28,50] if the child has parasitemia and any of the following:

· altered consciousness, hypoglycemia, jaundice, oliguria, or severe anemia;
· parasite count >100,000/mm^3 (>2% of red blood cells parasitized);
· vomiting or clinically acidotic.

Antimalarials for severe malaria (*Plasmodium falciparum*)

Question | For children with severe falciparum malaria including cerebral malaria, do the artemesinin derivatives compared with standard antimalarial regimens reduce mortality or morbidity?

Literature review | We found 16 RCTs and a Cochrane review[51] comparing parenteral or rectal artemisinin derivatives to standard therapy in adults and children with severe malaria, including cerebral malaria. We found 5 RCTs of artemisinin derivatives in children with severe malaria.[52–56] We found 4 RCTs of artemisinin derivatives in children with cerebral malaria.[57–60]

A Cochrane review[51] found 16 trials (2653 adult and child patients) that compared artemisinin drugs with quinine for severe malaria, including cerebral malaria. Artemisinin drugs were associated with better survival for severe malaria (mortality OR 0.61, 95% CI 0.46–0.82) and also for cerebral malaria. Hypoglycemia was more likely if adults with cerebral malaria were treated with quinine than with artemesisins.[51] We found five studies of artemesinin derivatives in children with severe malaria, which found that they were no better and no worse than conventional treatment with quinine.[52–56] Three studies comparing rectal artemether with parenteral therapy found that rectal artemether was as effective as parenteral therapy using artemether or quinine.[54–56]

We found four studies of parenteral artemether in cerebral malaria in children. They found that artemesinins were no better and no worse than conventional therapy, and hypoglycemia was equally common.[57–60] Artemether suppositories were as effective as parenteral therapy in two studies.[61,62]

In children with malaria and severe anemia, chloroquine-resistant *P. falciparum* should be assumed to be the infective agent. We recommend

establishing intravenous access, starting antimalarial treatment, and seeking expert advice.[28,50] The recommended dose of artesunate comes from a large study showing reduced mortality compared to quinine in Southeast Asia.[63]

For treating children with severe malaria, we recommend using artemesenin derivatives if they are available.

We recommend:

artesunate 2.4 mg/kg IV, on admission, repeated after 12 and 24 hours, then once daily until oral therapy is possible OR
artesunate suppository 10 mg/kg, rectally, once daily until oral therapy possible OR
quinine dihydrochloride 20 mg/kg loading dose in 5% dextrose IV over 4 hours, then 10 mg/kg IV over 4 hours, 8-hourly (max 1800 mg/day), commencing 4 hours after loading regimen is completed and continuing until the child can tolerate oral treatment

An initial loading dose of quinine should be given unless the patient has received three or more doses of quinine or quinidine in the previous 48 hours, or mefloquine prophylaxis in the previous 24 hours, or a mefloquine treatment dose within the previous 3 days. Frequent measurements of blood pressure and blood glucose are recommended, because quinine stimulates insulin secretion and can cause hypoglycemia.

When the child can tolerate oral therapy, give a full course of oral antimalarials, as for uncomplicated *P. falciparum* malaria (see p. 259).

If IV quinine is required for longer than 48 hours, seek expert advice, as a dose adjustment may be necessary especially in patients with renal impairment.

Adjunctive therapy for severe malaria (*Plasmodium falciparum*)

UK guidelines have been published on the management of severe malaria in children, and give important detail on the importance of monitoring for and treating hypoglycemia, the diagnosis and management of shock, the diagnosis and management of seizures and raised intracranial pressure, and the management of disturbances of electrolytes and acid–base balance.[62]

Fluid therapy for severe malaria (*Plasmodium falciparum*)

Symptomatic severe malarial anemia has a high fatality rate of 30–40%, and most deaths occur early.[64–66] Children with severe malaria with anemia may have been given inadequate fluid resuscitation in the past for fear of heart failure, while children with cerebral malaria are fluid restricted for fear of cerebral edema. This dogma has been challenged recently. Studies in Kenya suggest that children with severe malaria with acidosis have hypovolemia.[64,65] A preliminary study of children with severe malaria with anemia examined the safety of pretransfusion management (PTM) by volume expansion. Kenyan children with severe falciparum anemia (hemoglobin <5 g/dL) and respiratory distress were randomly assigned to 20 mL/kg of 4.5% albumin or 0.9% saline or maintenance only (control) while awaiting blood transfusion.[65] PTM was apparently safe, since it did not lead to the development of pulmonary edema or other adverse events. The number of children requiring emergency interventions was significantly greater in the control group, 4 of 18 (22%) than the saline group 0 of 20 ($p = 0.03$).[65]

A subsequent RCT compared 4.5% albumin with normal saline for children with severe malaria and metabolic acidosis (base deficit >8 mmol/L).[66] There was no significant difference in the resolution of acidosis between the groups, but the mortality rate was significantly lower among patients who received albumin (3.6%, 2 of 56 patients) than among those who received saline (18%, 11 of 61; RR 5.5, 95% CI 1.2–24.8, $p = 0.013$). Larger studies are under way, but these data are convincing enough to recommend albumin in preference to normal saline for resuscitation of children with severe malaria and acidosis.

A recommendation[62] to transfuse all children with severe malaria and a hemoglobin <10 g/dL is somewhat controversial. A Cochrane review[67] found only two RCTs in 230 children. The reviewers could not reach a conclusion for or against transfusion, because the transfusion group had a non-significant trend toward fewer deaths (RR 0.41, 95% CI 0.06–2.70) but also a trend toward more severe adverse events (RR 8.60, 95% CI 1.11–66.43).[67] The lower the hemoglobin the greater the need for transfusion, but albumin can safely be used while awaiting blood.[65,66]

Treatment of malaria due to *Plasmodium vivax*, *Plasmodium malariae*, and *Plasmodium ovale*

Although there is widespread chloroquine resistance of *P. falciparum*, non-falciparum malaria parasites are generally sensitive to chloroquine in most parts of the world. This is true even for places like Thailand, where all *P. falciparum* are chloroquine resistant.[68] However, in 1989, chloroquine-resistant *P. vivax* was described in Indonesian Papua New Guinea,[69] and it has been described since in Indonesia, Myanmar, India, and Guyana in South America.[70] In Indonesia, mefloquine has been shown to be an effective alternative to chloroquine for treating *P. vivax* infection.[71] To treat non-falciparum malaria, unless contracted in an area of chloroquine-resistant *P. vivax*, we recommend:

chloroquine 10 mg base/kg (max 620 mg base = 4 tablets) orally, initially, then 5 mg base/kg (max 310 mg base = 2 tablets) for three doses, one 6 hours later and one each on days 2 and 3

To treat non-falciparum malaria when chloroquine-resistant *P. vivax* is prevalent, we recommend:

mefloquine 15 mg/kg (max 750 mg) orally, initially, then 10 mg/kg (max 500 mg) 8–12 hours later

Artemether derivatives clear parasitemia rapidly and may be an alternative, but data are scanty.[72] We advise seeking expert advice for children with vivax malaria, who fail treatment with chloroquine.

Chloroquine and mefloquine act on the blood stages of the parasite, but do not eliminate the liver forms and relapse is fairly common. A 14-day course of primaquine is recommended by the WHO to reduce treatment failure or relapse.[73] In RCTs in India and Pakistan, 14 days of primaquine is 50–70% effective in preventing relapses.[74,75] Five days of primaquine is ineffective.[76] Primaquine-tolerant strains of *P. vivax* have been reported from Thailand, where up to 18% of people being treated with standard primaquine regimens relapse.[77]

To eliminate liver forms of *P. vivax* and *P. ovale* infections, we recommend adding to chloroquine or following within a few days with:

primaquine 0.3 mg/kg (max 15 mg) orally, daily with food for 14 days

[NB: Primaquine is not recommended for children <4 years old.[73] Patients should be tested for glucose-6-phosphate dehydrogenase (G6PD) deficiency before using primaquine, which should not be used in G6PD-deficient children, in whom it can cause severe hemolysis.[73]]

If the patient relapses after the primaquine treatment, it may be necessary, after treating the infection with chloroquine or mefloquine, to double the dose of primaquine or treat for longer. We recommend seeking expert advice.

If the patient is unable to tolerate oral therapy, which is best taken with food, we recommend treating as severe malaria as above and consulting an experienced specialist.

Prevention of malaria

Insecticide-treated bed nets

Question | For children in malarious areas, do insecticide-treated bed nets (ITNs) compared with no nets or untreated nets reduce the frequency of episodes of malaria and reduce mortality?
Literature review | We found 22 trials and a Cochrane review.[78]

Insecticide-treated bed nets are highly effective in reducing childhood mortality and morbidity from malaria. A Cochrane review[78] found 14 cluster randomized trials (where clusters or groups of children, such as villages, were randomized to ITNs or no ITNs), and eight RCTs where individual children were randomized. ITNs reduced deaths in children by 17–23% and episodes of malaria by about 50%. ITNs can save 5–6 lives each year for every 1000 children protected with ITNs.[78]

Vector avoidance
Other vector-avoidance measures apart from ITNs are recommended,[28] and although dictated by common sense, have not been studied in trials. These are:

· using topical insect repellent;
· wearing long trousers and long-sleeved shirts in the evening and the early morning;
· not going outdoors between the evening and the early morning;
· avoiding perfumes and aftershave.

Chemoprophylaxis

Question | For children living in or visiting malarious areas, does regular chemoprophylaxis with antimalarials compared with no prophylaxis or placebo reduce the frequency of attacks of malaria?
Literature review | We found four RCTs of regular prophylaxis and a Cochrane meta-analysis[79] of prophylaxis and intermittent treatment.

Because of the relatively low rate of malaria in visitors and for ethical reasons, it would be difficult to study the efficacy of chemoprophylaxis for visitors to malarious areas in an RCT. It is possible, however, to study chemoprophylaxis in young children who live in those areas. Children living in areas where malaria is endemic acquire natural immunity to malaria by 7–10 years of age.[80,81] Before this age, children living in malarious areas have inadequate immunity to malaria, which is why most of the 1 million malaria deaths that occur each year in endemic areas of sub-Saharan Africa occur in this age group.[27]

A Cochrane review of antimalarials in children up to 6 years old living in malarious areas found 18 eligible RCTs, all in Africa.[79] Eight studies examined episodes of clinical malaria as an outcome: four RCTs of regular chemoprophylaxis and four RCTs of intermittent treatment for episodes of presumed malaria (sometimes called "febrifuge"). Chemoprophylaxis reduced the number of episodes by 43% (RR 0.57, 95% CI 0.33–1.00, 2806 participants). Intermittent treatment had a similar effect, and when the eight trials were combined, antimalarial drugs were statistically significantly better than placebo at preventing clinical malaria (RR 0.52, 95% CI 0.35–0.77). Severe anemia was also reduced by about half. An analysis of nine trials (7929 participants) did not detect a significant difference in mortality (RR 0.82, 95% CI 0.65–1.04) but the confidence intervals do not exclude a potentially important difference. None of the trials reported serious adverse events.[79] It appears that there is good evidence to support chemoprophylaxis or intermittent treatment for children living in malarious areas, and this adds weight to recommendations for giving chemoprophylaxis to children visiting malarious areas.

Web sites for advice on antimalarial prophylaxis for children

The development of widespread multidrug-resistant strains of *P. falciparum* throughout the world, particularly Southeast Asia, complicates recommendations for prophylaxis. Useful information regarding the malaria risk and the drug susceptibility profile for specific geographic locations is available from the CDC[82] and WHO[48,83,84] Web sites.

· Centers for Disease Control and Prevention. Travelers' Health Information for Health Care Providers: Preventing Malaria in Infants and Children. Available at http://www.cdc.gov/travel/mal_kids_hc.htm.

· World Health Organization. International Travel and Health, 2005. Available at http://www.who.int/ith/en/ and click on malaria pdf. The most recent version at time of publication of this book is http://whqlibdoc.who.int/publications/2005/9241580364_chap7.pdf, which gives general information on antimalarials, including children. http://www.who.int/ith/countries/en/index.html gives the recommendations for antimalarials by country.

Travel medicine clinics, travel advisory services, and other experts can also provide appropriate information.

Recommendations on antimalarial prophylaxis for children

No drug regimen is completely safe and effective. The decision to use chemoprophylaxis must, therefore, weigh the risk of disease against the efficacy and toxicity of the drugs. The risk of acquiring malaria depends on factors such as the country visited, whether the visit is to urban or rural areas, the time of year, the duration of visit, and the type of activities undertaken. In some places, notably many major cities and tourist resorts in malaria-endemic countries, the risk of malaria is low and the risk of prophylaxis outweighs the risk of malaria. In this case, travelers should be advised against prophylaxis.

There are problems with chemoprophylaxis for children of availability of appropriate drugs and of adherence. Doxycycline can cause rash and esophagitis, and is not recommended for children 8 years or younger. Mefloquine can cause neuropsychiatric problems and is contraindicated in epilepsy.[83] Chloroquine and proguanil have been widely used as prophylaxis in children, but can no longer be relied on in most areas, including Africa, Southeast Asia, and the Pacific Islands. However, chloroquine may confer some benefit in selected areas with chloroquine-resistant malaria, especially for longer stay situations.

It is usual to start chemoprophylaxis a few days before traveling, in case of adverse events. Persons taking doxycycline, however, may not develop a sunsensitive rash until they are exposed to the sun when traveling. Antimalarials should be continued after returning because of the risk of delayed onset of disease.

Travelers to malarious areas should be advised that chemoprophylaxis is not always effective. A child who develops fever while traveling in a malarious area or after returning should see a doctor urgently, and the doctor should be told of the travel history.

Areas with chloroquine-sensitive malaria

For prophylaxis in those few areas with chloroquine-sensitive malaria (Central America, North of Panama, and the Middle East), we recommend:

chloroquine 5 mg base/kg (max 310 mg base or 2 tablets) orally, weekly (start 1 week before leaving and continue until 4 weeks after returning)

Areas with chloroquine-resistant malaria

Question | For travelers to chloroquine-resistant areas, is there evidence that one prophylactic regimen compared to other regimens is more effective at preventing malaria or safer?

Literature review | We found five RCTs in travelers,[85–89] of which three were in children.[86,88,89]

We found five RCTs, all of atovaquone-proguanil. Three compared atovaquone-proguanil to placebo,[86–88] and one each to mefloquine[85] and chloroquine-proguanil.[89] Atovaquone-proguanil was 96–100% effective in preventing *P. falciparum* malaria in adult and child travelers,[85–89] and was 84% effective against *P. vivax* in travelers to Papua New Guinea.[87] Both mefloquine[85] and chloroquine-proguanil[89] were as effective as atovaquone-proguanil, but caused more serious adverse events, including neuropsychiatric ones with mefloquine.

For prophylaxis in areas with chloroquine-resistant malaria (including Africa, China, the Indian subcontinent, the Pacific Islands, Southeast Asia, and South America), we recommend:

atovaquone+proguanil:
11–20 kg: 1 tablet of 62.5 + 25 mg pediatric formulation
21–30 kg: 2 tablets of 62.5 + 25 mg pediatric formulation
31–40 kg: 3 tablets of 62.5 + 25 mg pediatric formulation
>40 kg: 1 tablet of 250 + 100 mg adult formulation
orally, with fatty food, daily (starting 1–2 days before entering, and continuing until 7 days after leaving malarious area) OR
doxycycline: child >8 years: 2.5 mg/kg (max 100 mg) orally, daily (starting 2 days before entering, and continuing until 4 weeks after leaving malarious area) OR
mefloquine 5–9 kg: 31.25 mg (1/8 of 250 mg tablet); 10–19 kg: 62.5 mg (1/4 tablet); 20–29 kg: 125 mg (1/2 tablet); 30–44 kg: 187.5 mg (3/4 tablet) orally, weekly (starting 2–3 weeks before entering, and continuing until 4 weeks after leaving malarious area)

Alternatively, for limited areas of Africa, some authorities recommend:

chloroquine 5 mg base/kg (max 310 mg base or 2 tablets) orally, weekly (starting 1 week before and continuing until 4 weeks after leaving malarious area) PLUS
proguanil <2 years: 50 mg; 2–6 years: 100 mg; 7–10 years: 150 mg; >10 years: 200 mg, orally, daily (starting 1 week before entering, and continuing until 4 weeks after leaving malarious area)

Areas with mefloquine-resistant malaria

For prophylaxis in areas with mefloquine-resistant malaria (including parts of Southeast Asia), we recommend atovaquone+proguanil or doxycycline (see below).

Emergency treatment of malaria (febrifuge)

Some authorities recommend that travelers who elect to not use chemoprophylaxis, or who elect to use chloroquine for chemoprophylaxis in areas with chloroquine-resistant malaria, can be given a "standby" course of artemether+lumefantrine or atovaquone+proguanil, or a single dose of mefloquine for self-treatment of fever if medical care is not likely to be available within 24 hours (see pp. 259–61). However, travelers should be warned that uncertain diagnosis is a potential problem. Treatment courses of antimalarial drugs can often be bought without a prescription in tropical countries, but counterfeit products are common.

16.5 Melioidosis

Melioidosis is caused by the soil saprophyte, *Burkholderia pseudomallei*.[90] It occurs mainly in tropical parts of the Asia-Pacific region[91,92] and in northern Australia,[93] but also in Brazil,[94] and cases have been reported from Puerto Rico[95] and the West Indies.[96] Melioidosis may present in returned travelers, sometimes months or years after exposure.

Adult diabetics and alcoholics are at particular risk of developing severe illness,[90,93] but children can be affected. Children either develop a septicemic illness, with or without pneumonia and splenic abscesses, or they have localized disease with ulcers or abscesses in the skin, soft tissues, and lymph nodes.[90–93] Parotitis and pharyngocervical diseases are seen in Thailand,[92] and encephalomyelitis in Australia.[93]

There is an association with chronic granulomatous disease.[95,96] Neonatal cases have occurred and have been ascribed to breast milk transfer.[97]

Selective culture media, serology, and a PCR test assist diagnosis.[90]

We found 16 RCTs and a Cochrane review on treatment of melioidosis.[98] Only one study included children.[99] All studies, including the one involving children,[99] showed that ceftazidime halved mortality in acute severe melioidosis, while the addition of other drugs did not help. For initial intensive therapy, we recommend:

ceftazidime 50 mg/kg (max 2 g) IV, 6-hourly for at least 14 days

Granulocyte colony-stimulating factor therapy has been used in northern Australia, and in an historical observational study,[100] its introduction was associated with a fall in mortality from 95 to 10%.

After the initial intensive therapy, eradication is recommended. Two RCTs have shown that triple therapy with trimethoprim, sulfamethoxazole, and doxycycline is better tolerated than quadruple therapy using the three drugs plus chloramphenicol[101] and more effective than ciprofloxacin plus azithromycin.[102] We recommend:

trimethoprim+sulfamethoxazole 8 + 40 mg/kg (max 320 + 1600 mg) orally, 12-hourly for at least a further 3 months PLUS (if >8 years) **doxycycline 2.5 mg/kg (max 100 mg) orally, 12-hourly for at least a further 3 months**

16.6   Q fever

Q fever is caused by the intracellular rickettsial organism, *Coxiella burnetii*. It is a zoonosis, acquired most often from sheep, goats, and cows, although mammals, including cats, dogs, rodents, and marsupials, and birds can also transmit infection to humans. High numbers of *C. burnetii* are present in the placenta of infected parturient animals, and are shed in the environment following labor or abortion. Humans acquire the infection mainly by inhaling contaminated aerosolized particles or ingesting unpasteurized dairy products, including milk and cheese.[103,104] Outbreaks have been reported following exposure to birth products of cats, dogs, and rabbits.[103]

Most infections are asymptomatic. Pediatric cases are rarely reported: a review found only 46 published cases in children.[105] Acute self-limited febrile illness and pneumonia are the most common manifestations of acute Q fever in children,[105,106] but meningitis, hepatitis, and hemolytic-uremic syndrome have also been reported.[106] Chronic disease, manifesting as endocarditis and osteomyelitis, is very rarely reported in children.[105,106]

Culture is hazardous to laboratory staff and is not usually attempted. Diagnosis is by serology or PCR.[107,108] An immunofluorescent antibody (IFA) test has been shown to perform better than an ELISA or CFT.[107] The use of both PCR and IFA improves diagnostic accuracy.[108]

We found only one RCT of treatment of Q fever pneumonia, in which doxycycline resulted in more rapid resolution of fever than did erythromycin.[109] Chloramphenicol had been used, but we could find no trials. In observational studies, adult patients treated with clarithromycin and moxifloxacin defervesced as quickly as those given doxycycline, and may be alternatives.[110]

We recommend:

doxycycline >8 years: 2.5 mg/kg (max 100 mg) orally, 12-hourly for 14 days OR
clarithromycin 12.5 mg/kg (max 500 mg) orally 12-hourly for 14 days OR
moxifloxacin 10 mg/kg (max 400 mg) orally or IV, daily for 14 days

Chronic disease, particularly endocarditis, is rare, and the organism is extremely difficult to eradicate, requiring prolonged therapy usually with at least two drugs.[104,105,111]

16.7   Schistosomiasis (bilharziasis)

Schistosomiasis (bilharziasis) is a disease caused by trematode worms of the genus *Schistosoma*. Humans are the principal host, and certain fresh-water snails are the intermediate hosts. Eggs excreted into fresh water in the stool (*S. mansoni*, *S. japonicum*) or urine (*S. haematobium*) hatch into motile miracidia, which infect snails. The organism develops in the snail into infecting larvae or cercariae, which can penetrate human skin.

About 200 million people are infected worldwide, almost all in tropical countries.[112] *S. mansoni* occurs in tropical Africa, the Caribbean, Brazil, Venezuela, Surinam, and the Arabian peninsula. *S. haematobium* occurs in Africa and the eastern Mediterranean. *S. japonicum* occurs in China, Indonesia, and the Philippines.

Acute schistosomiasis is mostly seen in travelers after primary infection. *S. mansoni* and *S. japonicum* can cause Katayama fever, usually 4–8 weeks after exposure, with fever, malaise, nausea, abdominal pain, diarrhea (which can be bloody and mucoid in heavy infestation), cough, rash, lymphadenopathy, and sometimes hepatomegaly.[112,113] Eosinophilia is common.[113] Swimmer's itch is not caused by human strains, but by non-pathogenic avian and mammalian species of Schistosoma.

Chronic schistosomiasis affects mainly individuals with long-standing infections in poor, rural areas. Immunopathological reactions against schistosome eggs trapped in the tissues lead to inflammatory and obstructive disease of the urinary system (*S. haematobium*) or intestinal disease, hepatosplenic inflammation, and liver fibrosis (*S. mansoni* and *S. japonicum*). Untreated, these can lead to hematuria, to calcification of the bladder and lower ureters, resulting in hydroureter and hydronephrosis, and to bladder cancer (*S. haematobium*) or can lead to cirrhosis of the liver (*S. mansoni* and *S. japonicum*).

The microscopic examination of stool or urine for ova is the gold standard for the diagnosis of schistosomiasis.[112] Antibody-based assays are sensitive and are important for diagnosis in travelers, migrants, and other occasionally exposed people.[112,114] They cannot distinguish past exposure from active infection; and can cross-react with other helminths, so are not useful in field conditions.

Because of the risk of chronic schistosomiasis and the ease of treatment, we recommend screening migrants from endemic areas, using stool and urine microscopy or serology, and treating those who are infected.[115]

A Cochrane review of 13 trials found that both praziquantel, an acylated quinoline-pyrazine active against all schistosome species, and oxamniquine were active against *S. mansoni*.[116] However, oxamniquine is not active against other Schistosoma species and is only used in Brazil. Praziquantel is less toxic than oxamniquine, cheap, and effective in children,[117,118] and is the recommended treatment of choice. Adverse effects are usually mild, although occasionally a child who is heavily infested will develop colic, vomiting, diarrhea (sometimes bloody), urticaria, and edema within hours of taking praziquantel, probably provoked by massive worm shifts and antigen release.[112,119]

Katayama fever is often treated with corticosteroids to suppress the hypersensitivity reaction together with praziquantel to eliminate the already matured worms, although there are no RCTs.[113]

Praziquantel should be administered with great caution in neurocystercicosis[120] because of the danger of convulsions. Corticosteroids and anticonvulsants are possible adjuvant therapies to reduce the risk.[112] The management of neurocysticercosis is complex, and we recommend expert advice.

For infection with *S. haematobium* and *S. mansoni*, we recommend:

praziquantel 20 mg/kg orally, after food, and a second dose 4 hours later

The child's urine and/or stools should be checked 6 weeks later to make sure the treatment has been successful, and the course repeated if ova persist.

Infections with *S. japonicum* and *S. mekongi* are somewhat more resistant.[110] We recommend:

praziquantel 20 mg/kg orally, for three doses after food, 4 hours apart

References

1 Matyas Z, Fujikura T. Brucellosis as a world problem. *Dev Biol Stand* 1984;56:3–20.

2 al-Eissa YA, Kambal AM, al-Nasser MN, al-Habib SA, al-Fawaz IM, al-Zamil FA. Childhood brucellosis: a study of 102 cases. *Pediatr Infect Dis J* 1990;9:74–9.

3 Shaalan MA, Memish ZA, Mahmoud SA et al. Brucellosis in children: clinical observations in 115 cases. *Int J Infect Dis* 2002;6:182–6.

4 Almuneef M, Memish ZA, Al Shaalan M, Al Banyan E, Al-Alola S, Balkhy HH. Brucella melitensis bacteremia in children: review of 62 cases. *J Chemother* 2003;15:76–80.

5 Araj GF, Lulu AR, Mustafa MY, Khateeb MI. Evaluation of ELISA in the diagnosis of acute and chronic brucellosis in human beings. *J Hyg (Lond)* 1986;97:457–69.

6 Nimri LF. Diagnosis of recent and relapsed cases of human brucellosis by PCR assay. *BMC Infect Dis* 2003;3:5.

7 Al-Nakkas A, Mustafa AS, Wright SG. Large-scale evaluation of a single-tube nested PCR for the laboratory diagnosis of human brucellosis in Kuwait. *J Med Microbiol* 2005;54(pt 8):727–30.

8 Lubani MM, Dudin KI, Sharda DC et al. A multicenter therapeutic study of 1100 children with brucellosis. *Pediatr Infect Dis J* 1989;2:75–8.

9 Solera J, Medrano F, Rodriguez M, Geijo P, Paulino J. A comparative therapeutic and multicenter trial of rifampicin and doxycycline versus streptomycin and doxycycline in human brucellosis. *Med Clin (Barc)* 1991;96:649–53.

10 Solera J, Rodriguez-Zapata M, Geijo P et al. Doxycycline-rifampin versus doxycycline-streptomycin in treatment of human brucellosis due to Brucella melitensis. The GECMEI Group. Grupo de Estudio de Castilla-la Mancha de Enfermedades Infecciosas. *Antimicrob Agents Chemother* 1995;39:2061–7.

11 Ariza J, Gudiol F, Pallares R et al. Treatment of human brucellosis with doxycycline plus rifampin or doxycycline plus

streptomycin. A randomized, double-blind study. *Ann Intern Med* 1992;117:25–30.

12 Lang R, Dagan R, Potasman I, Einhorn M, Raz R. Failure of ceftriaxone in the treatment of acute brucellosis. *Clin Infect Dis* 1992;14:506–9.

13 Roushan MR, Gangi SM, Ahmadi SA. Comparison of the efficacy of two months of treatment with co-trimoxazole plus doxycycline vs. co-trimoxazole plus rifampin in brucellosis. *Swiss Med Wkly* 2004;134:564–8.

14 Hasanjani Roushan MR, Mohraz M, Hajiahmadi M, Ramzani A, Valayati AA. Efficacy of gentamicin plus doxycycline versus streptomycin plus doxycycline in the treatment of brucellosis in humans. *Clin Infect Dis* 2006;42:1075–80.

15 Pappas G, Seitaridis S, Akritidis N, Tsianos E. Treatment of brucella spondylitis: lessons from an impossible meta-analysis and initial report of efficacy of a fluoroquinolone-containing regimen. *Int J Antimicrob Agents* 2004;24:502–7.

16 American Academy of Pediatrics. Brucellosis. In: Pickering LK (ed.), *Red Book: 2003 Report of the Committee on Infectious Diseases*, 26th edn. Elk Grove Village, IL: American Academy of Pediatrics, 2003:222–4.

17 Nasseri Moghaddam S, Abrishami A, Malekzadeh R. Percutaneous needle aspiration, injection, and reaspiration with or without benzimidazole coverage for uncomplicated hepatic hydatid cysts. *The Cochrane Database of Systematic Reviews* 2006;(2):Art No CD003623.

18 Chaouachi B, Nouri A, Ben Salah S, Lakhoua R, Saied H. Hydatid cyst of the lung in children. Apropos of 643 cases. *Pediatrie* 1988;43:769–73.

19 Turgut M. Hydatidosis of central nervous system and its coverings in the pediatric and adolescent age groups in Turkey during the last century: a critical review of 137 cases. *Childs Nerv Syst* 2002;18:670–83.

20 Khuroo MS, Wani NA, Javid G et al. Percutaneous drainage compared with surgery for hepatic hydatid cysts. *N Engl J Med* 1997;337:881–7.

21 Dziri C, Haouet K, Fingerhut A. Treatment of hydatid cyst of the liver: where is the evidence? *World J Surg* 2004;28:731–6.

22 Khuroo MS, Dar MY, Yatto GN. Percutaneous drainage versus albendazole therapy in hepatic hydatidosis: a prospective, randomized study. *Gastroenterology* 1993;104:1452–9.

23 Teoh L, Kerrigan A, May M, Van Asperen P. Pseudo food allergy. *J Paediatr Child Health* 2005;41:63–4.

24 Kanat F, Turk E, Aribas OK. Comparison of pulmonary hydatid cysts in children and adults. *ANZ J Surg* 2004;74:885–9.

25 Fitzgerald D, Harvey J, Isaacs D, Kilham H. The case of the persistent pleural effusion. *Pediatr Infect Dis J* 1991;10:475, 479–80.

26 Dogru D, Kiper N, Ozcelik U, Yalcin E, Gocmen A. Medical treatment of pulmonary hydatid disease: for which child? *Parasitol Int* 2005;54:135–8.

27 Snow RW, Guerra CA, Noor AM et al. The global distribution of clinical episodes of *Plasmodium falciparum* malaria. *Nature* 2005;434:214–7.

28 Stauffer WM, Kamat D. Special challenges in the prevention and treatment of malaria in children. *Curr Infect Dis Rep* 2003;5:43–52.

29 Brabin BJ, Ganley Y. Imported malaria in children in the UK. *Arch Dis Child* 1997;77:76–81.

30 Stauffer W, Fischer PR. Diagnosis and treatment of malaria in children. *Clin Infect Dis* 2003;37:1340–8.

31 Molyneux ME, Taylor TE, Wirima JJ et al. Clinical features and prognostic indicators in paediatric cerebral malaria: a study of 131 comatose Malawian children. *QJM* 1989;71:441–59.

32 Maroushek SR, Aguilar E. Asymptomatic malaria in Liberian children. *Pediatr Res* 2002;51:193A.

33 Centers for Disease Control Web site. Treatment of malaria. *Guidelines for Clinicians*. Available at http://www.cdc.gov/malaria/diagnosis_treatment/tx_clinicians.htm. (accessed October 10, 2006).

34 McIntosh HM, Olliaro P. Artemisinin derivatives for treating uncomplicated malaria. *The Cochrane Database of Systematic Reviews* 1999;(2):Art No CD000256.

35 Adjuik M, Babiker A, Garner P, Olliaro P, Taylor W, White N. Artesunate combinations for treatment of malaria: meta-analysis. *Lancet* 2004;363:9–17.

36 Myint HY, Tipmanee P, Nosten F et al. A systematic overview of published antimalarial drug trials. *Trans R Soc Trop Med Hyg* 2004;98:73–81.

37 Adjuik M, Agnamey P, Babiker A et al. Amodiaquine-artesunate versus amodiaquine for uncomplicated *Plasmodium falciparum* malaria in African children: a randomised, multicentre trial. *Lancet* 2002;359:1365–72.

38 von Seidlein L, Milligan P, Pinder M et al. Efficacy of artesunate plus pyrimethamine-sulphadoxine for uncomplicated malaria in Gambian children: a double-blind, randomised, controlled trial. *Lancet* 2000;355:352–7.

39 Mayxay M, Khanthavong M, Lindegardh N et al. Randomized comparison of chloroquine plus sulfadoxine-pyrimethamine versus artesunate plus mefloquine versus artemether-lumefantrine in the treatment of uncomplicated falciparum malaria in the Lao People's Democratic Republic. *Clin Infect Dis* 2004;39:1139–47.

40 Stohrer JM, Dittrich S, Thongpaseuth V et al. Therapeutic efficacy of artemether-lumefantrine and artesunate-mefloquine for treatment of uncomplicated *Plasmodium falciparum* malaria in Luang Namtha Province, Lao People's Democratic Republic. *Trop Med Int Health* 2004;9:1175–83.

41 Mutabingwa TK, Anthony D, Heller A et al. Amodiaquine alone, amodiaquine+sulfadoxine-pyrimethamine, amodiaquine+artesunate, and artemether-lumefantrine for outpatient treatment of malaria in Tanzanian children: a four-arm randomised effectiveness trial. *Lancet* 2005;365:1474–80.

42 Koram KA, Abuaku B, Duah N, Quashie N. Comparative efficacy of antimalarial drugs including ACTs in the treatment of uncomplicated malaria among children under 5 years in Ghana. *Acta Trop* 2005;95:194–203.

43 van den Broek IV, Maung UA, Peters A et al. Efficacy of chloroquine+sulfadoxine—pyrimethamine, mefloquine+artesunate and artemether+lumefantrine combination therapies to treat *Plasmodium falciparum* malaria in the

Chittagong Hill Tracts, Bangladesh. *Trans R Soc Trop Med Hyg* 2005;99:727–35.

44 Meremikwu M, Alaribe A, Ejemot R et al. Artemether-lumefantrine versus artesunate plus amodiaquine for treating uncomplicated childhood malaria in Nigeria: randomized controlled trial. *Malar J* 2006;5:43.

45 Guthmann JP, Cohuet S, Rigutto C et al. High efficacy of two artemisinin-based combinations (artesunate+amodiaquine and artemether+lumefantrine) in Caala, Central Angola. *Am J Trop Med Hyg* 2006;75:143–5.

46 Smithuis F, Kyaw MK, Phe O et al. Efficacy and effectiveness of dihydroartemisinin-piperaquine versus artesunate-mefloquine in falciparum malaria: an open-label randomised comparison. *Lancet* 2006;367:2075–85.

47 Mayxay M, Thongpraseuth V, Khanthavong M et al. An open, randomized comparison of artesunate plus mefloquine vs. dihydroartemisinin-piperaquine for the treatment of uncomplicated *Plasmodium falciparum* malaria in the Lao People's Democratic Republic (Laos). *Trop Med Int Health* 2006;11:1157–65.

48 World Health Organization. International Travel and Health, 2005. Available at http://whqlibdoc.who.int/publications/2005/9241580364_chap7.pdf (accessed October 10, 2006).

49 Menard D, Madji N, Manirakiza A, Djalle D, Koula MR, Talarmin A. Efficacy of chloroquine, amodiaquine, sulfadoxine-pyrimethamine, chloroquine-sulfadoxine-pyrimethamine combination, and amodiaquine-sulfadoxine-pyrimethamine combination in Central African children with non-complicated malaria. *Am J Trop Med Hyg* 2005;72:581–5.

50 Maitland K, Nadel S, Pollard AJ, Williams TN, Newton CR, Levin M. Management of severe malaria in children: proposed guidelines for the United Kingdom. *BMJ* 2005;331;337–43.

51 McIntosh HM, Olliaro P. Artemisinin derivatives for treating severe malaria. *The Cochrane Database of Systematic Reviews* 2000;(2):Art No CD000527.

52 White NJ, Waller D, Crawley J et al. Comparison of artemether and chloroquine for severe malaria in Gambian children. *Lancet* 1992;339:317–21.

53 Adam I, Idris HM, Mohamed-Ali AA, Aelbasit IA, Elbashir MI. Comparison of intramuscular artemether and intravenous quinine in the treatment of Sudanese children with severe falciparum malaria. *East Afr Med J* 2002;79:621–5.

54 Cao XT, Bethell DB, Pham TP et al. Comparison of artemisinin suppositories, intramuscular artesunate and intravenous quinine for the treatment of severe childhood malaria. *Trans R Soc Trop Med Hyg* 1997;91:335–42.

55 Barnes KI, Mwenechanya J, Tembo M et al. Efficacy of rectal artesunate compared with parenteral quinine in initial treatment of moderately severe malaria in African children and adults: a randomised study. *Lancet* 2004;363:1598–605.

56 Karunajeewa HA, Reeder J, Lorry K et al. Artesunate suppositories versus intramuscular artemether for treatment of severe malaria in children in Papua New Guinea. *Antimicrob Agents Chemother* 2006;50:968–74.

57 van Hensbroek MB, Onyiorah E, Jaffar S et al. A trial of artemether or quinine in children with cerebral malaria. *N Engl J Med* 1996;335:69–75.

58 Murphy S, English M, Waruiru C et al. An open randomized trial of artemether versus quinine in the treatment of cerebral malaria in African children. *Trans R Soc Trop Med Hyg* 1996;90:298–301.

59 Olumese PE, Bjorkman A, Gbadegesin RA, Adeyemo AA, Walker O. Comparative efficacy of intramuscular artemether and intravenous quinine in Nigerian children with cerebral malaria. *Acta Trop* 1999;73:231–6.

60 Taylor TE, Wills BA, Courval JM, Molyneux ME. Intramuscular artemether vs intravenous quinine: an open, randomized trial in Malawian children with cerebral malaria. *Trop Med Int Health* 1998;3:3–8.

61 Hien TT, Arnold K, Vinh H et al. Comparison of artemisinin suppositories with intravenous artesunate and intravenous quinine in the treatment of cerebral malaria. *Trans R Soc Trop Med Hyg* 1992;86:582–3.

62 Aceng JR, Byarugaba JS, Tumwine JK. Rectal artemether versus intravenous quinine for the treatment of cerebral malaria in children in Uganda: randomised clinical trial. *BMJ* 2005;330:334.

63 Dondorp A, Nosten F, Stepniewska K, Day N, White N. South East Asian Quinine Artesunate Malaria Trial (SEAQUA-MAT) group. Artesunate versus quinine for treatment of severe falciparum malaria: a randomised trial. *Lancet* 2005;366:717–25.

64 Maitland K, Levin M, English M et al. Severe *P. falciparum* malaria in Kenyan children: evidence for hypovolaemia. *QJM* 2003;96:427–34.

65 Maitland K, Pamba A, English M et al. Pre-transfusion management of children with severe malarial anaemia: a randomised controlled trial of intravascular volume expansion. *Br J Haematol* 2005;128:393–400.

66 Maitland K, Pamba A, English M et al. Randomized trial of volume expansion with albumin or saline in children with severe malaria: preliminary evidence of albumin benefit. *Clin Infect Dis* 2005;40:538–45.

67 Meremikwu M, Smith HJ. Blood transfusion for treating malarial anaemia. *The Cochrane Database of Systematic Reviews* 1999;(4):Art No CD001475.

68 Vinetz JM. Emerging chloroquine-resistant *Plasmodium vivax* (Benign Tertian) malaria: the need for alternative drug treatment. *Clin Infect Dis* 2006;42:1073–4.

69 Rieckmann KH, Davis DR, Hutton DC. *Plasmodium vivax* resistance to chloroquine? *Lancet* 1989;2:1183–4.

70 Baird JK. Chloroquine resistance in *Plasmodium vivax*. *Antimicrob Agents Chemother* 2004;48:4075–83.

71 Maguire JD, Krisin, Marwoto H, Richie TL, Fryauff DJ, Baird JK. Mefloquine is highly efficacious against chloroquine-resistant Plasmodium vivax malaria and *Plasmodium falciparum* malaria in Papua, Indonesia. *Clin Infect Dis* 2006;42:1067–72.

72 Pukrittayakamee S, Imwong M, Looareesuwan S, White NJ. Therapeutic responses to antimalarial and antibacterial drugs in vivax malaria. *Acta Trop* 2004;89:351–6.

73 Bosman A, Delacollette C, Olumese P, Ridley G, Rietveld R, Shretta A. The use of antimalarial drugs. *Report of a WHO informal Consultation*. Geneva: World Health Organization, 2001.

74 Rajgor DD, Gogtay NJ, Kadam VS et al. Efficacy of a 14-day primaquine regimen in preventing relapses in patients with *Plasmodium vivax* malaria in Mumbai, India. *Trans R Soc Trop Med Hyg* 2003;97:438–40.

75 Leslie T, Rab MA, Ahmadzai H et al. Compliance with 14-day primaquine therapy for radical cure of vivax malaria—a randomized placebo-controlled trial comparing unsupervised with supervised treatment. *Trans R Soc Trop Med Hyg* 2004;98:168–73.

76 Yadav RS, Ghosh SK. Radical curative efficacy of five-day regimen of primaquine for treatment of *Plasmodium vivax* malaria in India. *J Parasitol* 2002;88:1042–4.

77 Looareesuwan S, Buchachart K, Wilairatana P et al. Primaquine-tolerant vivax malaria in Thailand. *Ann Trop Med Hyg* 1997;91:939–43.

78 Lengeler C. Insecticide-treated bed nets and curtains for preventing malaria. *The Cochrane Database of Systematic Reviews* 2004;(2):Art No CD000363.

79 Meremikwu MM, Omari AAA, Garner P. Chemoprophylaxis and intermittent treatment for preventing malaria in children. *The Cochrane Database of Systematic Reviews* 2005;(4):Art No CD003756.

80 Branch OH, Udhayakumar V, Hightower AW et al. A longitudinal investigation of IgG and IgM antibody responses to the merozoite surface protein-1 19-kiloDalton domain of *Plasmodium falciparum* in pregnant women and infants: associations with febrile illness, parasitemia, and anemia. *Am J Trop Med Hyg* 1998;58:211–9.

81 Warrell DA. To search and study out the secret of tropical diseases by way of experiment. *Lancet* 2001;358:1983–8.

82 Centers for Disease Control and Prevention. Travelers' health. Information for Health Care Providers: Preventing Malaria in Infants and Children. Available at http://www.cdc.gov/travel/mal_kids_hc.htm.

83 World Health Organization. International Travel and Health, 2005. Available at http://www.who.int/ith/en/

84 World Health Organization. International Travel and Health: Country list, 2005. Available at http://www.who.int/ith/countries/en/index.html.

85 Overbosch D, Schilthuis H, Bienzle U et al. Malarone international study team. Atovaquone-proguanil versus mefloquine for malaria prophylaxis in non-immune travelers: results from a randomized, double-blind study. *Clin Infect Dis* 2001;33:1015–21.

86 Lell B, Luckner D, Ndjave M, Scott T, Kremsner PG. Randomised placebo-controlled study of atovaquone plus proguanil for malaria prophylaxis in children. *Lancet* 1998;351:709–13.

87 Ling J, Baird JK, Fryauff DJ et al. Randomized, placebo-controlled trial of atovaquone/proguanil for the prevention of *Plasmodium falciparum* or *Plasmodium vivax* malaria among migrants to Papua, Indonesia. *Clin Infect Dis* 2002;35:825–33.

88 Faucher JF, Binder R, Missinou MA et al. Efficacy of atovaquone/proguanil for malaria prophylaxis in children and its effect on the immunogenicity of live oral typhoid and cholera vaccines. *Clin Infect Dis* 2002;35:1147–54.

89 Camus D, Djossou F, Schilthuis HJ et al. International malarone study team. Atovaquone-proguanil versus chloroquine-proguanil for malaria prophylaxis in non-immune pediatric travelers: results of an international, randomized, open-label study. *Clin Infect Dis* 2004;38:1716–23.

90 White NJ. Melioidosis. *Lancet* 2003;361:1715–22.

91 Sam IC, Puthucheary SD. Melioidosis in children from Kuala Lumpur, Malaysia. *Ann Trop Paediatr* 2006;26:219–24.

92 Lumbiganon P, Chotechuangnirun N, Kosalaraksa P. Clinical experience with treatment of melioidosis in children. *Pediatr Infect Dis J* 2004;23:1165–6.

93 Currie BJ, Fisher DA, Howard DM et al. Endemic melioidosis in tropical northern Australia: a 10-year prospective study and review of the literature. *Clin Infect Dis* 2000;31:981–6.

94 Rolim DB, Vilar DC, Sousa AQ et al. Melioidosis, northeastern Brazil. *Emerg Infect Dis* 2005;11:1458–60.

95 Dorman SE, Gill VJ, Gallin JI, Holland SM. *Burkholderia pseudomallei* infection in a Puerto Rican patient with chronic granulomatous disease: case report and review of occurrences in the Americas. *Clin Infect Dis* 1998;26:889–94.

96 Renella R, Perez JM, Chollet-Martin S et al. *Burkholderia pseudomallei* infection in chronic granulomatous disease. *Eur J Pediatr* 2006;165:175–7.

97 Ralph A, McBride J, Currie BJ. Transmission of *Burkholderia pseudomallei* via breast milk in northern Australia. *Pediatr Infect Dis J* 2004;23:1169–71.

98 Samuel M, Ti TY. Interventions for treating melioidosis. *The Cochrane Database of Systematic Reviews* 2002;(4):Art No CD001263.

99 White NJ, Dance DA, Chaowagul W, Wattanagoon Y, Wuthiekanun V, Pitakwatchara N. Halving of mortality of severe melioidosis by ceftazidime. *Lancet* 1989;2:697–701.

100 Cheng AC, Stephens DP, Anstey NM, Currie BJ. Adjunctive granulocyte colony-stimulating factor for treatment of septic shock due to melioidosis. *Clin Infect Dis* 2004;38:32–7.

101 Chaowagul W, Chierakul W, Simpson AJ et al. Open-label randomized trial of oral trimethoprim-sulfamethoxazole, doxycycline, and chloramphenicol compared with trimethoprim-sulfamethoxazole and doxycycline for maintenance therapy of melioidosis. *Antimicrob Agents Chemother* 2005;49:4020–5.

102 Chierakul W, Anunnatsiri S, Short JM et al. Two randomized controlled trials of ceftazidime alone versus ceftazidime in combination with trimethoprim-sulfamethoxazole for the treatment of severe melioidosis. *Clin Infect Dis* 2005;41:1105–13.

103 Maurin M, Raoult D. Q fever. *Clin Microbiol Rev* 1999;12:518–53.

104 Parker NR, Barralet JH, Bell AM. Q fever. *Lancet* 2006;367:679–88.

105 Maltezou HC, Raoult D. Q fever in children. *Lancet Infect Dis* 2002;2:686–91.

106 Maltezou HC, Constantopoulou I, Kallergi C et al. Q fever in children in Greece. *Am J Trop Med Hyg* 2004;70:540–4.

107 Slaba K, Skultety L, Toman R. Efficiency of various serological techniques for diagnosing *Coxiella burnetii* infection. *Acta Virol* 2005;49:123–7.

108 Fournier PE, Raoult D. Comparison of PCR and serology assays for early diagnosis of acute Q fever. *J Clin Microbiol* 2003;41:5094–8.

109 Sobradillo V, Zalacain R, Capelastegui A, Uresandi F, Corral J. Antibiotic treatment in pneumonia due to Q fever. *Thorax* 1992;47:276–8.

110 Morovic M. Q Fever pneumonia: are clarithromycin and moxifloxacin alternative treatments only? *Am J Trop Med Hyg* 2005;73:947–8.

111 Karakousis PC, Trucksis M, Dumler JS. Chronic Q fever in the United States. *J Clin Microbiol* 2006;44:2283–7.

112 Gryseels B, Polman K, Clerinx J, Kestens L. Human schistosomiasis. *Lancet* 2006;368:1106–18.

113 Bottieau B, Clerinx J, De Vega MR et al. Imported Katayama fever: clinical and biological features at presentation and during treatment. *J Infect* 2006;52:339–45.

114 Feldmeier H, Poggensee G. Diagnostic techniques in schistosomiasis control: a review. *Acta Trop* 1993;52:205–20.

115 Davidson N, Skull S, Chaney G et al. Comprehensive health assessment for newly arrived refugee children in Australia. *J Paediatr Child Health* 2004;40:562–8.

116 Saconato H, Atallah A. Interventions for treating schistosomiasis mansoni. *The Cochrane Database of Systematic Reviews* 1999;(3):Art No CD000528.

117 Olds GR, King C, Hewlett J et al. Double-blind placebo-controlled study of concurrent administration of albendazole and praziquantel in schoolchildren with schistosomiasis and geohelminths. *J Infect Dis* 1999;179:996–1003.

118 Tchuente LA, Shaw DJ, Polla L, Cioli D, Vercruysse J. Efficacy of praziquantel against *Schistosoma haematobium* infection in children. *Am J Trop Med Hyg* 2004;71:778–82.

119 Stelma FF, Talla I, Sow S et al. Efficacy and side effects of praziquantel in an epidemic focus of *Schistosoma mansoni*. *Am J Trop Med Hyg* 1995;53:167–70.

120 Fong GC, Cheung RT. Caution with praziquantel in neurocysticercosis. *Stroke* 1997;28:1648–9.

CHAPTER 17

Urinary tract infections

17.1 Acute urinary tract infection

Acute urinary tract infection (UTI) is common in children. Most UTIs in children result from ascending infections. Neonates with UTI are often septicemic, but that does not necessarily mean, as often stated, that neonatal UTI occurs due to hematogenous spread. It could be that UTI is due to ascending infection, but UTI is more likely to be complicated by septicemia in neonates. Indeed, neonatal UTI is often associated with urinary tract abnormality, implying local infection followed by bloodstream spread.[1–3] Boys are more susceptible to UTI than girls before the age of 3 months, because of a higher incidence of anatomic abnormalities. Thereafter, the incidence is substantially higher in girls. Estimates of the true incidence of UTI depend on rates of diagnosis and investigation. At least 8% of girls and 2% of boys will have a UTI in childhood.[1–3] Hospitalization is required in about 40% of cases, particularly in infancy.[4] Transient damage to the kidneys occurs in about 40% of affected children,[2] and about 5% suffer permanent damage,[5] sometimes even following a single infection. Symptoms are systemic and non-specific rather than localized in early childhood, consisting of fever, lethargy, anorexia, vomiting, and sometimes rigors.

Children who have had one infection are at risk of further infections: 30–40% of children who have had an initial UTI will have another UTI, and up to 30% will have recurrent UTIs.[6] The risk factors for recurrent infection are vesicoureteric reflux (VUR) leading to dilatation, bladder instability, and previous infections.[5,7] Recurrence of UTI is more common in girls than boys.[6,8] The major significance of UTI is the risk of renal damage, and this risk increases as the number of recurrences increases.[9]

The question of circumcision (see p. 277) and prophylactic antibiotics (see p. 278) to prevent UTI and reduce renal damage are considered below.

Definition of acute UTI

Urine is normally sterile. Girls may have asymptomatic bacteriuria, and an RCT showed that antibiotic treatment of schoolgirls with asymptomatic bacteriuria was not only of no benefit but caused more symptoms than did placebo.[10] In contrast, expert opinion is that children with symptomatic UTI benefit from antibiotics, although it would not be ethical to perform placebo-controlled trials to prove this.[1,2]

Traditionally, the definition of UTI has been a pure growth of 100,000 (10^5) colony-forming units (CFU) per milliliter from a voided specimen. This figure comes from Kass' studies, comparing voided specimens from women who were about to be catheterized with catheter specimens,[11] and has never been verified in children. Using this figure as the definition of UTI, a comparative study[7] arrived at the figures given in Table 17.1 to reach a definition of UTI when urine is collected by different methods.

UTI is caused by *Escherichia coli* in over 80% of cases.[13,14] Other organisms include *Proteus* (which is more common in boys and in children with renal stones), *Klebsiella, Enterococcus,* and coagulase-negative staphylococci.[13,14] The doubling time of *E. coli* in urine is less than an hour,[2,3] so urine that sits on the bench for any length of time may give a false-positive culture.

Table 17.1 Bacteriologic diagnostic criteria for acute UTI in children.[7,12]

Method of Urine Collection	Minimum Level of Bacteriuria for Diagnosis of UTI
Clean catch in girls	100,000 (10^5) CFU/mL (or 10^8/L)
Clean catch in boys	10,000 (10^4) CFU/mL (or 10^7/L)
Catheter	10,000 (10^4) CFU/mL (or 10^7/L)
Suprapubic aspiration	Gram-negative bacilli: any colonies Gram-positive cocci: 5000 CFU/mL (or 5×10^6/L)

CFU/mL = colony-forming units per mL (sometimes expressed as organisms/mL).

Method of urine collection

Urine can be collected by clean catch voiding, bag, pad, suprapubic aspiration (SPA), or catheterization. In an acute situation, when empiric antibiotics will be started regardless of urinalysis, it is important to get the specimen using a method which is both sensitive and specific, so as to be able to rely on the culture result as the basis for future decisions about investigation and ongoing management. On the other hand, if there is less urgency because treatment will not be started immediately, a less invasive test may be preferred, even it is much less specific.

Question | For children with suspected UTI, is one method of urine collection compared to others more sensitive, more specific, or more acceptable?

Literature review | We found seven studies[15–21] and a non-Cochrane systematic review[22] directly comparing different urine collection techniques.

Bag and pad specimens are contaminated (defined as 10^4–10^5 CFU/mL) in 16–29% of specimens.[15,16] Although this is sometimes said to be too inaccurate, these techniques are simple and minimally invasive. If the culture is negative, this excludes UTI and avoids more invasive tests. If the bag or pad culture grows an organism, the test can be repeated using a more specific collection method. On the other hand, the routine use of bag specimens to test urine from febrile children attending emergency departments tends to lead to overdiagnosis and overtreatment.[17] In one study, banning bag specimens reduced the number of urine specimens sent to the laboratory and reduced the number of children treated unnecessarily, without any reduction in the number of true UTIs diagnosed.[17]

Clean voided or clean catch urines often take time and patience to collect, and are contaminated in 2–15% of cases.[15,16]

Specimens collected by SPA or urethral catheter are very rarely contaminated, although an SPA can inadvertently puncture the bowel and a catheter specimen can be contaminated with perineal bowel organisms. A systematic review of rapid tests to diagnose UTI also looked at the accuracy of sampling techniques in terms of contamination.[22] Thirteen studies compared the results of culture from urine obtained by different sampling methods. When both clean voided urine samples and SPA urine samples were cultured (five stud-

ies), the agreement between the two sampling methods was good. Overall, there were insufficient data to draw any conclusions regarding the appropriateness of using urine samples obtained from bags (four studies) or pads/nappies (four studies).[22]

Invasive sampling procedures are not always successful. In one study, SPA yielded urine in only 62% of attempts, improving to 93% when ultrasound was used to locate the bladder.[18] Similarly, initial catheterization was successful in only 72% of children, but 93% if ultrasound was used first to make sure there was urine in the bladder.[19] We found two RCTs comparing SPA and catheterization.[20,21] In one study, at least 2 mL of urine was obtained from all 50 children randomized to catheterization, but only 46% of 50 who underwent SPA. After failed SPA, urethral catheterization was 100% successful.[20] A second small study found that an adequate urine sample was obtained from 66% with SPA and 83% with catheter, but that pain scores were significantly higher with SPA.[21]

Catheter urine samples are more likely to obtain urine and less painful than SPA, and are recommended as the method of choice when it is urgent to get a urine specimen.

Appearance of urine

Cloudy urine is often interpreted as meaning a definite UTI. In practice, about half of all symptomatic children with cloudy urine have a UTI.[23–25] If a symptomatic child has cloudy urine, the urine should be sent for culture, because it is important to know whether or not there is a true infection, which has major implications for investigation and management.

Some have claimed that a crystal clear appearance on visual inspection of urine excludes UTI.[23] This has been refuted by studies which found that 3–4% of crystal clear urine samples grew 10^5 organisms/mL or greater, and the patient was diagnosed as having a UTI.[24,25]

Urinalysis to detect UTI

It would be useful if urinalysis could predict whether a child was or was not likely to have a UTI, in terms of whether or not to send urine for culture and whether or not to start empiric therapy. A dipstick test would be the simplest rapid test, giving an answer in seconds. Microscopy for bacteria and/or white cells can be performed in the office but requires training and a bit more time.

Question | In febrile young children, does urinalysis reliably detect UTI?

Literature review | We found two non-Cochrane meta-analyses of urinalysis screening tests[26,27] and two non-Cochrane systematic reviews.[22,28]

A non-Cochrane meta-analysis of 26 studies[26] found that any organisms seen on gram stain had 93% sensitivity and 95% specificity for detecting UTI, and a dipstick test positive for both nitrite and leukocyte esterase performed almost as well, with a sensitivity of 88% and a specificity of 93%. These performed better than pyuria (defined as >10 white cells/mm^3), which was only 77% sensitive.

A subsequent non-Cochrane meta-analysis of 48 studies used a different technique, so-called receiver operator curves, to analyze sensitivity and specificity together, and concluded that pyuria (10 or more white cells per high-power field) and bacteriuria (any bacteria on gram stain) performed best.[27]

A non-Cochrane systematic review to determine the diagnostic accuracy of rapid tests for detecting UTI in children <5 years old found 70 studies, of which 39 evaluated dipstick tests.[22] The review concluded that either a dipstick positive for both nitrite and leukocyte esterase or microscopy positive for both pyuria and bacteriuria made UTI extremely likely. Similarly, they concluded that a dipstick negative for both nitrite and leukocyte esterase or microscopy negative for both pyuria and bacteriuria effectively excluded UTI.[22]

If rapid tests can identify children with UTI with a high degree of probability, they can be used as a basis for choosing children who should start empiric therapy. The best specificity (98%) in the two meta-analyses was for nitrite.[26,27] If specificity is high, false positives are rare, so a positive nitrite could be used as a basis to start empiric therapy.[28] It could be argued that if the child gets better with empiric antibiotics and the diagnosis of UTI does not mandate any investigations, there is no need to send urine for culture. We still recommend sending urine for culture, however, because of the need to know the antibiotic sensitivity of the bacteria and because we feel it is important to confirm UTI.

If rapid tests can identify children who are very unlikely to have UTI, the clinical options are to withhold antibiotics but send urine for culture or to decide that UTI has been effectively excluded and it is not necessary to send urine for culture. If both nitrite and leukocyte esterase are negative on dipstick, UTI is extremely unlikely. A clinical decision should be made whether to send urine for culture and withhold antibiotics, or to discard the urine and consider other diagnoses.[28]

Febrile children and urine culture

One study of over 4000 children <2 years attending an emergency department with fever compared culture with microscopy of catheter urines. There were 212 children with positive urine cultures. They found that the presence of pyuria had 95% sensitivity for UTI. If urine cultures had been performed only on specimens from children who had pyuria or who were managed presumptively with antibiotics, cultures of 2600 (61%) specimens would have been avoided, but 22 of 212 patients with positive urine cultures would not have been identified.[29] It is arguable whether the cost saved by not sending 2600 specimens justifies missing 22 UTIs.

Sending urine cultures routinely on febrile children with clinical evidence of respiratory infection or another focus of infection and who are not really suspected of having UTI is illogical. It will yield many false-positive urine cultures if a bag specimen is used, and is unnecessarily traumatic if invasive techniques are used.

Empiric antibiotic treatment for UTI

Question | In children with UTI, is oral antibiotic therapy compared to short-term intravenous followed by oral antibiotics effective in terms of immediate and long-term outcomes?

Literature review | We found 18 RCTs and a Cochrane review.[30]

The Cochrane review[30] was called "Antibiotics for Acute Pyelonephritis in Children." According to the Cochrane authors, acute pyelonephritis is the most severe form of UTI in children and is different from acute cystitis. They define acute cystitis and pyelonephritis as follows:

• *Acute cystitis*: This infection is limited to the urethra and bladder, seen most commonly in girls over 2 years of age, and presenting with localizing symptoms of dysuria (pain when passing urine), frequency, urgency, cloudy urine, and lower abdominal discomfort. Pyuria (white cells in the urine) and hematuria (blood in the urine) may also be found.[30]

· *Acute pyelonephritis*: This is infection of the kidney, associated with systemic features such as high fever, malaise, vomiting, abdominal and loin pain, and tenderness, poor feeding, and irritability in infants. Together with urine culture, diagnosis may be assisted by imaging using ^{99m}Tc-labeled dimercaptosuccinic acid (DMSA) renal scan and markers of inflammation in the blood, such as erythrocyte sedimentation rate and C-reactive protein.[30]

The Cochrane review included studies of children with UTI, who had one or more systemic symptoms.[30] The reviewers found 18 eligible trials (2612 children). No significant differences were found in persistent renal damage at 6 months (but based on only one trial, of 306 children: RR 1.45, 95% CI 0.69–3.03), or in duration of fever between oral cefixime therapy (14 days) and IV therapy (3 days) followed by oral therapy (10 days). Similarly, no significant differences in persistent renal damage (RR 0.99, 95% CI 0.72–1.37) were found between IV therapy (3–4 days) followed by oral therapy and IV therapy for 7–14 days. However, only two studies included neonates, a third of the studies did not include babies <3 months old, and it was not possible to look at outcome by age to see if younger children might benefit more from IV therapy. It is known that the incidence of septicemia with UTI is 4–10% overall, and is highest in younger children.[31–34]

We recommend treating children 3 months and older with acute pyelonephritis with oral cefixime or with short courses (2–4 days) of IV therapy followed by oral therapy.

We recommend commencing neonates and infants <3 months old on IV therapy, because the risk of septicemia is high[31–34] and it has not been shown that commencing with oral antibiotics is as effective as IV treatment at this age.

Question | In children with UTI, is short-course antibiotic treatment compared with 5 days or more of antibiotics effective in terms of immediate and long-term outcomes?

Literature review | We found a non-Cochrane meta-analysis comparing short-duration with long-duration antibiotics for acute cystitis in children,[35] and a non-Cochrane meta-analysis[36] and a Cochrane

review[37] comparing short course with standard duration for UTI in children.

A non-Cochrane meta-analysis found 22 studies that compared short-course antibiotics (up to 4 days) with 5 days or more for acute cystitis.[35] The overall difference in cure rates between short and conventional courses of therapy was significant (6.4%; 95% CI 1.9–10.9%), favoring the conventional course. Similar results were obtained when only studies comparing the same agents in the short and conventional courses were included. Short-course amoxicillin was inferior to conventional-length course (difference in cure rate, 13%; 95% CI 4–24%). No difference was found between short-course and conventional-length courses of trimethoprim-sulfamethoxazole (difference in cure rate, 6.2%; 95% CI 3.7–16.2%).

A non-Cochrane meta-analysis compared short-course antibiotics (from a single dose to 3 days) with standard duration (7–14 days) for UTI in children.[36] The meta-analysis found 16 studies, and concluded that long-course therapy was associated with fewer treatment failures. The difference remained significant if the analysis was restricted to studies of pyelonephritis. However, the review included single-dose treatment, which is used for acute cystitis in adult women. For studies that just compared 3-day therapy to long-course therapy, there was no significant difference in treatment failure or reinfection rates.[36]

A Cochrane review excluded single-dose studies, and compared 2–4 days of antibiotics with 7–14 days for UTI in children (with or without systemic symptoms).[37] The Cochrane reviewers identified 10 trials (652 children) with UTI. There was no significant difference in the frequency of positive urine cultures at 0–10 days after treatment. There was no significant difference between short- and standard-duration therapy in the development of resistant organisms, although there were trends to less resistance with short-course therapy at the end of treatment (one study: RR 0.57, 95% CI 0.32–1.01) or in recurrent UTI (three studies: RR 0.39, 95% CI 0.12–1.29). The reviewers conclude that a 2–4-day course of oral antibiotics appears to be as effective as 7–14 days in eradicating lower tract UTI in children.

We conclude that short courses of antibiotics longer than 1 day (i.e., 2–4 days) are no less effective than standard duration (7–14 days), and

can be recommended to treat uncomplicated UTI.

Aminoglycosides and UTI

Question | For children with UTI, is once daily administration of aminoglycosides compared with multiple daily dosing safer and more effective?
Literature review | We found four RCTs and a non-Cochrane meta-analysis.[38]

A non-Cochrane meta-analysis compared once daily with multiple daily dosing of aminoglycosides in a number of different clinical situations. There were 24 studies, including four RCTs where aminoglycosides were used to treat UTI.[38] Once daily dosing of aminoglycosides was at least as effective as multiple daily dosing, and was not associated with an increased incidence of oto- or nephrotoxicity. There was a suggestion of improved efficacy and reduced nephrotoxicity with once daily dosing in some trials. The available randomized evidence supports the general adoption of once daily dosing of aminoglycosides in pediatric clinical practice, to minimize cost, simplify administration, and to provide similar or even potentially improved efficacy and safety, compared with multiple dosing (see Appendix 2).

> **We recommend once daily dosing of aminoglycosides for treating children with acute UTI.**

Empiric antibiotic treatment for cystitis

Any of the following regimens can be expected to cure the majority of acute cystitis (acute uncomplicated lower UTI without systemic symptoms, usually in girls >2 years old):

> **cephalexin 25 mg/kg (max 1 g) orally, 8-hourly for 3 days** OR
> **trimethoprim 4 mg/kg (max 150 mg) orally, 12-hourly for 3 days** OR (if a trimethoprim liquid formulation is not available)
> **trimethoprim+sulfamethoxazole 4 + 20 mg/kg (max 160 + 800 mg) orally, 12-hourly for 3 days** OR
> **amoxicillin+clavulanate 12.5 + 3.1 mg/kg (max 500 + 125 mg) orally, 12-hourly for 3 days**

Empiric antibiotic treatment for acute pyelonephritis

For acute pyelonephritis (UTI with one or more systemic symptoms), we recommend either oral or IV therapy.

For initial oral therapy, we reviewed the literature and found 16 RCTs, which showed no significant differences in cure or relapse rates between many different oral antibiotics, including amoxicillin-clavulanate, cefaclor, cefadroxil, cefixime, cefprozil cephalexin, nitrofurantoin, and trimethoprim-sulfamethoxazole. Cefixime has been studied more thoroughly than other antibiotics. We recommend:

> **cefixime 4 mg/kg, orally, 12-hourly for 3 days** OR
> **cephalexin 25 mg/kg (max 1 g) orally, 8-hourly for 3 days** OR
> **amoxicillin+clavulanate 12.5 + 3.1 mg/kg (max 500 + 125 mg) orally, 12-hourly for 3 days** OR
> **trimethoprim 4 mg/kg (max 150 mg) orally, 12-hourly for 3 days** OR (if a trimethoprim liquid formulation is not available)
> **trimethoprim+sulfamethoxazole 4 + 20 mg/kg (max 160 + 800 mg) orally, 12-hourly for 3 days**

Fluoroquinolones should not be used as first-line drugs, as they are the only orally active drugs available for infections due to *Pseudomonas aeruginosa* and other multiresistant bacteria.

If resistance to all the above drugs is proven, however, suitable alternatives are:

> **norfloxacin 10 mg/kg (max 400 mg) orally, 12-hourly for 3 days** OR
> **ciprofloxacin 10 mg/kg (max 500 mg) orally, 12-hourly for 3 days**

Treatment failures are usually due to a resistant organism, reinfection with a similar organism, or an unsuspected underlying abnormality of the urinary tract for which further investigations should be considered.

For initial IV therapy, we recommend:

> **gentamicin <10 years: 7.5 mg/kg; ≥10 years: 6 mg/kg IV, daily** PLUS
> **amoxi/ampicillin 50 mg/kg (max 2 g) IV, 6-hourly**

In patients with penicillin allergy, gentamicin alone is usually effective.

Aminoglycosides are not recommended for patients with chronic renal failure. For such children, and in other situations where it is recommended not to use an aminoglycoside (e.g., chronic liver disease, hearing or vestibular problems, and neuromuscular disease; see Appendix 2), we recommend:

ceftriaxone 25 mg/kg (max 1 g) IV, daily OR
cefotaxime 25 mg/kg (max 1 g) IV, 8-hourly

[NB: This regimen does not provide adequate cover for *P. aeruginosa* or enterococci, which are inherently resistant to these third-generation cephalosporins.]

We recommend switching to oral therapy when the child is improving, usually after 3 days but often longer for infants. We suggest continuing IV antibiotics until neonates and infants have settled, which may take 7–10 days.

A follow-up urine culture is advised at least 48 hours after the conclusion of therapy.

Imaging following acute UTI

Diagnostic imaging to look for VUR and scarring has been performed for many years, in an attempt to prevent progression to renal damage as a result of chronic pyelonephritis.[39] The rationale has been that reflux plus infection may lead to renal scarring and chronic renal damage, and that preventing either reflux or infection or both might prevent renal damage.[39]

There is no clear consensus in the literature regarding imaging following acute UTI in infancy. In the past, it has been common to recommend micturating cystourethrogram (MCUG) to identify vesicoreflux, and ultrasound or ^{99m}Tc DMSA scan to identify renal tract anomalies and scarring.

Question | For a child presenting with a first UTI, can imaging of the urinary tract compared with no imaging identify children at risk of progressive renal damage?

Literature review | We found 73 observational studies, no RCTs, and two non-Cochrane systematic reviews[40,41] of imaging techniques following UTI. We found a non-Cochrane meta-analysis of MCUG after UTI.[42]

A non-Cochrane systematic review of routine diagnostic imaging following childhood UTI found 63 studies. All were descriptive, and only 10 were prospective.[40] Another systematic review that included 73 studies also noted the many methodological limitations of the studies.[41] The data did not support the use of less invasive tests such as ultrasound as an alternative to renal scintigraphy, either to rule out infection of the upper urinary tract or to detect renal scarring. Indeed, none of the tests accurately predicted the development of renal scarring. The reviewers concluded that the available evidence supports the consideration of contrast-enhanced ultrasound techniques for detecting VUR as an alternative to MCUG. They found no evidence to support the clinical effectiveness of routine investigation of children with confirmed UTI.[41]

Neonates with UTI, particularly boys, have a high rate of structural abnormalities, and post-erior urethral valves need to be excluded. In one study, 22 of 45 male neonates with UTI had abnormal MCUG and/or ultrasound, although 19 of them had VUR alone.[42] There is a continuum and no clear cut-off between neonates and older infants in terms of the incidence of abnormal findings.[40,41]

Micturating cystourethrogram

VUR is found in 8–40% of children being investigated for their first UTI,[43] and is a known risk factor for recurrent UTI.[5,7] A meta-analysis of patients found to have VUR by MCUG[42] showed that a positive MCUG increases the risk of renal damage in hospitalized UTI patients by about 20%, whereas a negative MCUG increases the chance of no renal involvement by just 8%. VUR is, hence, a weak predictor of renal damage in pediatric patients hospitalized with UTI. The authors concluded that physicians should be aware of the limitations of using MCUG-detected primary VUR as an effective screening test for renal damage in this population. The pathogenesis of renal damage in such patients is probably complex because renal damage often occurs without demonstrable VUR. It is estimated that about half of all renal damage identified is due to congenital renal dysplasia,[2,3,40] and may not be amenable to interventions that are aimed to prevent further renal damage.

VUR has a strong familial component. The incidence of reflux in siblings was 26% in a cohort of asymptomatic siblings and 86% in siblings with a history of UTI, but <1% in the normal population.[42] VUR tends to resolve with time: in a longitudinal study, 84% of children with UTI and VUR had spontaneous resolution after 5–15 years.[44]

Ultrasound

Renal ultrasound is a poor predictor of VUR. In one prospective study of children aged 0–5 years, ultrasound showed renal dilatation in only 17% of children found to have VUR by MCUG.[45] However, misssing mild-to-moderate reflux may not be important clinically, because the detection and treatment of lesser degrees of reflux has not been shown to confer benefit. One group has argued that the poor sensitivity of ultrasound to detect VUR may not matter.[46] They found that only 16% of kidneys with VUR had associated scarring, and 50% of scarred kidneys were not associated with VUR. The authors concluded that MCUG provided little additional information to ultrasound.[46]

Renal ultrasound will detect structural abnormalities of the kidneys (e.g., horseshoe kidney and duplex systems), and will detect obstuctive lesions that result in dilatation of the bladder (e.g., post-erior urethral valves), kidneys, or ureters (e.g., pelviureteric junction and vesicoureteric junction obstruction).

Renal ultrasound in young children may require sedation, but is less invasive than MCUG. It is a sensitive screening tool for low-prevalence serious conditions with an effective intervention (surgery). It is widely available, cheap, and non-invasive.

^{99m}Tc DMSA scan

DMSA scintigraphy is the most sensitive technique for diagnosing renal scarring. A systematic review of imaging in childhood UTI suggested that renal scarring, diagnosed by intravenous pyelogram or DMSA scan, occurs in 5–15% of children within 1–2 years of their first diagnosed UTI.[40] About a third of these scars are noted at the time of initial assessment, suggesting a high level of preexisting scarring, probably due to congenital renal dysplasia associated with high-grade VUR.[40,47] DMSA scans often show transient abnormalities and are too sensitive to be performed routinely to detect clinically relevant parenchymal abnormalities.[40,41,48]

Conclusion on imaging for child with UTI

We recommend that a routine ultrasound scan, if available, is performed on all neonates and children after their first UTI.

The need for further imaging will depend on the ultrasound result. If the ultrasound is normal, we do not recommend further imaging, because it is only likely to detect minor degrees of VUR (MCUG) or parenchymal abnormalities of little clinical significance (DMSA). If the ultrasound is abnormal, we recommend specialist consultation. Children with recurrent UTI may need further imaging to detect VUR and/or renal parenchymal defects (MCUG and/or DMSA scan), and specialist consultation on imaging is advised.

Preventing UTIs

Circumcision

Question | For boys with or without recurrent UTIs, does circumcision compared with no circumcision reduce the incidence of UTIs, and does circumcision cause harm?

Literature review | We found one RCT, seven case-control studies, four cohort studies, and a non-Cochrane systematic review.[49]

A non-Cochrane systematic review analyzed data on 402,908 children.[49] Circumcision was associated with a significantly reduced risk of UTI (OR 0.13, 95% CI 0.08–0.20) with the same odds ratio whatever the study design. The risk of UTI in normal boys is about 1%, so the number needed to treat (number of boys who would need to be circumcised to prevent one UTI) is 111. In boys with recurrent UTI or high-grade VUR, however, the risk of UTI recurrence is much higher at 10% and 30%, respectively, and so the respective numbers needed to treat are much lower at 11 and 4. About 2% of circumcisions are complicated by hemorrhage or infection.[49]

We do not recommend routine circumcision merely to prevent UTIs. In contrast, we recommend considering circumcision in boys with recurrent UTIs, high-grade VUR, or anatomic abnormalities putting them at high risk of UTIs.

Preventing chronic renal damage

A systematic review of diagnostic imaging reported on four longitudinal studies of scarring that followed children for at least 2 years.[40] New renal scars developed in 1.6–23% of children, and existing renal scars progressed in 6–34%. The highest rates of scarring were associated with the highest rates of recurrent UTI.[40] Scarring tends to occur early: children <2 years old are at greater risk for scarring than are older children.[50] In one study of children with normal DMSA scans at 3–4 years of age, 3% of 3-year-old and none of 179

4-year-old children developed scarring 2–11 years later, and 4 of the 5 who developed scarring had a history of ongoing recurrent UTI.[51]

One long-term follow-up study in the UK found that progressive renal damage occurred in children with both renal scarring and VUR, or in children with either renal scarring or VUR followed by documented UTI.[51] A combination of recurrent UTI, severe VUR, and the presence of renal scarring at first presentation is associated with the worst prognosis.[2] On the other hand, a longitudinal study of children with primary VUR, identified after fetal renal pelvic dilatation was diagnosed by fetal ultrasound, found that children with grades I–III reflux had no progression of renal damage.[52] Renal damage was strongly associated with grade IV–V reflux. Few children had UTI, and it appeared likely that most renal damage was due to pre-existing renal dysplasia rather than prior or ongoing UTIs.

Prophylactic antibiotics

Question | In children with a previous UTI, do long-term prophylactic antibiotics compared with no antibiotics or placebo reduce the frequency of recurrent UTIs, and do they prevent chronic renal damage? Is one antibiotic superior to other?

Literature review | We found eight RCTs, a Cochrane systematic review,[53] and a non-Cochrane systematic review.[54]

A Cochrane review[53] identified eight "poor-quality" studies (618 children), of which five (406 children) compared prophylactic antibiotics with placebo or no antibiotics. The duration of antibiotic prophylaxis varied from 10 weeks to 12 months. Antibiotics reduced the risk of repeat positive urine culture compared to placebo or no treatment (RR 0.44, 95% CI 0.19–1.00). No side effects were reported. Few studies looked at the emergence of antibiotic resistance during prophylaxis.

The authors of the Cochrane review pointed out that only one study differentiated symptomatic UTI from screen-detected, asymptomatic UTI, yet few doctors would treat asymptomatic bacteriuria.[53] They felt that the small number of poor-quality studies gave no reliable evidence of the effectiveness of antibiotics in preventing recurrent symptomatic UTI. They conclude that the evidence to support the widespread use of antibiotics to prevent recurrent symptomatic UTI is weak.[53]

One study reported nitrofurantoin was more effective than trimethoprim in preventing recurrent UTI (RR 0.48, 95% CI 0.25–0.92), but patients receiving nitrofurantoin were more than three times as likely to discontinue the antibiotic due to side effects (mainly, gastrointestinal). Nitrofurantoin prophylaxis altered neither the pattern of resistance nor the bacteriologic constellation, while patients receiving trimethoprim prophylaxis had 76% trimethoprim-resistant bacteria during prophylaxis.[55] Another study found that cefixime was as effective as nitrofurantoin in preventing recurrent UTI, but 62% of patients receiving cefixime and only 26% of patients receiving nitrofurantoin experienced an adverse reaction.[56]

The author of a non-Cochrane review interpreted the same data differently.[54] He concluded that prophylactic antibiotics seem to reduce recurrence of UTI. Because recurrent UTI is associated with new or progressive renal scarring in some children, he felt prophylaxis seemed sensible in two situations: (1) until a child's risk level is known (preinvestigation), and (2) after a child has been shown to have renal damage or increased risk. He suggested continuing antibiotics until reflux had largely resolved.[54]

A large, multicenter RCT published after both the above systematic reviews found that children with mild-to-moderate VUR randomized to prophylactic antibiotics had the same 1-year outcome as controls, who received placebo in respect to rate of recurrent UTI, type of recurrence, rate of subsequent pyelonephritis, and development of renal parenchymal scars.[57]

We feel the evidence for or against prophylactic antibiotics is weak.

We do not recommend prophylactic antibiotics for children with mild-to-moderate reflux following their first UTI. For children with grade IV–V reflux, we would recommend either commencing prophylaxis or waiting to see if the child has recurrence of UTI.

If it is decided to use prophylactic antibiotics, we recommend:

nitrofurantoin 1–2.5 mg/kg (max 100 mg) orally, at night OR

trimethoprim 4 mg/kg (max 150 mg) orally, at night OR (if a trimethoprim liquid formulation is not available)
trimethoprim+sulfamethoxazole 4 + 20 mg/kg (max 160 + 800 mg) orally, at night OR
cephalexin 12.5 mg/kg (max 500 mg) orally, at night

17.2 Catheter-associated bacteriuria and UTIs

Treatment of catheter-associated bacteriuria and UTIs

In patients with urinary catheters, asymptomatic bacteriuria and pyuria are common. Positive cultures may represent colonization, not infection, and are unreliable unless taken through a newly inserted catheter. Giving antibiotics in this situation, including bladder irrigation with antibiotics, is likely to select for antibiotic-resistant organisms.

Urinary culture and treatment of positive cultures is recommended only if the patient has signs of systemic infection, such as fever or rigors, risk factors such as neutropenia or kidney transplant, or before urological surgery.

Catheter-associated candiduria

Isolation of Candida from the urine is common, particularly in association with indwelling urinary catheters, and in most patients, it represents only colonization. Antifungal therapy is not usually indicated. Removal of urinary tract catheters and stents is often helpful. There is no good evidence to support bladder irrigation with amphotericin B desoxycholate.[58]

Candiduria may rarely be the source of subsequent dissemination or a marker of disseminated candidiasis in high-risk patients. We recommend considering treatment of candiduria in symptomatic patients and patients with neutropenia.

If it is decided to treat high-risk patients with localized infection due to *Candida albicans* and other susceptible species, we recommend:

fluconazole 6 mg/kg (max 300 mg) orally, daily for 7 days

Relapse after treatment is frequent, and this likelihood is increased by continued use of a urinary catheter.

For treatment of resistant or non-albicans species of Candida, see Chapter 9.

Prevention of catheter-associated UTIs

Prophylactic antibiotics and catheter-associated UTIs

A Cochrane review of antibiotics in adults who were catheterized short-term found six parallel-group RCTs that met the inclusion criteria.[59] There was weak evidence that antibiotic prophylaxis, compared to giving antibiotics when clinically indicated, reduced the rate of symptomatic UTI in female patients after abdominal surgery. There was limited evidence that giving antibiotics after surgery reduced the rate of bacteriuria, pyuria, and gram-negative isolates in patients' urine, but the benefits are uncertain. There was also limited evidence that prophylactic antibiotics reduced bacteriuria in non-surgical patients.[59] We found no studies in children.

We do not think the evidence is sufficient to justify giving prophylactic antibiotics to catheterized children.

Type of urethral catheter and catheter-associated UTIs

A variety of specialized urethral catheters have been designed to reduce the risk of infection, including antiseptic impregnated catheters and antibiotic impregnated catheters. We found a Cochrane review of the effect of type of indwelling urethral catheter on the risk of UTI in adults who undergo short-term urinary catheterization.[60] The review found 18 RCTs. Silver alloy indwelling catheters reduced the risk of catheter acquired UTI, but are expensive, and the authors recommended further economic evaluation. They found that catheters coated with a combination of minocycline and rifampin may also be beneficial in reducing bacteriuria in hospitalized men catheterized for less than 1 week, but this requires further testing. There was not enough evidence to suggest whether or not any standard catheter was better than another in terms of reducing the risk of UTI in hospitalized adults catheterized short-term.

A Cochrane review found evidence from 17 RCTs that suprapubic catheters have advantages over indwelling catheters in respect of bacteriuria, recatheterization, and discomfort.[61] The clinical significance of bacteriuria was uncertain, however, and there was no information about possible complications or adverse effects during catheter insertion.[61]

17.3 Intermittent catheterization and prophylactic antibiotics

Question | For children with neurogenic bladders using intermittent catheterization, do prophylactic antibiotics compared with giving antibiotics when clinically indicated reduce the frequency of UTIs or long-term renal tract morbidity?

Literature review | We found four RCTs and a Cochrane review.[62]

Children with neurogenic bladders are at risk of recurrent UTI, and often use intermittent catheterization. It is unclear whether prophylactic antibiotics are useful. A Cochrane review of urinary catheter policies found four trials, comparing antibiotic prophylaxis with giving antibiotics when microbiologically indicated.[62] For patients using intermittent catheterization, there was limited evidence that receiving antibiotics reduced the rate of bacteriuria (asymptomatic and symptomatic). There was weak evidence that prophylactic antibiotics were better in terms of fewer episodes of symptomatic bacteriuria. A subsequent RCT found that prophylactic antibiotics were associated with an increased risk of UTI, perhaps due to selection of resistant organisms.[63]

> **We do not recommend prophylactic antibiotics for children with neurogenic bladder using intermittent catheterization.**

References

1 Hellstrom A, Hanson E, Hansson S, Hjalmas K, Jodal U. Association between urinary symptoms at 7 years old and previous urinary tract infection. *Arch Dis Child* 1991;66: 232–4.

2 Larcombe J. Urinary tract infection in children. *Clin Evid* 2005;14:429–40. Available at http://www.clinicalevidence.com/ceweb/conditions/chd/0306/0306_background.jsp

3 Chang SL, Shortliffe LD. Pediatric urinary tract infections. *Pediatr Clin North Am* 2006;53:379–400.

4 Craig JC, Irwig LM, Knight JF, Sureshkumar P, Roy LP. Symptomatic urinary tract infection in preschool Australian children. *J Paediatr Child Health* 1998;34:154–9.

5 Coulthard MG, Lambert HJ, Keir MJ. Occurrence of renal scars in children after their first referral for urinary tract infection. *BMJ* 1997;315:918–9.

6 Winberg J, Bergstrom T, Jacobsson B. Morbidity, age and sex distribution, recurrences and renal scarring in symptomatic urinary tract infection in childhood. *Kidney Int Suppl* 1975;4:S101–6.

7 Hellerstein S. Recurrent urinary tract infections in children. *Pediatr Infect Dis* 1982;1:271–81.

8 Bergstrom T. Sex differences in childhood urinary tract infection. *Arch Dis Child* 1972;47:227–32.

9 Jodal U. The natural history of bacteriuria in childhood. *Infect Dis Clin North Am* 1987;1:713–29.

10 Cardiff-Oxford Bacteriuria Study Group. Sequelae of covert bacteriuria in schoolgirls. A four-year follow-up study. *Lancet* 1978;1:889–93.

11 Cohen SN, Kass EH. A simple method for quantitative urine culture. *N Engl J Med* 1967;277:176–80.

12 American Academy of Pediatrics. Practice parameter: the diagnosis, treatment, and evaluation of the initial urinary tract infection in febrile infants and young children. American academy of pediatrics. Committee on Quality Improvement. Sub-committee on Urinary Tract Infection. *Pediatrics* 1999;103:843–52.

13 Rushton HG. Urinary tract infections in children. Epidemiology, evaluation and management. *Pediatr Clin North Am* 1997;44:1133–69.

14 Twaij M. Urinary tract infection in children: a review of its pathogenesis and risk factors. *J R Soc Health* 2000;120:220–6.

15 Liaw LC, Nayar DM, Pedler SJ, Coulthard MG. Home collection of urine for culture from infants by three methods: survey of parents' preferences and bacterial contamination rates. *BMJ* 2000;320:1312–3.

16 Alam MT, Coulter JB, Pacheco J et al. Comparison of urine contamination rates using three different methods of collection: clean-catch, cotton wool pad and urine bag. *Ann Trop Paediatr* 2005;25:29–34.

17 Greaves J, Buckmaster A. Abolishing the bag: a quality assurance project on urine collection. *J Paediatr Child Health* 2001;37:437–40.

18 Ramage IJ, Chapman JP, Hollman AS, Elabassi M, McColl JH, Beattie TJ. Accuracy of clean-catch urine collection in infancy. *J Pediatr* 1999;135:765–7.

19 Chen L, Hsiao AL, Moore CL, Dziura JD, Santucci KA. Utility of bedside bladder ultrasound before urethral catheterization in young children. *Pediatrics* 2005;115:108–11.

20 Pollack CV, Jr, Pollack ES, Andrew ME. Suprapubic bladder aspiration versus urethral catheterization in ill infants: success, efficiency and complication rates. *Ann Emerg Med* 1994;23:225–30.

21 Kozer E, Rosenbloom E, Goldman D, Lavy G, Rosenfeld N, Goldman M. Pain in infants who are younger than 2 months during suprapubic aspiration and transurethral bladder catheterization: a randomized, controlled study. *Pediatrics* 2006;118:e51–6.

22 Whiting P, Westwood M, Watt I, Cooper J, Kleijnen J. Rapid tests and urine sampling techniques for the diagnosis of urinary tract infection (UTI) in children under five years: a systematic review. *BMC Pediatr* 2005;5:4.

23 Rawal K, Senguttuvan P, Morris M, Chantler C, Simmons NA. Significance of crystal clear urine. *Lancet* 1990;335:1228.

24 Tremblay S, Labbe J. Crystal-clear urine and infection. *Lancet* 1994;343:479–80.

25 Bulloch B, Bausher JC, Pomerantz WJ, Connors JM, Mahabee-Gittens M, Dowd MD. Can urine clarity exclude the diagnosis of urinary tract infection? *Pediatrics* 2000;106:E60.

26 Gorelick MH, Shaw KN. Screening tests for urinary tract infection: a meta-analysis. *Pediatrics* 1999;104:e54.

27 Huicho L, Campos-Sanchez M, Alamo C. Meta-analysis of urine screening tests for determining the risk of urinary tract infection in children. *Pediatr Infect Dis J* 2002;21:1–11.

28 Moyer VA, Craig JC. Acute urinary tract infection. In: Moyer VA (ed.), *Evidenc-based paediatrics and Child Health*, 2nd edn. London: BMJ Books, 2004:429–36.

29 Hoberman A, Wald ER, Reynolds EA, Penchansky L, Charron M. Is urine culture necessary to rule out urinary tract infection in young febrile children? *Pediatr Infect Dis J* 1996;15:304–9.

30 Bloomfield P, Hodson EM, Craig JC. Antibiotics for acute pyelonephritis in children. *The Cochrane Database of Systematic Reviews* 2005;(1):Art No CD003772.

31 Bachur R, Caputo GL. Bacteremia and meningitis among infants with urinary tract infections. *Pediatr Emerg Care* 1995;11:280–4.

32 Hoberman A, Wald ER, Hickey RW et al. Oral versus initial intravenous therapy for urinary tract infections in young febrile children. *Pediatrics* 1999;104:79–86.

33 Pitetti RD, Choi S. Utility of blood cultures in febrile children with UTI. *Am J Emerg Med* 2002;20:271–4.

34 Gauthier M, Chevalier I, Sterescu A, Bergeron S, Brunet S, Taddeo D. Treatment of urinary tract infections among febrile young children with daily intravenous antibiotic therapy at a day treatment center. *Pediatrics* 2004;114:e469–76.

35 Tran D, Muchant DG, Aronoff SC. Short-course versus conventional therapy for uncomplicated lower urinary tract infections in children: a meta-analysis of 1279 patients. *J Pediatr* 2001;139:93–9.

36 Keren R, Chan E. A meta-analysis of randomized, controlled trials comparing short- and long-course antibiotic therapy for urinary tract infections in children. *Pediatrics* 2002;109:E70.

37 Michael M, Hodson EM, Craig JC, Martin S, Moyer VA. Short versus standard duration oral antibiotic therapy for acute urinary tract infection in children. *The Cochrane Database of Systematic Reviews* 2003;(1):Art No CD003966.

38 Contopoulos-Ioannidis DG, Giotis ND, Baliatsa DV, Ioannidis JP. Extended-interval aminoglycoside administration for children: a meta-analysis. *Pediatrics* 2004;114:e111–8.

39 Jacobson S, Eklof O, Erikkson CG et al. Development of hypertension and uraemia after pyelonephritis in childhood: 27 year follow up. *BMJ* 1989;299:703–6.

40 Dick PT, Feldman W. Routine diagnostic imaging for childhood urinary tract infections: a systematic overview. *J Pediatr* 1996;128:15–22.

41 Westwood ME, Whiting PF, Cooper J, Watt IS, Kleijnen J. Further investigation of confirmed urinary tract infection (UTI) in children under five years: a systematic review. *BMC Pediatr* 2005;5:2.

42 Gordon I, Barkovics M, Pindoria S et al. Primary vesicoureteric reflux as a predictor of renal damage in children hospitalized with urinary tract infection: a systematic review and meta-analysis. *J Am Soc Nephrol* 2003;14:739–44.

43 Goldman M, Lahat E, Strauss S et al. Imaging after urinary tract infection in male neonates. *Pediatrics* 2000;105:1232–5.

44 Chertin B, Puri P. Familial vesicoureteral reflux. *J Urol* 2003;169:1804–8.

45 McKerrow W, Vidson-Lamb N, Jones PF. Urinary tract infection in children. *BMJ* 1984;289:299–303.

46 Zamir G, Sakran W, Horowitz Y, Koren A, Miron D. Urinary tract infection: is there a need for routine renal ultrasonography? *Arch Dis Child* 2004;89:466–8.

47 Moorthy I, Easty M, McHugh K, Ridout D, Biassoni L, Gordon I. The presence of vesicoureteric reflux does not identify a population at risk for renal scarring following a first urinary tract infection. *Arch Dis Child* 2005;90:733–6.

48 Piepsz A, Tamminen-Mobius T, Reiners C et al. Five-year study of medical and surgical treatment in children with severe vesico-ureteric reflux dimercaptosuccinic acid findings. International Reflux Study Group in Europe. *Eur J Pediatr* 1998;157:753–8.

49 Singh-Grewal D, Macdessi J, Craig J. Circumcision for the prevention of urinary tract infection in boys: a systematic review of randomised trials and observational studies. *Arch Dis Child* 2005;90:853–8.

50 Vernon SJ, Coulthard MG, Lambert HJ et al. New renal scarring in children who at age 3 and 4 years had had normal scans with dimercaptosuccinic acid: follow up study. *BMJ* 1997;315:905–8.

51 Merrick MV, Notghi A, Chalmers N et al. Long-term follow up to determine the prognostic value of imaging after urinary tract infections. Part 2: Scarring. *Arch Dis Child* 1995;72:393–6.

52 McIlroy PJ, Abbott GD, Anderson NG, Turner JG, Mogridge N, Wells JE. Outcome of primary vesicoureteric reflux detected following fetal renal pelvic dilatation. *J Paediatr Child Health* 2000;36:569–73.

53 Williams GJ, Wei L, Lee A, Craig JC. Long-term antibiotics for preventing recurrent urinary tract infection in children. *The Cochrane Database of Systematic Reviews* 2006;(3):Art No CD001534.

54 Larcombe J. Urinary tract infection in children. Prophylactic antibiotics. *Clin Evid* 2005. Available at http://www.clinicalevidence.com/ceweb/conditions/chd/0306/0306_I1.jsp

55 Brendstrup L, Hjelt K, Petersen KE et al. Nitrofurantoin versus trimethoprim prophylaxis in recurrent urinary tract infection in children. A randomized, double-blind study. *Acta Paediatr Scand* 1990;79:1225–34.

56 Leggten B, Troster K. Prophylaxis of recurrent urinary tract infections in children. Results of an open, controlled and randomized study about the efficacy and tolerance of cefixime compared to nitrofurantoin. *Klin Padiatr* 2002;214:353–8.

57 Garin EH, Olavarria F, Garcia Nieto V, Valenciano B, Campos A, Young L. Clinical significance of primary vesicoureteral reflux and urinary antibiotic prophylaxis after

acute pyelonephritis: a multicenter, randomized, controlled study. *Pediatrics* 2006;117:626–32.

58 Drew RH, Arthur RR, Perfect JR. Is it time to abandon the use of amphotericin B bladder irrigation? *Clin Infect Dis* 2005;40:1465–70.

59 Niel-Weise BS, van den Broek PJ. Antibiotic policies for short-term catheter bladder drainage in adults. *The Cochrane Database of Systematic Reviews* 2005;(3):Art No CD005428.

60 Brosnahan J, Jull A, Tracy C. Types of urethral catheters for management of short-term voiding problems in hospitalised adults. *The Cochrane Database of Systematic Reviews* 2004;(1):Art No CD004013.

61 Niël-Weise BS, van den Broek PJ. Urinary catheter policies for short-term bladder drainage in adults. *The Cochrane Database of Systematic Reviews* 2005;(3):Art No CD004203.

62 Niël-Weise BS, van den Broek PJ. Urinary catheter policies for long-term bladder drainage. *The Cochrane Database of Systematic Reviews* 2005;(1):Art No CD004201.

63 Clarke SA, Samuel M, Boddy SA. Are prophylactic antibiotics necessary with clean intermittent catheterization? A randomized controlled trial. *J Pediatr Surg* 2005;40:568–71.

CHAPTER 18

Viral infections

In this chapter, we will not try to cover all virus infections in children. Instead, we will concentrate on some general principles and on those important virus infections not covered elsewhere in the book and where the diagnosis or management is controversial or difficult.

18.1 Diagnosing virus infections

Virus infections may be diagnosed clinically, by detecting the virus or by serology. A **clinical diagnosis** may be adequate in most circumstances for virus infections with a characteristic rash, such as chicken pox, or where a definitive diagnosis is not informative, such as a common cold. **Viral culture** is definitive, but often slow. It is possible, however, to speed up the diagnosis by initiating viral culture by placing a clinical specimen in tissue culture, and then using rapid viral techniques, such as immunofluorescence or polymerase chain reaction (PCR) on the tissue culture cells to diagnose specific infections, e.g., shell vial cultures for detecting cytomegalovirus (CMV)[1] or other respiratory viruses.[2] Other rapid techniques include techniques that can detect antigen in clinical specimens, such as **immunofluorescence** or **ELISA**, or that can detect viral nucleic acid, such as **PCR**. Rapid techniques are particularly useful when a rapid diagnosis is needed for decisions about antiviral treatment, e.g., herpes simplex virus (HSV) in the neonatal period, or for decisions about antibiotics and infection control, e.g., respiratory syncytial virus (RSV) infection.

Serology can be helpful in certain infections, but has limitations. Even newborns are capable of mounting an IgM response to some infections, e.g., CMV and rubella. Other viruses, however, elicit a delayed IgM response even in older children, so that the usefulness of an immediate serum specimen to detect specific IgM can be limited. IgG responses generally take 2–3 weeks, which is why acute and convalescent sera are sent. In general, serology is more useful in older children, who mount a more vigorous immune response. It is best to detect RSV by rapid techniques or even culture, while RSV serology is almost never clinically useful.

18.2 Cytomegalovirus

CMV is a herpesvirus, and as such can cause congenital infection and primary infection, and can establish a latent infection and reactivate, especially if there is altered cellular immunity.

Congenital CMV infection

Congenital CMV infection is the most common congenital infection (3–12/1000 live births).[3] It is usually asymptomatic at birth, although 6–23% of asymptomatic and 22–65% of symptomatic babies with congenital CMV develop late sensorineural deafness.[3,4] About 10% of congenitally infected babies are symptomatic at birth, with one or more of intrauterine growth retardation, microcephaly, periventricular calcification, purpuric rash due to thrombocytopenia, chorioretinitis, hepatosplenomegaly, and jaundice.[3] The diagnosis is made by detecting CMV-specific IgM or by detecting CMV by viral culture or rapid diagnosis as early as possible, preferably within 1 week and certainly within 3 weeks of birth. This is because the incubation period for contracting CMV infection is 3–12 weeks. A retrospective diagnosis of congenital CMV infection can sometimes be made by using PCR to detect CMV DNA in dried blood on the filter paper from newborn screening cards.

Question | For babies with congenital CMV infection, does ganciclovir compared with no treatment improve outcome?

Literature review | We found case reports and observational studies (total 36 patients), two studies comparing doses (54 patients), one RCT (42 patients),[5] and an overview.[6]

All studies reported the use of IV ganciclovir for babies with symptomatic infection. The only RCT studied the effect of 6 weeks of IV ganciclovir, begun in the neonatal period, on hearing in 42 babies with central nervous system (CNS) infection.[5] The study found that ganciclovir therapy prevented hearing deterioration at 6 months (none of 25 versus 7 of 17 or 41%), and may prevent hearing deterioration at 1 year.[5] Almost two-thirds of treated infants, however, had significant neutropenia during therapy. There was one case report of a baby given IV ganciclovir followed by oral valganciclovir, to prevent hearing loss.[7] There are no RCTs on the use of ganciclovir for liver disease or pneumonitis. The neurological prognosis and survival of congenital CMV with microcephaly or intracranial calcification is poor,[8] which is important when making decisions about treatment. An overview concluded that studies of ganciclovir are promising but of insufficient number to make evidence-based recommendations about indications for treatment of congenital CMV.[6]

> **We do not recommend ganciclovir routinely for all babies with congenital CMV infection. We recommend considering ganciclovir for babies with significant liver or lung disease from congenital or acquired CMV infection.**
>
> **ganciclovir 5 mg/kg IV, 12-hourly for 2–3 weeks**

Acquired or reactivation CMV disease

Being a herpesvirus, CMV can cause disease by primary infection or by reactivation, even in normal children. The presentation depends on age, and whether or not the child is immunocompromised. Most acquired CMV infection is asymptomatic or mild and self-limiting. Manifestations in normal children include rash and fever or a mononucleosis-like syndrome in adolescents. Patients with defects of T-cell immunity are at risk of retinitis, pneumonitis, and colitis. CMV infection is associated with graft rejection in renal transplant patients,[9] and can cause severe disease in liver and bone marrow transplant patients and with human immunodeficiency virus (HIV) infection.

Treatment is not necessary in normal children, so recommendations about treatment and prevention apply essentially to immuncompromised children. There is no effective vaccine available. Prevention options include CMV immunoglobulin and long-term antiviral therapy. A Cochrane review of solid-organ transplant

Table 18.1 Treatment and prevention of opportunist CMV infections.[4–11]

Treatment	Prophylaxis
Ganciclovir 5 mg/kg IV, 12-hourly for 14–21 days	Ganciclovir 10 mg/kg IV, three times weekly or 5 mg/kg IV, five times weekly
Foscarnet 90 mg/kg IV, 12-hourly for 14–21 days (actual dose based on creatinine clearance; see product information)	Foscarnet 90–120 mg/kg/day IV, five times weekly (actual dose based on creatinine clearance; see product information)
Cidofovir 5 mg/kg IV, weekly for 2 weeks, given with probenecid and hydration (contraindicated if proteinuria >2+ or creatinine clearance <55 mL/min)	Cidofovir 5 mg/kg IV every 2 weeks, given with probenecid and hydration OR 3 mg/kg IV, once weekly (contraindicated if proteinuria >2+ or creatinine clearance <55 mL/min)
Valganciclovir 900 mg orally, 12-hourly for 14–21 days (for adolescents, no data in children)	Valganciclovir 900 mg orally, daily (for adolescents, no data in children)

recipients found that prophylaxis with acyclovir, ganciclovir, or valacyclovir compared with placebo or no treatment significantly reduced the risk for CMV disease (19 trials; RR 0.42, 95% CI 0.34–0.52) and all-cause mortality (17 trials; RR 0.63, 95% CI 0.43–0.92), primarily due to reduced mortality from CMV disease.[10] Treatment options include IV ganciclovir, oral valganciclovir, foscarnet, and cidofovir (see Table 18.1). We recommend specialist advice.

18.3 Epstein-Barr virus (EBV)

EBV is a herpesvirus, which is lymphotropic for B cells. EBV infection is often asymptomatic or unrecognized in infants and children. However, hospital-based series find that even very young children can present with an infectious mononucleosis-like syndrome, with fever, tonsillopharyngitis, lymphadenopathy, and hepatosplenomegaly.[12,13] Young children are more likely to have skin rash and upper eyelid edema than older children,[12] whereas older children are more likely to develop hepatitis.[11] Marked lymphocytosis with atypical lymphocytes is a consistent hematologic finding in all age groups.[11] Neurological manifestations include meningitis, meningoencephalitis, including the "Alice in Wonderland syndrome" (distortion in body image characterized by enlargement, diminution, or distortion of part of or the whole body, which the person knows is not real), cerebellitis, Guillain–Barré syndrome, and facial nerve palsy.[14] EBV can replicate in B cells, which viral replication is normally controlled by T cells and natural killer cells. EBV is oncogenic: it can cause Burkitt lymphoma, B-cell lymphoma (particularly in association with HIV infection), and nasopharyngeal carcinoma, and can disseminate to cause a lymphoproliferative syndrome in children post-transplant and children born with X-linked lymphoproliferative syndrome.

Although acyclovir has in vitro activity against EBV, it has little activity in vivo. It has not been shown to reduce symptoms of EBV infection in RCTs,[15,16] although in one of the studies acyclovir plus prednisone did reduce viral shedding.[16] Valacyclovir[17] and ganciclovir[18] have had no clinical or virologic effect in studies.

Parenteral corticosteroids are often recommended if there is imminent airways obstruction, although without formal evidence. We found no studies on the effect of corticosteroids on airways obstruction. We found one RCT on the effect of dexamethasone on pain in exudative tonsillitis due to infectious mononucleosis.[19] A single dose of dexamethasone 0.3 mg/kg (max 15 mg), orally, reduced pain at 12 hours, but not later. We found an observational study that reported that corticosteroids were given to 45% of patients with EBV infection, although only 8% qualified based on "traditional criteria."[20]

18.4 Herpes simplex virus

HSV is a double-stranded DNA herpesvirus. There are two major serotypes, HSV-1 and HSV-2.

Neonatal HSV

Neonatal HSV carries a high mortality if untreated. It is uncommon, with an incidence from 1 in 2500 live births in the USA to 1 in 60,000 in the UK.[21,22] HSV-1 is now responsible for around 50% of cases.[21,22] Neonatal HSV infection is acquired during the birth process in about 85% of cases, as the neonate comes in contact with the virus during passage through an infected birth canal.[21,22] Infection is probably post-natally acquired from contact with infected oral secretions from a caregiver in the remaining 15% of cases.[21,22]

Neonatal infection most commonly follows primary maternal genital HSV, because the baby is exposed to a high viral inoculum before there has been maternal seroconversion producing transplacental maternal IgG antibody that would protect the baby. Neonatal infection less commonly follows reactivation of maternal genital HSV when the high viral load presumably swamps any maternal antibody. The risk of neonatal infection is 33–50% if the mother develops primary genital HSV, and some authorities recommend empiric acyclovir for the baby of a mother with known primary genital HSV around delivery. Cesarean section reduces but does not eliminate the risk of neonatal infection in this setting.[21,22] However, only about a quarter of all women with primary genital HSV are themselves symptomatic at delivery.

If a woman with recurrent genital HSV without visible genital lesions is shedding the virus, the risk to the baby is <5%.[21,22]

True congenital HSV infection from intrauterine transfer with chorioretinitis, microcephaly, and skin lesions at birth is seen in <5% of cases.

Neonatal HSV disease usually presents in the first 3 weeks, but can be anything from day 1–4 weeks. Infection can manifest as localized disease, pneumonitis, encephalitis, or disseminated disease.[21,22] About half the babies now present with disease localized to the skin, eye, or mouth (SEM disease), with one or more of skin vesicles, conjunctivitis, and vesicles in the mouth. Viral pneumonitis with onset at 3–5 days is another recognized presentation, and early suspicion of the diagnosis is critical to outcome. Disseminated HSV presents at about 1 week of age with fever, shock, disseminated intravascular coagulopathy, jaundice with hepatitis, and sometimes with seizures from encephalitis.[21,22]

If localized HSV infection or pneumonitis is recognized and treated early, the prognosis is relatively good, with 10% long-term morbidity. If not, the risk of dissemination is as high as 70%.[21,22] Even with modern antiviral therapy, the mortality for babies with encephalitis is 15%, and over 65% of survivors have significant neurological impairment. For children with disseminated multiorgan disease, the mortality approaches 50% and over 50% of survivors have severe neurological impairment.[21,22]

Diagnosis needs to be made urgently, usually by rapid viral techniques, such as immunofluorescence or PCR on fluid from a vesicle, swabs from eyes or nasopharynx, and cerebrospinal fluid. If the baby has pneumonitis, a rapid diagnosis can be made using immunofluorescence or PCR on secretions from a nasopharyngeal or endotracheal aspirate. Serology is generally unhelpful in acute diagnosis. If rapid diagnosis is not available and HSV is suspected, we recommend taking samples for viral cultures and serum for HSV-specific IgM and treating empirically. Pharmacokinetic studies have shown that a high dose of acyclovir is needed for neonates.[22] We recommend:

acyclovir 20 mg/kg IV, 8-hourly (14 days for localized disease, 21 days for encephalitis or disseminated disease)

Primary HSV gingivostomatitis

Primary HSV infection can be asymptomatic, or can cause herpetic gingivostomatitis or genital herpes. Gingivostomatitis means inflammation of the gums and mouth. It mainly affects children aged 6 months to 2 years. The main features are painful ulcers on the gums, tongue, and pharynx, often with satellite vesicular lesions on the lips and cheeks where the child dribbles. The child is febrile, miserable, and drools saliva, which cannot be swallowed because of pain. There is often edema of the mouth and neck, and tender submandibular lymphadenopathy. The condition is extremely painful.[23]

We found one RCT, in which children with primary herpetic gingivostomatitis were randomized to acyclovir suspension 15 mg/kg (max 200 mg) five times a day for 7 days, or placebo.[24] Children receiving acyclovir had oral lesions for 4 days compared with 10 days for placebo, and had shorter duration of fever (1 versus 3 days), extraoral lesions around the mouth (0.0 versus 5.5 days), eating difficulties (4 versus 7 days), and drinking difficulties (3 versus 6 days). Viral shedding was significantly shorter in the group treated with acyclovir (1 versus 5 days).[22] The per kilogram dose of acyclovir in the study[24] is somewhat higher than that recommended by pharmacokinetic studies, and the maximum dose is lower.[25,26]

For treatment, depending on whether or not the child can drink, we recommend:

acyclovir 10 mg/kg (max 400 mg) orally, five times daily for 7 days OR
acyclovir 10 mg/kg (max 400 mg) IV, 8-hourly, until drinking, then oral as above

Recurrent herpes simplex labialis (cold sores)

About 20–40% of adults have recurrent cold sores, but onset is often in childhood.[21,27] Cold sores arise due to reactivation of chronic, latent HSV-1 infection from the ganglion of the trigeminal nerve, which can be spontaneous or precipitated by stress.[27] The frequency can range from more frequently than monthly to occasional cases every few years. Cold sores occur at the border of the lip and the skin.[27] Aphthous oral ulcers occur within the mouth and may be confused with recurrent mucosal herpetic lesions, but should not be confused with cold sores because of their position.[28] If necessary, a swab for HSV immunofluorescence and/or culture will confirm HSV infection.

Studies of topical agents have shown that early treatment can be effective. An RCT found that 15% idoxuridine in dimethyl sulfoxide (DMSO) cream shortened pain by 1.3 days and time to healing by 1.7 days.[29] Topical acyclovir ointment is ineffective in immunocompetent adults. However, both acyclovir cream[30] and topical penciclovir,[31,32] which is the prodrug for famciclovir, penetrate better and reduce the duration of lesions statistically significantly, but only by about 0.5 day.[30–32] Topical therapy has not been associated with significant resistance to antivirals.[33] The use of an iontophoretic applicator to improve skin penetration of topical acyclovir reduced the duration of lesions by 1.5 days in an RCT.[34]

Oral antivirals are effective, but frequent use is expensive and risks selecting for resistant HSV. A single dose of valacyclovir in adults reduces the duration of cold sores by 1 day.[35] Valacyclovir has not been studied in children.

We recommend that, if possible, acyclovir be given at the first sign of a recurrence, using an iontophoretic applicator. We recommend:

acyclovir 5% cream topically, 4-hourly while awake, for 5 days OR
penciclovir 1% cream topically, 2-hourly while awake, for 4 days OR
15% idoxuridine in DMSO cream, 3-hourly while awake, for 4 days

Prevention of recurrent HSV skin infections

For prevention of extremely frequent skin recurrences, we found only one RCT, a double-blind crossover study in adults with recurrent cold sores.[36] Regular oral acyclovir 400 mg 12-hourly reduced the mean number of recurrences per 4-month treatment period from 1.80 to 0.85 episodes per patient, and the mean number of virologically confirmed recurrences from 1.40 to 0.40 per patient.[36] There were no adverse events, although resistance was not studied. There are concerns about acyclovir resistance and expense with prolonged use, and the benefits are modest. We recommend only prophylactic oral acyclovir for children with extremely frequent and debilitating recurrences of HSV skin infections:

acyclovir 10 mg/kg (max 400 mg) orally, 12-hourly

Genital HSV

For primary genital herpes and for recurrent genital herpes, see p. 218.

Eczema herpeticum

Eczema herpeticum is a widespread HSV infection of inflamed skin, most often occurring in patients with atopic dermatitis.[37] It is sometimes called Kaposi's varicelliform eruption, but is caused by HSV, not varicella. Although it is sometimes suggested that it may result from excessive use of topical corticosteroids, a large retrospective review suggested that undertreatment of atopic dermatitis is a greater factor.[38] The HSV infection is equally likely to be primary or recurrent.[38]

The characteristic clinical pattern is an eruption of dome-shaped blisters and pustules in the eczematous lesions, along with severe systemic illness with fever and lymphopenia.[38] The diagnosis is made by immunofluorescent staining of skin swabs or PCR or culture.

Eczema herpeticum can be severe. Depending on severity, we recommend:

acyclovir 10 mg/kg (max 400 mg) orally, five times daily for 7–14 days OR
acyclovir 10 mg/kg (max 400 mg) IV, 8-hourly, until drinking, then oral as above

HSV infection in immunocompromised children

Immuncompromised children with defective T-cell function are at risk of severe and recurrent HSV infections. These are usually severe, local, mucocutaneous, or skin lesions, although disseminated infection with visceral or CNS involvement can occur.[39] Oral acyclovir is highly effective at preventing HSV infections

in immunocompromised children.[40] If HSV infections do occur in immunocompromised children, we recommend treating for longer:

acyclovir 10 mg/kg (max 400 mg) orally, five times daily for 14 days OR
acyclovir 10 mg/kg (max 400 mg) IV, 8-hourly, until drinking, then oral as above

18.5   Measles

Measles is an acute viral infection that is responsible for an estimated 800,000 deaths annually, almost all being children in developing countries.[41,42] The live attenuated vaccines are highly effective, so measles is a vaccine-preventable disease. Furthermore, measles affects only humans, and the vaccine is effective against all strains, so global elimination of measles is possible.[42]

In developing countries, the diagnosis is made clinically. In Brazil, where measles is common, a clinical case definition had 100% sensitivity compared with serum IgM.[43] In industrialized countries, where occasional cases of measles occur following introduction by a traveler or an unimmunized person, clinical diagnosis is far less reliable.[44] In this setting, a clinical diagnosis should be confirmed either by antigen detction (detecting measles virus antigen in nasopharyngeal secretions using an immunofluorescent stain) or by detecting serum IgM to measles. Immunization also causes a raised measles-specific IgM, so if a child who has recently been immunized against measles develops a suspicious rash, a raised serum IgM to measles does not distinguish between vaccine-acquired and wild-type measles.

There is no specific treatment for measles virus infection. In developing countries, children die because of acute measles pneumonia often complicated by secondary bacterial pneumonia, acute encephalitis, or because of immunosuppression that follows measles and leaves the child susceptible to diarrheal diseases for up to a year post-measles.[41,42] Children with HIV infection develop more severe measles and are more likely to die from measles.[45]

Treatment of measles

Measles and vitamin A treatment

It has been suggested that children in developing countries with low serum levels of retinol (vitamin A) who develop measles might benefit from being given vitamin A acutely. An RCT from South Africa found that 92% of children admitted with severe measles had low serum retinol levels.[46] Those randomized to receive retinyl palmitate (200,000 IU orally, daily for 2 days) recovered more rapidly from pneumonia and diarrhea, had less croup, and spent fewer days in the hospital. Of the 12 children who died, 10 were among those given placebo ($p = 0.05$). Overall, the risk of death or a major complication during the hospital stay was halved in children treated with vitamin A.[46]

A Cochrane review found eight RCTs of the use of vitamin A in acute measles.[47] There was no significant reduction in the risk of mortality in the vitamin A group when all the studies were pooled (RR 0.70, 95% CI 0.42–1.15). Using two doses of vitamin A (200,000 IU) on consecutive days was associated with a reduction in the risk of mortality in children <2 years old (RR 0.18, 95% CI 0.03–0.61) and a reduction in the risk of pneumonia-specific mortality (RR 0.33, 95% CI 0.08–0.92). The three studies using two doses were from areas where case fatality was more than 10%. There was no evidence that vitamin A in a single dose was associated with a reduced risk of mortality among children with measles. There was a reduction in the incidence of croup (RR 0.53, 95% CI 0.29–0.89), but no significant reduction in the incidence of pneumonia (RR 0.92, 95% CI 0.69–1.22) or diarrhea (RR 0.80, 95% CI 0.27–2.34) with two doses. There were no trials that directly compared a single dose with two doses. There has been no toxicity shown from this dose of vitamin A. Vitamin A given to vitamin A-deficient children with acute measles in Zambia reduces the risk of measles-related pneumonia.[48]

There has been only one study in an industrialized country, an RCT of 105 children in Japan that showed that vitamin A was associated with a reduction in duration from cough from 9.2 to 7.2 days, without toxicity.[49]

We support the WHO recommendation[50] that two doses of vitamin A (200,000 IU) be given to all children with measles in developing countries, especially to children under the age of 2 with severe measles, in addition to the standard management. For acute measles in a developing country, we recommend:

vitamin A (200,000 IU) orally, daily for 2 days

Measles and antibiotics

Measles virus can cause severe viral pneumonia, but children with measles are also at risk of develop-

ing bacterial pneumonia due to immunosuppression and superinfection. We found surprisingly few studies on the bacteria causing pneumonia in measles. One study performed endotracheal aspirates in children with measles, not the ideal specimen because the organisms grown may not be causing the pneumonia. Some of the organisms were probably commensals (e.g., *Streptococcus viridans*), but the study authors also reported growing Gram-negative bacilli, *Staphlyococcus aureus* and *Streptococccus pneumoniae*, which are more likely to have been pathogens.[51]

Treating children with severe measles pneumonia with antibiotics empirically might save lives. In a study designed to detect and treat pneumonia according to a WHO decision strategy, children in Nepal with a WHO clinical diagnosis of pneumonia were treated at home with 5 days of oral co-trimoxazole.[52] By the third year of the program, there was a 28% reduction in all-cause mortality, particularly among infants. In addition to reduction in deaths due to pneumonia, there was a significant reduction in deaths due to diarrhea and measles, indicating that reduction in pneumonia morbidity had considerable carryover effect. The longitudinal, observational nature of the study[52] does not provide strong evidence that empiric antibiotics improve mortality in measles.

A Cochrane review looked at all trials of antibiotics for children with measles, not just those with measles pneumonia.[53] Six trials with 1304 children were included. The reviewers felt that the quality of the trials reviewed was poor. All the trials were unblended except one, and randomization was either not described or was by alternate allocation. Four of the 764 children given antibiotics died compared with 1 of the 637 controls. The reviewers concluded that there was very weak evidence for giving "prophylactic" antibiotics to all children with measles, and that available evidence suggests that antibiotics should be given only if a child has clinical signs of pneumonia or other evidence of sepsis.[53] The Cochrane review has been withdrawn because the authors do not have time to update it. At least one writer has argued passionately that it is vitally important to perform RCTs to see whether or not all children with measles in developing countries should be given antibiotics, because the disease is so common with such a high mortality that if they are effective, prophylactic antibiotics could have a profound effect on outcome.[54] This letter writer feels that the existing evidence from the Cochrane review of controlled trials[53] suggests that prophylactic antibiotics are likely to reduce serious morbidity, and he argues that children in developing countries with measles should be given prophylactic antibiotics.[54] If it is decided to give antibiotics to a child in a developing country with measles, the choice may depend on availability, but we would advise antibiotics with activity against *S. aureus* and *S. pneumoniae* (see p. 188).

Micronutrients and measles

There is evidence from RCTs that giving antioxidants, vitamin C and vitamin E,[55] or giving zinc[56] does not improve the outcome of children with measles and pneumonia.

Prevention of measles

Measles immunization

Vaccine is the most effective way of preventing measles, and has been shown to be one of the most cost-effective public health interventions available.[57] Current measles vaccines use live, attenuated measles virus. They are generally contraindicated in immune-deficient children. Because measles is more severe in HIV infection and is common in developing countries, however, and because severe adverse events from measles vaccine are rare, it is recommended that HIV-infected children be immunized routinely with measles or measles–mumps–rubella (MMR) vaccine unless they are severely immunocompromised (defined as CD4 count <750 cells/μL or 750×10^9/L if <12 months, <500 aged 1–5 years, <200 aged >5 years; see Chapter 8).

In industrialized countries, because maternal antibody interferes with the response, the proportion of children responding to measles immunization depends on age. In the USA, 98% of children aged 15 months seroconverted to measles, compared with 95% vaccinated at 12 months and 87% vaccinated at 9 months.[58] There is a trade-off between early protection and the proportion seroconverting. In industrialized countries, the first dose of measles vaccine with or without mumps and rubella is given at 12–15 months. A booster is usually recommended at 5–12 years to improve coverage. In developing countries, in contrast, the first dose is recommended at 9 months because the morbidity and mortality are higher in the first year of life.

Immunization at 6 months is less successful,[42] although some have argued that a two-dose schedule with vaccine at 4–8 months followed by reimmunization saves more lives.[59,60] There is controversy about the relative merits of the standard Schwartz and the high-potency Edmonston–Zagreb strains.

Measles vaccine can be given directly into the respiratory tract, by intranasal aerosol. A non-Cochrane meta-analysis suggested that the intranasal respiratory route is at least as efficacious as the subcutaneous route for delivery of measles vaccine.[61] The intranasal route has the potential to decrease problems with interference from maternal antibody. However, more research is required on standardization of dosage, administration equipment, efficacy, and safety of aerosolized measles vaccine.[61]

Measles post-exposure prophylaxis

It is currently recommended that unimmunized or immunocompromised household and other close measles contacts be given measles vaccine or MMR within 72 hours of exposure or normal human immunoglobulin within 6 days of exposure, to prevent measles or reduce the severity.[62] Immunoglobulin is recommended for those who are least likely to respond to vaccine (infants <1 month), for those who might get disseminated disease from the vaccine (severely immunocompromised persons), and for pregnant women (because of the potential but unknown risk of the vaccine to the fetus).[62]

The evidence for these recommendations is sparse. In a measles outbreak in California, primary measles immunization was 95% protective against infection; i.e., previously immunized children were well protected.[63] In contrast, it was not possible to show that either post-exposure vaccination (protection 4%) or immunoglobulin (protection 8%) prevented infection, although severity of measles was not measured, so either vaccine or immunoglobulin may have reduced severity.[63] A Japanese study found that commercially available normal human immunoglobulin had variable measles antibody titers, and 57% of children receiving immunoglobulin with a titer of 16 IU/mL or lower developed clinical measles.[64]

Primary immunization is clearly superior to secondary prevention.

Prophylactic vitamin A and measles

There is good evidence that vitamin A improves outcome when given to children with acute measles.

Mainly on this basis, the WHO has recommended vitamin A prophylaxis be given at the time of immunization to children in developing countries when vitamin A deficiency is likely. It has been argued that prophylactic vitamin A, which is extremely cheap, will reduce mortality from diarrhea and reasonable evidence that it will reduce mortality from measles and malaria.[65]

We could find no convincing evidence that vitamin A supplementation prevents diarrhea (see p. 81). We found one study suggesting that vitamin A suplementation was associated with lower measles antibody titers,[66] although a subsequent study found that vitamin A-supplemented children had equal or higher measles titers.[67,68] An RCT in Ghana found a lower incidence of measles in vitamin A-supplemented children (23.6/1000 child-years) than in children given placebo (28.9/1000 child-years), but the difference was not statistically significant[69] and measles case fatality was no different (15.4% versus 14.5%, respectively).[69] A large RCT in Ghana, India, and Peru found that vitamin A supplementation was safe, but had no measurable benefits in terms of severe morbidity or mortality.[70]

18.6 Varicella zoster virus (VZV)

VZV is a herpesvirus that can cause primary infections (varicella or chicken pox) and can reactivate (zoster or shingles). The name is confusing; it used to be thought that varicella virus and herpes zoster were different viruses causing different syndromes, and VZV is a composite name.

Chicken pox

Most chicken pox is mild, but because almost all children get chicken pox and occasional cases are severe, the overall effect in terms of morbidity and mortality of chicken pox in an unimmunized population is great.[71,72]

Recovery from VZV is dependent on cellular (T-cell) immunity. Chicken pox and zoster are both far more severe in immunocompromised patients with defective T-cell immunity. In contrast, boys with X-linked agammaglobulinemia who cannot make antibodies recover normally from acute chicken pox. Nevertheless, previously healthy children with no demonstrable immunodeficiency sometimes get severe and even fatal chicken pox.[71,72]

Diagnosis in primary care is usually clinical. When definitive diagnosis is important, the most useful technique is rapid diagnosis using immunofluorescent staining to detect antigen in scrapings of lesions. PCR, if available, is highly sensitive.[73] Antibody testing for specific IgM is less reliable, while viral culture and a rise in specific IgG both give delayed results.

Antiviral treatment of varicella

Antiviral treatment is not recommended routinely in normal, otherwise healthy children with varicella.[74,75] In a placebo-controlled RCT, previously healthy children with varicella given acyclovir defervesced sooner than the placebo group (median 1 versus 2 days), their lesions healed quicker (median 3 versus 2 days), and they had fewer skin lesions (median 500 versus 336). However, acyclovir did not significantly change the rate of complications of varicella (10% versus 13.5%), and acyclovir recipients had lower geometric mean serum antibody titers to VZV than their placebo counterparts 4 weeks after the onset of illness, suggesting acyclovir may impair the immune response.[76] The modest benefits do not justify the cost, possible adverse effects, and risk of acyclovir resistance.

Antiviral therapy should be reserved for children with or at risk of severe disease, and the dose and route should be determined by the circumstances, such as the age and immune status of the child, and the timing and severity of infection.[74,75]

In immunocompromised patients with significant T-cell deficiency, with or without severe chicken pox, and in normal patients with complications of varicella (e.g., pneumonitis or encephalitis), we recommend:

acyclovir 10 mg/kg IV, 8-hourly until all lesions crusted and healed (usually 7–14 days)

Zoster (shingles)

Zoster (herpes zoster, shingles) is caused by reactivation of VZV from where it lies dormant in dorsal root ganglia. Generally, primary varicella tends to occur in childhood, whereas herpes zoster is a disease of adults, with most patients being over 45 years old.[77,78] The age-adjusted incidence rates of herpes zoster are lowest (0.45/1000 person-years) in children 0–14 years of age and highest (4.2–4.5/1000 person-years) in people 75 years and older.[79] In the pediatric population, the incidence is lowest from 0 to 5 years of age (20/100,000 person-years) and highest in adolescents (63/100,000 person-years).[80]

Antigen-specific T cells are believed to be the principal gatekeepers of latent VZV. Conditions in which cellular responses are lost or diminished by immunosuppression pose a risk for reactivation of VZV and recurrent disease manifestation as herpes zoster. Herpes zoster in the elderly is associated with loss of VZV-specific cellular immunity.[81] Zoster in children is particularly associated with immunosuppression due to chemotherapy or HIV infection. The mechanism in chemotherapy is suppression of cellular immunity, whereas zoster occurs in HIV infection due to viral destruction of T cells.

Acquisition of herpes zoster in healthy immunocompetent children in early childhood or during intrauterine exposure has been attributed to immaturity of the immune system. If zoster occurs in a previously well child whose physical examination is normal apart from the rash, the child almost never has an underlying malignancy or other systemic disease.[82−84] There is an association between maternal chicken pox in pregnancy and the child developing zoster in the first year of life.[82] Zoster in infancy can also follow post-natal chicken pox.[83,84] It has been suggested that in infancy the presence of maternal antibody modifies primary infection and that subclinical primary infection may predispose to herpes zoster.[83]

Post-herpetic neuralgia is age dependent. In a large, observational study, severe post-herpetic neuralgia occurred only in adults >60 years old.[85] For patients <50 years old, only 1.5% had mild pain after 3 months and 98.5% had no pain.[85] Zoster almost never causes post-herpetic neuralgia in children. In an observational study of 118 children and adolescents with 121 episodes of zoster, no child had pain after 1 month, even though none received antivirals.[86]

Ophthalmic zoster is potentially sight-threatening at any age. Without antiviral therapy, approximately 50% of patients will have ocular complications (e.g., keratopathy, episcleritis, iritis, or stromal keratitis), some of which are potentially sight-threatening.[87,88] Oral antiviral therapy reduces the frequency of late ocular complications from about 50% to 20–30%.[88−90] Systemic antivirals are advisable in severe cases. It is advised that patients with herpes zoster ophthalmicus should be evaluated by an ophthalmologist who is experienced in the management of corneal diseases.[88]

Antivirals are also recommended for immunosuppressed children with zoster, as zoster infection can be fatal.[72,91]

We do not recommend antivirals for immunocompetent children with zoster.

For immuncompromised children with zoster and for any child with ophthalmic zoster, we recommend antivirals. The route and duration will depend on severity and risk, which is a function of degree of immunosuppression. We recommend:

acyclovir 10 mg/kg (max 400 mg) IV, 8-hourly (until healed, usually 7–14 days) OR
acyclovir 20 mg/kg (max 800 mg) orally, five times daily OR
famciclovir 250 mg orally, 8-hourly (>12 years) OR
famciclovir 500 mg orally, 8-hourly (>12 years and immunocompromised) OR
valacyclovir 1 g orally, 8-hourly (>12 years)

Prevention of varicella zoster infections
Immunization against VZV

It is possible to reduce the incidence of varicella using universal childhood immunization with live, attenuated VZV vaccines, and this has been shown to reduce morbidity and mortality in the USA.[92,93] It is controversial whether or not universal varicella vaccine is cost-effective. Because of the relatively high cost of the vaccine, a number of cost-effectiveness analyses have found that the cost-effectiveness is marginal.[94−99] Universal VZV vaccine has been introduced in Australia, as well as the USA. In the UK, universal VZV vaccine has been opposed,[100] because mathematical modeling suggests that universal VZV vaccine might lead to a temporary rise in zoster in the elderly. This is because elderly persons in contact with young children have less zoster than those with less contact,[101] which has been interpreted as being due to natural boosting of immunity from children with chicken pox[100] (although other interpretations of the reason for reduced zoster are possible, such as the emotional benefits of contact with children).

In countries without universal immunization, individuals can be protected by the use of VZV vaccine from 1 year. This is only about 85% protective against infection, but virtually 100% protective against severe varicella.[102−104]

VZV vaccines are not recommended usually for children with immunodeficiency. The vaccine has been shown, however, to be safe and immunogenic in children with HIV infection, who are not profoundly immunosuppressed (CD4 count $>200/\mu$L)[105,106] (see Section 8.5, p. 107).

VZV vaccine is recommended for susceptible health-care workers, provided they are not immunocompromised.[107]

Post-exposure prophylaxis against varicella zoster infection

Varicella is spread by air and is highly infectious, although the duration and nature of exposure that constitute a significant risk are unknown and controversial. About 90% of non-immune household contacts develop varicella.[107] Possible ways to prevent or ameliorate varicella infection post-exposure are by active immunization with varicella vaccine, by passive use of immunoglobulin or by using antivirals.

Post-exposure immunization with VZV vaccine

Data from the USA and Japan from household, hospital, and community settings indicate that varicella vaccine is effective in modifying varicella severity if used up to 3 days, and possibly up to 5 days after exposure.[108-111] In an RCT,[111] 22 children given VZV vaccine following household exposure had the same rate of varicella infection as 20 children given placebo (RR 1.1, 95% CI 0.55–2.21), but the risk of developing moderate to severe disease was eight times greater in the placebo group, indicating an 80% protective effect against moderate to severe disease.[111]

The US Advisory Committee on Immunization Practices recommends the use of VZV vaccine in susceptible persons aged 1 year or older following exposure to varicella.[107] If exposure to varicella does not cause infection, post-exposure immunization should induce protection against subsequent exposure. If the exposure results in infection, there is no evidence that administration of VZV vaccine during the presymptomatic or prodromal stage of illness increases the risk for vaccine-associated adverse events.[111]

Post-exposure immunoglobulin for protection against varicella

Immunoglobulin with high-titer antibodies against VZV provides passive protection against varicella, and is most useful when active immunization is likely to be ineffective or dangerous because of age (e.g., neonates, high-risk infants <1 year old) or impaired T-cell immunity. Immunoglobulin is expensive, in scarce supply, and provides only temporary protection. It should be given only to prevent varicella in exposed patients who cannot be given VZV vaccine.

Studies conducted in 1969 indicated that zoster immune globulin (ZIG), which is prepared from patients recovering from herpes zoster and contains high levels of VZV antibody, prevented clinical varicella in susceptible, healthy children if administered within 72 hours of exposure.[112] ZIG also lowered attack rates among immunocompromised persons if administered no later than 96 hours after exposure.[112]

Varicella zoster immune globulin (VZIG; prepared from plasma obtained from healthy, volunteer blood donors who are identified by routine screening to have high antibody titers to VZV) became available in 1978. Both serologic and clinical evaluations have demonstrated that the product is equivalent to ZIG in preventing or modifying clinical illness in susceptible, immunocompromised persons who are exposed to varicella.

Subsequent studies have shown that, like VZV vaccine, ZIG does not always prevent infection but does reduce the severity in immunosuppressed household contacts[113] and in neonates whose mothers have perinatal chicken pox.[114]

The duration of protection is unknown, but should be at least one half-life or approximately 3 weeks. It is recommended that susceptible high-risk persons for whom varicella vaccination is contraindicated and who are again exposed 3 weeks or more after a dose of VZIG should receive another full dose of VZIG.[107]

VZIG has no effect in *treating* clinical varicella or herpes-zoster infection.[107]

We do not recommend treating children with active chicken pox or zoster with ZIG.

VZIG is supplied in 125 U and 625 U vials. The recommended dose is 125 U/10 kg, up to a maximum of 625 U. The minimum dose is 125 U; fractional doses are not recommended. VZIG should be administered intramuscularly as directed by the manufacturer, and never intravenously.

VZIG prophylaxis is generally recommended for certain groups of children at high risk of severe varicella, shown in Box 18.1, and the rationale is discussed below.

Box 18.1 Children for whom prophylaxis with ZIG is recommended[74,107,115] following significant exposure.

· Neonate whose mother develops chicken pox 5 days or fewer before delivery (some say 7 days or fewer)[115] to 2 days after delivery
· Premature infants < 28 weeks' gestation or who weigh 1000 g or less at birth, regardless of maternal history
· Premature infants 28 weeks' gestation or more with no history of maternal chicken pox or no VZV-specific IgG
· Immunocompromised child (with impaired T-cell immunity), with no prior history of varicella or VZV immunization and no VZV-specific IgG
*The definition of a significant exposure to VZV is controversial, and not based on strong evidence.[74]

Neonates and VZIG
The attack rate in healthy neonates is highest in babies exposed to maternal chicken pox, when transmission is mainly transplacental. Neonates whose mothers develop chicken pox 5 days or fewer before delivery and up to 2 days after birth are the highest risk group, because the babies are exposed to large amounts of virus before maternal IgG can cross the placenta. The neonatal mortality was as high as 30% for untreated babies, who developed neonatal chicken pox after being exposed to maternal chicken pox in this high-risk time period.[114,115] The advent of VZIG has changed this. The rate of neonatal chicken pox in babies given VZIG after birth is 30–40%, which is not substantially different from neonates not given VZIG.[116] However, the occurrence of complications and fatal outcomes is substantially lower for neonates who are treated with VZIG than for those who are not, and VZIG is recommended for high-risk neonates.[116,117] VZIG is probably not necessary for neonates whose mothers develop varicella more than 5 days before delivery, because those infants should be protected from severe varicella by transplacentally acquired maternal antibody, although some authorities extend the recommendation for VZIG out to 7 days before delivery, because antibody levels in the baby are sometimes low if mother's varicella was within 7 days.[116–119]

Transmission of varicella to neonates in the hospital nursery following post-natal exposure is rare, because most neonates are protected by maternal antibody. Premature infants who have substantial postnatal exposure should be evaluated on an individual basis. The risk of post-natally acquired varicella in premature infants is unknown. Because the immune systems of premature infants may be compromised, administration of VZIG to those who are exposed and born to susceptible mothers may be prudent. These infants should be considered at risk for as long as they are hospitalized. Premature infants <28 weeks' gestation or who weigh 1000 g or less at birth, who are exposed to VZV, should receive VZIG, regardless of maternal history, because such infants are born before they have acquired adequate maternal antibody transplacentally.[118,119] Most premature infants of 28 weeks' gestation or greater born to immune mothers have enough transplacental antibody to protect them from severe disease and complications.

Although infants are at higher risk for serious and fatal complications than older children,[118,119] the risk for healthy, full-term infants who develop varicella following post-natal exposure is substantially less than for infants whose mothers were infected 5 days before to 2 days after delivery. VZIG is not generally recommended for healthy, full-term neonates or infants who are exposed post-natally, even if their mothers have no history of varicella infection.[74,107]

Neonates who develop chicken pox despite being given VZIG are at less risk of severe infection than are untreated babies,[116,117] but can still develop severe infection despite VZIG.[118,119] For this reason, many authorities recommend treating such babies with intravenous acyclovir.

Immunocompromised children and VZIG
Following household exposure, attack rates among immunocompromised children and adolescents given VZIG are 33–50%.[107] Data are not available for immunocompromised, susceptible persons who were not given VZIG. The risk for varicella following close contact (e.g., contact with playmates) or hospital exposure is approximately 20% of the risk occurring from household exposure.[107]

VZIG is recommended for passive immunization of susceptible, immunocompromised children after substantial exposure to varicella or herpes zoster, including children who (a) have primary and acquired immunodeficiency disorders, (b) have neoplastic diseases, and (c) are receiving immunosuppressive treatment.[74,107]

Immunocompromised children who have a positive past history of varicella (except for bone marrow transplant recipients) can be considered immune. A non-Cochrane meta-analysis suggests that children with acute lymphoblastic leukemia can be expected to mount an adequate immune response, even if they have undetectable antibody, provided they are not too immunosuppressed.[120]

The CDC recommends that children who receive hematopoietic stem cell transplants should be considered susceptible, regardless of whether they or their donors have a prior history of varicella or varicella vaccination.[74,107] In contrast, some authorities feel that children with VZV-specific IgG are protected and do not routinely recommend prophylaxis.[121]

Post-exposure prophylaxis with acyclovir

We found three studies on the prophylactic use of acyclovir in susceptible, immunocompetent children following household exposure to varicella.[122–124] Prophylaxis given in the second week after exposure (7–14 days) was 73–93% protective against clinical varicella.[122–124] Prophylaxis in the first week after exposure was less protective against clinical disease. The major disadvantage was that about 15% of children failed to seroconvert and remained susceptible. On the other hand, the advantage was that acyclovir could be used at a time after exposure when VZV vaccine and immunoglobulin are no longer effective.

There are case reports but no trials of acyclovir prophylaxis for immuncompromised children[125] and neonates.[126] Post-exposure use of acyclovir may be an alternative to VZIG in some cases, and is likely to be beneficial for high-risk patients when VZIG is unavailable or if exposure was more than 4 days earlier.

References

1 Pancholi P, Wu F, Della-Latta P. Rapid detection of cytomegalovirus infection in transplant patients. *Expert Rev Mol Diagn* 2004;4:231–42.

2 Weinberg A, Brewster L, Clark J, Simoes E; ARIVAC consortium. Evaluation of R-Mix shell vials for the diagnosis of viral respiratory tract infections. *J Clin Virol* 2004;30:100–5.

3 Pass RF. Congenital cytomegalovirus infection and hearing loss. *Herpes* 2005;12:50–5.

4 Fowler KB, Boppana SB. Congenital cytomegalovirus (CMV) infection and hearing deficit. *J Clin Virol* 2006; 35:226–31.

5 Kimberlin DW, Lin CY, Sanchez PJ et al. Effect of ganciclovir therapy on hearing in symptomatic congenital cytomegalovirus disease involving the central nervous system: a randomized, controlled trial. *J Pediatr* 2003;143:16–25.

6 Smets K, De Coen K, Dhooge I et al. Selecting neonates with congenital cytomegalovirus infection for ganciclovir therapy. *Eur J Pediatr* 2006;165:885–90.

7 Meine Jansen CF, Toet MC, Rademaker CM, Ververs TF, Gerards LJ, van Loon AM. Treatment of symptomatic congenital cytomegalovirus infection with valganciclovir. *J Perinat Med* 2005;33:364–6.

8 Jones CA, Isaacs D. Predicting the outcome of symptomatic congenital cytomegalovirus infection. *J Paediatr Child Health* 1995;31:70–1.

9 Helantera I, Koskinen P, Finne P et al. Persistent cytomegalovirus infection in kidney allografts is associated with inferior graft function and survival. *Transpl Int* 2006;19:893–900.

10 Hodson EM, Barclay PG, Craig JC et al. Antiviral medications for preventing cytomegalovirus disease in solid organ transplant recipients. *The Cochrane Database of Systematic Reviews* 2005;(4):Art No CD003774.

11 American Academy of Pediatrics. Antiviral drugs for non-human immunodeficiency virus infections. In: Pickering LK (ed.), *Red Book: 2003 Report of the Committee on Infectious Diseases*, 26th edn. Elk Grove Village, IL: American Academy of Pediatrics, 2003:729–32.

12 Kanegane H, Kanegane C, Yachie A, Miyawaki T, Tosato G. Infectious mononucleosis as a disease of early childhood in Japan caused by primary Epstein-Barr virus infection. *Acta Paediatr Jpn* 1997;39:166–71.

13 Chan CW, Chiang AK, Chan KH, Lau AS. Epstein-Barr virus-associated infectious mononucleosis in Chinese children. *Pediatr Infect Dis J* 2003;22:974–8.

14 Hausler M, Ramaekers VT, Doenges M, Schweizer K, Ritter K, Schaade L. Neurological complications of acute and persistent Epstein-Barr virus infection in paediatric patients. *J Med Virol* 2002;68:253–63.

15 van der Horst C, Joncas J, Ahronheim G et al. Lack of effect of peroral acyclovir for the treatment of acute infectious mononucleosis. *J Infect Dis* 1991;164:788–92.

16 Tynell E, Aurelius E, Brandell A et al. Acyclovir and prednisolone treatment of acute infectious mononucleosis: a multicenter, double-blind, placebo-controlled study. *J Infect Dis* 1996;174:324–31.

17 Cox AJ, Gleeson M, Pyne DB, Saunders PU, Clancy RL, Fricker PA. Valtrex therapy for Epstein-Barr virus reactivation and upper respiratory symptoms in elite runners. *Med Sci Sports Exerc* 2004;36:1104–10.

18 Humar A, Hebert D, Davies HD et al. A randomized trial of ganciclovir versus ganciclovir plus immune globulin for prophylaxis against Epstein-Barr virus related posttransplant

lymphoproliferative disorder. *Transplantation* 2006;81:856–61.

19 Roy M, Bailey B, Amre DK, Girodias JB, Bussieres JF, Gaudreault P. Dexamethasone for the treatment of sore throat in children with suspected infectious mononucleosis: a randomized, double-blind, placebo-controlled, clinical trial. *Arch Pediatr Adolesc Med* 2004;158:250–4.

20 Thompson SK, Doerr TD, Hengerer AS. Infectious mononucleosis and corticosteroids: management practices and outcomes. *Arch Otolaryngol Head Neck Surg* 2005;131:900–4.

21 Kimberlin DW. Herpes simplex virus infections in neonates and early childhood. *Semin Pediatr Infect Dis* 2005;16:271–81.

22 Whitley R. Neonatal herpes simplex virus infection. *Curr Opin Infect Dis* 2004;17:243–6.

23 Kolokotronis A, Doumas S. Herpes simplex virus infection, with particular reference to the progression and complications of primary herpetic gingivostomatitis. *Clin Microbiol Infect* 2006;12:202–11.

24 Amir J, Harel L, Smetana Z, Varsano I. Treatment of herpes simplex gingivostomatitis with acyclovir in children: a randomised double blind placebo controlled study. *BMJ* 1997;314:1800–3.

25 Sullender WM, Arvin AM, Diaz PS et al. Pharmacokinetics of acyclovir suspension in infants and children. *Antimicrob Agents Chemother* 1987;31:1722–6.

26 Eksborg S. The pharmacokinetics of antiviral therapy in paediatric patients. *Herpes* 2003;10:66–71.

27 Spruance SL, Kriesel JD. Treatment of herpes simplex labialis. *Herpes* 2002;9:64–9.

28 Akintoye SO, Greenberg MS. Recurrent aphthous stomatitis. *Dent Clin North Am* 2005;49:31–47, vii–viii.

29 Spruance SL, Stewart JC, Freeman DJ et al. Early application of topical 15% idoxuridine in dimethyl sulfoxide shortens the course of herpes simplex labialis: a multicenter placebo-controlled trial. *J Infect Dis* 1990;161:191–7.

30 Spruance SL, Nett R, Marbury T, Wolff R, Johnson J, Spaulding T. Acyclovir cream for treatment of herpes simplex labialis: results of two randomized, double-blind, vehicle-controlled, multicenter clinical trials. *Antimicrob Agents Chemother* 2002;46:2238–43.

31 Spruance SL, Rea TL, Thoming C, Tucker R, Saltzman R, Boon R. Penciclovir cream for the treatment of herpes simplex labialis: a randomized, multicenter, double-blind, placebo-controlled trial. Topical Penciclovir Collaborative Study Group. *JAMA* 1997;277:1374–9.

32 Raborn GW, Martel AY, Lassonde M et al. Effective treatment of herpes simplex labialis with penciclovir cream: combined results of two trials. *J Am Dent Assoc* 2002;133:303–9.

33 Sarisky RT, Bacon TH, Boon RJ et al. Profiling penciclovir susceptibility and prevalence of resistance of herpes simplex virus isolates across eleven clinical trials. *Arch Virol* 2003;148:1757–69.

34 Morrel EM, Spruance SL, Goldberg DI; Iontophoretic Acyclovir Cold Sore Study Group. Topical iontophoretic administration of acyclovir for the episodic treatment of herpes

labialis: a randomized, double-blind, placebo-controlled, clinic-initiated trial. *Clin Infect Dis* 2006;43:460–7.

35 Spruance SL, Jones TM, Blatter MM et al. High-dose, short-duration, early valacyclovir therapy for episodic treatment of cold sores: results of two randomized, placebo-controlled, multicenter studies. *Antimicrob Agents Chemother* 2003;47:1072–80.

36 Rooney JF, Straus SE, Mannix ML et al. Oral acyclovir to suppress frequently recurrent herpes labialis: a double-blind, placebo-controlled trial. *Ann Intern Med* 1993;118:268–72.

37 Wollenberg A, Zoch C, Wetzel S, Plewig G, Przybilla B. Predisposing factors and clinical features of eczema herpeticum: a retrospective analysis of 100 cases. *J Am Acad Dermatol* 2003;49:198–205.

38 Niimura M, Nishikawa T. Treatment of eczema herpeticum with oral acyclovir. *Am J Med* 1988;85:49–52.

39 Straus SE, Rooney JF, Sever JL, Seidlin M, Nusinoff-Lehrman S, Cremer K. NIH Conference: herpes simplex virus infection: biology, treatment, and prevention. *Ann Intern Med* 1985;103:404–19.

40 Gluckman E, Lotsberg J, Devergie A et al. Prophylaxis of herpes infections after bone-marrow transplantation by oral acyclovir. *Lancet* 1983;2:706–8.

41 Centers for Disease Control and Prevention (CDC). Vaccine preventable deaths and the Global Immunization Vision and Strategy, 2006–2015. *MMWR* 2006;55:511–5.

42 de Quadros CA. Is global measles eradication feasible? *Curr Top Microbiol Immunol* 2006;304:153–63.

43 Oliveira SA, Camacho LA, Pereira AC, Setubal S, Nogueira RM, Siqueira MM. Assessment of the performance of a definition of a suspected measles case: implications for measles surveillance. *Rev Panam Salud Publica* 2006;19:229–35.

44 Hutchins SS, Papania MJ, Amler R et al. Evaluation of the measles clinical case definition. *J Infect Dis* 2004;189(suppl 1):S153–9.

45 Perry RT, Mmiro F, Ndugwa C, Semba RD. Measles infection in HIV-infected African infants. *Ann N Y Acad Sci* 2000;918:377–80.

46 Hussey GD, Klein M. A randomized, controlled trial of vitamin A in children with severe measles. *N Engl J Med* 1990;323:160–4.

47 Huiming Y, Chaomin W, Meng M. Vitamin A for treating measles in children. *The Cochrane Database of Systematic Reviews* 2005;(4):Art No CD001479.

48 Rosales FJ. Vitamin A supplementation of vitamin A deficient measles patients lowers the risk of measles-related pneumonia in Zambian children. *J Nutr* 2002;132:3700–3.

49 Kawasaki Y, Hosoya M, Katayose M, Suzuki H. The efficacy of oral vitamin A supplementation for measles and respiratory syncytial virus (RSV) infection. *Kansenshogaku Zasshi* 1999;73:104–9.

50 WHO. *A Guide to the Treatment and Prevention of Vitamin A Deficiency and Xerophthalmia*, 2nd edn. Geneva: WHO, 1997.

51 Berkowitz FE, Cotton MF. Endotracheal aspiration for the bacteriological diagnosis of nosocomial- and measles-associated pneumonia. *Ann Trop Paediatr* 1988;8:217–21.

52 Pandey MR, Daulaire NM, Starbuck ES, Houston RM, McPherson K. Reduction in total under-five mortality in western Nepal through community-based antimicrobial treatment of pneumonia. *Lancet* 1991;338:993–7.

53 Shann F, D'Souza RM, D'Souza R. Antibiotics for preventing pneumonia in children with measles. *The Cochrane Database of Systematic Reviews* 2000;(4):Art No CD001477.

54 Chalmers I. Why we need to know whether prophylactic antibiotics can reduce measles-related morbidity. *Pediatrics* 2002;109:312–5.

55 Mahalanabis D, Jana S, Shaikh S et al. Vitamin E and vitamin C supplementation does not improve the clinical course of measles with pneumonia in children: a controlled trial. *J Trop Pediatr* 2006;52:302–3.

56 Mahalanabis D, Chowdhury A, Jana S et al. Zinc supplementation as adjunct therapy in children with measles accompanied by pneumonia: a double-blind, randomized controlled trial. *Am J Clin Nutr* 2002;76:604–7.

57 Edejer TT, Aikins M, Black R, Wolfson L, Hutubessy R, Evans DB. Cost effectiveness analysis of strategies for child health in developing countries. *BMJ* 2005;331:1177.

58 Redd SC, King GE, Heath JL, Forghani B, Bellini WJ, Markowitz LE. Comparison of vaccination with measles-mumps-rubella vaccine at 9, 12, and 15 months of age. *J Infect Dis* 2004;189(suppl 1):S116–22.

59 Aaby P, Andersen M, Sodemann M, Jakobsen M, Gomes J, Fernandes M. Reduced childhood mortality after standard measles vaccination at 4–8 months compared with 9–11 months of age. *BMJ* 1993;307:1308–11.

60 Garly ML, Bale C, Martins CL et al. Measles antibody responses after early two dose trials in Guinea-Bissau with Edmonston-Zagreb and Schwarz standard-titre measles vaccine: better antibody increase from booster dose of the Edmonston-Zagreb vaccine. *Vaccine* 2001;19:1951–9.

61 Hiremath GS, Omer SB. A meta-analysis of studies comparing the respiratory route with the subcutaneous route of measles vaccine administration. *Hum Vaccin* 2005;1:30–6.

62 Centers for Disease Control and Prevention (CDC). Post-exposure prophylaxis, isolation, and quarantine to control an import-associated measles outbreak—Iowa, 2004. *MMWR* 2004;53:969–71.

63 King GE, Markowitz LE, Patriarca PA, Dales LG. Clinical efficacy of measles vaccine during the 1990 measles epidemic. *Pediatr Infect Dis J* 1991;10:883–8.

64 Endo A, Izumi H, Miyashita M, Taniguchi K, Okubo O, Harada K. Current efficacy of post-exposure prophylaxis against measles with immunoglobulin. *J Pediatr* 2001;138:926–8.

65 Jones G, Steketee R, Black RE, Bhutta ZA, Morris SS; Bellagio Child Survival Study Group. How many child deaths can we prevent this year? *Lancet* 2003;62:65–71.

66 Semba RD, Munasir Z, Beeler J et al. Reduced seroconversion to measles in infants given vitamin A with measles vaccination. *Lancet* 1995;345:1330–2.

67 Benn CS, Aaby P, Bale C et al. Randomised trial of effect of vitamin A supplementation on antibody response to measles vaccine in Guinea-Bissau, West Africa. *Lancet* 1997;350:101–5.

68 Benn CS, Balde A, George E et al. Effect of vitamin A supplementation on measles-specific antibody levels in Guinea-Bissau. *Lancet* 2002;359:1313–4.

69 Dollimore N, Cutts F, Binka FN, Ross DA, Morris SS, Smith PG. Measles incidence, case fatality, and delayed mortality in children with or without vitamin A supplementation in rural Ghana. *Am J Epidemiol* 1997;146:646–54.

70 WHO/CHD Immunisation-Linked Vitamin A Supplementation Study Group. Randomised trial to assess benefits and safety of vitamin A supplementation linked to immunisation in early infancy. *Lancet* 1998;352:1257–63.

71 Lieu TA, Cochi SL, Black SB et al. Cost-effectiveness of a routine varicella vaccination program for US children. *JAMA* 1994;271:375–81.

72 Chant KG, Sullivan EA, Burgess MA et al. Varicella-zoster virus infection in Australia. *Aust N Z J Public Health* 1998;22:413–8.

73 Sauerbrei A, Eichhorn U, Schacke M, Wutzler P. Laboratory diagnosis of herpes zoster. *J Clin Virol* 1999;14:31–6.

74 American Academy of Pediatrics. Varicella zoster infections. In: Pickering LK (ed.), *Red Book: 2003 Report of the Committee on Infectious Diseases*, 26th edn. Elk Grove Village, IL: American Academy of Pediatrics, 2003:672–86.

75 Balfour HH, Jr, Kelly JM, Suarez CS et al. Acyclovir treatment of varicella in otherwise healthy children. *J Pediatr* 1990;116:633–9.

76 Committee on Infectious Diseases, American Academy of Pediatrics. The use of oral acyclovir in otherwise healthy children with varicella. *Pediatrics* 1993;91:674–6.

77 Shishov AS, Smirnov IuK, Kulikova VA. Clinical picture and treatment of herpes zoster in children [in Russian]. *Zh Nevrol Psikhiatr Im S S Korsakova* 1983;83:1467–71.

78 Bharija SC, Kanwar AJ, Singh G. Ophthalmic zoster in infancy: a case report. *Indian J Dermatol* 1983;28:173–4.

79 Ragozzino MW, Melton LJ, III, Kurland LT, Chu CP, Perry HO. Population-based study of herpes zoster and its sequelae. *Medicine (Baltimore)* 1982;61:310–6.

80 Donahue JG, Choo PW, Manson JE. The incidence of herpes zoster. *Arch Intern Med* 1995;155:1605–9.

81 Berger R, Florent G, Just M. Decrease in the lymphoproliferative response to varicella-zoster virus antigen in the aged. *Infect Immun* 1981;32:24–7.

82 Enders G, Miller E, Cradock-Watson J, Bolley I, Ridehalgh M. Consequences of varicella and herpes zoster in pregnancy: prospective study of 1739 cases. *Lancet* 1994;343:1548–51.

83 Baba K, Yabuuchi H, Takahashi M, Ogra PL. Increased incidence of herpes zoster in normal children infected with varicella zoster virus during infancy: community-based follow-up study. *J Pediatr* 1986;108:372–7.

84 Kurlan JG, Connelly BL, Lucky AW. Herpes zoster in the first year of life following postnatal exposure to varicella-zoster virus: four case reports and a review of infantile herpes zoster. *Arch Dermatol* 2004;140:1268–72.

85 Helgason S, Petursson G, Gudmundsson S, Sigurdsson JA. Prevalence of post-herpetic neuralgia after a first episode of herpes zoster: prospective study with long term follow up. *BMJ* 2000;321:794–6.

86 Petursson G, Helgason S, Gudmundsson S, Sigurdsson JA. Herpes zoster in children and adolescents. *Pediatr Infect Dis J* 1998;17:905–8.

87 Cobo M, Foulks GN, Liesegang T et al. Observations on the natural history of herpes zoster ophthalmicus. *Curr Eye Res* 1987;6:195–9.

88 Gnann JW, Jr, Whitley RJ. Clinical practice. Herpes zoster. *N Engl J Med* 2002;347:340–6.

89 Cobo LM, Foulks GN, Liesegang T et al. Oral acyclovir in the treatment of acute herpes zoster ophthalmicus. *Ophthalmology* 1986;93:763–70.

90 Opstelten W, Zaal MJ. Managing ophthalmic herpes zoster in primary care. *BMJ* 2005;331:147–51.

91 Preblud SR. Varicella: complications and costs. *Pediatrics* 1986;78:728–35.

92 Seward JF, Watson BM, Peterson CL et al. Varicella disease after introduction of varicella vaccine in the United States, 1995–2000. *JAMA* 2002;287:606–11.

93 Nguyen HQ, Jumaan AO, Seward JF. Decline in mortality due to varicella after implementation of varicella vaccination in the United States. *N Engl J Med* 2005;352:450–8.

94 Thiry N, Beutels P, Van Damme P et al. Economic evaluations of varicella vaccination programmes: review of the literature. *Pharmacoeconomics* 2003;21:13–38.

95 Lieu TA, Cochi SL, Black SB et al. Cost-effectiveness of a routine varicella vaccination program for US children. *JAMA* 1994;271:375–81.

96 Beutels P, Clara R, Tormans G et al. Costs and benefits of routine varicella vaccination in Geman children. *J Infect Dis* 1996;174(suppl 3):S335–41.

97 Scuffham PA, Lowin AV, Burgess MA. The cost-effectiveness of varicella vaccine programs for Australia. *Vaccine* 2000; 18:407–15.

98 Coudeville L, Paree F, Lebrun T et al. The value of varicella vaccination in healthy children: cost-benefit analysis of the situation in France. *Vaccine* 1999;17:142–51.

99 Brisson M, Edmunds WJ. The cost-effectiveness of varicella zoster virus (VZV) vaccination in Canada. *Vaccine* 2002;20:1113–25.

100 Brisson M, Edmunds WJ. Varicella vaccination in England and Wales: cost-utility analysis. *Arch Dis Child* 2003;88: 862–9.

101 Thomas SL, Wheeler JG, Hall AJ. Contacts with varicella or with children and protection against herpes zoster in adults: a case-control study. *Lancet* 2002;360:678–82.

102 Brisson M, Edmunds WJ, Gay NJ, Law B, De Serres G. Analysis of varicella vaccine breakthrough rates: implications for the effectiveness of immunisation programmes. *Vaccine* 2000;18:2775–8.

103 Kuter B, Matthews H, Shinefield H et al. Ten year follow-up of healthy children who received one or two injections of varicella vaccine. *Pediatr Infect Dis J* 2004;23: 132–7.

104 Hambleton S, Gershon AA. Preventing varicella-zoster disease. *Clin Microbiol Rev* 2005;18:70–80.

105 Armenian SH, Han JY, Dunaway TM, Church JA. Safety and immunogenicity of live varicella virus vaccine in children with human immunodeficiency virus type 1. *Pediatr Infect Dis J* 2006;25:368–70.

106 Levin MJ, Gershon AA, Weinberg A et al. Administration of live varicella vaccine to HIV-infected children with current or past significant depression of CD4 (+) T cells. *J Infect Dis* 2006;194:247–55.

107 CDC. Prevention of varicella: recommendations of the Advisory Committee on Immunization Practices (ACIP). *MMWR* 1996;45(RR-11):21.

108 Asano Y, Nakayama H, Yazaki T, Kato R, Hirose S. Protection against varicella in family contacts by immediate inoculation with varicella vaccine. *Pediatrics* 1977;59:3–7.

109 Arbeter AM, Starr SE, Plotkin SA. Varicella vaccine studies in healthy children and adults. *Pediatrics* 1986;78(suppl):748–56.

110 Salzman MB, Garcia C. Post-exposure varicella vaccination in siblings of children with active varicella. *Pediatr Infect Dis J* 1998;17:256–7.

111 Mor M, Harel L, Kahan E, Amir J. Efficacy of post-exposure immunization with live attenuated varicella vaccine in the household setting—a pilot study. *Vaccine* 2004;23:325–8.

112 CDC. Varicella zoster immune globulin for the prevention of chickenpox. *MMWR* 1984;33:84–90, 95–100.

113 Zaia JA, Levin MJ, Preblud SR et al. Evaluation of varicella-zoster immune globulin: protection of immunosuppressed children after household exposure to varicella. *J Infect Dis* 1983;147:737–43.

114 De Nicola LK, Hanshaw JB. Congenital and neonatal varicella. *J Pediatr* 1979;94:175–6.

115 Erlich RM, Turner JAP, Clarke M. Neonatal varicella. *J Pediatr* 1958;53:139–47.

116 Miller E, Cradock-Watson JE, Ridehalgh MK. Outcome in newborn babies given anti-varicella-zoster immunoglobulin after perinatal maternal infection with varicella-zoster virus. *Lancet* 1989;2:371–3.

117 Heuchan AM, Isaacs D. The management of varicella-zoster virus exposure and infection in pregnancy and the newborn period. Australasian sub-group in paediatric infectious diseases of the Australasian Society for infectious diseases. *Med J Aust* 2001;174:288–92.

118 Hanngren K, Grandien M, Granstrom G. Effect of zoster immunoglobulin for varicella prophylaxis in the newborn. *Scand J Infect Dis* 1985;17:343–7.

119 Rubin L. Disseminated varicella in the neonate and implications for immunoprophylaxis in neonates exposed to varicella. *Pediatr Infect Dis J* 1986;56:100–2.

120 van Tilburg CM, Sanders EA, Rovers MM, Wolfs TF, Bierings MB. Loss of antibodies and response to (re-)vaccination in children after treatment for acute lymphocytic leukemia: a systematic review. *Leukemia* 2006;20: 1717–22.

121 Weinstock DM, Boeckh M, Boulad F et al. Post-exposure prophylaxis against varicella-zoster virus infection among

recipients of hematopoietic stem cell transplant: unresolved issues. *Infect Control Hosp Epidemiol* 2004;25:603–8.

122 Asano Y, Yoshikawa T, Suga S et al. Post-exposure prophylaxis of varicella in family contacts by oral acyclovir. *Pediatrics* 1993;92:219–22.

123 Suga S, Yoshikawa T, Ozaki T, Asano Y. Effect of oral acyclovir against primary and secondary viraemia in incubation period of varicella. *Arch Dis Child* 1993;69: 639–42.

124 Lin TY, Huang YC, Ning HC, Hsueh C. Oral acyclovir prophylaxis of varicella after intimate contact. *Pediatr Infect Dis J* 1997;16:1162–5.

125 Ishida Y, Tauchi H, Higaki A, Yokota-Outou Y, Kida K. Post-exposure prophylaxis of varicella in children with leukemia by oral acyclovir. *Pediatrics* 1996;97:150–1.

126 Huang YC, Lin TY, Lin YJ, Lien RI, Chou YH. Prophylaxis of intravenous immunoglobulin and acyclovir in perinatal varicella. *Eur J Pediatr* 2001;160:91–4.

APPENDIX 1

Renal impairment and antimicrobials

Renal impairment is mainly important for antimicrobials or their metabolites excreted by the kidneys, e.g., aminoglycosides. These may necessitate dose adjustments in terms of the starting dose or duration of an antimicrobial (see Appendix 2).

A.1.1 Creatinine clearance

Serum creatinine is not an accurate enough measure of renal function and can be normal in renal failure. Creatinine clearance, which provides a measure of glomerular filtration rate (GFR), is preferred. The most accurate measures of creatinine clearance use the excretion of radioactive-labeled tracers, e.g., technetium Tc99m-labeled DTPA scanning. Schwartz and colleagues developed an equation for children based on their serum creatinine and body length.[1,2] The Schwartz equation

has been evaluated in comparison to radioactive techniques and is more sensitive than serum creatinine in detecting impaired renal function.[3,4] The Schwartz equation tends to overestimate creatinine clearance, but to a neglible extent when renal function is mildly impaired (GFR 50–90 mL/min). When renal function is moderately impaired (GFR 15–50 mL/min) GFR is overestimated only by about 10%, but by 164% when GFR is <15 mL/min.[4]

The Schwartz equation is inaccurate in critically ill children,[5,6] but is useful in children who are about to undergo hematopoietic stem cell transplantation, being most accurate if they are <5 years old.[7]

The Schwartz equation is sufficiently accurate to provide an estimate of creatinine clearance to make dose adjustments. We recommend the Schwartz equation for estimating creatinine clearance in children unless they are critically ill (see Table A.1.1).

Table A.1.1 Schwartz formula for calculating creatinine clearance in children.

Age	Formula for Creatinine Clearance in mL/min/1.73 m²
Preterm neonate	29 × length (cm)/[serum creatinine (mmol/L) × 1000] **OR**
	0.33 × length (cm)/serum creatinine (mg/100 mL)
1 month to <1 year	40 × height (cm)/[serum creatinine (mmol/L) × 1000] **OR**
	0.45 × length (cm)/serum creatinine (mg/100 mL)
1 year to <12 year	49 × height (cm)/[serum creatinine (mmol/L) × 1000] **OR**
	0.55 × length (cm)/serum creatinine (mg/100 mL)
12 years or older (female)	49 × height (cm)/[serum creatinine (mmol/L) × 1000] **OR**
	0.55 × length (cm)/serum creatinine (mg/100 mL)
12 years or older (male)	62 × height (cm)/[serum creatinine (mmol/L) × 1000] **OR**
	0.7 × length (cm)/serum creatinine (mg/100 mL)

A.1.2 Dose or interval adjustment of antimicrobials in renal insufficiency

Antimicrobial therapy can be altered in renal impairment by reducing the dose or by extending the interval between doses. We found two different tables giving recommendations on dose or interval adjustments in children.[8,9] The recommendations were quite different and neither publication gave the primary data for making the recommendations.[8,9] One paper said its table was based on pharmaceutical company drug information sheets, PICU dosing guidelines, publications, an electronic database, and extrapolation from adult doses.[9] We are unable to recommend one of these tables in preference to the other because of lack of data, and recommend consulting the product information sheet for dose or interval adjustment when prescribing an antimicrobial for a patient with impaired renal function.

References

1 Schwartz GJ, Haycock GB, Edelmann CM, Jr, Spitzer A. A simple estimate of glomerular filtration rate in children derived from body length and plasma creatinine. *Pediatrics* 1976;58:259–63.

2 Schwartz GJ, Brion LP, Spitzer A. The use of plasma creatinine concentration for estimating glomerular filtration rate in infants, children, and adolescents. *Pediatr Clin North Am* 1987:34:571–91.

3 Springate JE, Christensen SL, Feld LG. Serum creatinine level and renal function in children. *Am J Dis Child* 1992;146: 1232–5.

4 Seikaly MG, Browne R, Bajaj G, Arant BS, Jr. Limitations to body length/serum creatinine ratio as an estimate of glomerular filtration in children. *Pediatr Nephrol* 1996;10:709–11.

5 Kwong MB, Tong TK, Mickell JJ, Chan JC. Lack of evidence that formula-derived creatinine clearance approximates glomerular filtration rate in pediatric intensive care population. *Clin Nephrol* 1985;24:285–8.

6 Pong S, Seto W, Abdolell M et al. 12-hour versus 24-hour creatinine clearance in critically ill pediatric patients. *Pediatr Res* 2005;58:83–8.

7 Kletzel M, Pirich L, Haut P, Cohn RA. Comparison of Tc-99 measurement of glomerular filtration rate vs. calculated creatinine clearance to assess renal function pretransplant in pediatric patients undergoing hematopoietic stem cell transplantation. *Pediatr Transplant* 2005;9:584–8.

8 Therapeutic Guidelines Ltd. *Therapeutic Guidelines: Antibiotic*, 13th edn. Melbourne: Therapeutic Guidelines Ltd, 2006.

9 Daschner M. Drug dosage in children with reduced renal function. *Pediatr Nephrol* 2005;20:1675–86.

APPENDIX 2

Aminoglycosides: dosing and monitoring blood levels

A.2.1 Aminoglycosides

Aminoglycosides are antibiotics that are rapidly bactericidal against aerobic Gram-negative bacilli. They also have some activity against *Staphylococcus aureus* and coagulase negative staphylococci, which is potentially useful in neonatal sepsis when aminoglycosides are used with an antistaphylococcal antibiotic. Aminoglycosides are associated with a phenomenon called the post-antibiotic effect where bacteria continue to be killed even after blood levels have fallen below the minimum inhibitory concentration (MIC) of the organism. This is probably because aminoglycosides are still present and active in the intracellular environment where they block protein synthesis at the ribosome but are not detectable in the extracellular space. Killing of bacteria by aminoglycosides is thought to be concentration-dependent, and to depend more on the total amount of antibiotic, the "area under the curve," in contrast to beta-lactams like penicillin, whose optimal killing depends on maintaining blood levels above the MIC of the organism for as long as possible.[1-3]

Aminoglycosides accumulate in renal tissue and otolymph,[4] and are nephrotoxic and ototoxic. Almost all patients develop some nephrotoxicity with prolonged use of aminoglycosides, even if serum aminoglycoside levels are within the designated therapeutic range.[1-3] For this reason, prolonged use should be avoided and aminoglycosides should be stopped within 7 days whenever possible.[1-3]

There are very few absolute contraindications to aminoglycosides. We recommend that an alternative antibiotic be used if possible, however, or at least that aminoglycoside be stopped within 3 days for children with any of the conditions shown in Table A.2.1, which are known to predispose to aminoglycoside toxicity.[1-3,5-7]

Table A.2.1 Preexisting conditions that predispose to aminoglycoside toxicity.

- Chronic renal failure or deteriorating renal function[5]
- Chronic liver disease[6]
- Severe cholestasis[6]
- Significant conductive hearing problems[1-3]
- Vestibular problems (e.g., dizziness, vertigo, or tinnitus)[7]

We recommend monitoring aminoglycoside levels and renal function regularly, at least every 2–3 days, if patients need to be on aminoglycosides for prolonged periods. We also recommend warning the child and/or parents of the potential risks of aminoglycosides and discussing any possible alternatives. We advise monitoring children on prolonged aminoglycosides clinically for hearing and balance problems, and considering formal vestibular function testing and high-frequency audiometric testing, if available, for older children, e.g., children with endocarditis (see Section 3.1, p. 14).

A.2.2 Starting doses of aminoglycosides

The recommended starting dose depends on the volume of distribution and renal clearance, which are related to body weight and renal function. Aminoglycosides are excreted by the kidneys and so renal function is critical. A guide to calculating creatinine clearance in children is given in Table A.1.1.

Initial doses of aminoglycosides for patients with normal renal function are given in Table A.2.2 and are derived from References 2, 3, and 7. Low-dose aminoglycosides are used for synergy in endocarditis (see Section 3.1, p. 17).

Table A.2.2 Aminoglycoside starting doses for patients with normal renal function.

Age	Starting Dose for Gentamicin, Tobramycin	Starting Dose for Amikacin
Neonates < 34 weeks	2.5 mg/kg/dose 18–24-hourly	7.5 mg/kg/dose 12–24-hourly
Neonates ≥34 weeks	2.5–7.5 mg/kg/day	7.5–10 mg/kg/dose 8–12-hourly
< 10 years	7.5 mg/kg/day	30 mg/kg/day
10 years and older	6 mg/kg/day	24 mg/kg/day
Any age: streptococcal and enterococcal endocarditis	Gentamicin 1 mg/kg/dose, 8-hourly (see Section 3.1)	Not recommended

Some doses are given in mg/kg/dose and then the dose interval, others are given as mg/kg/day which is the total daily dose given once or three times per day.

Adapted from Reference 8, with permission.

For children with impaired renal function, **either** starting doses should be reduced (see Table A.2.3) **or** the interval between doses should be increased (see Table A.2.4). Whichever is chosen, aminoglycoside levels and renal function should be monitored very closely.

A.2.3 Dosing interval of aminoglycosides

Question | In neonates and children, is once-daily aminoglycoside compared with multiple-daily dosing safe and effective?

Literature review | We found a non-Cochrane meta-analysis of 16 studies in neonates,[9] a non-Cochrane meta-analysis of 24 studies in children of all ages,[10] and a Cochrane systematic review of 4 studies in children with cystic fibrosis.[11]

Table A.2.3 Reduced aminoglycoside starting doses for patients with impaired renal function.

Creatinine Clearance		Starting Dose (% of Usual Recommended Dose)
mL/s/1.73 m²	mL/min/1.73 m²	
> 1.1	> 66	100
0.9–1.1	54–66	85
0.7–0.9	42–54	70
0.5–0.7	30–42	55
0.35–0.5	21–30	40
< 0.35	< 21	Seek specialist advice

Use either the method in Table A.2.3 above or the prolonged interval method in Table A.2.4, not both.

Adapted from Reference 8, with permission.

A non-Cochrane meta-analysis in neonates found 16 studies, mostly of good quality, which compared extended interval dosing (once daily or less frequent) with multiple-daily dosing.[9] Extended interval dosing of aminoglycosides in neonates was found to be safe and effective, with no increase in nephrotoxicity or ototoxicity and with a reduced risk of serum drug concentrations outside the therapeutic range.[9]

The non-Cochrane meta-analysis[10] in children of all ages compared once-daily with multiple-daily dosing in different clinical settings: neonatal intensive care unit 6 studies; cystic fibrosis 3 studies; cancer 5 studies; urinary tract infections 4 studies; diverse infectious indications 5 studies; pediatric intensive care unit 1 study.[10] Aminoglycosides used were gentamicin (11 studies), amikacin (9), tobramycin (2), netilmicin (2), and tobramycin or netilmicin (1). There was no significant difference between once-daily and multiple-daily dosing in clinical failure rate, in microbiologic failure rate, and in combined clinical or microbiologic failure rates, but trends favored once-daily dosing consistently.[10] There was no difference in ototoxicity, and no difference in nephrotoxicity as measured by serum creatinine, but urinary excretion of proteins or phospholipids, which were called secondary nephrotoxicity outcomes, significantly favored once-daily dosing.[10]

For children with cystic fibrosis, the Cochrane systematic review[11] found 11 studies, but only 4 eligible RCTs. The efficacy was similar but once-daily dosing was less nephrotoxic than multiple-daily dosing in children (although not in adults).[11]

Table A.2.4 Aminoglycoside starting doses and prolonged intervals for patients with impaired renal function.*

Creatinine Clearance		Starting Dose and Initial Interval*	Starting Dose and Initial Interval*
mL/sec/1.73 m²	mL/min/1.73 m²	for Gentamicin and Tobramycin	for Amikacin
> 1.0	> 60	5 mg/kg every 24 hours	20 mg/kg every 24 hours
0.7–1.0	40–60	5 mg/kg every 36 hours	20 mg/kg every 36 hours
0.5–0.7	30–40	5 mg/kg every 48 hours	20 mg/kg every 48 hours
< 0.5	< 30	5 mg/kg, once, then seek specialist advice	20 mg/kg, once, then seek specialist advice

Use either the increased dose interval method in Table A.2.4 above or the reduced dose method in Table A.2.3, not both.
*Interval may need adjustment according to aminglycoside level after first dose.
Adapted from Reference 8, with permission.

We found one RCT that showed that once-daily dosing is safe and effective in malnourished children.[12]

Once-daily dosing has been shown to be as effective as multiple-daily dosing in most clinical settings, and if anything less nephrotoxic. It is also easier to give aminoglycosides once daily in clinical practice.

We recommend once-daily (or less frequent) dosing of aminoglycosides in most clinical settings.

We do not recommend once-daily dosing for children in situations where unconventional kinetics are likely (e.g., patients with burns and others with large volumes of distribution). In addition, there is insufficient evidence currently to say whether once-daily dosing is preferred to multiple-daily dosing for the treatment of endocarditis.

A.2.4 Monitoring plasma levels of aminoglycosides

It is recommended to monitor plasma levels for all patients in whom it is anticipated that aminoglycosides will be given for more than 48 hours. Neonates are often started on empiric therapy with a beta-lactam and an aminoglycoside, but only about 10% have bacteremia and need to continue antibiotics beyond 48–72 hours. It is necessary to measure levels only for babies who continue aminoglycosides unless they have renal problems.

Once-daily or less frequent dosing

For once-daily or less frequent dosing of aminoglycosides, the reasons for measuring aminoglycosides may be to measure total therapeutic dose, in which case an area-under-the-curve method is appropriate, or to detect accumulation, in which case a trough level would be needed.

Area-under-the-curve methods

The most accurate way to measure the "area under the curve" (i.e., to estimate the total amount of aminoglycoside in the plasma between doses) is to measure the plasma aminoglycoside level twice, once about an hour after the dose was given that will be near the peak, and another after 6–14 hours. The 24-hour area under the curve (AUC) can then be calculated using a computer program, which also recommends the appropriate dose or interval adjustment. When computer-based methods are not available, graphical methods can be used instead.[4,8,13-15] An example of a nomogram is given in Figure A.2.1 and the calculation in Table A.2.5. Nomograms have been studied mainly in adults. The advantage is that they need only a single measurement and are easy to calculate, but somewhat less accurate. The nomogram recommended in *Therapeutic Guidelines*[8] (see Figure A.2.1) has been compared with a manual method and two computer programs.[16] The *Therapeutic Guidelines* nomogram works well for patients with normal or mildly impaired renal function (creatinine clearance [CrCl] 60–90 mL/min/1.73 m²). For patients with moderate renal impairment (CrCl 30–60), the nomogram estimates lower doses than the computer programs.[16]

For once-daily dosing of gentamicin or tobramycin, up to 7 mg/kg/day, a single measurement of plasma concentration should be made between 6 and 14 hours

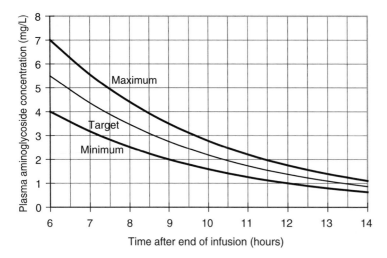

Figure A. 2.1 Nomogram for plasma aminoglycoside plasma concentration using once-daily dosing. (From Reference 8, with permission.)

after the end of the infusion. When using the dose adjustment method, the plasma concentration is compared to the graph in Figure A.2.1.

If the plotted plasma concentration is between the maximum and minimum lines on the graph, no dose adjustment is needed. If the plasma concentration is above the maximum line or below the minimum line, a proportional decrease or increase in dose is recommended (see Table A.2.5).

The level should be measured after the first dose and the dose adjusted if necessary. It should be repeated daily if the clinical state, especially renal function, is unstable and otherwise every 3–5 days.

Table A.2.5 Calculating dose adjustment from nomogram.

Dose of aminoglycoside*	= 5 mg/kg
Actual concentration at 9 hours	= 5.4 mg/L
Target concentration, calculated from the midpoint of the two lines	= 2.7 mg/L
Next dose	= Target concentration/actual concentration × initial dose
	= 2.7/5.4 × 5 mg/kg
	= 2.5 mg/kg

*This method of dose adjustment applies to gentamicin, netilmicin, and tobramycin. For once-daily amikacin dosing, divide the measured actual concentration by 4 and use the same graph. From Reference 8, with permission.

An alternative method that involves altering the dosing interval according to a nomogram instead of altering the dose of aminoglycoside has not been evaluated and we cannot recommend it.[8]

Trough measurements for once-daily dosing

The recommended trough levels when using once-daily dosing are <1 mg/L for gentamicin or tobramycin and <5 mg/L for amikacin.

Multiple-daily dosing

The commonest method for monitoring multiple-daily dosing (usually 8- or 12-hourly doses) of aminoglycosides is by measuring peak and trough plasma levels.

Trough levels, taken just before the next dose is due, are measured to prevent drug accumulation and reduce risk of toxicity. They should be repeated at least every 3–5 days and more frequently if there is impaired renal function.

Peak levels are measured to ensure that the dose of aminoglycoside is adequate. Blood is collected 30 minutes after completion of the infusion of a dose of aminoglycoside.

The usual recommended target trough and peak levels are in Table A.2.6. It is not appropriate to apply these peak and trough levels to once-daily dosing.

For monitoring 8-hourly low-dose (1 mg/kg) gentamicin use in endocarditis, we recommend

Table A.2.6 Recommended aminoglycoside trough and peak levels for multiple-daily dosing.

Aminoglycoside	Recommended Trough level (mg/L)	Recommended Peak Level (mg/L)
Amikacin	< 10	20–30
Gentamicin and tobramycin	< 2	5–10
Gentamicin in endocarditis	< 1	None recommended

performing trough levels and keeping the level < 1 mg/L to avoid toxicity.

References

1 Craig WA. Once-daily versus multiple-daily dosing of aminoglycosides. *J Chemother* 1995;7(suppl 2):47–52.

2 Lacy MK, Nicolau DP, Nightingale CH, Quintiliani R. The pharmacodynamics of aminoglycosides. *Clin Infect Dis* 1998;27:23–7.

3 Turnidge J. Pharmacodynamics and dosing of aminoglycosides. *Infect Dis Clin North Am* 2003;17:503–28.

4 Tran Ba Huy P, Bernard P, Schacht J. Kinetics of gentamicin uptake and release in the rat: comparison of inner ear tissues and fluids with other organs. *J Clin Invest* 1986;77:1492–500.

5 Rougier F, Claude D, Maurin M, Maire P. Aminoglycoside nephrotoxicity. *Curr Drug Targets Infect Disord* 2004;4:153–62.

6 Lucena MI, Andrade RJ. Extrahepatic cholestasis as a distinct factor predisposing to gentamicin nephrotoxicity. *Am J Med* 1990;89:698–9.

7 Minor LB. Gentamicin-induced bilateral vestibular hypofunction. *JAMA* 1998;279:541–4.

8 Therapeutic Guidelines Ltd. *Therapeutic Guidelines: Antibiotic*, 13th edn. Melbourne: Therapeutic Guidelines Ltd, 2006:338–48.

9 Nestaas E, Bangstad HJ, Sandvik L, Wathne KO. Aminoglycoside extended interval dosing in neonates is safe and effective: a meta-analysis. *Arch Dis Child Fetal Neonatal Ed* 2005;90:F294–300.

10 Contopoulos-Ioannidis DG, Giotis ND, Baliatsa DV, Ioannidis JP. Extended-interval aminoglycoside administration for children: a meta-analysis. *Pediatrics* 2004;114:e111–8.

11 Smyth AR, Tan KH. Once-daily versus multiple-daily dosing with intravenous aminoglycosides for cystic fibrosis. *The Cochrane Database of Systematic Reviews* 2006;(3): Art No CD002009.

12 Khan AM, Ahmed T, Alam NH, Chowdhury AK, Fuchs GJ. Extended-interval gentamicin administration in malnourished children. *J Trop Pediatr* 2006;52:179–84.

13 Nicolau DP, Freeman CD, Belliveau PP, Nightingale CH, Ross JW, Quintiliani R. Experience with a once-daily aminoglycoside program administered to 2184 adult patients. *Antimicrob Agents Chemother* 1995;39:650–5.

14 Gilbert DN, Lee BL, Dworkin RJ et al. A randomized comparison of the safety and efficacy of once-daily gentamicin or thrice-daily gentamicin in combination with ticarcillin-clavulanate. *Am J Med* 1998;105:182–91.

15 Prins JM, Weverling GJ, de Blok K, van Ketel RJ, Speelman P. Validation and nephrotoxicity of a simplified once-daily aminoglycoside dosing schedule and guidelines for monitoring therapy. *Antimicrob Agents Chemother* 1996;40:2494–9.

16 Mohan M, Batty KT, Cooper JA, Wojnar-Horton RE, Ilett KF. Comparison of gentamicin dose estimates derived from manual calculations, the Australian "Therapeutic Guidelines: Antibiotic" nomogram and the SeBA-GEN and DoseCalc software programs. *Br J Clin Pharmacol* 2004;58:521–7.

APPENDIX 3
Antimicrobial drug dose recommendations

Table A.3.1 Antimicrobial drug dose recommendations

Antimicrobial	Indication(s)	Dose (Do Not Exceed Adult Dose)	Notes
Acyclovir	Usual dose, e.g., herpes simplex labialis (cold sores), herpetic whitlow	5–10 mg/kg (max 400 mg) orally, 5 times daily	
	Eczema herpeticum, herpes simplex virus (HSV) encephalitis (except neonatal), ophthalmic herpes zoster, severe mucocutaneous HSV infections, severe varicella	10 mg/kg (max 400 mg) IV, 8-hourly or 1.5 g/m^2/day in three divided doses	Monitor renal function
	Neonatal HSV infection, including disseminated disease, encephalitis, hepatitis, pneumonitis, skin lesions	20 mg/kg IV, 8-hourly (14 days for localized disease, 21 days for encephalitis or disseminated disease)	Monitor renal function
Albendazole (6 months or older)	Community worm programs, hookworm, roundworm, threadworm	≤10 kg: 200 mg, > 10 kg: 400 mg orally, as a single dose	Only recommended for children > 6 months old
	Cutaneous larva migrans, strongyloidiasis, whipworm	≤10 kg: 200 mg, > 10 kg: 400 mg orally, daily	
	Microsporidiosis	≤10 kg: 200 mg, > 10 kg: 400 mg orally, 12-hourly	
	Hydatid disease	> 6 years: 7.5 mg/kg (max 400 mg) 12-hourly, orally	
Amikacin	Term neonates ≤7 days	15 mg/kg IV, daily *OR* 7.5 mg/kg IV, 12-hourly	See Appendix 2 for preterm neonates
	Term neonates > 7 days	22.5 mg/kg IV, daily *OR* 7.5 mg/kg IV, 8-hourly	See Appendix 2 for preterm neonates
	Single daily dose	24 mg/kg (max 1 g) IV, daily	Single daily dosing regimen not recommended for patients with renal impairment or cancer monitor drug levels: for once-daily dosing, take level at 6–14 hours and use nomogram (Appendix 2); or trough < 5 mg/L
	Three times a day	7.5 mg/kg (max 300 mg) IV, 8-hourly	Monitor levels: aim for trough: < 10 mg/L peak: 20–30 mg/L

Table A.3.1 (*Continued*)

Antimicrobial	Indication(s)	Dose (Do Not Exceed Adult Dose)	Notes
Amoxicillin	Usual dose	15 mg/kg (max 500 mg) orally, 8-hourly	
	Cholera	10 mg/kg (max 250 mg) orally, 6-hourly	
	Community-acquired pneumonia	25 mg/kg (max 1 g) orally, 8-hourly	
	Gonococcal conjunctivitis	75 mg/kg (max 3 g) orally, as a single dose	
	Typhoid and paratyphoid fevers	25 mg/kg (max 1 g) orally, 6-hourly	
	Pyelonephritis	25 mg/kg (max 1 g) IV, 6-hourly	
	Severe sepsis	50 mg/kg (max 2 g) IV, 6-hourly	
	Enterococcal endocarditis, meningitis	50 mg/kg (max 2 g) IV, 4-hourly	
	Endocarditis prophylaxis	50 mg/kg (max 2 g) orally or IV, as a single dose	
	Post-splenectomy prophylaxis	<2 years: 20 mg/kg, ≥2 years: 250 mg orally, daily	
Amoxicillin+ clavulanate	Usual dose	22.5 + 3.2 mg/kg (max 875 + 125 mg) orally, 12-hourly	
	Severe infection, e.g., bacterial sinusitis, pneumonia	22.5 + 3.2 mg/kg (max 875 + 125 mg) orally, 8-hourly	
Amphotericin B desoxycholate (conventional)	Candidal sepsis, fungal pneumonia	1 mg/kg IV, daily	
Amphotericin (liposomal)	Systemic aspergillosis, systemic candidiasis, mould infections (*Fusarium*, Zygomycetes)	3 mg/kg IV, daily for candidiasis 3–5 mg/kg IV, daily for aspergillosis 5 mg/kg IV, daily for mould infections	Use instead of conventional amphotericin B if preexisting renal impairment, nephrotoxicity, or severe infusion-related toxicity (dose 1 mg/kg) (see p. 123)
Ampicillin	Usual dose	25 mg/kg (max 1 g) IV, 6-hourly	
	Pyelonephritis	25 mg/kg (max 1 g) IV, 6-hourly	
	Severe sepsis	50 mg/kg (max 2 g) IV, 6-hourly	
	Enterococcal endocarditis, meningitis	50 mg/kg (max 2 g) IV, 4-hourly	
	Endocarditis prophylaxis	50 mg/kg (max 2 g) IV, as a single dose	

(*Continued*)

Table A.3.1 (*Continued*)

Antimicrobial	Indication(s)	Dose (Do Not Exceed Adult Dose)	Notes
Ampicillin-sulbactam	Usual dose	30 mg/kg (max 2 g) of ampicillin IV, 6-hourly	Not licensed for infants and children
	Severe infection	50–100 mg/kg (max 4 g) of ampicillin IV, 6-hourly	
Atovaquone+ proguanil	Uncomplicated *Plasmodium falciparum* malaria	11–20 kg: 1 tablet, 21–30 kg: 2 tablets, 31–40 kg: 3 tablets, > 40 kg: 4 tablets orally, daily (atovaquone+proguanil 250 + 100 mg strength)	Only recommended for children > 10 kg
Azithromycin	*Mycobacterium avium* complex	15 mg/kg (max 600 mg) orally, daily	Only recommended for children > 6 kg
	Pneumonia	10 mg/kg orally, daily	
	Chlamydia trachomatis conjunctivitis, post-sexual assault prophylaxis, gonorrhea, chlamydia	20 mg/kg (max 1 g) orally, as a single dose	
	Salmonella or shigella enteritis	20 mg/kg (max 1 g) orally on the first day, followed by 10 mg/kg (max 500 mg) orally, daily	
	Typhoid	20 mg/kg orally or IV, daily for 5 days	
	Pertussis, cat scratch disease	10 mg/kg (max 500 mg) orally on day 1, then 5 mg/kg orally, daily for 4 days	
	Early syphilis	50 mg/kg (max 2 g) orally, as a single dose	
Aztreonam	Usual dose	30 mg/kg (max 1.2 g) IV, 6–8-hourly	Modify dose in renal failure
	Severe infection	50 mg/kg (max 2 g) IV, 6–8-hourly	
Benzathine penicillin	Rheumatic fever prophylaxis	900 mg (1.5 million U) IM, every 3–4 weeks	Mix 2 mL in syringe with 0.5-mL lignocaine
	Early syphilis	30 mg (50,000 U)/kg (max 1.2 g or 2 million U) IM, as a single dose	
	Late latent syphilis	30 mg (50,000 U)/kg (max 1.2 g or 2 million U) IM, once weekly	For three doses
Benzylpenicillin	Usual dose	30 mg (50,000 U)/kg (max 1.2 g or 2 million U) IV, 4–6-hourly	
	Severe infection, e.g., meningitis, endocarditis, necrotizing fasciitis, tertiary syphilis	60 mg (100,000 U)/kg (max 2.4 g or 4 million U) IV, 4-hourly	

Table A.3.1 (*Continued*)

Antimicrobial	Indication(s)	Dose (Do Not Exceed Adult Dose)	Notes
	Congenital syphilis	30 mg (50,000 U)/kg IV, 12-hourly	For 10 days
	Gonococcal ophthalmia	15 mg/kg IV, 12-hourly during the first week of life, then 7.5 mg/kg 6-hourly	
	Presumptive meningococcal meningitis or sepsis (first dose)	< 1 year: 300 mg (500,000 U); 1–9 years: 600 mg (1 million U); 10 years or more: 1200 mg (2 million U) IV/IM	
Cefaclor	Otitis media	10 mg/kg (max 250 mg) orally, 8-hourly	Second or third line choice
Cefadroxil	Otitis media	15 mg/kg (max 600 mg) orally, 12-hourly	
Cefazolin	Usual dose	15 mg/kg (max 600 mg) IV, 8-hourly	
	Serious staphylococcal infections	25 mg/kg (max 1 g) IV, 8-hourly	
Cefdinir	Streptococcal sore throat	7 mg/kg (max 300 mg) orally, 12-hourly	
Cefixime	Urinary tract infection	4 mg/kg (max 160 mg) orally, 12-hourly	
	Gonorrhea	20 mg/kg (max 800 mg) orally, as a single dose	
Cefepime	Hospital-acquired pneumonia, *Pseudomonas sepsis*, febrile neutropenia	50 mg/kg (max 2 g) IV, 8-hourly	Modify dose in renal failure
Cefotaxime	Usual dose	25 mg/kg (max 1 g) IV, 6–8-hourly	Cefotaxime has no useful activity against *Pseudomonas* modify dose in renal failure
	Severe infection, e.g., brain abscess, meningitis	50–75 mg/kg (max 3 g) IV, 6-hourly	
	Gonorrhea	25 mg/kg (max 1 g) IM, as a single dose	
Cefotetan	Severe infections, pelvic inflammatory disease	40 mg/kg (max 2 g) IV, 12-hourly	Modify dose in renal failure
Cefoxitin	Severe infections	40 mg/kg (max 2 g) IV, 6-hourly	Modify dose in renal failure
Cefpirome	*Pseudomonas sepsis*	50 mg/kg (max 2 g) IV, 12-hourly	Modify dose in renal failure
Cefpodoxime proxetil	Usual dose, e.g., streptococcal sore throat, pneumonia, urinary tract infection	5 mg/kg (max 200 mg) orally, 12-hourly	Modify dose in renal failure
	More severe infection	8 mg/kg (max 320 mg) orally, 12-hourly	
Cefprozil	Otitis media	15 mg/kg (max 600 mg) orally, 12-hourly	Modify dose in renal failure

(*Continued*)

Table A.3.1 (*Continued*)

Antimicrobial	Indication(s)	Dose (Do Not Exceed Adult Dose)	Notes
Ceftazidime	Febrile neutropenia, *Pseudomonas sepsis*	50 mg/kg (max 2 g) IV, 8-hourly	Modify dose in renal failure
	Melioidosis	50 mg/kg (max 2 g) IV, 6-hourly	Modify dose in renal failure
Ceftibuten	Otitis media	9 mg/kg (max 400 mg) orally, daily	Modify dose in renal failure
Ceftriaxone	Usual dose	50 mg/kg (max 2 g) IV, daily	Not recommended in neonates: displaces bilirubin from albumin
	Severe infection, e.g., brain abscess, meningitis	50 mg/kg (max 2 g) IV, 12-hourly *OR* 100 mg/kg (max 4 g) IV, daily	
	Endophthalmitis, presumed meningococcal infection	50 mg/kg (max 2 g) IV, as a single dose	
	Haemophilus influenzae type b meningitis prophylaxis	50 mg/kg (max 2 g) IM, daily for 4 days	
	Typhoid and paratyphoid fevers	75 mg/kg (max 3 g) IV, daily	
	Neisseria gonorrhoeae infection	≤45 kg: 125 mg, >45 kg: 250 mg IM, as a single dose	
	N. meningitidis meningitis prophylaxis	125 mg IM, as a single dose	
Cefuroxime	Otitis media, sinusitis	10–15 mg/kg (max 500 mg) orally, 12-hourly	Modify dose in renal failure
Cephalexin	Usual dose	25 mg/kg (max 1 g) orally, 8-hourly	Modify dose in renal failure
	Epididymoorchitis, cystitis	12.5 mg/kg (max 500 mg) orally, 12-hourly	
	Recurrent urinary tract infection prophylaxis	12.5 mg/kg (max 500 mg) orally, nightly	
	Endocarditis prophylaxis	50 mg/kg (max 2 g) orally, as a single dose	As an alternative if allergic to amoxicillin
Cephalothin	Usual dose	25 mg/kg (max 1 g) IV, 6-hourly	Modify dose in renal failure
	Severe infection	50 mg/kg (max 2 g) IV, 6-hourly	
	Surgical prophylaxis	50 mg/kg (max 2 g) IV, as a single dose	
Cephazolin	Usual dose	25 mg/kg (max 1 g) IV, 6-hourly	Modify dose in renal failure
	Severe sepsis	50 mg/kg (max 1 g) IV, 8-hourly	
	Surgical prophylaxis	25 mg/kg (max 1 g) IV, as a single dose	

Table A.3.1 *(Continued)*

Antimicrobial	Indication(s)	Dose (Do Not Exceed Adult Dose)	Notes
Cephradine	Usual dose	25 mg/kg (max 1 g) orally, 12-hourly	Modify dose in renal failure
	Severe infection	25 mg/kg (max 1 g) IV, 6-hourly	
Chloramphenicol	Rickettsial infections	12.5 mg/kg (max 500 mg) orally/IV, 6-hourly	Because of risk of aplastic anemia use only if no better alternative
	Typhoid and paratyphoid fevers	25 mg/kg (max 750 mg) orally or IV, 6-hourly	
Chloroquine	Malaria prophylaxis	5 mg base/kg orally, weekly	
	Plasmodium vivax, *P. malariae*, and *P. ovale* malaria	10 mg base/kg orally, then 5 mg base/kg 6 hourly later and on days 2 and 3	
Ciprofloxacin	Usual dose	10 mg/kg (max 500 mg) orally, 12-hourly	Caution family about possible risk of Achilles tendonitis
	Severe infection, e.g., *Pseudomonas sepsis*	15 mg/kg (max 600 mg) IV or orally, 12-hourly	
	Cholera	25 mg/kg (max 1 g) orally, as a single dose	
	Endophthalmitis, penetrating eye injuries	15 mg/kg (max 750 mg) orally, as a single dose	
	Typhoid and paratyphoid fevers	15 mg/kg (max 500 mg) orally, 12-hourly *OR* 10 mg/kg (max 400 mg) IV, 12-hourly	
Clarithromycin	Cervical lymphadenitis, *Mycobacterium avium* complex infection, *M. marinum* infection	12.5 mg/kg (max 500 mg) orally, 12-hourly	
	Pertussis	7.5 mg/kg (max 300 mg) orally, 12-hourly	
Clindamycin	Usual dose	10 mg/kg (max 450 mg) IV 8-hourly, then same dose orally 8-hourly	
	Severe infection	15 mg/kg (max 600 mg) IV, 8-hourly	
	Endocarditis prophylaxis	15 mg/kg (max 600 mg) orally/IV, as a single dose	
Cloxacillin	Usual dose	25 mg/kg (max 1 g) orally, 6-hourly	
Co-trimoxazole	See trimethoprim-sulfamethoxazole		

(Continued)

Table A.3.1 (*Continued*)

Antimicrobial	Indication(s)	Dose (Do Not Exceed Adult Dose)	Notes
Dapsone	*Pneumocystis jiroveci* pneumonia (PCP) treatment	2 mg/kg (max 100 mg) orally, daily	
	PCP prophylaxis	2 mg/kg (max 100 mg) orally, daily *OR* 4 mg/kg (max 200 mg) orally, weekly	
Dicloxacillin	Usual dose	12.5 mg/kg (max 500 mg) orally, 6-hourly	
	Moderate infection	25 mg/kg (max 1 g) orally, 6-hourly	
	Severe infection	50 mg/kg (max 2 g) IV, 6-hourly	
	Endocarditis	50 mg/kg (max 2 g) IV, 4-hourly	
	Surgical prophylaxis	50 mg/kg (max 2 g) IV, as a single dose	
Diloxanide furoate	Amebiasis	7 mg/kg (max 500 mg) orally, 8-hourly	
Doxycycline (9 years or older)	Usual dose	2.5 mg/kg (max 100 mg) orally, 12-hourly	
	Malaria prophylaxis	2.5 mg/kg (max 100 mg) orally, daily	
	Bacterial sinusitis	4 mg/kg (max 200 mg) orally, as a single dose, then 2 mg/kg (max 100 mg) orally, daily	
Erythromycin (doses are expressed in terms of erythromycin base. For products containing erythromycin ethyl succinate, multiply the dose by 1.6)	*Chlamydia trachomatis* conjunctivitis, pneumonia	10 mg/kg orally, 6-hourly	
	Campylobacter enteritis, pertussis	10 mg/kg (max 500 mg) orally, 6-hourly	
	Impetigo, cat scratch disease	10 mg/kg (max 500 mg) orally, 12-hourly	
	Severe infection, e.g., pneumonia	10 mg/kg (max 500 mg) IV, 6-hourly	
	Post-splenectomy prophylaxis	250 mg orally, daily	
	Recurrent rheumatic fever prevention	250 mg orally, 12-hourly	Use only if allergic to penicillin

Table A.3.1 (*Continued*)

Antimicrobial	Indication(s)	Dose (Do Not Exceed Adult Dose)	Notes
Ethambutol (6 years or older)	Tuberculosis	15 mg/kg orally, daily *OR* 30 mg/kg orally, three times a week	>6 years old only, and check vision
	Mycobacterium kansasii	25 mg/kg orally, daily	
	M. avium complex infection	25 mg/kg orally, daily for 2 months, then 15 mg/kg daily	
	M. marinum infection	15 mg/kg orally, daily	
Flucloxacillin	Usual dose	12.5 mg/kg (max 500 mg) orally, 6-hourly	
	Moderate infection	25 mg/kg (max 1 g) orally, 6-hourly	
	Severe infection	50 mg/kg (max 2 g) IV, 6-hourly	
	Endocarditis	50 mg/kg (max 2 g) IV, 4-hourly	
	Surgical prophylaxis	50 mg/kg (max 2 g) IV, as a single dose	
Fluconazole	Usual dose, e.g., oral candidiasis	4 mg/kg (max 150 mg) orally, daily	
	Mucocutaneous candidiasis	6 mg/kg (max 300 mg) orally, daily	
	Candida sepsis	6 mg/kg (max 300 mg) IV daily, then same dose orally	
	Cryptococcal pneumonia or meningitis	12 mg/kg (max 800 mg) orally or IV for one dose, then 6 mg/kg (max 400 mg) orally, daily	
Flucytosine	Cryptococcal pneumonia or meningitis	25 mg/kg IV or orally, 6-hourly	Modify dose in renal failure
Foscarnet	CMV retinitis, colitis, or esophagitis	60 mg/kg IV, 8-hourly or continuous infusion	
	Acyclovir-resistant HSV infection	60 mg/kg IV, 12-hourly	
Fusidate sodium or fusidic acid suspension	MRSA osteomyelitis or septic arthritis, recurrent staphylococcal skin infection	12 mg/kg (max 500 mg) orally or IV, 12-hourly fusidic acid suspension 18 mg/kg (max 750 mg) orally, 12-hourly (fusidate sodium 500 mg is equivalent to fusidic acid suspension 750 mg)	Not recommended as sole antibiotic, because of rapid emergence of resistance monitor blood levels and adjust dose
Ganciclovir	Cytomegalovirus colitis, retinitis, or esophagitis	5 mg/kg IV, 12-hourly	

(*Continued*)

Table A.3.1 (*Continued*)

Antimicrobial	Indication(s)	Dose (Do Not Exceed Adult Dose)	Notes
Gentamicin	Term neonates ≤7 days	5 mg/kg IV, daily *OR* 2.5 mg/kg IV, 12-hourly	See Appendix 2 for preterm neonates
	Term neonates >7 days	7.5 mg/kg IV, daily *OR* 2.5 mg/kg IV, 8-hourly	See Appendix 2 for preterm neonates
	Usual dose	< 10 years: 7.5 mg/kg IV daily, 10 years or older: 6 mg/kg IV daily (daily regimen) or 2.5 mg/kg IV 8-hourly (8-hourly regimen)	Modify dose in renal failure single daily dosing regimen not recommended for patients with renal impairment or cancer monitor drug levels: for once-daily dosing, take level at 6–14 hourly and use nomogram (Appendix 2); or trough < 1 mg/L for 8-hourly dosing: aim for peak 5–10 mg/L and trough < 2 mg/L
	Cystic fibrosis	2.5–4 mg/kg (max 80 mg) IV, 8-hourly	Higher doses because of abnormal metabolism
	Brucellosis (< 8 years)	2.5 mg/kg IV, 8-hourly	
	Endocarditis treatment	1 mg/kg IV, 8-hourly	
	Endocarditis prophylaxis	2.5 mg/kg IV, as a single dose	
	Endophthalmitis, penetrating eye injuries	5 mg/kg IV, as a single dose	
	Surgical prophylaxis	2 mg/kg IV, as a single dose	
Griseofulvin	Fungal infections	Ultramicrosize 10 mg/kg (max 750 mg) orally, daily microsize: 10 mg/kg (max 500 mg) orally, 12-hourly	
Imipenem-cilastatin	*Acinetobacter baumanii* pneumonia, melioidosis	25 mg/kg (max 1 g) IV, 6-hourly (dose does not include the cilastatin component)	May cause seizures in meningitis or predisposed children
Isoniazid	Tuberculosis	10 mg/kg (max 300 mg) orally daily *OR* 15 mg/kg (max 600 mg) orally, three times a week	
	Mycobacterium kansasii, tuberculosis chemoprophylaxis	10 mg/kg (max 300 mg) orally daily	
Itraconazole	Usual dose	2.5–5 mg/kg (max 200 mg) orally, 12-hourly	Improved absorption if taken with acid drink, e.g., coca cola
	Pulmonary aspergillosis	7.5 mg/kg (max 300 mg) orally as the capsule, 12-hourly for 3 days, then 5 mg/kg (max 200 mg) orally, 12-hourly	

Table A.3.1 (*Continued*)

Antimicrobial	Indication(s)	Dose (Do Not Exceed Adult Dose)	Notes
Ivermectin (> 5 years)	Crusted (Norwegian) scabies, cutaneous larva migrans	200 µg/kg orally, as a single dose	
Lamivudine	HIV, post-needlestick injury, HIV prophylaxis	4 mg/kg (max 150 mg) orally, 12-hourly	See Chapter 8
	Chronic hepatitis B	3 mg/kg (max 100 mg) orally, daily	
Linezolid	Resistant staphylococcal and enterococcal infections	10 mg/kg (max 400 mg) orally or IV, 8-hourly	May cause myelosuppression
Liposomal amphotericin	See amphotericin (liposomal)		
Loracarbef	Otitis media	15 mg/kg (max 600 mg) orally, 12-hourly	
Mebendazole	Threadworm	Up to 10 kg: 50 mg; > 10 kg: 100 mg, orally, as a single dose	
	Hookworm, roundworm, whipworm	Up to 10 kg: 50 mg, > 10 kg: 100 mg orally, 12-hourly	
Mefloquine	Uncomplicated *Plasmodium falciparum* malaria	15 mg/kg (max 750 mg) orally, then 10 mg/kg (max 500 mg) 6–8 hourly later, both as single doses	
	Malaria prophylaxis	15–19 kg: 1/4 tablet, 20–30 kg: 1/2 tablet, 31–40 kg: 3/4 tablet orally, weekly (mefloquine 250-mg tablets)	
Meropenem	*Acinetobacter baumanii* pneumonia, melioidosis	25 mg/kg (max 1 g) IV, 8-hourly	
	Hospital-acquired meningitis	40 mg/kg (max 2 g) IV, 8-hourly	
Methicillin	Usual dose	25 mg/kg (max 1 g) orally, 6-hourly	
	Moderate infection	40 mg/kg (max 1.6 g) orally, 6-hourly	
	Severe infection	50 mg/kg (max 2 g) IV, 6-hourly	
	Endocarditis	50 mg/kg (max 2 g) IV, 4-hourly	
	Surgical prophylaxis	50 mg/kg (max 2 g) IV, as a single dose	
Metronidazole	Usual dose	10 mg/kg (max 400 mg) orally, 12-hourly	
	Severe sepsis	12.5 mg/kg (max 500 mg) IV, 8–12-hourly	
	Antibiotic-associated diarrhea, *Dientamoeba fragilis* diarrhea, giardiasis (see also single daily dose regimen below)	10 mg/kg (max 400 mg) orally, 8-hourly	

(*Continued*)

Table A.3.1 (*Continued*)

Antimicrobial	Indication(s)	Dose (Do Not Exceed Adult Dose)	Notes
	Giardiasis (single daily dose regimen)	30 mg/kg (max 2 g) orally, daily	
	Amebiasis	15 mg/kg (max 600 mg) orally, 8-hourly	
	Post-sexual assault prophylaxis	50 mg/kg (max 2 g) orally, as a single dose	
	Surgical prophylaxis	12.5 mg/kg (max 500 mg) IV, as a single dose	
Moxifloxacin	Pneumonia	10 mg/kg (max 400 mg) orally or IV, daily	Alternative to penicillin if allergic to penicillin
Nafcillin	Usual dose	25 mg/kg (max 1 g) orally, 6-hourly	
	Moderate infection	40 mg/kg (max 1.6 g) orally, 6-hourly	
	Severe infection	50 mg/kg (max 2 g) IV, 6-hourly	
	Endocarditis	50 mg/kg (max 2 g) IV, 4-hourly	
	Surgical prophylaxis	50 mg/kg (max 2 g) IV, as a single dose	
Nelfinavir	HIV infection	30 mg/kg (max 1.25 g) orally, 8-hourly	
	HIV prophylaxis for high-risk exposures	< 13 years: 55 mg/kg (max 2 g) orally, 12-hourly; > 12 years 1250 mg orally, 12-hourly	For 4 weeks or until source shown to be HIV negative
Nitrofurantoin	Recurrent urinary tract infection prophylaxis	1–2.5 mg/kg (max 100 mg) orally, nightly	
Norfloxacin	Usual dose	10 mg/kg (max 400 mg) orally, 12-hourly	
Nystatin	Oral candidiasis	1 mL of 100,000 units/mL suspension orally, 6-hourly	
Oxacillin	Usual dose	25 mg/kg (max 1 g) orally, 6-hourly	
	Moderate infection	40 mg/kg (max 1.6 g) orally, 6-hourly	
	Severe infection	50 mg/kg (max 2 g) IV, 6-hourly	
	Endocarditis	50 mg/kg (max 2 g) IV, 4-hourly	
	Surgical prophylaxis	50 mg/kg (max 2 g) IV, as a single dose	
Penicillin	See benzathine penicillin or benzylpenicillin or phenoxymethylpenicillin or procaine penicillin		
Pentamidine	PCP treatment	4 mg/kg IV, daily	
	PCP prophylaxis	4 mg/kg IV or nebulized, every 2–4 weeks	

Table A.3.1 (*Continued*)

Antimicrobial	Indication(s)	Dose (Do Not Exceed Adult Dose)	Notes
Phenoxymethyl penicillin	Pharyngitis, tonsillitis	10 mg/kg (max 500 mg) orally, 12-hourly	
	Balanitis, cellulitis, erysipelas, impetigo	10 mg/kg (max 500 mg) orally, 6-hourly	
	Post-splenectomy prophylaxis	<2 years: 125 mg; 2 years or older: 250 mg orally, 12-hourly	
	Recurrent rheumatic fever prevention	250 mg orally, 12-hourly	
Piperacillin	Severe sepsis, including *Pseudomonas*	100 mg/kg (max 4 g) IV, 8-hourly	
Piperacillin+ tazobactam	Severe sepsis, including *Pseudomonas*	100 + 12.5 mg/kg (max 4 + 0.5 g) IV, 8-hourly	
Praziquantel	*Schistosoma haematobium* infection, *S. mansoni* infection	20 mg/kg orally (two doses, 4 hourly apart)	
	S. japonicum infection, *S. mekongi* infection	20 mg/kg orally (three doses, 4 hourly apart)	
	Beef tapeworm, pork tapeworm	10 mg/kg orally, as a single dose	
	Dwarf tapeworm	25 mg/kg orally, as a single dose	
Primaquine	*Plasmodium vivax* (acquired outside Southeast Asia and the Pacific Islands), *P. ovale*	0.3 mg/kg (max 15 mg) orally, daily	
	P. vivax (acquired in Southeast Asia or the Pacific Islands)	0.5 mg/kg (max 30 mg) orally, daily with food *OR* if nausea occurs, 0.25 mg/kg (max 15 mg) orally, 12-hourly	
Procaine penicillin	Congenital or early syphilis	30 mg (50,000 U)/kg (max 1.5 g or 2.4 million U) IM, daily	For 10 days
	Tertiary syphilis	60 mg (100,000 U)/kg (max 2.4 g or 4 million U) IM, daily	For 14 days
	Cellulitis, erysipelas	50 mg (80,000 U)/kg (max 1.5 g or 2.4 million U) IM, daily	
	Bites and clenched fist injuries	50 mg (80,000 U)/kg (max 1.5 g or 2.4 million U) IM, as a single dose	
Proguanil	Malaria prophylaxis	<2 years: 50 mg, 2–6 years: 100 mg, 7–10 years: 150 mg, >10 years: 200 mg orally, daily	
Pyrantel	Threadworm	10 mg/kg (max 750 mg) orally, as a single dose	
	Hookworm, roundworm	20 mg/kg (max 750 mg) orally, as a single dose	

(*Continued*)

Table A.3.1 (*Continued*)

Antimicrobial	Indication(s)	Dose (Do Not Exceed Adult Dose)	Notes
Pyrazinamide	Tuberculosis	25 mg/kg (max 1 g) orally daily OR 50 mg/kg (max 2 g) orally, thrice weekly	
Pyrimethamine	Toxoplasma encephalitis or cysts	2.5 mg/kg (max 100 mg) orally, then 1 mg/kg (max 25 mg) orally, daily	Give daily folinic acid 5 mg (adult dose) or folic acid supplementation
Pyrimethamine+ sulfadoxine	*Plasmodium falciparum* malaria	6 weeks to < 1 year: 1/4 tablet, 1–3 years: 1/2 tablet, 4–8 years: 1 tablet, 9–14 years: 2 tablets orally, as a single dose (pyrimethamine+sulfadoxine 25 + 500 mg)	
Quinine dihydrochloride	Severe *Plasmodium falciparum* malaria	**Loading dose:** 20 mg/kg (max 1.4 g) in 5% dextrose IV over 4 hourly OR 7 mg/kg (max 500 mg) IV over 30 min followed immediately by 10 mg/kg (max 700 mg) over 4 hourly **Maintenance dose:** 10 mg/kg (max 700 mg) IV, 8-hourly over 4 hourly	
Quinine sulfate	Uncomplicated *Plasmodium falciparum* malaria	10 mg/kg (max 600 mg) orally, 8-hourly	
Quinupristin/ dalfopristin	Vancomycin-resistant enterococcal infection	7.5 mg/kg IV, 8-hourly	
Rifabutin	*M. avium* complex infection	5 mg/kg (max 300 mg) orally, daily	
Rifampin or rifampicin	Usual dose	10 mg/kg (max 600 mg) orally daily	Not recommended as sole antibiotic, because of rapid emergence of resistance
	Tuberculosis	10 mg/kg (max 600 mg) orally, daily OR 15 mg/kg (max 600 mg) orally, thrice weekly	
	Haemophilus influenzae type b meningitis prophylaxis	< 1 month: 10 mg/kg; ≥1 month: 20 mg/kg (max 600 mg) orally, daily for 4 days	
	Neisseria meningitidis prophylaxis	< 1 month: 5 mg/kg; ≥1 month: 10 mg/kg (max 600 mg) orally, 12-hourly for 2 days	
	Brucellosis	15 mg/kg (max 600 mg) orally, daily	
Roxithromycin	Usual dose	4 mg/kg (max 150 mg) orally, 12-hourly	
Sulfadiazine	Toxoplasma encephalitis or cysts	50 mg/kg (max 1.5 g) orally, 6-hourly	
Teicoplanin	*Staphylococcus aureus* infections	10 mg/kg (max 400 mg) IV, 12-hourly for three doses, then 6 mg/kg (max 400 mg) IV, daily	
	Endocarditis prophylaxis	10 mg/kg (max 400 mg) IV, as a single dose	

Table A.3.1 *(Continued)*

Antimicrobial	Indication(s)	Dose (Do Not Exceed Adult Dose)	Notes
Terbinafine	Tinea capitis, tinea corporis, tinea cruris, tinea pedis, tinea unguium	< 20 kg: 62.5 mg, 20–40 kg: 125 mg, ≥40 kg: 250 mg orally, daily	
Ticarcillin	Severe sepsis, including *Pseudomonas*	50 mg/kg (max 3g) IV, 6-hourly	
Ticarcillin+ clavulanate	Usual dose for sepsis	50 + 1.7 mg/kg (max 3 + 0.1 g) IV, 6-hourly	
	Pseudomonas sepsis	50 + 1.7 mg/kg (max 3 + 0.1 g) IV, 4-hourly	
Tinidazole	Giardiasis, Trichomonas, post-sexual assault prophylaxis	50 mg/kg (max 2 g) orally, as a single dose	
	Amebiasis	50 mg/kg (max 2 g) orally, daily	
Tobramycin	*Pseudomonas sepsis*	< 10 years: 7.5 mg/kg, ≥10 years: 6 mg/kg IV, daily	Modify dose in renal failure monitor drug levels: for once-daily dosing, take level at 6–14 hourly and use nomogram (Appendix 2); and/or trough < 1 mg/L; for 8-hourly dosing: aim for peak 5–10 mg/L and trough < 2 mg/L
	Cystic fibrosis	< 5 years: 40 mg, 5–10 years: 80 mg, > 10 years: 160 mg nebulized 12-hourly	
Trimethoprim	Recurrent urinary tract infection prophylaxis	2 mg/kg (max 150 mg) orally, nightly	
	Cystitis, epididymoorchitis, pyelonephritis	4 mg/kg (max 150 mg) orally, 12-hourly	
Trimethoprim+ sulfamethoxazole (co-trimoxazole)	Usual dose	4 + 20 mg/kg (max 160 + 800 mg) orally, 12-hourly	
	PCP treatment	5 + 25 mg/kg IV, 6-hourly	
	PCP prophylaxis	4 + 20 mg/kg (max 80 + 400 mg) or 8 + 40 mg/kg (max 160 + 800 mg) orally, daily or 4 + 20 mg/kg (max 80 + 400 mg) orally, thrice weekly	
	Isospora belli gastroenteritis	4 + 20 mg/kg (max 160 + 800 mg) orally, 6-hourly	
	Listeria monocytogenes meningitis	5 + 25 mg/kg (max 160 + 800 mg) IV, 6-hourly	
	Melioidosis	8 + 40 mg/kg (max 320 + 1600 mg) orally or IV, 12-hourly	

(Continued)

Table A.3.1 (*Continued*)

Antimicrobial	Indication(s)	Dose (Do Not Exceed Adult Dose)	Notes
Vancomycin	Usual dose, e.g., methicillin-resistant *Staphylococcus aureus* or *S. epidermidis* infections	25 mg/kg [child < 12 years 30 mg/kg] (max dose 1 g) IV, 12-hourly *OR* 15 mg/kg (max 600 mg) IV, 8-hourly	
	Severe infection, e.g., brain abscess, pneumococcal meningitis, severe sepsis	15 mg/kg (max 1 g) IV, 6-hourly *OR* 30 mg/kg (max 2 g) IV, 12-hourly	
	Pseudomembranous colitis	10 mg/kg (max 125 mg) orally, 6-hourly	
	Endocarditis prophylaxis, endophthalmitis, eye injuries	20 mg/kg (max 1 g) IV, as a single dose	
	Surgical prophylaxis	15 mg/kg (max 1 g) IV, as a single dose	
Voriconazole	Invasive pulmonary aspergillosis	6 mg/kg IV, 12-hourly for two doses, then 4 mg/kg IV or orally, 12-hourly	
Zidovudine	HIV infection	10 mg/kg (max 300 mg) orally, 12-hourly	

Index

Acetaminophen, 61–62
Acinetobacter baumanii, 140
Acquired immunodeficiency syndrome (AIDS), 102
Actinomycosis, 160
Activated protein C
  in severe sepsis, 247
Acute bronchitis, 185
Acute diskitis, 159–160
Acute disseminated encephalomyelitis (ADEM),
  146–147
Acute gastroenteritis, 74–82
  antibiotics and, 79–80
  antiemetics in, 80
  dehydration in, 74–75
  diet in, 80–81
    breast-feeding, 80
    soy fiber in, 81
    vitamin A in, 81
    zinc in, 81
  management guidelines, 82
  nitazoxanide in, 82
  ORS in, 78
  probiotics in, 81–82
  rehydration in, 75–77
    calculations of, 76*b*
    IV fluids for, 79
Acute laryngotracheobronchitis, 180–181
Acute osteomyelitis, 156–159
  antibiotic therapy in, 158–159
    delivery mode in, 159
    duration of, 159
  bone scan in, 157
  clinical features of, 156
  CT scans, 157
  diagnosis of, 156–157
  imaging in, 156–157
  laboratory tests in, 156–157
  MRI in, 157
  organisms in, 157–158

Acute otitis media (AOM), 166–169
  antibiotics for, 167–169
  diagnosis of, 166
  organisms in, 166–167
  recurrent, 169
  treatment of, 167–169
Acute phase reactants, 59–60
Acute rheumatic fever, 22–26
  antibiotic prophylaxis of, 25–26
  diagnosis of, 24
  prevention of, 24–25
  treatment of, 25
Acute tonsillitis, 176–180
Acyclovir, 44, 145, 186, 218, 286, 287, 290, 291,
  294
ADEM. *See* Acute disseminated encephalomyelitis
Adenovirus, 43
ADH. *See* Antidiuretic hormone
Agropyron caninum, 229
AIDS. *See* Acquired immunodeficiency syndrome
Albendazole, 95, 230, 257
Algorithms
  bacterial meningitis management, 135*f*
  febrile child management, 58*f*
Amebiasis, 88–89
Amebic dysentery, 88–89
Amebic liver abscess, 89
American Medical Association, 21
Amikacin, 50
Aminoglycosides, 17, 21, 119, 159, 171–172, 275
Amoxicillin, 12, 40, 41, 134, 168–169, 169, 175, 176, 187, 189,
  193, 219, 225, 237, 238, 243, 275
Amoxicillin-clavulanate, 10, 12, 158, 162, 170
Amphotericin, 20, 50, 123, 149, 192–193
Amphotericin B, 122
Ampicillin, 134, 219, 225
Ancylostoma braziliense, 229
Ancylostoma duodenale, 95, 229
Anthrax, 226

Antibiotics, 60–61, 146. *See also specific types*
    broad-spectrum, 9–10, 11–12
    bronchiectasis, 195
    cystic fibrosis, 197
    diarrhea associated with, 82–83
    dose and duration, 10, 12
    febrile neutropenia and, 118–120
    for AOM, 167–169
    for bacterial meningitis, 134–137, 138*t*
    for bites, 224–225
    for bronchiectasis, 195
    for bronchiolitis, 184
    for common cold, 173–174
    for community-acquired pneumonia, 186–187
    for cystic fibrosis, 195–196
    for cystitis, 275
    for GAS, 177–178
    for necrotizing skin infections, 232–233
    for OME, 170
    for pyelonephritis, 275–276
    for severe sepsis, 243–244
    for sore throat, 177
    for UTIs, 278–279
    in acute gastroenteritis, 79–80
    in acute osteomyelitis, 158–159
    in cellulitis, 229
    in cervical lymphadenopathy, 33
    in erysipelas, 229
    in fever management, 60–61
    intermittent catheterization and, 280
    measles and, 288–289
    mucosal penetration, 11
    multiple, 12
    narrow-spectrum, 9–10, 11–12
    oral, 12
    parenteral, 12
    population use of, 10
    prehospital treatment of, 249–250
    prevention, 12
    reducing use of, 11
    resistance, 9–12
    single, 12
    topical, 10–11, 12
Antidiuretic hormone (ADH), 79
Antiemetics, in acute gastroenteritis, 80
Antifungals, 121, 122, 123
Antihistamines, 169
    common cold and, 174
    for chronic OME, 171
Antimicrobials, 12, 16, 33, 51, 67, 148
Antipyretics, in fever management, 61–62
AOM. *See* Acute otitis media
Artemether, 259

Artesunate, 260
Arthritis, 162
Aspergillus, 142, 191
    allergic bronchopulmonary, 191
    invasive pulmonary, 191–192
Aspirin, 25, 65–66
Asplenia, 125–126
    antibiotic prophylaxis for, 126
    immunization for, 126
    reducing risk of, 127*t*
Atovaquone-proguanil, 264
Azithromycin, 25, 34, 48, 67, 83, 84, 86, 88, 178, 182, 186, 187, 203, 213, 217, 219, 220

Bacillus anthracis, 226–228
Bacitracin, 43, 44, 45, 47, 49
Bacterial meningitis, 132–141
    algorithms for management of, 135*f*
    antibiotics for, 134–137
    aseptic, 144
    chemoprophylaxis, 138–139
    clinical diagnosis of, 132
    cochlear implants, 140
    corticosteroids for, 137–138
    IV fluids for, 138
    recurrent, 140
    skull fracture and, 139–140
    treatment of, 134–138
        in neonates, 134–136
Bacterial vaginosis, 214
Balanitis, 211
Balanoposthitis, 211
Bartonella, 20, 66–67, 157
BCG vaccine, 199
Benzathine penicillin, 26, 178, 179, 217, 231
Benzyl benzoate, 235
Benzylpenicillin, 17, 35, 36, 37, 60, 61, 142, 143, 147, 186, 187, 189, 193, 217, 249*t*, 250, 252
    streptococci-resistance to, 18
Beta-lactam, 10, 119
Bilharziasis, 265–266
Bites, 224–226
    immunization and, 225–226
    prophylactic antibiotics for, 224–225
Blastocystis, 82, 89
Blepharokeratoconjunctivitis, 48
Blood cultures, 15, 20, 49, 63, 124, 142, 156, 196
Boils, 226–228
Bordetella parapertussis, 181
Bordetella pertussis, 181
Borrelia burgdorferi, 67–68, 147
Brain abscesses, 142–143
Brazilian purpuric fever, 43

Breast-feeding
    gastroenteritis and, 80
    in TB, 202
    MTCT and, 110–111
Bronchiectasis, 195
    antibiotics for, 195
    physical therapy for, 195
Bronchiolitis, 182–185
    antibiotics for, 184
    bronchodilators for, 183
    chest physiotherapy for, 184
    corticosteroids for, 183–184
    epinephrine for, 183
    palivizumab, 184–185
    ribavirin for, 183
    RSV immunoglobulin, 184
    surfactant for, 184
    treatment of, 183–184
Bronchodilators
    for bronchiolitis, 183
Brucellosis, 256
Budesonide, 180
Burkholderia cepacia, 197
Burkholderia pseudomallei, 264

C-reactive protein (CRP), 156, 159
Caesarean section, 110
Campylobacter enteritis, 83
Campylobacter jejuni, 150
Candida, 15, 20, 47, 123, 192, 211
Candidosis, 123
Carbuncles, 226–228
Cardiac infections, 14–25
Case-control studies, 3
Cat scratch disease, 34, 66–67
Catheter-associated bacteriuria, 279–280
Catheter-associated candiduria, 279
Cefazolin, 40, 41, 49
Cefdinir, 170, 179, 187
Cefepime, 190
Cefixime, 213, 215, 275
Cefotaxime, 14, 36, 40, 41, 45, 61, 134, 136, 142, 147, 172,
    184, 186, 189, 194, 213, 215, 225, 226, 236, 243, 244,
    250
Cefotetan, 219
Cefpodoxime, 168, 170, 176, 178–179, 187
Ceftazidime, 50, 119, 141, 142, 158
Ceftriaxone, 17, 40, 41, 45, 61, 68, 86, 136, 139, 142, 143, 147,
    189, 213, 215, 220, 225, 250, 251, 264
Cefuroxime, 40, 170, 176, 178, 186, 187, 188, 189
Cellulitis, 228–229. *See* Periocular cellulitis
    antibiotic treatment of, 229
    perianal, 233–234

Cephalexin, 33, 40, 49, 158, 178, 215, 228, 231, 275
Cephalothin, 162, 188, 229, 234, 237, 238, 244, 252
Cephazolin, 162, 188, 229, 234, 237, 238, 244, 252
Cerebrospinal fluid (CSF), 60
    glucose, 134
    lactate, 134
    microscopy, 144
    organisms in, 134
    PCR testing, 144–145
    pleocytosis, 144*b*
    protein, 134
    rapid bacterial assays on, 134
    white count, 134
Cervical infections, 29–37
Cervical intraepithelial neoplasia (CIN), 218
Cervical lymphadenopathy, 29–34
    acute presentation of, 29–30
    bilateral, 30
    causes of, 29, 30*t*
    chronic presentation of, 29–30
    examination of, 31–32
    fine needle aspiration in, 32, 33
    hematology in, 32
    history, 29–31
        age, 31
        cat contact, 30–31
        dental infections, 31
        exposure, 31
    investigation of, 32
    neck swelling in, 30
    PCR in, 33
    treatment of, 33–34
        antibiotic, 33
        cat scratch disease, 34
        daily regimen, 34
        for atypical mycobacterial infections, 34
        surgical, 33
    tuberculin skin testing in, 32–33
    unilateral, 30
Cervicofacial actinomycosis, 35
CGD. *See* Chronic granulomatous disease
Chalazion, 48–49
Chemoprophylaxis
    in bacterial meningitis, 138–139
    in infective endocarditis, 21–22, 23*t*
Chest physiotherapy, for bronchiolitis, 184
Chest radiography, 60, 147, 257
Chicken pox, 290
Chlamydia, 181, 213
Chloramphenicol, 45
Chloroquine, 259, 261, 264
    resistance to, 263–264
Cholera, 83–84

Chorioretinitis, 50
   cytomegalovirus, 50–51
   toxoplasma, 51
Chronic bronchitis, 185
Chronic dacryocystitis, 47
Chronic granulomatous disease (CGD), 227
Chronic osteomyelitis, 160
Chronic recurrent multifocal osteomyelitis (CRMO),
     160–161
Chronic renal damage, 277–278
Chronic suppurative otitis media (CSOM),
     171–172
Cilastatin, 190
CIN. *See* Cervical intraepithelial neoplasia
Ciprofloxacin, 11, 45, 48, 50, 83, 84, 86, 88, 137, 139, 158, 162,
     172, 196, 225, 226, 236, 244, 250, 251
Clarithromycin, 34, 182, 186, 187, 203, 237, 265
Clavulanate, 162, 173, 176, 189, 225, 238
Clindamycin, 10, 33, 36, 37, 40, 41, 51, 91, 158, 162,
     188, 193, 225, 227, 228, 229, 231, 232, 234, 238, 244,
     252
Clinical Evidence, 2
Clostridium difficile, 11, 82
Clostridium perfringens, 231
Clotrimazole, 214
CNS shunt infections, 140–141
Cochlear implants, bacterial meningitis and, 140
Cochrane Collaboration, 1–2
Cochrane Library, 1–2, 4*f*
Cochrane reviews, 2, 3–5, 21, 25, 43
Cochrane, Archie, 1
Cohort studies, 2–3
Colony-stimulating factors
   febrile neutropenia and, 124–125
   in severe sepsis, 247
Common cold, 173–175
   antibiotics for, 173–174
   antihistamines and, 174
   decongestants and, 174
   vitamin C and, 174
   zinc and, 174–175
Computed tomography (CT), 232
   in acute osteomyelitis, 156–157
   in hepatic hydatid cysts, 257
   in mastoiditis, 172–173
   in recurrent bacterial meningitis, 140
Conjunctivitis, 41–45
   acute hemorrhagic, 42
   chemical, 45
   chlamydia, 46
   chronic, 47–48
   clinical features of, 42–43
   from *S. aureus,* 46–47
   gonococcal, 42

HSV, 42
   neonatal, 46
   meningococcal, 42
   organisms causing, 41–42
   treatment of, 43–45
      bacterial, 44–45
      gonococcal, 45
      HSV, 44
      meningococcal, 45
      viral, 44
Conjunctivitis-otitis syndrome, 42
Corticosteroids, 25, 146
   for bacterial meningitis, 137–138
   for bronchiolitis, 183–184
   for OME, 170
   for PCP, 191
   in KD, 65–66
   in meningococcal infection, 250–251
   in septic shock, 246
   TB and, 202
Corynebacterium diphtheriae, 20
CRMO. *See* Chronic recurrent multifocal osteomyelitis
Crotamiton, 235
Croup, 180–181
CRP. *See* C-reactive protein
Cryptococcal meningitis, 149
Cryptococcus neoformans
   pneumonia, 192–193
Cryptosporidium, 82, 89–90, 102
CSF. *See* Cerebrospinal fluid
CSOM. *See* Chronic suppurative otitis media
CT. *See* Computed tomography
Cutaneous larva migrans, 229–230
Cyclic neutropenia, 70
Cystic fibrosis, 195–196
   elective admission for, 196–197
   hypertonic saline for, 198
   nebulized antibiotics for, 197
   physical therapy for, 198
   rhDNase for, 198
Cystitis, 273–274
   antibiotic treatment for, 275
Cytokines, 251
Cytomegalovirus, 283–284
   opportunistic, 284*t*
Cytomegalovirus chorioretinitis, 50–51

Dacryoadenitis, 49
Dacryocystitis, 49
Decongestants, 169
   common cold and, 174
   for chronic OME, 171
Deep neck infections, 35–36
   clinical features of, 35*t*

Dehydration
  in acute gastroenteritis, 74–75
    replacement fluids, 76*b*
    severe, 77
Dental infections
  in cervical lymphadenopathy, 31
Dexamethasone, 137, 156, 162, 172, 173, 180
Di/flucl/oxa/nafcillin, 17, 19, 21, 33, 40, 41, 49, 61, 143,
    158, 162, 187, 188, 227, 229, 231, 234, 237, 238, 243,
    252
Diagnosis
  evidence about, 3
  searching for queries about, 7–8
Diarrhea
  antibiotic-associated, 82–83
  traveler's, 86–88
Diet
  in acute gastroenteritis, 80–81
Dihydroartemisinin-piperaquine, 259
Diloxanide furoate, 89
Dimercaptosuccinic acid (DMSA), 274, 277
Directly observed therapy (DOT), 201
  TB, 202
DMSA. *See* Dimercaptosuccinic acid
DOT. *See* Directly observed therapy
Doxycycline, 19, 68, 84, 215, 219, 256, 259, 264, 265

EBM. *See* Evidence-based medicine
EBV. *See* Epstein-Barr virus
Echinococcus granulosus, 95, 257
Echocardiography, 16*b*
  in infective endocarditis, 15
  in KD, 64
ECMO. *See* Extracorporeal membrane oxygenation
Eczema herpeticum, 287
EHEC enteritis. *See* Enterohemorrhagic *E. coli* enteritis
EIA. *See* Enzyme immunoassay
Endophthalmitis, 49–50
Entamoeba, 82, 88–89
Enterobius, 212
Enterobius vermicularis, 95
Enterococcus faecalis, 18, 140
Enterococcus faecium, 18
Enterohemorrhagic *E. coli* (EHEC) enteritis, 84
Enteropathogenic *E. coli* (EPEC) enteritis, 84
Enterotoxigenic *E. coli* (ETEC), 87
Enzyme immunoassay (EIA), 67
EPEC enteritis. *See* Enteropathogenic *E. coli* enteritis
Epididymo-orchitis, 214–215
Epinephrine, 180
  for bronchiolitis, 183
Epstein-Barr virus (EBV), 284–285
Erysipelas, 229, 232
Erythromycin, 10, 26, 46, 83, 84, 182, 186

ESBL. *See* Extended spectrum betalactamase
Escherichia coli, 10, 49, 140. *See also* Enterohemorrhagic *E. coli*
    enteritis; Enteropathogenic *E. coli* enteritis;
    Enterotoxigenic *E. coli*
ETEC. *See* Enterotoxigenic *E. coli*
Ethambutol, 148, 203, 237
Evidence-based medicine (EBM), 1
  diagnosis in, 3
  etiology in, 3
  framing questions in, 3
  hierarchy in, 2–3
  prognosis in, 3
  searching literature in, 3–8
Evidence-based practice, 1–8
Extended spectrum betalactamase (ESBL), 9
Extracorporeal membrane oxygenation (ECMO)
  in severe sepsis, 247
Eye infections, 40–51

Famciclovir, 44, 218, 291
Familial Hibernian fever (FHF), 70
Familial Mediterranean fever (FMF), 69–70
Febrifuge, 264
Febrile neutropenia, 117–125
  clinical features, 117
  duration of treatment, 120
  empiric antibiotic treatment of, 118–120
  laboratory markers of, 117–118
  organisms causing, 117
  outpatient management, 120
  persistent fever and, 120–124
  preventive therapy for, 124–125
    colony-stimulating factors to, 124–125
Fever, 55–70
  acute phase reactants in, 59–60
  age and, 56–57
  chest radiograph in, 60
  clinical assessment of, 57
  comparative features of, 69*t*
  CSF in, 60
  defined, 55
  focus of infection in, 59
  height of, 56
  investigation of, 59–60
  management, 60–62
    antibiotics in, 60–61
    antipyretics in, 61–62
    recommendations, 62*b*
  management algorithm, 58*f*
  measuring, 55–56
  of unknown origin, 68
  physical reduction methods for, 62
  prolonged, 68
    neutropenia and, 120–124

Fever (*Cont.*)
  recurrent, 68–70
  toxicity and, 57–58, 59*b*
  urinalysis and urine culture in, 60
  UTI and, 273
  white blood count in, 59
  with petechial rash, 62–63
  with purpura, 62–63
FHF. *See* Familial Hibernian fever
Fine needle aspiration (FNA)
  for mycobacterial infection, 33
  in cervical lymphadenopathy, 32
Fluconazole, 121, 122, 123, 149, 192, 193, 214, 279
Flucytosine, 20, 149, 193
Fluid requirements, 75*t*, 76*b*
Fluid therapy
  for malaria, 261–262
  in severe sepsis, 244–245
Flumethasone, 173
FMF. *See* Familial Mediterranean fever
FNA. *See* Fine needle aspiration
Folliculitis, 230
Framycetin, 10, 45, 172, 173
Furuncles, 226–228
Fusidate sodium, 158
Fusidic acid, 12
Fusobacterium necrophorum, 37

Ganciclovir, 51, 284
GAS infection. *See* Group A streptococcal
Gastrointestinal infections, 74–95
GBS. *See* Group B streptococcal
GCS. *See* Glasgow Coma Score
Gentamicin, 10, 17, 18, 19, 20, 21, 60, 91, 143, 144, 173, 186,
    189, 190, 196, 197, 219, 237, 238, 275
Giardia, 82, 90
Glandular fever, 179
Glasgow Coma Score (GCS), 133
Globe, infections of, 49–51
Glycemic control, in severe sepsis, 246
Glycopeptides, 21, 123–124
Gonococcal ophthalmia neonatorum, 45–46
Gramicidin, 172, 173
Group A streptococcal (GAS) infection, 22, 24, 176
  antibiotics for, 177–178
  rapid diagnosis of, 177
  vulvovaginitis, 212
Group B streptococcal (GBS) infection, 212
Guillain-Barré syndrome, 150

H. aegyptius, 43
H. influenzae, 41, 137, 140, 157, 166, 172, 176, 178, 194, 195
HAART. *See* Highly active antiretroviral therapy
HACEK organisms, 15
Head lice, 233

Helicobacter pylori, 91
Hematology, in cervical lymphadenopathy, 32
Hepatic hydatid cysts, 257
Hepatitis A, 92
Hepatitis B, 92–94
  babies born to mothers with, 93
  immunization, 92–93
  post-exposure prophylaxis, 93–94, 220
  prevention of, 92–94
  treatment of, 94
Hepatitis C, 94
Herpes simplex virus (HSV), 285–287
  conjunctivitis, 42, 44, 46
  encephalitis, 145–146
  genital infection, 218
  gingivostomatitis, 286
  in immunocompromised children, 287
  neonatal, 285–286
  prevention of, 286–287
  recurrent, 286–287
Highly active antiretroviral therapy (HAART), 102–103,
    104–106
  combinations, 105–106
  drug interactions, 105
  in children, 106*t*
  when to start, 104–105
HIV infection, 29, 89–90, 102–113, 137, 216, 217, 225
  clinical presentation of, 102–103
  diagnosis of, 103–104
  IgG antibodies and, 103
  IgM antibodies and, 104
  immunization, 107
  management issues, 107
  MTCT and, 108–111
  needlestick exposure to, 112
  PCP prophylaxis in, 106–107
  PCR and, 104
  post-exposure prophylaxis, 111–113
  prophylaxis, 220
  sexual exposure to, 112
  slow progressors, 102
  tests for, 103*t*
  transmission risks, 111
  treating opportunistic infections in, 107
  viral antigen, 103
  viral culture, 103
  web sites on, 113
Hookworms, 95, 229
HPV. *See* Human papillomavirus
HSV. *See* Herpes simplex virus
HSV encephalitis, 145–146
Human papillomavirus (HPV), 218–219
Hydatid disease, 257
Hyperbaric oxygen, 233
Hyperimmunoglobulin D (hyper-IgD) syndrome, 70

Hypernatremia, 75
Hypertonic saline, for cystic fibrosis, 198

IgG antibodies, 103–104
Imipenem, 190
Immune deficiency, 117–127
Immune reconstitution syndrome (IRS), 102–103
Immunization, 12
    asplenia, 126
    bites and, 225–226
Immunofluorescent antibodies (IFA), 67, 283
Impetigo, 230–231
Infants, febrile, 56–57
Infectious mononucleosis, 179
Infective endocarditis, 14–22
    chemoprophylaxis for, 21–22, 23t
    clinical presentation of, 14
    complicated, 18
    diagnosis of, 15–16
        blood cultures, 15
        echocardiography, 15
    organisms causing, 14–15
    risk for, 22t
    treatment of, 16–21
        antimicrobials, 16–17
        blood parameters in, 21
        cat scratch, 19
        culture-negative, 20
        empiric, 17
        enterococcal, 18–19
        fungal, 20
        HACEK group, 19
        penicillin allergy and, 20
        prosthetic material, 19–20
        S. aureus, 19
        streptococcal, 17–18
        surgical, 16
Influenza, 181
Inotropes, 245–246
Insecticide-treated bed nets, 262
Interferon-gamma assays, and TB, 200
Intermittent catheterization, 280
Intracranial pressure (ICP), 133
Intravenous immunoglobulin (IVIG), 66, 146, 150
    for necrotizing skin infections, 233
    in KD, 64
    in severe sepsis, 246
Intravenous therapy (IVT), 77
Iodonoquil, 89
Iridocyclitis, 50
Isoniazid, 34, 200, 201, 203
Isospora belli, 91
Itraconazole, 122, 191, 214
Ivermectin, 95, 230, 236
IVIG. *See* Intravenous immunoglobulin

Janeway lesions, 14
Juvenile idiopathic arthritis (JIA), 70

Kawasaki disease (KD), 63–64
    aspirin in, 65
    corticosteroids in, 65–66
    diagnostic criteria for, 64b
    echocardiography in, 64
    investigations in, 64b
    IVIG in, 64
    laboratory tests for, 63–64
    management of, 64
        in treatment-resistant children, 66
KD. *See* Kawasaki disease
Keratoconjunctivitis, 48
Kingella kingae, 157
Klebsiella, 49, 91, 160, 193

Lactose-free formula, 80
Lamivudine, 108, 220
Lateral pharyngeal abscess, 36
Legionella, 20
Lemierre syndrome, 37, 193
Leukemia, 125
Liposomal amphotericin, 121, 122
Listeria monocytogenes, 49, 134
Liver abscesses, 91
Lopinavir, 220
Lower respiratory tract infections, 182–203
Ludwig angina, 36–37
Lumbar puncture (LP), 132–134
    delayed, 133–134
Lumefantrine, 259, 264
Lung abscess, 193
Lyme disease, 67–68
Lyme meningitis, 147

MAC. *See Mycobacterium avium* complex
Macrolide, 10, 197–198
Magnetic resonance imaging (MRI)
    in acute osteomyelitis, 157
Malaria, 257–264
    adjunctive therapy for, 260
    antimalarials for severe, 260
    chemoprophylaxis, 262–263
        recommendations on, 263
    chloroquine-resistant, 263–264
    emergency treatment of, 264
    fluid therapy for, 261–262
    prevention of, 262–264
    treatment of, 258–262
Malassezia, 230
Mastoiditis, 172–173
    acute, 172
    chronic-173, 172

McIsaac scoring system, 177*b*
MDR organisms. *See* Multi-drug-resistant organisms
Measles, 287–290
  immunization, 289
  post-exposure prophylaxis, 289
  prevention of, 289–290
  treatment of, 287–289
    antibiotics, 288–289
    vitamin A, 287–288, 289–290
Mebendazole, 95, 212
Medline, 2, 6
Mefloquine, 261, 264
Meibomian abscess, 49
Melioidosis, 264–265
Meningitis, 132–151
Meningococcal infection, 63
  antibiotic treatment of, 249–250
  chemoprophylaxis for, 251
  clinical diagnosis of, 248–249
  corticosteroids in, 250–251
  immunization, 251–252
  management of, 248–252
Meropenem, 119, 136, 141, 190, 232
Meta-analysis, 2
  searching for, 6
Methicillin-resistant *S. aureus* (MRSA), 189
Metronidazole, 36, 37, 83, 89, 142, 143, 193, 214, 219, 220, 225, 238
Microsporidium, 91
Micturating cystourethrogram, 276
Modified Duckett Jones criteria, 24
Modified Duke criteria, 15–16
  simplified, 16*b*
Monoclonal antibodies
  in meningococcal infection, 251
  in systemic sepsis, 247
  meningococcal infection in, 251
Moraxella, 47, 166, 178
Mother-to-child-transmission (MTCT), 102, 106, 108–110
Moxifloxacin, 137, 189, 265
MRI. *See* Magnetic resonance imaging
MRSA. *See* Methicillin-resistant *S. aureus*
MTCT. *See* Mother-to-child-transmission
Mucosal penetration, 10
Multi-drug-resistant (MDR) organisms, 189
Munchausen syndrome, 140
Mupirocin, 230
Mycobacterial infection, 32–33
  fine needle aspiration for, 33
  non-tuberculous, 202–203
Mycobacterium avium, 29, 32
Mycobacterium avium complex (MAC), 202–203
  disseminated, 203

Mycobacterium kansasii, 203
Mycobacterium marinum, 236–237
Mycobacterium pneumoniae, 193
Mycobacterium scrofulaceum, 29, 32
Mycobacterium tuberculosis, 32, 33, 103, 142, 193
Mycoplasma meningoencephalitis, 146

Naloxone, in severe sepsis, 247
Naproxen, 25
Nasogastric tube feeds, 78
National Health Service (NHS), 2
Necator americanus, 95, 229
Necrotizing skin infections, 231–233
  antibiotics for, 232–233
  clinical features of, 231–232
  diagnosis of, 231–232
  hyperbaric oxygen for, 233
  IVIG for, 233
  treatment of, 232–233
Neisseria gonorrhoeae, 20, 212–213, 215
Neisseria meningitidis, 49, 140
Nelfinavir, 220
Neomycin, 45
Neonatal eye infections, 45–47
Neonates
  bacterial meningitis in, 134–136
  cervical lymphadenopathy and, 31
  febrile, 56
  HSV in, 285–286
Neurocystercicosis, 266
Neurosyphilis, 218
Nevirapine, 108
NHS. *See* National Health Service
Nitazoxanide, 90
  in acute gastroenteritis, 82
Nitric oxide antagonists, 247
Nitrofurantoin, 10, 278
Nocardia, 142
Nocardiosis, 35
Non-randomized studies
  searching for, 7
Non-tuberculous mycobacterial infection, 202–203
Non-typhoid Salmonella enteritis, 84–85
Norfloxacin, 88, 215, 275
Nucleic acid detection
  TB and, 200
Nystatin, 214

Obsessive compulsive disorder, 151
Ofloxacin, 86
OME. *See* Otitis media with effusion
Open fractures, 162

Opportunist infections, 107
Oral feeds, 78
Oral hydration therapy (ORT), 77
    in acute gastroenteritis, 78
ORT. *See* Oral hydration therapy
Oseltamivir, 181
Osler nodes, 14
Osteomyelitis, 156–162
Otitis externa, 173
Otitis media with effusion (OME), 166
    antibiotics in, 170
    antihistamines for, 171
    chronic, 169–171
    corticosteroids, 170
    decongestants for, 171
    diagnosis, 169–170
    ventilation tubes for, 170–171
Oxacillin, 11, 19

P. jiroveci, 106–107, 190–191
    corticosteroids for, 191
    mild to moderate, 190
    prophylaxis against, 126–127
    severe, 190–191
Palivizumab
    for bronchiolitis, 184–185
PANDAS, 150–151
Papua New Guinea (PNG), 138
Paratyphoid fevers, 85–86
Paromomycin, 89
Pasteurella multocida, 224
PCR. *See* Polymerase chain reaction
Pediculosis capitis, 233
Pelvic inflammatory disease, 219
Penciclovir, 286
Penicillin, 12
Perianal cellulitis, 233–234
Periocular cellulitis, 40–41
    bacteremia-associated, 41
    deep orbital, 40–41
    local, 40
Periodic fever, aphthous stomatitis, pharyngitis, and adenitis
        (PFAPA) syndrome, 70
Peritonsillar abscess, 36
Permethrin, 25, 235, 236
Pertussis, 181–182
    prevention of, 182
    prophylaxis against, 182
    treatment of, 181–182
Petechiae
    fever with, 62–63
PFAPA syndrome. *See* Periodic fever, aphthous stomatitis,
        pharyngitis, and adenitis syndrome

Pharyngitis, 176–179
    recurrent, 179–180
Pharyngoconjunctival fever, 43
Phenoxymethyl penicillin, 26, 178, 179, 211, 212, 226–228, 229,
        231
Physical therapy
    for bronchiectasis, 195
    for cystic fibrosis, 198
Pinworms, 95, 211, 212, 233
Piperacillin, 158, 162, 173, 190, 225, 237
Plasmapharesis, 146, 147
Plasmodium falciparum, 258–259, 260
Pleural empyema, 193–194
    antibiotic treatment of, 194
    diagnosis of, 194
    operative therapy for, 194–195
Pneumonia, 185–193
    aspiration, 193
    Candida, 192
    community-acquired, 185–187
        antibiotic treatment of, 186–187
        investigations of, 186
    Cryptococcus, 192–193
    diagnosis, 185
    fungal, 191–193
    hospital-acquired, 188–190
    in immunocompromised child, 190
    staphylococcal, 188
PNG. *See* Papua New Guinea
Polymerase chain reaction (PCR), 212, 283
    CSF testing, 144–145
    HIV and, 104
    in cervical lymphadenopathy, 33
    on CSF, 134
Polymyxin, 45
Post-sexual assault prophylaxis, 219–220
    antibiotic, 220
    HBV, 220
    HIV, 220
Praziquantel, 266
Prednisolone, 149, 170, 180
Prednisone, 180
Pregnancy
    in TB, 202
    syphilis and, 216–217
Primaquine, 262
Probiotics
    in acute gastroenteritis, 81–82
Procaine penicillin, 217, 225, 229
Prognosis
    evidence about, 3
Proguanil, 264
Propionibacterium, 141

Protozoal infections, 88–91
Pseudomonas aeruginosa, 10, 20, 46–47, 49, 118–119, 158, 195, 230
    exacerbations of, 197
    initial colonization, 196
Pseudomonas fluorescens, 224
PubMed, 2, 6, 7
    clinical queries page, 6*f*
    home page, 5*f*
Pulmonary hydatid disease, 257
Purpura
    fever with, 62–63
Purulent rhinitis, 173–175
Pyelonephritis, 274
    antibiotics for, 275–276
Pyomyositis, 234
Pyrantel, 95, 212
Pyrazinamide, 34, 148, 201
Pyrimethamine, 51

Q fever, 265
Quinine, 259
Quinolone, 10

Radionuclide scans, 157
Rapid IV rehydration, 77
RCT, 1, 2, 21, 25, 43
Recurrent eyelid swelling, 41
Recurrent furuncles, 227–228
Red Book, 199
Rehydration
    in acute gastroenteritis, 75–77
    rapid IV, 77
Respiratory tract infections, 162–203
Retropharyngeal abscess, 36
RhDNase, for cystic fibrosis, 198
Ribavirin
    for bronchiolitis, 183
    for hepatitis C, 94
Rifabutin, 203
Rifampicin, 12, 19, 34, 105, 139, 148, 158, 188, 201, 203, 228, 237, 251, 256
Rifampin, 139, 158, 203
Rifaximin, 88
Ritonavir, 220
Rochester criteria, 57*b*
Roundworms, 229
Roxithromycin, 12, 178, 187, 215
RSV immunoglobulin, for bronchiolitis, 184

S. agalactiae, 134
S. anginosus, 142
S. haematobium, 265, 266
S. japonicum, 266

S. mansoni, 266
S. milleri, 193
S. pyrogenes, 26, 172, 176, 178, 194, 211, 230
Saccharomyces boulardii, 81
Salmonella, 160
Sarcoptes scabiei, 234
SARS. *See* Severe acute respiratory syndrome
Scabies, 234–236
    crusted, 236
    in babies, 235
    oral treatment for, 235–236
    topical treatment for, 235
Scedosporium, 142
Schistosomiasis, 265–266
Searching
    Cochrane reviews, 3–5
    for diagnosis queries, 7–8
    for meta-analysis, 6
    for non-randomized studies, 7
    for RCTs, 7
    question type in, 7*t*
    systematic reviews, 5–6
Sepsis bundles, 247–248
Sepsis, severe
    activated protein C, 247
    antibiotics, 243–244
    colony-stimulating factors, 247
    ECMO, 247
    fluid therapy, 244–245
    glycemic control, 246
    IVIG, 246
    naloxone, 247
    nitric oxide antagonists, 247
Septic arthritis, 161–162
Septic shock, 245–246
Serology, 283
Severe acute respiratory (SARS), 198
Severe sepsis. *See* sepsis, severe
Sexual abuse, 212
Sexually transmitted infections, 211–220
    post-sexual assault prophylaxis for, 219–220
Shigellosis, 86
Shingles, 290–294
SIADH. *See* Syndrome of inappropriate antidiuretic hormone secretion
Sinusitis, 175–176
Skin infections, 224–238
Skin sepsis, 24–25
Skull fracture, and bacterial meningitis, 139–140
Soft tissue infections, 224–238
Sore throat, 24
    antibiotics for, 177
    McIsaac scoring system for, 177*b*
SPA. *See* Suprapubic aspiration

Spinal epidural abscess, 143–144
Splenectomy, 125–126
Splenomegaly, 14
Staphylococcal toxic shock syndrome, 252
Staphylococcus aureus, 9, 14, 15, 49, 62, 91, 141, 157, 160, 172, 193, 194, 224, 230, 233, 234, 288
    endocarditis, 19
    methicillin-resistant, 189
    methicillin-sensitive, 227–228
    neonatal conjunctivitis from, 46–47
Streptococcal tonsillopharyngitis, 177
Streptococcal toxic shock syndrome, 252
Streptococci
    in infective endocarditis, 17–18
        benzylpenicillin-resistance, 18
Streptococcus pneumoniae, 10, 11, 29, 41, 47, 59, 62, 125, 134, 166, 172, 195
Streptococcus viridans, 288
Strongyloides stercoralis, 95
Strongyloidiasis, 95
Stye, 49
Subdural empyema, 142
Sulbactam, 225
Sulfadiazine, 51
Sulfur, 235
Suprapubic aspiration (SPA), 272
Syndrome of inappropriate antidiuretic hormone secretion (SIADH), 79
Syphilis, 215–218
    early, 217
    late latent, 217–218
    pregnancy and, 216–217
    tertiary, 218
    treatment of, 216
Systematic reviews, 2, 5–6
Systemic sepsis, 243–252
    activated protein C in, 247
    antibiotic therapy for, 243–244
    colony stimulating factors, 247
    ECMO in, 247
    fluid therapy in, 244–245
    glycemic control, 246
    goal-directed therapy in, 247
    IVIG in, 246
    management of, 248
    monoclonal antibodies in, 247
    naloxone in, 247
    nitric oxide antagonists in, 247

Tapeworm, 95
Tazobactam, 162, 173, 190
TB. *See* Tuberculosis
TBM. *See* Tuberculosis meningitis
Teicoplanin, 21

Thiabendazole, 230
Threadworms, 95, 212
Ticarcillin, 162, 173, 189, 190, 225, 237
Tinidazole, 89, 90, 91, 214, 220
TMP-SMX. *See* Trimethoprim-sulfamethoxazole
TNF. *See* Tumor necrosis factor
Tobramycin, 196, 197
Tourette syndrome, 151
Toxicity
    in febrile children, 57, 59*b*
Toxoplasma chorioretinitis, 51
Toxoplasma gondii, 51, 142
Trachoma, 47–48
Transverse myelitis, 149–150
Traveler's diarrhea, 86–88
    prevention of, 87
    treatment of, 87–88
Treatment, clinical questions about, 4*f*
Treponema pallidum, 216
Trichuris trichiura, 95
Trimethoprim, 215, 275
Trimethoprim-sulfamethoxazole, 10, 51, 86, 88, 127, 191, 265
Trimethoprim-sulfamethoxazole (TMP-SMX), 106–107, 127, 256
Tropical infections, 256–266
TST. *See* Tuberculin skin testing
Tuberculin skin testing (TST), 32–33, 199
Tuberculosis (TB), 102, 198–202
    corticosteroids and, 202
    diagnosis, 199
    DOT, 202
    extrapulmonary, 201–202
    in breast-feeding, 202
    in pregnancy, 202
    interferon-gamma assays and, 200
    nucleic acid detection, 200
    prevention of, 202
    treatment of, 200–202
    TST and, 199
Tuberculosis meningitis (TBM), 147–149
    clinical presentation of, 147
    diagnosis of, 147–148
    treatment of, 148–149
        corticosteroids in, 148–149
Tumor necrosis factor (TNF), 70
Tympanocentesis, 166
Tympanometry, 166
Typhoid fevers, 85–86

Ultrasound
    abdominal, for prolonged fever, 68
    in acute osteomyelitis, 156
    in cellulitis, 229
    in epididymo-orchitis, 214–215

Ultrasound (*Cont.*)
   in hepatic hydatid cysts, 257
   in UTI, 276–277
Upper respiratory tract infections (URTIs), 10, 11, 166–182
Urinalysis
   in acute epididymo-orchitis, 215
   in fever, 60
   in UTI, 60, 272–273
Urinary tract infection (UTI), 271–279
   aminoglycosides and, 275
   antibiotic treatment for, 273–284
   catheter-associated, 279–280
   definition of, 271
   fever and, 273
   imaging following, 276–277
   preventing, 277–279
   prophylactic antibiotics, 278–279
   urinalysis for, 272–273
   urine in, 272
URTIs. *See* Upper respiratory tract infections
UTI. *See* Urinary tract infection
Uveitis, 50

Valaciclovir, 44, 218, 291
Valganciclovir, 51
Vancomycin, 11, 18, 19, 20, 21, 50, 83, 134, 136, 137, 141, 142, 144, 172, 188, 190, 194, 229, 234, 237, 238, 243, 252
Varicella zoster immune globulin (VZIG), 292, 293–294
Varicella zoster virus (VZV), 230, 290–294
   antiviral treatment of, 290
   immunization, 291–292
   ophthalmic, 43
   post-exposure immunization, 292
   prevention, 291–294
Vasopressors, 245–246
Vector avoidance, 262
Ventilation tubes, for chronic OME, 170–171
Viral culture, 283
Viral encephalitis, 145

Viral infections, 283–294
   diagnosing, 283
Viral meningitis, 144–145
   clinical features of, 144
   CSF microscopy, 144
   CSF-PCR testing in, 144–145
   serology, 145
   treatment of, 145
   viral culture in, 145
Vitamin A, 289–290
   in gastroenteritis, 81
   measles and, 287–288, 289–290
Vitamin C
   common cold and, 174
Voriconazole, 121, 123, 192
Vulvovaginal candidiasis, 213–214
Vulvovaginitis, 211–214
   enterobius and, 212
   foreign bodies and, 212
   GAS, 212
   GBS, 212
   non-specific, 211–212
   trichomonas, 214
VZIG. *See* Varicella zoster immune globulin
VZV. *See* Varicella zoster virus

Water-related infections, 236–237
Whipworm, 95
White blood count, 58, 59
Worms, 95, 211, 212, 229, 233
Wound infections, 237–238
   clean, 238
   contaminated, 238
   post-traumatic, 238

Zanamivir, 181
Zidovudine, 108, 109
ZIG. *See* Zoster immune globulin
Zinc, 81, 174–175
Zoster immune globulin (ZIG), 292, 293*b*